THE DYSTONIAS

SERIES EDITOR
Eva Feldman, MD, PhD, FAAN, FANA
Russell N. DeJong Professor of Neurology
University of Michigan

Contemporary Neurology Series

74 NEUROLOGIC COMPLICATIONS OF CRITICAL ILLNESS
Third Edition
Eelco F. M. Wijdicks, MD, PhD, FACP

75 CLINICAL NEUROPHYSIOLOGY
Third Edition
Jasper R. Daube, MD, and Devon I. Rubin, MD, Editors

76 PERIPHERAL NEUROPATHIES IN CLINICAL PRACTICE
Steven Herskovitz, MD, Stephen N. Scelsa, MD, and Herbert H. Schaumburg, MD

77 CLINICAL NEUROPHYSIOLOGY OF THE VESTIBULAR SYSTEM
Fourth Edition
Robert W. Baloh, MD, FAAN, and Kevin A. Kerber, MD

78 THE NEURONAL CEROID LIPOFUSCINOSES (BATTEN DISEASE)
Second Edition
Sara E. Mole, PhD, Ruth D. Williams, MD, and Hans H. Goebel, MD, Editors

79 PARANEOPLASTIC SYNDROMES
Robert B. Darnell, MD, PhD, and Jerome B. Posner, MD

80 JASPER'S BASIC MECHANISMS OF THE EPILEPSIES
Jeffrey L. Noebels, MD, PhD, Massimo Avoli, MD, PhD, Michael A. Rogawski, MD, PhD, Richard W. Olsen, PhD, and Antonio V. Delgado-Escueta, MD

81 MYASTHENIA GRAVIS AND MYASTHENIC DISORDERS
Second Edition
Andrew G. Engel, MD, Editor

82 MOLECULAR PHYSIOLOGY AND METABOLISM OF THE NERVOUS SYSTEM
Gary A. Rosenberg, MD

83 SEIZURES AND EPILEPSY
Second Edition
Jerome Engel, Jr., MD, PhD

84 MULTIPLE SCLEROSIS
Moses Rodriguez, MD, Orhun H. Kantarci, MD, and Istvan Pirko, MD

85 FRONTOTEMPORAL DEMENTIA
Bruce L. Miller, MD

86 AUTONOMIC NEUROLOGY
Eduardo E. Benarroch, MD

87 EVALUATION AND TREATMENT OF MYOPATHIES
Second Edition
Emma Ciafaloni, MD, Patrick F. Chinnery, FRCP, FMedSci, and Robert C. Griggs, MD, Editors

88 MOTOR NEURON DISEASE IN ADULTS
Mark Bromberg, MD

89 HYPERKINETIC MOVEMENT DISORDERS
Roger M. Kurlan, MD, Paul E. Green, MD, and Kevin M. Biglan, MD, MPH

90 THE NEUROLOGY OF EYE MOVEMENTS
Fifth Edition
R. John Leigh, MD, FRCP, and David S. Zee, MD

91 MIGRAINE
Third Edition
David W. Dodick, MD, and Stephen D. Silberstein, MD, FACP, FAHS, FAAN

92 CLINICAL NEUROPHYSIOLOGY
Fourth Edition
Devon Rubin, MD and Jasper Daube, MD, Editors

93 PLUM AND POSNER'S DIAGNOSIS AND TREATMENT OF STUPOR AND COMA
Fifth Edition
Jerome B. Posner, MD, Clifford B. Saper, MD, PhD, Nicholas D. Schiff, MD, and Jan Claassen, MD, PhD

94 NEUROIMMUNOLOGY
Fifth Edition
Bibiana Bielekova, MD, Gary Birnbaum, MD, and Robert P. Lisak, MD, FRCP

95 CLINICAL NEUROPHYSIOLOGY
Fifth Edition
Devon I. Rubin, MD, Editor

96 PARKINSON DISEASE
Roger L. Albin, MD

97 NEUROLOGIC COMPLICATIONS OF CRITICAL ILLNESS
Fourth Edition
Eelco F. M. Wijdicks, MD, PhD, FACP

98 JASPER'S BASIC MECHANISMS OF THE EPILEPSIES
Fifth Edition
Jeffrey L. Noebels, MD, PhD, Massimo Avoli, MD, PhD, Michael A. Rogawski, MD, PhD, Annamaria Vezzani, PhD, Antonio V. Delgado-Escueta, MD, Editors

THE DYSTONIAS

Dr. H. A. Jinnah

Professor in Departments of Neurology, Pediatrics, & Human Genetics, Emory University School of Medicine, Atlanta, USA

Dr. Bettina Balint

Assistant Professor for Clinical Research on Complex Movement Disorders and Parkinson's Disease,, Department of Neurology, University Hospital Zurich, Switzerland

Dr. Victor S. C. Fung

Professor of Neurology and Motor Control, Sydney Medical School, The University of Sydney
Director of the Movement Disorders Unit, Department of Neurology, Westmead Hospital, Sydney, Australia

OXFORD
UNIVERSITY PRESS

OXFORD
UNIVERSITY PRESS

Oxford University Press is a department of the University of Oxford. It furthers the University's objective of excellence in research, scholarship, and education by publishing worldwide. Oxford is a registered trade mark of Oxford University Press in the UK and certain other countries.

Published in the United States of America by Oxford University Press
198 Madison Avenue, New York, NY 10016, United States of America.

Library of Congress Cataloging-in-Publication Data
Names: Jinnah, H. A., author. | Balint, Bettina, author. | Fung, Victor S. C., author.
Title: The Dystonias / H. A. Jinnah, Bettina Balint, and Victor S. C. Fung.
Description: New York, NY : Oxford University Press, [2025] |
Series: Contemporary neurology series |
Includes bibliographical references and index.
Identifiers: LCCN 2024044867 | ISBN 9780197631966 (hardback) |
ISBN 9780197631980 (epub) | ISBN 9780197631973 | ISBN 9780197631997
Subjects: LCSH: Dystonia.
Classification: LCC RC935.D8 J56 2024 | DDC 616.8/3—dc23/eng/20241207
LC record available at https://lccn.loc.gov/2024044867

DOI: 10.1093/med/9780197631966.001.0001

Printed by Marquis Book Printing, Canada

FSC www.fsc.org MIX Paper | Supporting responsible forestry FSC® C103567

Contents

Figures

Preface

The dystonias encompass a large family of very heterogeneous disorders, with hundreds of varied clinical presentations and etiologies. Because of this heterogeneity, the dystonias are among the most frequently misdiagnosed disorders. Over the past few decades, our knowledge regarding the clinical features and biological basis for the many different types of dystonia has grown dramatically. There has been a rapid growth in the number of publications (Figure P.1) as well as an ever-increasing number of electronic and online resources and platforms for learning the latest news. The explosion of information can make it challenging to find the most relevant information quickly.

Considering the marked growth in knowledge regarding the dystonias, it is surprising that the information has not been assembled into a single comprehensive but easy-to-use resource. Over the years, only a few books devoted to dystonia have been produced. Two books of the same title (*Handbook of Dystonia*, Dekker, 1995; *Handbook of Dystonia*, Informa, 2007) provide good resources for the reader who is not an expert in dystonia. However, much of the material in these books is now out-dated. Four books have appeared in the *Advances in Neurology* series (*Dystonia 1*, *Dystonia 2*, *Dystonia 3*, and *Dystonia 4*). The last of this series appeared in 2004, and each was organized according to the agenda of an international meeting on dystonia, with selected coverage of trending topics. Two more recent books were published, including *Dystonia & Dystonic Syndromes* (Springer, 2015) and *Treatment of Dystonia* (Cambridge, 2018). Both were aimed at experts in movement disorders, with coverage of select topics based on the proceedings of international meetings. Most recently, a book focusing on the neurobiological basis of the dystonias was published (*International Review of Neurobiology*, Elsevier, 2023), but it did not cover clinical topics. A modern and ready-to-reach resource is clearly needed for clinicians who encounter individuals with dystonia.

The audience of potential readers for the book is quite varied. On the one hand, there is a need for a resource that is practical and easily accessible to healthcare providers who are not specialists because they may participate in diagnosis and referral to appropriate specialists. A practical resource also is needed for trainees such as medical students, residents, or fellows. At the same time, there is a need for a more comprehensive resource for general neurologists, subspecialists in movement disorders, pediatric neurologists, neurosurgeons, rehabilitation medicine specialists, ophthalmologists, otolaryngologists, orthopedic surgeons, mental health providers, physical and occupational therapists, and others. This book was prepared with this broad audience in mind.

The dystonias are a big topic, with many potential ways to lump and split the material. The organizational plan includes 32 chapters divided into five main sections: I, introductory material; II, syndromes where dystonia is the sole or main problem; III, syndromes where dystonia is combined with other clinical problems; IV, etiology and pathogenesis as it relates to clinical application; and V, medical and surgical management. Dystonia affects individuals of all ages from infancy to older adults, with extensively overlapping needs over the lifespan. Rather than present separate chapters on children or adults, each chapter includes information relevant for all age groups.

During preparation of this book, close attention was paid to several issues. One of these issues was citations. In addition to the most recent and relevant citations, careful thought was given to some of the earliest or most comprehensive references from the past so that useful classics can be found more readily.

Another area that received careful attention was illustrations. In some cases, original data from the classic or the most comprehensive articles have been converted into graphical format so that key information can be seen at a glance. In other cases, data have been systematically collected across articles and presented in a summary graph. The authors express deep gratitude to Deniz Boz for collecting these data and preparing many graphs. Regarding illustrations of people with dystonia, it is customary to include pictures or videos of patients depicting specific clinical phenomena. This strategy can be

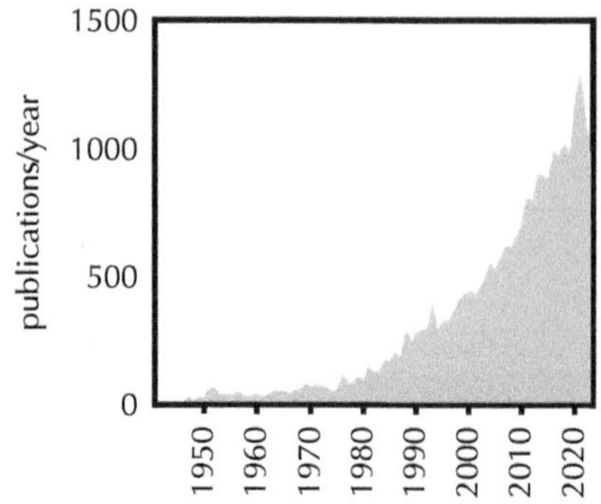

Figure P.1. Number of citations retrieved from the PubMed database with "dystonia" as a keyword, according to year.

misleading because a representative example must be selected from an enormous number of possible variants. As a result, a different approach was used for illustrating clinical features. Multiple pictures of a similar phenomenon were collected, and a professional illustrator was asked to distill the essence of the problem into a single illustration. For this, the authors express sincere thanks to Loren Bergantini (https://www.lorenbergantini.studio/), who did a remarkable job preparing these illustrations. Finally, special thanks go to Gamze Kilic-Berkmen, who reviewed all the chapters and figures and helped enormously to keep this project on track.

The cover illustration shows a painting from the artist Amedeo Modigliani. This image is often shown by lecturers as an illustration of cervical dystonia, with a sensory trick touching the cheek. However, it is not clear that this painting reflects cervical dystonia. Real photographs of the woman in the painting do not show the neck postures Modigliani depicted, and he has several other paintings of people who show similarly abnormal neck postures. These observations suggest these postures reflect his preferred style of painting.

SECTION I

Introduction to the Dystonias

Chapter 1

A Brief History of the Concept of Dystonia and Its Evolution

INTRODUCTION

Historical reports describing what is probably dystonia date back to 10 BC, and depictions of dystonia in art and literature preceded its recognition as a neurological condition. In Dante Alighieri's *Divine Comedy*, moaners walk with their heads twisted backward, as a punishment for having tried to descry the future.[49] In *David Copperfield*, Charles Dickens described a man who "had no voice, but spoke in a whisper," like a patient with spasmodic dysphonia, or another man with "a way of carrying his head on one side, as if it were a little too heavy for him," suggestive of cervical dystonia.[15] The term *torticollis*, which we still use for a subtype of cervical dystonia, was introduced by the French Renaissance writer and physician François Rabelais in his book *Pantagruel*.[35]

Other famous personalities, including the musician and composer Robert Schumann or the philosopher and physician Albert Schweitzer, suffered from dystonia without knowing it. After initial success as piano player, increasing technical difficulties due to an isolated and painless loss of control of the right middle finger prevented Schumann from becoming a concert pianist.[3] Schweitzer wrote profusely on theology, music theory, and philosophy. He also suffered from severe and painful muscle cramps in the right arm triggered by handwriting.[45] Today we recognize these symptoms as characteristic of focal task-specific musician's dystonia or writer's cramp, respectively (see Chapter 10, "Musician's and Other Task-Specific Dystonias"), but the concept of dystonia and the recognition of its variants developed only later.

William Hammond (1828–1900) coined the term *athetosis* to describe three individuals "in which the most characteristic symptoms are an inability to retain the fingers and toes in any position in which they may be placed, and their continual motion."[18] This term evolved over the years to include more proximal writhing movements. Athetosis is now considered part of the dystonia spectrum, describing a more mobile dystonia, though the term is only infrequently used in modern dystonia literature.[33,42] Gowers called the dystonic postures in hands and feet in two siblings affected by Wilson disease "tetanoid chorea."[17]

Lacking the framework of a name, these many different observations were not recognized as a single entity.[5,35] The schematic in Figure 1.1

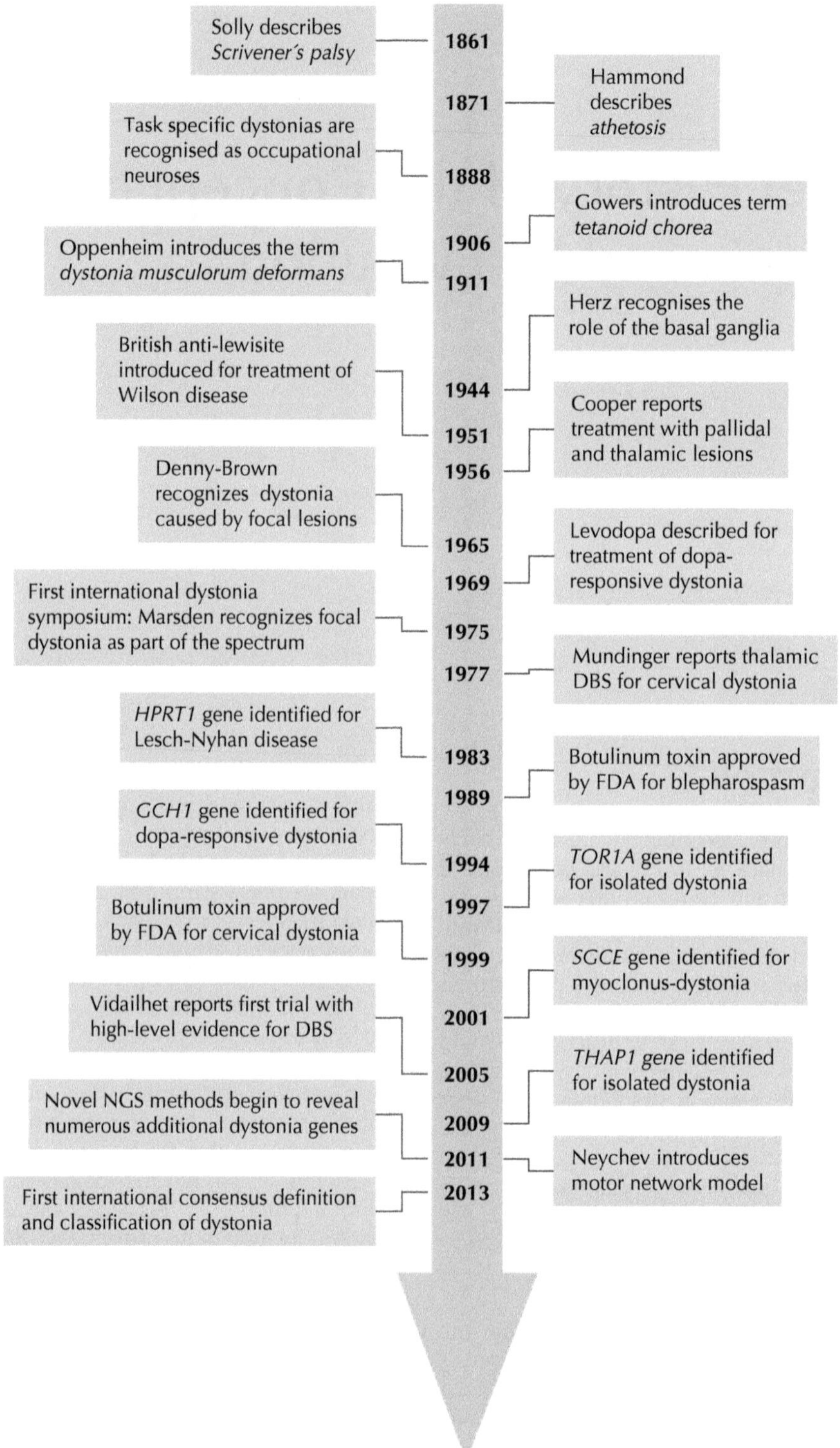

Figure 1.1. Timeline for selected events in the history of dystonia. Abbreviations: DBS, deep brain stimulation; FDA, Food and Drug Administration of the United States of America; NGS, next generation sequencing.

shows some of the key events in the history of the concept of dystonia, discoveries of its biological underpinnings, and its treatments.

EARLY CONCEPT OF DYSTONIA

Hermann Oppenheim (1858–1919) introduced the term *dystonia* or, more precisely, *dystonia musculorum deformans*, when describing four unrelated Jewish children with what is sometimes called *Oppenheim's dystonia*.[28,38] He noted profound fluctuations in muscle tone, from hypotonia at rest to hypertonia with voluntary action. He viewed these children as having a disorder of central control of muscle tone (Figure 1.2). In fact, the term dystonia is derived from ancient Greek, δύς- or *dys*- ("bad" or "wrong") and τόνος or *tonos* ("tone"). Oppenheim himself was convinced of the organic nature of the condition, but his discovery was made at a time when the concepts of psychology and the psychiatric schools of Freud and Charcot prevailed, and dystonia was considered a psychiatric disorder.

Over the years, others described additional disorders that were grouped under the heading of dystonia, including disorders where resting muscle tone was not abnormal. Indeed, shortly after Solly described *scrivener's palsy* in 1864,[43] numerous cases were later described as writer's cramp.[40] Gowers grouped it as an occupational neurosis together with other task-specific dystonias, including *pianoforte player's cramp, telegraphist's cramp*, and similar conditions among violin or zither players, harpists, seamstresses, tailors, knitters, engravers, milkers, painters, cigarette makers, money counters (see Chapter 10).[16]

For many years, individuals with dystonia suffered the hardship of being called hysterical and their symptoms were attributed to psychiatric disease.[34] Some particular characteristics of dystonia reinforced this viewpoint. Dystonia worsens with stress and is sometimes relieved by certain unusual maneuvers (*geste antagoniste*). The phenomenology of eye closure (blepharospasm) or head turning (torticollis) offers seemingly self-evident psychopathological explanations, such as not wanting to see or face reality. Another layer of difficulty in grasping the organic nature of dystonia in the early days came from the lack of any obvious anatomical, physiological, or biochemical abnormality.[32] Nonetheless, a paradigm shift toward the current concept of dystonia as a neurological disease was paved by reports of failure of psychotherapy in dystonia,[18] association with basal ganglia lesions,[7] and animal models with dystonia based on brain lesions.[9]

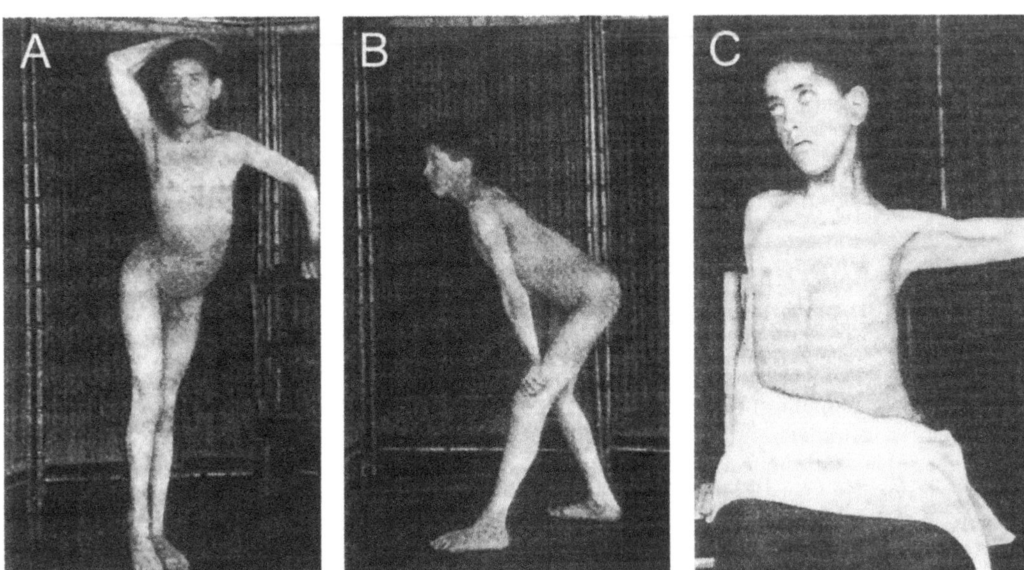

Figure 1.2. Photos from Oppenheim's original paper. In the original report, Panels A and B were labeled "figure 1" and Panel C was labeled "figure 2." All panels show the same individual (modified from English translation[28]). No figure legends were given in the original article.

DYSTONIA AS A NEUROLOGICAL DISORDER

Historically, Hammond hypothesized that the cause of athetosis was a striatal lesion,[9] and Herz already noted from autopsy studies that dystonia could be associated with lesions in various basal ganglia regions such as putamen, caudate, and pallidum.[19] Similarly, Denny-Brown concluded, after his landmark experiments in the 1960s, that lesions in different anatomical structures, including the cortex, might eventually result in dystonia,[9] therefore laying the basis for the network hypothesis. A little later, Zeman introduced the distinction of dystonia secondary to overt basal ganglia pathology or dystonia without any obvious pathology as potential disorders of biochemistry or function.[52]

Based on these insights, the First International Symposium on Dystonia in 1975 provided a forum to integrate many previous observations and implemented the recognition of the full clinical spectrum of dystonia (Figure 1.1).[13] This implementation recognized generalized dystonia as well as the many focal occupational cramps as *formes frustes* of dystonia. Dystonia was also recognized as an etiologically heterogeneous condition that may arise as a consequence of a visible brain lesion but also of biochemistry or function without visible lesions. This symposium laid the foundations for a better understanding of the many clinical manifestations of dystonia. The defining features of dystonia and formal classification system of the many clinical manifestations into specific subgroups were presented at the Fifth International Symposium on Dystonia in 2013[1] and revised in 2025[2]).

EVOLVING CONCEPT OF PATHOGENESIS FOR DYSTONIA

In parallel with advances in the recognition of the many clinical manifestations of dystonia were advances in understanding its biological basis (Figure 1.1). Although a role for inheritance was recognized very early, the identification of dystonia genes came much later. The first discoveries in genetics depend on how a dystonia gene is defined (see Chapter 22, "Dystonia Genetics"). The first gene associated with a disorder that included dystonia was described in 1983.[27] Jolly and colleagues described *HPRT1* as the causal gene for Lesch-Nyhan disease, an X-linked recessive disorder with a classic phenotype in which all affected individuals have severe generalized dystonia along with chorea, spasticity, cognitive dysfunction, and behavioral problems.[26] Later, variant clinical phenotypes were recognized in which generalized or focal dystonia might be the main presenting feature without the other neurological or behavioral problems.[24] The first gene associated with a disorder where dystonia is the main defining feature was described in 1994; Ichinose and colleagues described autosomal dominant gene variants in *GCH1*, leading to a decrease in the activity of the enzyme GTP-cyclohydrolase, as the cause of dopa-responsive dystonia.[20] Many affected individuals present with dystonia as the sole feature, although many also have parkinsonism.[51] In 1997, Ozelius and colleagues identified the *TOR1A* gene as the cause of early-onset isolated dystonia,[39] where dystonia is consistently the main problem.[29]

The subsequent development of next-generation sequencing methods led to a rapid increase in the number of genes associated with dystonia, beginning in 2011. Most of these genes were associated with clinical phenotypes where dystonia occurs along with other neurological or medical problems. The current number of genes depends on how a dystonia gene is defined. Only a small number of genes are associated with isolated dystonia, but some databases such as Online Mendelian Inheritance in Man list more than 500 genes where dystonia may occur (see Chapter 22). When considering all types of genes where dystonia may occur, it has become possible to identify common biological processes responsible for dystonia, including derangements of dopamine signaling, ion channel function, heavy metal accumulation, intracellular trafficking, and others.[11,12,47]

There have also been major changes in the evolution of concepts regarding the neuroanatomical substrates of dystonia. The role of the basal ganglia was recognized very early, so dystonia was initially considered to be a basal ganglia disorder.[19] However, many subsequent observations pointed to other brain regions, too. The concept that dystonia was due to a disorder of a broader sensorimotor network came following synthesis of the many insights from clinical observations, neuroimaging studies, animal experiments, and neurophysiology.[36] Dystonia is now viewed as a network disorder involving the basal ganglia along with other regions including the cerebellum, cerebral cortex, thalamus, midbrain/brainstem, and potentially other regions as well.[8,25,41]

SOME KEY ADVANCES IN TREATMENT

There have been several pivotal advances in the treatment of dystonia (Figure 1.1). In 1951, Denny-Brown and Porter described the use of British anti-lewisite (2,3-dimercaptopropanol) for the treatment of Wilson disease,[10] where dystonia is a frequent problem.[31,44] These observations provided a precedent that there may be special life-altering treatments addressing biological mechanisms which are useful only in certain conditions. Following on these ideas, Walshe described the use of penicillamine for copper chelation to treat Wilson disease in 1956.[50] The value of levodopa for dopa-responsive dystonia came later,[6,37] followed more recently by recognition of approximately 30 disorders where special treatments could be useful (see Chapter 28, "Symptom-Targeted Oral Medications for Dystonia").[23]

Oral therapies play a central role for treatment, but only for a limited number of rare subtypes of dystonia. The development of the botulinum toxins provided enormous relief as a symptomatic treatment for much larger numbers of individuals with dystonia, regardless of underlying cause. Onabotulinumtoxin A was approved by the US Food and Drug Administration (FDA) for use in blepharospasm in 1989,[3] and, 10 years later, in 1999, for cervical dystonia. These early studies paved the way for application of additional botulinum toxin preparations for many different types of dystonia (see Chapter 30, "Botulinum Toxin Treatment for Dystonia").[21]

There have been similar advances in surgical treatments for dystonia, which initially focused on resection of muscles or nerves most responsible for abnormal movements.[30] Cooper began to describe a brain lesion approach to dystonia in the 1950s,[7] Mundinger first reported deep brain stimulation of the thalamus in 1977, and Vidailhet reported the first double-blind clinical trial of pallidal stimulation in 2005.[48] More recently, the network model has inspired efforts to target other brain regions (see Chapter 31, "Surgical Treatments for Dystonia").

SYNOPSIS AND FUTURE PROSPECTS

History has witnessed a substantial evolution in the clinical concept of dystonia, including its core clinical features and how they are classified.[22] While the core features of dystonia have been outlined, there are some areas where current defining characteristics used for dystonia overlap with other disorders. For example, there are overlapping features between dystonia and tremor (see Chapter 12, "Dystonia and Tremor"), dystonia and parkinsonism (see Chapter 13, "Dystonia and Parkinsonism"), dystonia and myoclonus (see Chapter 15, "Dystonia and Myoclonus"), and some other disorders that may mimic dystonia (see Chapter 26, "Pseudodystonia and Differential Diagnosis"). These overlaps mean that there are still some gray areas where the borders between dystonia and other disorders are sometimes not clear, so further refinement of the clinical criteria used to define dystonia may be expected in the future.

History has seen a similar evolution in concepts relating to the etiology of dystonia, beginning with the belief that it was largely a psychological or psychiatric disorder. Efforts to define its biological basis initially focused only on the basal ganglia and later recognized a broader network (see Chapter 23, "The Neuroanatomical Substrates of Dystonia").[8] These scientific advances have raised new possibilities for surgical treatments of dystonia.[4,46]

Initial ideas regarding the inheritance of dystonia focused on one or a few genes affecting a specific biological pathway in the brain. The identification of hundreds of different genes with very different functions has raised awareness of the remarkable etiological heterogeneity of dystonia as well as the realization that effective therapies may be relevant for specific types of dystonia or specific groups of dystonia sharing a similar mechanism.[11,12,47] It is likely that additional genes and pathways will be discovered, but existing scientific advances have already opened the door to development of mechanism-specific treatments for some dystonias and the possibility to develop biomarkers to aid in diagnosis.

REFERENCES

1. Albanese A, Bhatia K, Bressman SB, DeLong MR, Fahn S, Fung VSC, et al. Phenomenology and

classification of dystonia: A consensus update. Mov Disord 2013;28:863–873.

2. Albanese A, Bhatia K, Fung V, Hallett M, Jankovic J, et al. Definition and Classification of Dystonia, 2025 (first presented at the International Dystonia Symposium in 2023).
3. Altenmüller E. Robert Schumann's focal dystonia. In: Bogousslavsky J, Boller F, eds. *Frontiers in Neurology and Neuroscience.* Karger, 2005: 179–188.
4. Cajigas I, Morrison MA, Luciano MS, Starr PA. Cerebellar deep brain stimulation for the treatment of movement disorders in cerebral palsy. J Neurosurg 2023:1–10.
5. Camargo CH, Teive HA. Evolution of the concept of dystonia. Arq Neuropsiquiatr 2014;72:559–561.
6. Coleman MP, Barnet A. L-dopa reversal of muscle spasm, vomiting and insomnia in a patient with an atypical form of familial dystonia. Trans Am Neurol Assoc 1969;94:91–95.
7. Cooper IS. Dystonia musculorum deformans: Natural history and neurosurgical alleviation. J Pediatr 1969;74:585–592.
8. Corp DT, Morrison-Ham J, Jinnah HA, Joutsa J. The functional anatomy of dystonia: Recent developments. Int Rev Neurobiol 2023;169:105–136.
9. Denny-Brown D. The nature of dystonia. Bull N Y Acad Med 1965;41:858–869.
10. Denny-Brown D, Porter H. The effect of BAL (2,3-dimercaptopropanol) on heptatolenticular degeneration (Wilson's disease). Trans Am Neurol Assoc 1951;56:79–84.
11. Di Fonzo A, Albanese A, Jinnah HA. The apparent paradox of phenotypic diversity and shared mechanisms across dystonia syndromes. Curr Opin Neurol 2022;35:502–509.
12. Di Fonzo A, Jinnah HA, Zech M. Dystonia genes and their biological pathways. Int Rev Neurobiol 2023;169:61–103.
13. Eldridge R, Fahn S. Dystonia, Advances in Neurology, vol 14; Raven Press, NY1976.
14. Eldridge R, Riklan M, Cooper IS. The limited role of psychotherapy in torsion dystonia. Experience with 44 cases. JAMA 1969;210:705–708.
15. Garcia-Ruiz PJ, Slawek J, Sitek EJ, Martinez Castrillo JC. Art and dystonia. J Neurol Sci 2015;356:49–54.
16. Gowers WR. *A Manual of Diseases of the Nervous System.* Churchill, 1888.
17. Gowers WR. On tetanoid chorea and its association with cirrhosis of the liver. Rev Neurol Psychiatry 1906;4:249–258.
18. Hammond WA. *A Treatise on Diseases of the Nervous System.* D. Appleton, 1871.
19. Herz E. Dystonias, part 3: Pathology and conclusions. Arch Neurol Psychiatr 1944;52:20.
20. Ichinose H, Ohye T, Takahashi E, Seki N, Hori T, Segawa M, et al. Hereditary progressive dystonia with marked diurnal fluctuation caused by mutation in the GTP-cyclohydrolase I gene. Nature Genet 1994;8:232–242.
21. Jabbari B. History of botulinum toxin treatment in movement disorders. Tremor Other Hyperkinet Mov 2016;6:394.
22. Jinnah HA, Albanese A. The new classification for the dystonias: Why was it needed and how was it accomplished? Mov Disord Clin Pract 2014;1:280–284.
23. Jinnah HA, Albanese A, Bhatia KP, Cardoso F, Da Prat G, de Koning TJ, et al. Treatable inherited rare movement disorders. Mov Disord 2018;33:21–35.
24. Jinnah HA, Ceballos-Picot I, Torres RJ, Visser JE, Schretlen D, Verdu A, et al. Attenuated variants of Lesch-Nyhan disease. Brain 2010;133:671–689.
25. Jinnah HA, Neychev V, Hess EJ. The anatomical basis for dystonia: The motor network model. Tremor Other Hyperkinet Mov 2017;7:506.
26. Jinnah HA, Visser JE, Harris JC, Verdu A, Larovere L, Ceballos-Picot I, et al. Delineation of the motor disorder of Lesch-Nyhan disease. Brain 2006;129:1201–1217.
27. Jolly DJ, Okayama H, Berg P, Esty AC, Filpula D, Bohlen P, et al. Isolation and characterization of a full-length expressible cDNA for human hypoxanthine phosphoribosyltransferase. Proc Natl Acad Sci (USA) 1983;80:477–481.
28. Klein C, Fahn S. Translation of Oppenheim's 1911 paper on dystonia. Mov Disord 2013;28:851–862.
29. Lange LM, Junker J, Loens S, Baumann H, Olschewski L, Schaake S, et al. Genotype-phenotype relations for isolated dystonia genes: MDSGene systematic review. Mov Disord 2021;36:1086–1103.
30. Loher TJ, Pohle T, Krauss JK. Functional stereotactic surgery for treatment of cervical dystonia: Review of the experience from the lesional era. Stereotact Funct Neurosurg 2004;82:1–13.
31. Machado A, Chien HF, Deguti MM, Cancado E, Azevedo RS, Scaff M, Barbosa ER. Neurological manifestations in Wilson's disease: Report of 119 cases. Mov Disord 2006;21:2192–2196.
32. Marsden CD. The problem of adult-onset idiopathic torsion dystonia and other isolated dyskinesias in adult life (including blepharospasm, oromandibular dystonia, dystonic writer's cramp, and torticollis, or axial dystonia). Adv Neurol 1976;14:259–276.
33. Morris JG, Jankelowitz SK, Fung VS, Clouston PD, Hayes MW, Grattan-Smith P. Athetosis I: Historical considerations. Mov Disord 2002;17:1278–1280.
34. Munts AG, Koehler PJ. How psychogenic is dystonia? Views from past to present. Brain 2010;133:1552–1564.
35. Newby RE, Thorpe DE, Kempster PA, Alty JE. A history of dystonia: Ancient to modern. Mov Disord Clin Pract 2017;4:478–485.
36. Neychev VK, Gross R, Lehericy S, Hess EJ, Jinnah HA. The functional neuroanatomy of dystonia. Neurobiol Dis 2011;42:185–201.
37. Nygaard TG, Marsden CD, Fahn S. Dopa-responsive dystonia: Long-term treatment response and prognosis. Neurology 1991;41:174–181.
38. Oppenheim H. Uber eineeigenartige Krampfkrankheit des kind-lichen und jugendlichen Alters (Dysbasia lordotica lordotica progressive, Dystonia musculorum deformans). Neurol CBL 1911;30:1090–1107.
39. Ozelius LJ, Hewett JW, Page CE, Bressman SB, Kramer PL, Shalish C, et al. The early-onset torsion dystonia gene (DYT1) encodes an ATP-binding protein. Nature Genet 1997;17:40–48.
40. Poore GV. An analysis of ninety-three cases of writers' cramp and impaired writing power; making, with seventy-five cases previously reported, a total of one hundred and sixty-eight cases. Medico-Chirurg Trans 1887;70:301–333.
41. Prudente CN, Hess EJ, Jinnah HA. Dystonia as a network disorder: What is the role of the cerebellum? Neuroscience 2014;260:23–35.
42. Salam-Adams M, Adams RD. Athetotic syndromes. In: Vinken PJ, Bruyn GW, Klawans HL, eds. *Handbook of Clinical Neurology 49: Extrapyramidal Disorders.* Elsevier Science, 1997: 381–389.

43. Solly S. Clinical lectures on scriveners' palsy, or the paralysis of writers. Lancet 1864;84:709–711.
44. Svetel M, Kozic D, Stefanova E, Semnic R, Dragasevic N, Kostic VS. Dystonia in Wilson's disease. Mov Disord 2001;16:719–723.
45. Tacik P, Schrader C, Weber E, Dressler D. Albert Schweitzer: A patient with writer's cramp. Parkinsonism Relat Disord 2012;18:453–457.
46. Tai CH, Tseng SH. Cerebellar deep brain stimulation for movement disorders. Neurobiolo Dis 2022;175:105899.
47. Thomsen M, Lange LM, Zech M, Lohmann K. Genetics and pathogenesis of dystonia. Annu Rev Pathol 2024;19:99–131.
48. Vidailhet M, Vercueil L, Houeto JL, Krystkowiak P, Benabid AL, Cornu P, et al. Bilateral deep-brain stimulation of the globus pallidus in primary generalized dystonia. N Engl J Med 2005;352:459–467.
49. Villarejo A. Neurological references in the Divine Comedy. Neurosci History 2014;2:170–175.
50. Walshe JM. Penicillamine, a new oral therapy for Wilson's disease. Amer J Med 1956;21:487–495.
51. Weissbach A, Pauly MG, Herzog R, Hahn L, Halmans S, Hamami F, et al. Relationship of genotype, phenotype, and treatment in dopa-responsive dystonia: MDSGene review. Mov Disord 2021;2022:237–252.
52. Zeman W. Pathology of the torsion dystonias (dystonia musculorum deformans). Neurology 1970;20:79–88.

Chapter 2

Defining the Clinical Features of Dystonia

INTRODUCTION

Historically, the term *dystonia* was used in different ways: as a descriptor for a type of abnormal movement, as an abnormal movement syndrome, as an etiology, or as a group of diseases with dystonic movements (see Chapter 1, "A Brief History of the Concept of Dystonia and Its Evolution"). Modern usage of the term emphasizes its clinical phenomenology and syndromic qualities. Dystonia currently is defined as *a movement disorder characterized by sustained or intermittent abnormal movements, postures, or both. Dystonic movements and postures are typically patterned and repetitive, and may be tremulous or jerky.*[1] This definition provides a starting place to describe the most characteristic features of dystonia. The approach to a patient with dystonia follows three diagnostic levels:

Level 1: Establish the presence of dystonia and rule out other movement disorders that may mimic dystonia (see Chapter 26, "Pseudodystonia and Differential Diagnosis").

Level 2: Define a specific dystonia syndrome based on the movement disorder(s) identified and other neurological and non-neurological features. For example, dystonia may occur as sole feature (isolated dystonia, see Chapter 3, "Classification and Diagnostic Strategy for Dystonia") or combined with other problems, such as parkinsonism or myoclonus (see Chapter 18, "Dystonias Combined with Other Features").

Level 3: Delineate potential etiologies based on the clinical syndrome. At this stage, diagnostic tests may be used to ascertain or refute conditions. Such tests may include magnetic resonance imaging, genetic testing, and other tests of blood or urine (see Chapter 27, "Workup of Dystonia").

The aim of this chapter is to address the main defining clinical features of dystonia (Level 1), and briefly introduce relevant concepts pertaining to dystonia syndromes (Level 2) and their etiologies (Level 3). Dystonia syndromes and their etiologies are covered in more detail in subsequent chapters.

DEFINING FEATURES OF DYSTONIA (LEVEL 1)

Abnormal Movements and Postures

The most characteristic features of dystonia include abnormal movements and postures. Movements and postures may range in severity from very subtle to very obvious. Many abnormal movements have a slow or twisting quality, but they may also be very quick. Whether slow or fast, a key feature of dystonic movements is that they are often patterned, occurring in a stereotyped fashion. The same task or action will lead to the same posture or movement. In some cases, performing one voluntary action will trigger one pattern of dystonia, but another voluntary action will trigger an alternative pattern. In an individual with foot dystonia, for example, walking may cause stereotyped intorsion of a foot during the swing phase, but external rotation just before the stance phase. The pattern may repeat at each gait cycle in the same leg.

Although dystonic movements and postures are typically patterned, severity can vary for a single individual at different times under different conditions. For example, an individual with blepharospasm with prominent spasms may appear normal during consultation in the outpatient clinic, but there may be severe eye closing spasms driving home or when trying to read. Some forms of dystonia are diurnal, occurring mostly in the evenings. Dystonia also worsens with stress and anxiety.[10]

Worsening by Voluntary Action

Dystonic movements are typically most evident on action, with sometimes little or no abnormalities at rest. For example, in an individual with cervical dystonia, turning of the neck may only be observed when the arms are outstretched or only with walking. Similarly, foot dystonia may become only apparent on walking and may not be visible when resting.

For some cases, the task that triggers dystonia may be highly specific. Task-specific dystonias occur only when certain actions are performed. Common examples include writing in writer's cramp or playing an instrument like the piano in musician's dystonia. Other examples include occupational cramps or sports-related cramps (see Chapter 10, "Musician's and Other Task-Specific Dystonias"). Such task-specific dystonias typically develop with repetitive, highly practiced movements. Similarly, sometimes dystonic posturing or tremor become evident only when adopting certain postures or positions.

Associated Movements

It is not uncommon for a voluntary movement to produce extra movements remote from the intended movement. The term *overflow* refers to a spread of movements to an adjacent region.[32] For example, individuals with writer's cramp might have obvious difficulties with the hand and distal arm muscles when writing, but there may be additional elbow flexion or shoulder elevation. In this example, activation of hand muscles during writing spreads inappropriately to involve activation of upper arm muscles. Overflow is a common feature of many types of dystonia, but it is not universal.

Mirroring refers to a phenomenon where voluntary movements on one side of the body trigger unintentional movement on the contralateral side.[7,16,32] Some experts discriminate *mirror movements* from *mirror dystonia*.[7,16,32] In mirror movements, tasks performed on one side of the body are unintentionally reproduced in a similar pattern on the opposite side. In mirror dystonia, tasks performed on the unaffected side reproduce dystonic movements on the affected side, but they are often less prominent and sometimes quite subtle. The mirror dystonia movements reproduce the dystonic pattern in the affected limb, but they do not always replicate the movements being conducted by the unaffected side. In writer's cramp, for example, individuals may experience not only dystonic posturing of the hand while writing, but also dystonic movements of the same hand when writing with the other hand.

A related phenomenon is *homolateral synkinesis*, a term used to describe voluntary movements on one side of the body that trigger similar unintentional movements ipsilaterally. A common example is that voluntarily tapping the hand may trigger synchronized tapping of the ipsilateral foot. In children who are learning to write, there is often subtle posturing of the ipsilateral face.

While overflow is a clinically useful sign that is relatively specific for dystonia, mirroring and homolateral synkinesis are less specific. Mirroring and homolateral synkinesis are commonly seen in cerebral palsy, in other movement disorders, or after stroke.[7,16] They can also be transient benign findings in normal children during development.

Geste Antagoniste or Sensory Trick

A highly characteristic feature of dystonia is the *geste antagoniste* or *sensory trick* or *alleviating maneuvre*.[22] This phenomenon refers to an action that alleviates dystonic postures or movements. A common example is touching the cheek to suppress abnormal head movements in cervical dystonia or touching the brow to alleviate blepharospasm. The touch is relatively light, rather than a forceful suppression of the dystonic movement. Sometimes, improvement of the dystonic posture can be seen even before the actual touch, or even by imagining the *geste antagoniste*.

Tremor

Dystonia may coexist with other movement abnormalities, most commonly tremor. The relationship between dystonia and tremor is complex, as described in more detail in Chapter 12, "Dystonia and Tremor." On the one hand, a typical tremor may coexist with dystonia. About half of all individuals with dystonia also have a tremor, but the frequency of their coexistence varies according to the type of dystonia.[29] In some cases, dystonia may begin years before tremor emerges. In other cases, the tremor starts first.

In addition to typical tremors, dystonic movements may mimic a tremor when they are rapid and repetitive. The term *dystonic tremor* historically referred to this type of tremor-like dystonic movement, which could be distinguished from other tremors by several features, including irregular amplitude and/or rhythm, a jerky quality, a null point where the tremor abates, and a *geste antagoniste*. Although the term *dystonic tremor* is often applied, it may be preferable to refer to this type of movement as "jerky dystonia," rather than tremor.[3,9]

The term *dystonic tremor* has also been used to describe any tremor occurring in the same body region where there also was dystonia.[4] As a result of this dual use of the same term, the literature regarding dystonic tremor can be confusing. It may be preferable to avoid use of the dystonic tremor and use more descriptive language such as *dystonia with tremor* or *dystonia-tremor syndrome*.

DIFFERENTIAL DIAGNOSIS

Other Involuntary Movements

There are several distinct types of abnormal movements. Their clinical features differ in many aspects (Table 2.1). *Chorea* tends to be more variable rather than patterned. Movements in chorea may appear almost random, moving from one body part to another. They are often very brief, in contrast to dystonic movement which are more often sustained or repetitive.

Athetosis was originally used to describe slow and writhing movements of the trunk and limbs. This usage overlapped with dystonia, but its definition has evolved over the years.[20] This term is used much less in the modern literature, and now it is chiefly used to describe subtle movements of the fingers or toes.

Table 2.1 **Distinguishing different movement disorders**

Movement disorder	Description
Dystonia	Sustained or intermittent muscle contractions causing abnormal, often repetitive movements, postures, or both. Dystonic movements are typically patterned and twisting, and may be tremulous.
Chorea	Usually brief and irregular, purposeless movements which seem to flow from one body part to another.
Tics	Involuntary stereotyped movements or vocalizations that are often suppressible or associated with a premonitory urge.
Myoclonus	Sudden and rapid jerk-like movements which may come in isolation or in groups.

Myoclonus refers to a sudden shock-like movement.[36] Dystonic movements are usually slower and/or more sustained, but they can also be fast and jerky. In these cases, it can be difficult to discriminate dystonia from myoclonus, as described further in Chapter 15, "Dystonia and Myoclonus."

Tics can resemble dystonia. Like dystonia, tics are patterned. However, tics can usually be discriminated from dystonia by a premonitory urge and by the ability to suppress the movement. Dystonic movements usually do not have a premonitory urge, and they cannot be voluntarily suppressed.

Parkinsonism is a syndrome that typically combines a paucity of movements that are often slowed, along with other features such as resting tremor and gait disability (see Chapter 13, "Dystonia and Parkinsonism"). It is usually easy to discriminate dystonia from parkinsonism, but they may coexist. Movements in dystonia may be slow, but slowing usually only affects the dystonic body region. Tremor in dystonia is often action-induced, while tremor in parkinsonism more often occurs at rest. The gait disorder of dystonia often looks quite different from the gait disorder of parkinsonism.

Although dystonia can usually be discriminated from other abnormal movements, it is not uncommon to see different types of abnormal movements combined. Dystonia is frequently combined with tremor, parkinsonism, chorea, or myoclonus. In some cases, multiple movement disorders coexist.

Disorders of Muscle Tone

Abnormal postures due to increased muscle activity are not specific for dystonia but can be found in other disorders of muscle tone, most notably the *spasticity* of cerebral palsy and other disorders affecting the corticospinal pathways. Increased muscle tone also occurs in *rigidity* associated with Parkinson disease and related disorders.[11,26]

Careful clinical examination helps in the differentiation of disorders of muscle tone (Table 2.2). In general, dystonia may have a normal or reduced muscle tone at rest and on passive movements, but the tone increases with voluntary action. Spasticity, in contrast, is described by an increased tone at rest that may increase with passive flexion. It typically includes a rate-dependent catch (*spastic catch*), often associated with other corticospinal signs like hyperreflexia, clonus, and pathological reflexes like Babinski, Gordon, or Oppenheim reflex. Rigidity has a uniformly increased tone at rest and with passive movement, where there may also be some cogwheeling or lead-pipe rigidity.

Paratonia (or *Gegenhalten*, "to go against") refers not to a disorder of resting tone but to an increase in resistance when movements are produced by the examiner.[14] This resistance is

Table 2.2 **Distinguishing disorders of muscle tone**

Clinical feature	Dystonia	Spasticity	Rigidity	Paratonia
Abnormal postures at rest	Sometimes; postures vary according to type of dystonia	Often; postures dominated by flexors in arm and leg or plantar flexion and inversion of ankle	Sometimes, slight flexion of upper limbs	No or variable
Increased tone with voluntary action	Yes	Yes	No	No
Increased resistance to passive limb movements	Sometimes	Yes	Yes	Variable
Rate-dependent catch	No	Yes	No	Variable
Hypotonia at rest	Sometimes	No	No	Variable
Other helpful features	*Geste antagoniste*	Other corticospinal signs	Cogwheeling, other parkinsonian signs	Associated often with dementia; tone can normalize with distraction

often proportional to the strength of the stimulus applied, and it is most frequently seen in dementia. However, given that paratonia does not produce an abnormal tone or postures at rest or with voluntary activities, it is usually easy to discriminate from dystonia. Other higher motor disorders that can lead to abnormal movements include disorders of disinhibition, motor intention, and alien limb syndromes. Those are typically not patterned, and patients report a lack of sense of agency or a loss of control over the affected limb.[14]

Although abnormalities of muscle tone in dystonia can be distinguished from related disorders of muscle tone, it is not uncommon to see some overlap. For example, many children with cerebral palsy have a combination of spasticity and dystonia, as described in more detail in Chapter 16, "Dystonia and Cerebral Palsy."

DYSTONIA SYNDROMES (LEVEL 2)

The Strategy of Syndromic Patterns

The main focus of this chapter is to describe the defining clinical features of dystonia and how to discriminate dystonia from related motor abnormalities. Once the presence of dystonia is established, as outlined above, the next step is to delineate a syndrome.

There are many different clinical manifestations of dystonia and hundreds of specific syndromes where dystonia may occur. Because there are so many different syndromes, it is useful to have a strategy for lumping and splitting them into subgroups. The most useful factors for classifying the many types of dystonia are described in more detail in the next chapter, "Classification and Diagnostic Strategy for Dystonia." In brief, these factors include some of the clinical manifestations of dystonic movements themselves, age at onset, body region affected, manner of onset, progression over time, and any relevant additional neurological or systemic features. The identification of a specific syndrome narrows the list of potential etiologies to consider.

Some Well-Recognized Dystonia Syndromes

Dystonia can affect individuals of all ages, in nearly any body region. However, there are some commonly recognized syndromes. This section provides a short overview of these common syndromes, each of which is covered in more details in other chapters.

CERVICAL DYSTONIA

Cervical dystonia may be the most common manifestation of dystonia, as described in detail in Chapter 5, "Cervical Dystonias."[2] It can affect individuals of any age, but more commonly arises in adults. It is usually gradual in onset, emerging over several weeks or months, often with a pulling sensation and neck discomfort, eventually with more persistent deviation of the head and neck.

The most frequent manifestation is *torticollis*, which involves rotating the head to the right or left. Other variations are *laterocollis* (tilt of one ear toward the shoulder), *retrocollis* (neck extension), and *anterocollis* (neck flexion). Abnormal postures may also relate to the position of the head in relation to the neck, with a similar nomenclature (e.g., torticaput, laterocaput, retrocaput, and anterocaput).[8,13] Temporary remissions may occur, but they are uncommon. Many individuals have tremor of the head or hands as well.

CRANIOFACIAL DYSTONIA

Dystonia affecting the craniofacial region may present as blepharospasm, oromandibular dystonia, or a combination of both.[27,28] Like cervical dystonia, craniofacial dystonias are more common in adults than in children.

The first symptoms in blepharospasm may be a feeling of discomfort in the eyes and abnormal sensitivity to bright light, before increased blinking or more sustained spasms of eye closure develop. Symptoms are aggravated by fatigue, stress, reading, and bright lights. Conversely, symptoms usually improve with mental concentration or speaking. They may therefore appear distractable, or they may be absent during clinical consultation.

Oromandibular dystonia manifests as jaw opening, jaw closing, jaw retraction or protrusion, lip pursing, tongue deviations, and/or platysma overactivity. Affected individuals have difficulties chewing and speaking but only rarely have trouble swallowing. The craniofacial dystonias are described further in Chapter 6, "Craniofacial Dystonias."

WRITER'S CRAMP

Writer's cramp is a task-specific dystonia, described further in Chapter 10, "Musician's and Other Task-Specific Dystonias." Affected individuals describe difficulties when writing. They use excessive force often with obvious abnormal postures of fingers or hand, or they may describe cramping and soreness of the muscles of the hand or forearm. There are increasing difficulties as writing continues. Sometimes difficulties begin even when attempting to pick up or hold a pen.

In many cases, the problem evolves over time, and dystonia is not limited to writing but becomes also obvious in other activities like using cutlery, brushing teeth, or buttoning shirts. Similar dystonic "cramps" may occur wherever repetitive, stereotyped movements are performed and have been described in musicians, typists, and many others. Similarly, the lower limbs may be affected in dancers, runners, or sewing-machine workers.

LARYNGEAL DYSTONIA

The laryngeal dystonias are another form of task-specific dystonia, triggered usually by speaking (see Chapter 7, "Laryngeal Dystonias"). Two main types are recognized. Adductor laryngeal dystonia has a characteristically strained voice and frequent voice breaks. Abductor laryngeal dystonia is characterized by a whispering or breathy quality. Laryngeal dystonias, like other dystonias, might be aggravated by anxiety and stress, and they are therefore often mistaken as expression of psychological issues.

CEREBRAL PALSY

Cerebral palsy is probably one of the most common syndromes where dystonia may occur (see Chapter 16, "Dystonia and Cerebral Palsy"). Several subtypes of cerebral palsy are defined by the predominant motor problem (spastic, dyskinetic, ataxic), although most cases have a mixed picture.[18] Dystonia is the main problem in dyskinetic cerebral palsy, which accounts for 10–15% of all cases. However, the most careful studies of the motor problems across all types of cerebral palsy have indicated that at least 80% of all cases have at least some dystonia.[24] The syndrome is not progressive.

Historically, this label was used to imply prenatal or perinatal brain damage due to intrauterine infection, extreme preterm birth, birth asphyxia, stroke, or other causes. The term has also been applied to individuals with a similar clinical syndrome even when the cause is not known. Recently, it has become increasingly clear that cerebral palsy is a mix of different syndromes with different etiologies.[12,19,37]

OTHER DYSTONIA SYNDROMES

There are numerous other well-recognized dystonia syndromes that include dystonia combined with other neurological features such as parkinsonism (see Chapter 13, "Dystonia and Parkinsonism"), ataxia (see Chapter 14, "Dystonia and Ataxia"), or myoclonus (see Chapter 15, "Dystonia and Myoclonus"). There are also numerous other inherited syndromes where dystonia may occur (see Chapter 18, "Dystonias Combined with Other Features").

DYSTONIA ETIOLOGIES (LEVEL 3)

Once the existence of dystonia has been established (Level 1) and a dystonia syndrome has been identified (Level 2), the next step is to consider potential etiologies that may require diagnostic testing. The overall strategy for workup and the value of different types of tests are described in Chapter 27, "Workup of Dystonia."

Briefly, the workup depends greatly on the age at which dystonia began. For most adult-onset dystonias, little or no diagnostic testing is required. The vast majority of adult-onset cases are idiopathic, even after extensive laboratory evaluations. Diagnostic testing rests on recognition of a typical dystonia syndrome, and additional tests are warranted only if there are clinical features that point to a specific cause.

In contrast, some workup is essential for nearly all early-onset cases of dystonia. Unless there is documented evidence for an acquired cause such as cerebral palsy, neuroimaging is usually conducted. Blood and other tests to rule out conditions with specific mechanism-based treatments may also be needed.

SYNOPSIS AND FUTURE PROSPECTS

Dystonia is a movement disorder defined by abnormal, often repetitive movements, postures, or both. These movements are typically patterned and twisting. Typical features of dystonia comprise overflow, mirroring, and the *geste antagoniste*. Tremor or tremor-like movements also are common. A large number of different terms are used in the dystonia literature, and some of the most common ones are listed in Table 2.3.

The diagnosis of dystonia is based on clinical identification of its characteristic features and the exclusion of other movement disorders (such as chorea or tics) or disorders that may mimic dystonia (such as pseudodystonias). Helpful clues to recognizing common dystonia syndromes include age at onset, body distribution, specific characteristics of dystonic movements, temporal pattern, and any relevant associated features.

Currently, the diagnosis of dystonia and its discrimination from other disorders is based on clinical recognition. At some point in the future, diagnosis may be aided by more objective biological measures. Dystonia currently cannot be definitively diagnosed by routine clinical tests such as brain imaging or electromyography. In a small portion of cases, genetic testing can be informative, but many dystonia genes may also cause other movement disorders, so

Table 2.3 **Glossary of dystonia terms**

Term	Explanation
Blepharospasm	Dystonia affecting the orbicularis oculi muscles leading to excessive blinking and spasms
Camptocormia	Forward bending of the trunk, sometimes caused by dystonia or orthopedic problems
Dyskinesia	A generic term which means "abnormal movement"
Dystonic seizure	Seizure with tonic or twisting movements that resemble dystonia
Dystonic tic	Tic with tonic or twisting movements that resemble dystonia
Dystonic tremor	A tremor or tremor-like movement occurring with dystonia
Functional dystonia	A psychiatric disorder with abnormal movements resembling dystonia, also known as psychogenic dystonia
Geste antagoniste	Something the individual does to alleviate dystonia; also known as *sensory trick* or *alleviating maneuver*
Homolateral synkinesis	Voluntary movements on one side of the body trigger similar unintentional movements ipsilaterally
Meige syndrome	Combination of blepharospasm with oromandibular dystonia
Mirror dystonia	Voluntary movements on the unaffected side of the body trigger dystonic movements on the affected side
Mirror movements	Voluntary movements on one side of the body provoke similar involuntary movements on the opposite side of the body
Myoclonic dystonia	Dystonic movements with a rapid and jerky quality resembling myoclonus
Myoclonus-dystonia	Syndrome that combines both myoclonus and dystonia
Oculogyric crisis	Involuntary conjugate deviation of the eyes, usually upward and laterally
Opisthotonus	Dystonic backward arching of the trunk
Overflow	Contractions of muscles spread to nearby muscles that are not required for movement
Pisa syndrome	Sideways bending of the trunk, caused by dystonia or orthopedic issues
Pseudodystonia	Abnormal movements or postures that are not true dystonia
Psychogenic dystonia	A neuro-psychiatric disorder with movements resembling dystonia, also known as functional dystonia
Sensory trick	Something the individual does to alleviate dystonia; also known as *geste antagoniste* or *alleviating maneuver*
Spasmodic dysphonia	Laryngeal dystonia with characteristic voice breaks
Spastic dystonia	Spasticity combined with dystonia, as in cerebral palsy
Striatal toe	Extensor movement of the great toe that resembles the Babinski reflex; also known as *dystonic toe*
Tardive dystonia	Subtype of tardive dyskinesias caused by dopamine antagonists
Task-specific dystonia	Dystonia triggered only by a specific task, such as writing
Writer's cramp	Task-specific dystonia triggered by writing

identification of a "dystonia gene" does not mean the abnormal movement is always dystonia.

Recent attempts to recognize the movements of dystonia have involved kinematic strategies,[5,21,25,30,31] digital analysis of video recordings,[6,23,34] or electromyography.[15,17] Some studies have suggested that different types of dystonia can be diagnosed using software algorithms that detect microstructural anomalies on brain MRI,[35] and recent studies have hinted that blood-based biomarkers may be available in the future.[33] Further development of these tools may aid clinical recognition of dystonia and its many subtypes in the future.

REFERENCES

1. Albanese A, Bhatia K, Fung V, Hallett M, Jankovic J, et al. Definition and Classification of Dystonia, 2025 (first presented at the International Dystonia Symposium in 2023).
2. Albanese A, Bhatia KP, Cardoso F, Comella C, Defazio G, Fung VSC, et al. Isolated cervical dystonia: Diagnosis and classification. Mov Disord 2023;38:1367–1348.
3. Asmus F, Langseth A, Doherty E, Nestor T, Munz M, Gasser T, et al. "Jerky" dystonia in children: Spectrum of phenotypes and genetic testing. Mov Disord 2009;24:702–709.
4. Bhatia KP, Bain P, Bajaj N, Elble RJ, Hallett M, Louis ED, et al. Consensus statement on the classification of tremors. from the task force on tremor of the International Parkinson and Movement Disorder Society. Mov Disord 2018;33:75–87.
5. Boccagni C, Carpaneto J, Micera S, Bagnato S, Galardi G. Motion analysis in cervical dystonia. Neurol Sci 2008;29:375–381.
6. Chen Q, Vu JP, Cisneros E, Benadof CN, Zhang Z, Barbano RL, et al. Postural directionality and head tremor in cervical dystonia. Tremor Other Hyperkinet Mov 2020;10. doi:10.7916/tohm.v0.745.
7. Cox BC, Cincotta M, Espay AJ. Mirror movements in movement disorders: A review. Tremor Other Hyperkinet Mov (N Y) 2012;2:tre-02-59-398-1.
8. Finsterer J, Maeztu C, Revuelta GJ, Reichel G, Truong D. Collum-caput (COL-CAP) concept for conceptual anterocollis, anterocaput, and forward sagittal shift. J Neurol Sci 2015;355:37–43.
9. Ghika J, Bogousslavsky J, Henderson J, Maeder P, Regli F. The "jerky dystonic unsteady hand": A delayed motor syndrome in posterior thalamic infarctions. J Neurol 1994;241:537–542.
10. Jahanshahi M. Factors that ameliorate or aggravate spasmodic torticollis. J Neurol Neurosurg Psychiatry 2000;68:227–229.
11. Jethwa A, Mink J, Macarthur C, Knights S, Fehlings T, Fehlings D. Development of the Hypertonia Assessment Tool (HAT): A discriminative tool for hypertonia in children. Dev Med Child Neurol 2010;52:e83–87.
12. Jonsson U, Eek MN, Sunnerhagen KS, Himmelmann K. Cerebral palsy prevalence, subtypes, and associated impairments: A population-based comparison study of adults and children. Dev Med Child Neurol 2019;61:1162–1167.
13. Jost WH, Tatu L, Pandey S, Slawek J, Druzdz A, Biering-Sorensen B, et al. Frequency of different subtypes of cervical dystonia: A prospective multicenter study according to Col-Cap concept. J Neural Transm 2020;127:45–50.
14. Kojovic M, Bhatia KP. Bringing order to higher order motor disorders. J Neurol 2019;266:797–805.
15. Kwon YT, Lee Y, Kilic-Berkmen G, Lim HR, Scorr L, Jinnah HA, Yeo WH. Soft materials-enabled, active wireless, thin-film bioelectronics for quantitative diagnostics of cervical dystonia. Adv Mater Technol 2019;4:1900458.
16. Liu P, Yuan Y, Zhang N, Liu X, Yu L, Luo B. Mirror movements in acquired neurological disorders: A mini-review. Front Neurol 2021;12:736115.
17. Mahmood M, Kwon S, Kilic-Berkmen G, Kim YS, Scorr L, Jinnah HA, Yeo WH. Soft nanomembrane sensors and flexible hybrid bioelectronics for wireless quantification of blepharospasm. IEEE Trans Biomed Engineer 2020;67:3094–3100.
18. Monbaliu E, Himmelmann K, Lin JP, Ortibus E, Bonouvrie L, Feys H, et al. Clinical presentation and management of dyskinetic cerebral palsy. Lancet Neurol 2017;16:741–749.
19. Moreno-De-Luca A, Millan F, Pesacreta DR, Elloumi HZ, Oetjens MT, et al. Molecular diagnostic yield of exome sequencing in patients with cerebral palsy. JAMA 2021;325:467–475.
20. Morris JG, Jankelowitz SK, Fung VS, Clouston PD, Hayes MW, Grattan-Smith P. Athetosis I: Historical considerations. Mov Disord 2002;17:1278–1280.
21. Nowak DA, Dafotakis M, Fink GR. Kinematic analysis of grasping in focal dystonia of the face and neck. Neuroscience 2013;237:216–222.
22. Patel N, Hanfelt J, Marsh L, Jankovic J, Coalition on Motion Disorders. Alleviating manoeuvres (sensory tricks) in cervical dystonia. J Neurol Neurosurg Psychiatry 2014;85:882–884.
23. Peterson DA, Littlewort GC, Bartlett MS, Macerollo A, Perlmutter JS, Jinnah HA, et al. Objective, computerized video-based rating of blepharospasm severity. Neurology 2016;87:2146–2153.
24. Rice J, Skuza P, Baker F, Russo R, Fehlings D. Identification and measurement of dystonia in cerebral palsy. Dev Med Child Neurol 2017;59:1249–1255.
25. Samotus O, Lee J, Jog M. Personalized botulinum toxin type A therapy for cervical dystonia based on kinematic guidance. J Neurol 2018;265:1269–1278.
26. Sanger TD, Delgado MR, Gaebler-Spira D, Hallett M, Mink JW, Task F. Classification and definition of disorders causing hypertonia in childhood. Pediatrics 2003;111:89–97.
27. Scorr L, Cho HJ, Kilic-Berkmen G, McKay JL, Hallett M, Klein C, et al. Clinical features and evolution of blepharospasm: A multicenter international cohort and systematic literature review. Dystonia 2022;1:10359.
28. Scorr LM, Factor SA, Perez-Parra S, Kaye R, Paniello RC, Norris SA, et al. Oromandibular dystonia: A clinical examination of 2,020 cases. Front Neurol 2021;12:700714.
29. Shaikh AG, Beylergil SB, Scorr L, Kilic-Berkmen G, Freeman A, Klein C, et al. Dystonia & tremor: A cross-sectional study of the Dystonia Coalition cohort. Neurology 2021;96:e563–e574.

30. Shaikh AG, Wong AL, Zee DS, Jinnah HA. Keeping your head on target. J Neurosci 2013;33:11281–11295.
31. Shaikh AG, Zee DS, Jinnah HA. Oscillatory head movements in cervical dystonia: Dystonia, tremor, or both? Mov Disord 2015;30:834–842.
32. Sitburana O, Wu LJ, Sheffield JK, Davidson A, Jankovic J. Motor overflow and mirror dystonia. Parkinsonism Relat Disord 2009;15:758–761.
33. Timsina J, Dinasarapu AR, Kilic-Berkmen G, Wang L, Budde J, Sung YJ, et al. Blood-based proteomics for adult-onset focal dystonias. Ann Neurol 2024;96:110–120.
34. Trotta GF, Pellicciari R, Boccaccio A, Brunetti A, Cascarano GD, Manghisi VM, et al. A neural network-based software to recognise blepharospasm symptoms and to measure eye closure time. Comput Biol Med 2019;112:103376.
35. Valeriani D, Simonyan K. A microstructural neural network biomarker for dystonia diagnosis identified by a DystoniaNet deep learning platform. Proc Natl Acad Sci 2020;117:26398–26405.
36. van der Veen S, Caviness JN, Dreissen YEM, Ganos C, Ibrahim A, Koelman J, et al. Myoclonus and other jerky movement disorders. Clin Neurophysiol Pract 2022;7:285–316.
37. Zech M, Jech R, Boesch S, Skorvanek M, Weber S, Wagner M, et al. Monogenic variants in dystonia: An exome-wide sequencing study. Lancet Neurol 2020;19:908–918.

Chapter 3

Classification and Diagnostic Strategy for Dystonia

INTRODUCTION

The dystonias have widely varying clinical manifestations (see Chapter 2, "Defining the Clinical Characteristics of Dystonia")[11,15] and hundreds of different etiologies.[3] With so many different clinical manifestations and causes, it is useful to have a plan for separating them into meaningful subgroups. The design of any plan for lumping and splitting groups depends on the goals of making the subgroups. For the dystonias, there are two goals. One goal is to aid clinicians in grouping clinical features into meaningful categories that guide diagnosis and management. The other goal is to aid basic scientists in organizing knowledge regarding the underlying biology into categories that guide understanding of pathogenesis and aid in the design of new therapies.

Strategies for classifying the dystonias have evolved over the years (Table 3.1) in keeping with the steadily growing appreciation of their varied clinical manifestations and causes.[16] One of the earliest strategies divided the dystonias into two broad groups according to etiology: primary (idiopathic) and secondary (due to a known cause). This simple and intuitive approach was eventually discarded. One of the major reasons for discarding this dichotomy is that subsequent classification strategies introduced the concept that primary dystonias were phenotypically relatively pure, while secondary dystonias more typically had additional neurological features mixed into the phenotype. Thus a dichotomy initially based on etiology was merged with one based on clinical features. Because the correspondence between causes and clinical features was imperfect, this evolution of the original classification system led to different opinions, idiosyncratic applications of the classification plans, and frequent calls for revision.[16]

Although the simple dichotomy of primary (pure dystonia) and secondary (dystonia combined with other problems) is still sometimes found in the literature, a more broadly accepted classification plan was introduced by an international panel of experts in 2013.[1] This plan classified the dystonias according to two separate axes.[1] Axis I was based on clinical manifestations, and Axis II was based on etiology (Figure 3.1). This proposal was widely adopted,[29] with demonstrated applicability in both children[23] and adults.[35] The two-axis plan was also adapted for tremor.[4] In the years following the introduction of the two-axis plan, a few

Table 3.1 **History of dystonia classification**

Fahn & Eldridge 1976	Fahn 1988[12]	Fahn 1998	Bressman 2004	Albanese 2011
Primary hereditary sporadic	Idiopathic	Primary hereditary sporadic	Primary hereditary sporadic	Primary pure dystonia plus paroxysmal
Secondary heredodegenerative environmental	Symptomatic	Dystonia plus	Secondary dystonia plus degenerative complex acquired	Heredodegenerative
Psychological		Heredodegenerative Acquired		Secondary

This table shows some of the dystonia classification strategies most commonly used over the years.

Source: Jinnah HA, Albanese A. The new classification for the dystonias: Why was it needed and how was it accomplished? Mov Discord Clin Pract 2014;1:280–284.

shortcomings were recognized.[23,35] Therefore, the classification plan was revised in 2025.[2] The relevant clinical features of Axis I were clarified and expanded to include new items. The etiologies of Axis II were also expanded to be more inclusive of any potential biological contributors to etiology or pathogenesis (Figure 3.2). Only the most recent classification plan is summarized below.

CLASSIFICATION ACCORDING TO CLINICAL MANIFESTATIONS (AXIS I)

Body Area Affected

One important factor is based on the body areas affected with dystonia (Figure 3.2). *Focal dystonia* refers to involvement of one region of the body. The most commonly affected regions are the neck (cervical dystonia or torticollis), eye region (blepharospasm), one limb (such as writer's cramp or foot dystonia), or larynx (laryngeal dystonia or spasmodic dysphonia). However, nearly any region of the body can be affected, such as a single finger or toe, the tongue, shoulder, trunk, or pelvis.

Segmental dystonia refers to involvement of two or three contiguous body regions. A common example is simultaneous involvement of the eye region along with the oromandibular region. This combination is sometimes called *Meige syndrome*, although the more modern term is *craniofacial dystonia*.[22] Multifocal *dystonia* refers to involvement of two or three noncontiguous body regions, such as writer's cramp combined with blepharospasm, or one hand combined with the opposite foot.

Generalized dystonia refers to broader involvement of the body. The 2013 Consensus plan required the trunk and at least two additional body regions, but the 2025 plan acknowledges a more flexible combination of body regions (e.g., three limbs). *Hemidystonia* might be considered a subtype of multifocal dystonia when there is involvement of the ipsilateral arm and leg. Alternatively, it might be considered a subtype of generalized dystonia if the ipsilateral arm and leg are combined with neck and/or trunk.[36]

It is important to appreciate that the classification system provides guidelines, not strict rules, and some clinical judgment is needed. For example, the discrimination of focal from segmental dystonia is sometimes ambiguous because of the lack of precise criteria regarding what defines a single body region. One common example is cervical dystonia, where the shoulder is very commonly involved because some muscles jointly move the head/neck and shoulder. Even though the shoulder is a distinct body region, involvement of the neck and shoulder is still usually considered a focal dystonia.[21] A similar ambiguity exists for the face, where upper (eye region) and lower (mouth region) are sometimes considered one or two body regions, leading to the label of focal or segmental dystonia.[19] There are also variations in the application of the term hemidystonia.[36]

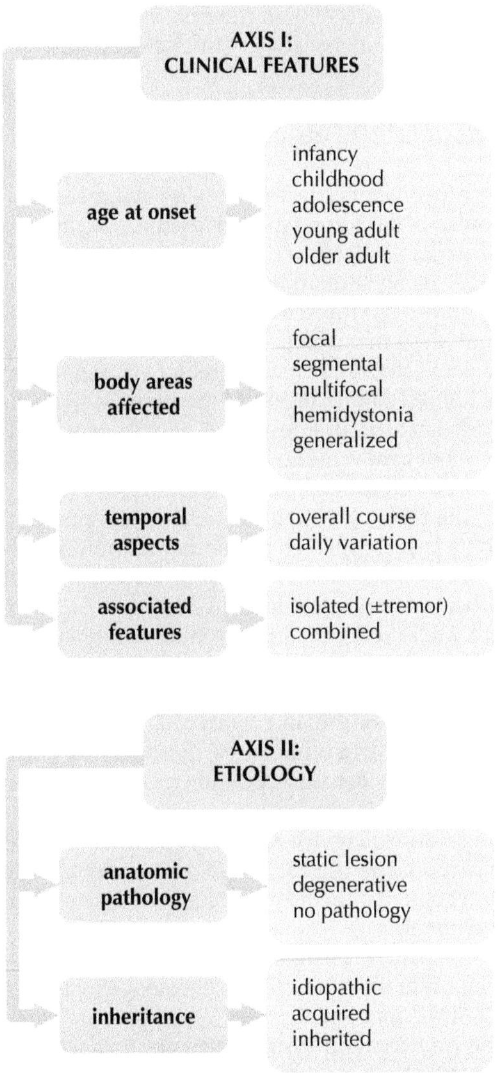

Figure 3.1. Classification plan for the many types of dystonia in 2013.

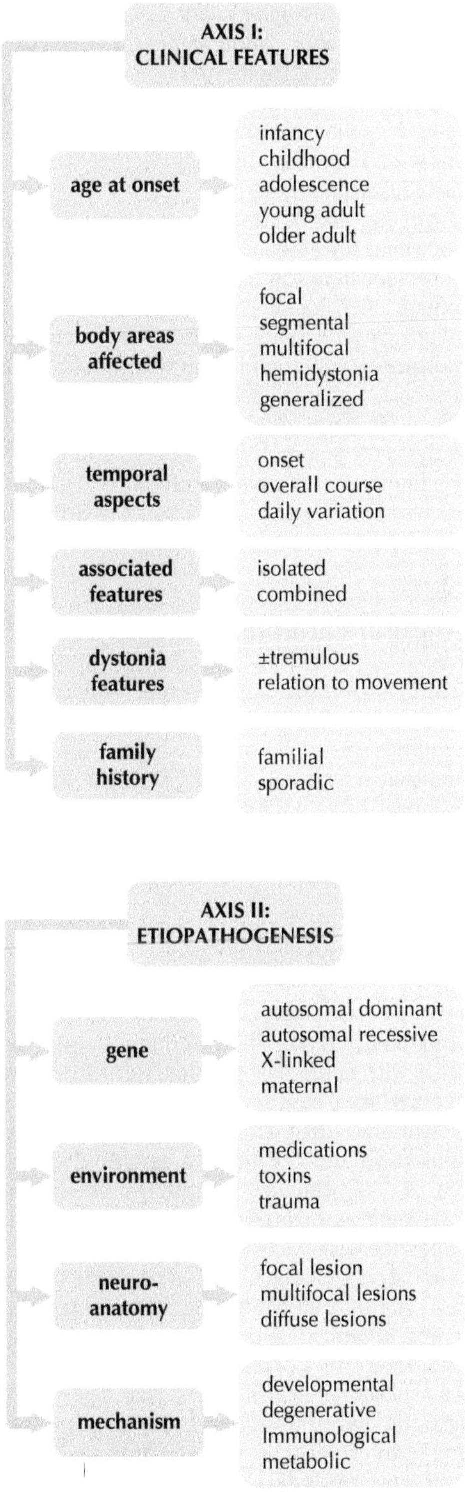

Figure 3.2. Abbreviated classification plan for the many types of dystonia in 2025.

Guidelines are currently lacking for discriminating focal versus segmental dystonia for the upper limb, which includes the shoulder, upper and lower arm, and the hand. However, recent studies have implied that these regions should be combined as one when it comes to defining focal or segmental.[5]

Age at Onset

Another important clinical aspect for classifying the dystonias is the age when it began (Figure 3.2).

The age groups include infancy (<2 years), childhood (3–12 years), adolescence (13–20 years), early adulthood (21–40 years), and late adulthood (>40 years). These groups are not specific to the dystonias, but they are based on conventions widely used for other neurological and non-neurological disorders.

A precise age of onset is sometimes difficult to pinpoint for early-onset neurodevelopmental disorders, where motor delay might be the first problem, with insidious emergence of dystonic posturing over months or years.[23,35] For complex syndromes that combine dystonia with other features, it may be necessary to stipulate the age at onset for each problem separately. For example, dystonia is combined with myoclonus in the myoclonus-dystonia syndrome, but one problem may be appreciated years before the other one emerges.

Temporal Variables

A third important clinical aspect for classifying the dystonias involves temporal variables, including speed of onset, short-term variations that may occur during a single day, and the longer-term course of the disorder (Figure 3.2). The speed of onset is relevant since most types of dystonia evolve over a period of many months or years. A few types of dystonia reach peak severity over a much shorter time frame of a few days or weeks. Sudden onset is a red flag for a psychogenic (functional) neurological disorder (see Chapter 25, "Psychogenic [Functional] Dystonia"). Sudden onset also occurs with acute dystonic reactions from neuroleptics (see Chapter 19, "Dystonia Induced by Medications, Illicit Drugs, and Environmental Exposures") and certain rare genetic disorders such as rapid-onset dystonia-parkinsonism or dystonia associated with disorders of acute striatal necrosis.

Short-term changes in severity also are relevant. The diurnal worsening of dystonia in the evening is typical of dopa-responsive dystonia, while intermittent attacks of dystonia indicate a paroxysmal dyskinesia (see Chapter 17, "Dystonia and the Paroxysmal Dyskinesias"). Long-term changes in severity may also occur. Many types of dystonia progress slowly or in a stepwise fashion, often over many months or years. Others remain relatively static over the years. The dystonia of cerebral palsy shows a period of worsening in the first year or two, but usually remains relatively static thereafter.

Associated Features

Another clinical factor for classifying the dystonias is based on whether dystonia is the only problem (isolated, or pure) or combined with other relevant neurological or medical problems (Figure 3.2). The term *isolated dystonia* means that dystonia is the sole neurological feature. Isolated dystonia does not refer to dystonia that is limited to one region of the body. Individuals with isolated dystonia may have broader patterns of involvement, including segmental, multifocal, and generalized.

The term *combined dystonia* means that dystonia is accompanied by another relevant movement disorder, other neurological features, or other systemic features. In some cases, there are well-recognized syndromic combinations, such as dystonia with parkinsonism, or dystonia with myoclonus (see Chapter 13, on "Dystonia and Parkinsonism" or Chapter 15, "Dystonia and Myoclonus"). In other cases, dystonia may coexist with another very common problem, such as age-related neuropathy or migraines. Whether these other features should be considered part of a more specific combined dystonia syndrome or a coincidental disorder requires some clinical judgment.

The place of tremor in the classification of dystonia remains a matter of debate (see Chapter 12, "Dystonia and Tremor").[26] On the one hand, the classification system suggests that isolated dystonia may include coexisting tremor because the combination of dystonia with tremor is very common.[31] On the other hand, tremor and dystonia are also considered distinct movement disorders, so dystonia with tremor might be classified among the combined disorders. A good example of the conundrum regarding tremor and dystonia is the very common combination of cervical dystonia with hand tremors. This combination is most often viewed as an isolated focal dystonia of the neck with a coincidental but separate movement disorder of hand tremor. However, if the hand tremors are considered a part of a broader dystonia syndrome, then the same combination would be classified as a multifocal dystonia.[20,25] Further work therefore is needed to clarify the best approach to classifying combinations of dystonia with tremor.

Dystonia Characteristics

In the 2025 revision of the dystonia classification plan, certain characteristics of dystonia were added because they have important implications for diagnosis or treatment.[2] These include the relationship to voluntary movement and tremor-like movements.

The relationship of dystonia to voluntary movement is an important characteristic. Attempted voluntary movements often exaggerate the abnormal postures and movements of most types of dystonia. Some types of dystonia are triggered only by a single task, such as writing in writer's cramp (see Chapter 10, "Musician's and Other Task-Specific Dystonias").[28,32] Other types of dystonia are triggered by multiple tasks, such as an upper limb dystonia that is triggered by writing, buttoning a shirt, or reaching for a cup. Sometimes, dystonic movements or postures may even occur at rest, without any voluntary action.[9] In these cases, attempted voluntary activity often worsens the dystonia. Abnormal postures that are relatively immobile or fixed may occur with long-standing severe dystonia and sometimes reflect permanent contractures. This relationship between dystonia and voluntary movement may evolve over time. It is not uncommon for an individual to begin with writer's cramp, progress to dystonia of the same limb with multiple activities, and then experience abnormal movements or postures even at rest. If untreated, relatively fixed abnormal postures may eventually appear.

Another important characteristic relates to the speed of dystonic movements. Dystonic movements often have a slow and twisting quality. However, dystonic movements can also be quick.[11] Dystonic jerks may resemble myoclonus or tics (see Chapter 15). When multiple jerks appear in a semi-rhythmical manner, they may resemble tremor. In some cases, these repetitive movements may be sufficiently regular to look like a tremor. Therefore, tremor and other tremor-like movements are also important characteristics.

Family History

The presence of a family history has obvious implications for potential etiologies for dystonia. Dystonia genes are inherited in many ways, including autosomal dominant, autosomal recessive, X-linked, and maternal (see Chapter 22, "Dystonia Genetics").

It is important to appreciate that patterns of inheritance may be difficult to determine, especially when the family is small. Additionally, some genes have complex patterns of inheritance that may be misleading. Some genes are only partly penetrant (e.g., *TOR1A* and *THAP1*), some are subject to imprinting (e.g., *SGCE*), and many are sporadic with no family history. These conditions are summarized in more detail in other chapters, including Chapter 22.

CLASSIFICATION ACCORDING TO BIOLOGICAL BASIS (AXIS II)

From Etiology to Pathogenesis

In the 2013 classification plan, Axis II referred to etiology, with only two main subgroups. One related to whether there was a detectable neuroanatomical lesion and the other related to patterns of inheritance that might imply a genetic cause (Figure 3.1). At the time this plan was proposed, it was recognized that there were limited data to develop a more sophisticated plan, and the plan would be further elaborated as more was learned.[1,16] Since then, there have been enormous advances in knowledge regarding the biology of dystonia.[3] As a result, the 2025 classification approach to Axis II has been expanded. Axis II now contains categories for many major fields in biology. Some of these are relevant for clinicians seeking an etiological diagnosis, while others may be more relevant for biologists looking for common themes among the many different subtypes of dystonia.

Etiology

Most adult-onset focal dystonias will fall into the idiopathic category because an underlying cause often cannot be found, even with extensive laboratory testing (see Chapter 27, "Workup of Dystonia"). On the other hand, the most common dystonia of children probably occurs with cerebral palsy, which often is combined with spasticity and often acquired from early brain injury (see Chapter 16, "Dystonia in Cerebral Palsy"). There are numerous additional potential acquired causes for both children and adults including exposure to drugs or toxins, vascular events, infections or immune-related processes, trauma, and others.

There also are many genes that can cause dystonia (see Chapter 22). They may be subgrouped by patterns of inheritance as autosomal dominant or recessive, X-linked, and maternal. These patterns can sometimes be hard to recognize when families are small or the gene is subject to partial penetrance or imprinting. It also is valuable to recognize that genetic dystonias are not always inherited, and a substantial proportion may be sporadic.

Pathogenesis

Knowledge regarding the pathogenesis of dystonia is growing rapidly. This knowledge may be grouped according to major fields with biology (molecular, anatomical, and physiological).

Some of the known etiologies (both acquired and genetic) affect specific shared molecular or cellular mechanisms. There are numerous reviews of this topic, each recognizing certain types of dystonia that have shared mechanisms.[10,18,34,37] The most common shared mechanisms include abnormalities in dopamine neurotransmission, failure of energy sources including mitochondrial disorders, toxic accumulation of metals, abnormalities of channels that transport specific ions or metals, DNA transcription and repair, intracellular trafficking (nuclear envelope, endoplasmic reticulum, lysosomes) and/or intracellular stress, and others. Each of these molecular or cellular mechanisms may apply to a select subgroup of dystonias, although they may also intersect in some cases. Appreciating differences among these molecular mechanisms has obvious clinical implications since some of them have specific treatments (see Chapter 28, "Symptom-Targeted Oral Medications for Dystonia").[17]

The molecular and cellular mechanisms also are relevant for specific regions of the nervous system responsible for triggering dystonia. Neuroanatomical pathology might be delineated either by routine clinical neuroimaging procedures (e.g., CT or MRI scan), by postmortem histopathological evaluation of the nervous system, or by knowledge of the regional specificity of certain molecular mechanisms.[8] For many types of dystonia, there are no obvious structural defects in neuroimaging or autopsy studies. In some types of dystonia, there may be evidence for a neurodevelopmental or neurodegenerative cause or evidence for an acquired lesion, such as stroke or tumor. Historically, dystonia was linked with neuroanatomical pathology in the basal ganglia. However, it is now known that the responsible pathology may occur in many regions of the brain (see Chapter 23, "The Neuroanatomical Substrates of Dystonia"). Most of these regions are components of the brain's network for motor control, and they include the basal ganglia, sensorimotor cortex, cerebellum, midbrain, brainstem, and sometimes the spinal cord.[8,24] Knowing these different anatomical substrates for dystonia has obvious implications for diagnosis and treatment. More importantly, they have substantial implications for understanding the underlying biological mechanisms regardless of the original inciting etiology.

There are also some shared physiological themes, even when the etiology may remain unknown (see Chapter 24, "Dystonia Physiology").[7,13] An imbalance of inhibitory and excitatory processes has been established for numerous types of dystonia, at many levels of the nervous system. Maladaptive plasticity may play an important role for a subgroup of dystonias, too, such as the task-specific dystonias. Certain abnormal physiological processes may emerge within specific regions of the motor network responsible for dystonia. In the basal ganglia, for example, there may be an imbalance between the direct and indirect pathways and an imbalance between striosome and matrix compartments, or rate or rhythm abnormalities of pallidal output. In the cerebellum, a common abnormality underlying dystonia has been a change in the normal firing of Purkinje neurons from a steady tempo to a bursting pattern.[6,27] These physiological findings are receiving increasing attention as potential therapeutic targets.

THE DIAGNOSTIC APPROACH USING AXIS I AND AXIS II

There are two separate axes separating clinical features and biological underpinnings. However, both axes are envisioned to be used together. The goal of defining the clinical features in Axis I is to delineate a syndromic pattern that aids in the consideration of possible biological underpinnings in Axis II. The clinical factors in Axis I were chosen because they were viewed as the most useful aids to reaching an etiological diagnosis or to directing treatment toward pathogenic mechanisms of Axis II.

For example, delineating the body regions affected guides both clinical diagnosis and management. Individuals with generalized dystonia are more likely to have a discoverable cause than those with focal dystonia, especially in adults. Some specific patterns of body involvement are also useful. For example, opisthotonos and retrocollis may occur in older adults, but they are uncommon. When they occur in an adult, tardive dystonia should be considered (see Chapter 19). Similarly, lingual protrusion dystonia may occur in adults, but it is not common. The occurrence of prominent tongue dystonia in an adult should also raise concern for a tardive syndrome. Hemidystonia is also relatively uncommon in adults.[36] It may raise concern for a contralateral brain lesion or Parkinson disease. In children, opisthotonos and retrocollis may be viewed as red flags for certain genetic metabolic or degenerative disorders, such as neurodegeneration with brain iron accumulation.[33] Lingual dystonia similarly raises concern for certain genetic metabolic disorders.[30] Regarding treatment, individuals with focal dystonia are most often treated with local injection of botulinum toxin. On the other hand, local injections may not provide adequate relief for individuals with broader patterns of involvement. Instead, they may need other treatment options, such as deep brain stimulation surgery.

The different age groups also are relevant for clinical management, prognosis, and etiology. For example, most individuals with onset of dystonia in late adulthood are focal, idiopathic, and have only limited progression. Even within the adult-onset group there are relevant age differences. Writer´s cramp occurs typically with a peak in the fourth decade, cervical dystonia manifests in the fourth or fifth decade, cranial dystonia occurs around the sixth decade. In these adult-onset cases, additional signs and symptoms are usually coincidental and not part of the dystonia syndrome. Most cases are idiopathic. In contrast to cases with dystonia onset in adulthood, a larger proportion of individuals with onset of dystonia in late childhood or early adolescence have a genetic etiology, with greater risk of spread to other parts of the body. Individuals with onset in infancy are most likely to have a metabolic cause, often with a dire prognosis. Many of these childhood-onset dystonias are combined with other neurological or medical problems.

Temporal aspects also guide clinical diagnosis and management. For example, insidious onset with slow or stepwise progression is typical of most adult-onset focal dystonias as well as genetic dystonias associated with genes such as *TOR1A* or *THAP1*. By contrast, sudden onset with a relatively static course is typical of certain other disorders such as psychogenic (functional) disorders, and certain rare inherited disorders such as those due to glutaric aciduria or genetic variants in *ATP1A3*. Subacute onset is also indicative of more specific syndromes, such as a reaction to a drug or toxin (see Chapter 19), autoimmune dystonia (see Chapter 21, "Dystonia and Autoimmunity"), or several inherited metabolic disorders associated with acute striatal necrosis (see Chapter 22). Regular diurnal variations in dystonia severity point to dopa-responsive dystonia, while episodic attacks of dystonia characterize the paroxysmal dyskinesias.

Whether or not dystonia is isolated or combined with other relevant neurological or medical problems also is relevant for etiological diagnosis and treatment. There are many inherited and acquired causes where dystonia is combined with parkinsonism, ataxia, spasticity, or myoclonus. Each of these syndromes is covered in separate chapters. Dystonia may also be combined with systemic defects, such as liver dysfunction in Wilson disease. Many of these are described in the Chapter 18, "Dystonia Combined with Other Features." Knowledge of syndromic patterns narrows the differential diagnosis for subsequent laboratory testing.

Certain clinical features of the dystonia itself have diagnostic value, such as whether abnormal postures are mobile or fixed, relationship to voluntary movement, and whether movements are slow, jerky, or tremulous. It is very likely that the biological underpinnings of these different types of movements are quite distinct and may require different approaches to treatment.

It is important to recognize that individuals may be classified in different ways as their disorder progresses. For example, it is not unusual for a focal isolated dystonia to evolve into a segmental or generalized pattern. Similarly, an individual with isolated dystonia may be reclassified as combined dystonia when additional phenotypic elements emerge over time.

SYNOPSIS AND FUTURE PROSPECTS

The many different clinical features and biological contributors to the dystonias are currently classified using a two-axis strategy. Axis I addresses the clinical manifestations according to body area affected, age at onset, temporal features, certain characteristics of dystonic movements, and associated nondystonic features. Axis II addresses the known or presumed biological basis.

It is valuable to appreciate that the two-axis strategy is a guideline for lumping and splitting relevant features. Classification of the dystonias into subgroups aids in differential diagnosis and in guiding what etiologies might be considered. However, the two-axis strategy should not be viewed as an algorithmic flow chart to be used to reach a specific diagnosis, and varied interpretations or conclusions are expected.[35]

The two-axis classification plan introduced in 2013 has been largely successful, and some shortcomings were addressed in the 2025 revision. How well the 2025 plan will fare remains to be determined. Of course, it is likely that this most recent plan will require revision again in the future as more is learned about the clinical manifestations and biological basis for this very complex group of disorders.

REFERENCES

1. Albanese A, Bhatia K, Bressman SB, DeLong MR, Fahn S, Fung VSC, et al. Phenomenology and classification of dystonia: A consensus update. Mov Disord 2013;28:863–873.
2. Albanese A, Bhatia K, Fung V, Hallett M, Jankovic J, et al. Definition and Classification of Dystonia, 2025 (first presented at the International Dystonia Symposium in 2023).
3. Albanese A, Bhatia K, Jinnah HA. *Dystonia*. Elsevier, 2023.
4. Bhatia KP, Bain P, Bajaj N, Elble RJ, Hallett M, Louis ED, et al. Consensus statement on the classification of tremors. from the task force on tremor of the International Parkinson and Movement Disorder Society. Mov Disord 2018;33:75–87.
5. Boz D, Kilic-Berkmen G, Perlmutter JS, Norris SA, Wright LJ, Klein C, et al. An empirical comparison of commonly universal rating scales for dystonia. Mov Disord Clin Pract 2023;10:1777–1786.
6. Brown AM, van der Heijden ME, Jinnah HA, Sillitoe RV. Cerebellar dysfunction as a source of dystonic phenotypes in mice. Cerebellum 2023;22:719–729.
7. Conte A, Rocchi L, Latorre A, Belvisi D, Rothwell JC, Berardelli A. Ten-year reflections on the neurophysiological abnormalities of focal dystonias in humans. Mov Disord 2019;34:1616–1628.
8. Corp DT, Morrison-Ham J, Jinnah HA, Joutsa J. The functional anatomy of dystonia: Recent developments. Int Rev Neurobiol 2023;169:105–136.
9. Defazio G, Ercoli T, Erro R, Pellicciari R, Mascia MM, Fabbrini G, et al. Idiopathic non-task-specific upper limb dystonia, a neglected form of dystonia. Mov Disord 2020;35:2038–2045.
10. Di Fonzo A, Jinnah HA, Zech M. Dystonia genes and their biological pathways. Int Rev Neurobiol 2023;169:61–103.
11. Fahn S. The varied clinical expressions of dystonia. Neurol Clinics 1984;2:541–554.
12. Fahn S. Concept and classification of dystonia. Adv Neurol 1988;50:1–8.
13. Fischer P, Pina-Fuentes D, Kassavetis P, Sadnicka A. Physiology of dystonia: Human studies. Int Rev Neurobiol 2023;169:137–162.
14. Fung VS, Jinnah HA, Bhatia K, Vidailhet M. Assessment of the patient with dystonia: An update on dystonia syndromes. Mov Disord 2013;28:889–898.
15. Jinnah HA. The dystonias. Continuum 2019;25:976–1000.
16. Jinnah HA, Albanese A. The new classification for the dystonias: Why was it needed and how was it accomplished? Mov Disord Clin Pract 2014;1:280–284.
17. Jinnah HA, Albanese A, Bhatia KP, Cardoso F, Da Prat G, de Koning TJ, et al. Treatable inherited rare movement disorders. Mov Disord 2018;33:21–35.
18. Jinnah HA, Sun YV. Dystonia genes and their biological pathways. Neurobiol Dis 2019;129:159–168.
19. Kilic-Berkmen G, Defazio G, Hallett M, Berardelli A, Ferrazzano G, Belvisi D, et al. Diagnosis and classification of blepharospasm: Recommendations based on empirical evidence. J Neurol Sci 2022;439:120319.
20. Kilic-Berkmen G, Jinnah HA. Cervical dystonia with tremor: One movement disorder or two? Mov Disord Clin Pract 2022;9:719–720.
21. Kilic-Berkmen G, Pirio Richardson S, Perlmutter JS, Hallett M, Klein C, Wagle-Shukla A, et al. Current guidelines for classifying and diagnosing cervical dystonia: Empirical evidence and recommendations. Movement Disorders Clinical Practice 2021;9:183–190.
22. LeDoux MS. Meige syndrome: What's in a name? Parkinsonism Relat Disord 2009;15:483–489.
23. Lumsden DE, Gimeno H, Lin JP. Classification of dystonia in childhood. Parkinsonism Relat Disord 2016;33:138–141.
24. Neychev VK, Gross R, Lehericy S, Hess EJ, Jinnah HA. The functional neuroanatomy of dystonia. Neurobiol Dis 2011;42:185–201.
25. Pandey S, Jost WH. Classification and diagnosis of cervical dystonia: Revived call for consensus. Movement Disorders Clinical Practice 2022;15:717–718.
26. Panyakaew P, Jinnah HA, Shaikh AG. Clinical features, pathophysiology, treatment, and controversies of tremor in dystonia. J Neurol Sci 2022;435:120199.
27. Rey Hipolito AG, van der Heijden ME, Sillitoe RV. Physiology of dystonia: Animal studies. Int Rev Neurobiol 2023;169:163–215.
28. Sadnicka A, Kassavetis P, Parees I, Meppelink AM, Butler K, Edwards M. Task-specific dystonia: Pathophysiology and management. J Neurol Neurosurg Psychiatry 2016;87:968–974.
29. Sasikumar S, Albanese A, Krauss JK, Fasano A. Implementation of the current dystonia classification from 2013 to 2018. Mov Disord Clin Pract 2019;6:250–253.

30. Schneider SA, Aggarwal A, Bhatt MH, Dupont E, Tisch S, Limousin P, et al. Severe tongue protrusion dystonia: Clinical syndromes and possible treatment. Neurology 2006;67:940–943.
31. Shaikh AG, Beylergil SB, Scorr L, Kilic-Berkmen G, Freeman A, Klein C, et al. Dystonia & tremor: A cross-sectional study of the Dystonia Coalition cohort. Neurology 2021;96:e563–e574.
32. Stahl CM, Frucht SJ. Focal task specific dystonia: A review and update. J Neurol 2017;264:1536–1541.
33. Stamelou M, Lai SC, Aggarwal A, Schneider SA, Houlden H, Yeh TH, et al. Dystonic opisthotonus: A "red flag" for neurodegeneration with brain iron accumulation syndromes? Mov Disord 2013;28:1325–1329.
34. Thomsen M, Lange LM, Zech M, Lohmann K. Genetics and pathogenesis of dystonia. Annu Rev Pathol 2024;19:99–131.
35. van Egmond ME, Contarino MF, Lugtenberg CHA, Peall KJ, Brouwer OF, Fung VSC, et al. Variable Interpretation of the dystonia consensus classification items compromises its solidity. Mov Disord 2019;34:317–320.
36. Vizcarra JA, Jinnah HA. What is hemidystonia? Movement Disord Clin Pract 2023;10:477–481.
37. Weisheit CE, Pappas SS, Dauer WT. Inherited dystonias: Clinical features and molecular pathways. Handb Clin Neurol 2018;147:241–254.

Chapter 4

Epidemiology of the Dystonias

INTRODUCTION

Dystonia is regarded as a rare disorder. However, there are no globally accepted definitions for what constitutes a rare disorder.[19] The US Food and Drug Administration defines "rare" as a disease or condition that affects fewer than 200,000 citizens. In the European Union, "rare" is defined as a prevalence of 50 or fewer cases per 100,000 people. The relative rarity of dystonia makes exact estimates of prevalence (the proportion of persons who have dystonia) and incidence (the proportion of persons who will develop a condition during a particular time period) challenging. The challenge is further increased because there are no diagnostic tests, and diagnosis relies on expert clinical assessment.

Most epidemiological studies of the prevalence of dystonia are based on counting patients receiving medical services or participants entered into research databases for diagnosis or treatment. These studies are likely to underestimate total numbers of cases because many affected individuals may not seek medical attention or are misdiagnosed as having another disorder. Far fewer studies are community-based because they require a labor-intensive effort in interviewing and examining all individuals in a community. Even for these types of studies, the lack of widely accepted diagnostic criteria for many common types of dystonia sometimes renders uncertain results.

Finally, the vast majority of epidemiological studies have addressed disorders where dystonia is the only problem, with very little data available for dystonias that may be combined with other problems. Most have used the older classification and terminology (e.g., primary dystonia) rather than modern classification and terminology (e.g., isolated dystonia) for diagnosis.[1] These two terms are only roughly equivalent, so this chapter summarizes the epidemiology of dystonia according to the terms used in the original studies.

PREVALENCE OF ISOLATED OR PRIMARY DYSTONIAS

Two meta-analyses have attempted to combine results across many different epidemiological studies. The first meta-analysis included 16 epidemiological studies of primary dystonia published from 1985 to 2010.[23] Most studies came from Europe, with a few from Asia and one from the United States. The majority reported on prevalence, with 12 service-based studies and 3 population-based studies. The overall prevalence of all types of primary dystonia was 16.4 cases per

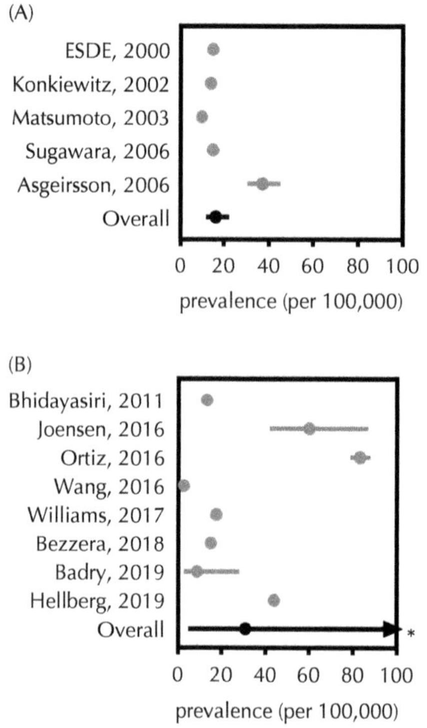

Figure 4.1. Epidemiological studies of primary or isolated dystonias. Panel A is adapted from an early meta-analysis when the term *primary dystonia* was used.[23] Panel B is adapted from a second meta-analysis after the term *isolated dystonia* was adopted.[13] For both panels, the points give the prevalence estimates and the bars show confidence intervals. Abbreviation: ESDE, epidemiological study of dystonia in Europe.

100,000 with a 95% confidence interval (CI) of 12.1–22.3 (Figure 4.1). The vast majority of these cases were adult-onset focal or segmental dystonias, with an overall prevalence of 15.4 cases per 100,000 (Table 4.1). For the most common subtypes, the overall prevalences per 100,000 were 5.0 (CI, 3.6–6.9) for cervical dystonia, 4.2 (CI, 2.9–6.2) for blepharospasm, 1.2 (CI, 0.4–4.4) for limb dystonia, 1.6 (CI, 0.9–3.0) for writer's cramp, and 1.5 (CI, 0.6–3.6) for laryngeal dystonia. Generalized dystonia was the least common, with a prevalence of only 0.4 (CI, 0.3–0.7) cases per 100,000.

A second meta-analysis in 2022 included 17 additional epidemiological studies of isolated dystonia published between 2010 and 2022 from Europe, North and South America, Asia, and Africa. The overall prevalence of all types of isolated dystonia was 30.8 cases per 100,000 with a 95% CI of 5.1–187.7 (Figure 4.1).[13] The apparent increase in prevalence between the 2012 and 2022 meta-analyses was not statistically significant (Table 4.1). Similar to the first meta-analysis, the most common subtypes had overall prevalence rates per 100,000 of 10.0 (CI, 3.5–28.2) for cervical dystonia, 2.8 (CI, 1.1–7.1) for blepharospasm, 1.3 (CI, 0.4–4.5) for upper limb, 0.6 (CI, 0.2–2.2) for oromandibular, and 0.4 (CI, 0.1–1.8) for laryngeal dystonia. There were significant geographical differences in the prevalence of specific subtypes of dystonia, but these differences may reflect differences in methods of ascertainment rather than real geographical differences.

The topographic expression of isolated dystonia is significantly influenced by age. An early meta-analysis of 84 reports of all types of isolated dystonia revealed significant differences in the average age at onset across different types of primary dystonias.[15] For example, individuals with focal hand dystonia tend to present in early adulthood, while those with blepharospasm tend to present later (Table 4.2). This early finding has been corroborated by numerous subsequent reports (Figure 4.2). Individuals with monogenic dystonia tend to present even earlier,

Table 4.1 **Prevalence of primary or isolated dystonia**

Type of dystonia	1985–2010 Primary dystonia (95% confidence interval)	2010–2022 Isolated dystonia (95% confidence interval)	Statistical comparison (p-value)
All types	16.4 (12.1–22.3)	30.8 (5.1–187.7)	0.46
Cervical dystonia	5.0 (3.6–6.9)	10.0 (3.5–28.2)	0.22
Blepharospasm	4.2 (2.9–6.2)	2.8 (1.1–7.1)	0.42
Upper limb dystonia	2.2 (1.3–3.8)	1.3 (0.4–4.5)	0.42
Laryngeal dystonia	1.5 (0.6–3.6)	0.4 (0.1–1.8)	0.13
Oromandibular dystonia	0.5 (0.2–1.5)	0.6 (0.2–2.2)	0.90

Adapted from Medina et al. 2022.[13]

Table 4.2 **Age at onset among focal isolated dystonias**

Type of dystonia	Studies reviewed (N)	Cases included (N)	Mean age at onset (yrs)	95% confidence interval (yrs)
Writer's cramp	13	280	38.4	36.9–39.3
Cervical dystonia	28	2673	40.8	40.3–41.2
Spasmodic dysphonia	13	921	43.0	42.2–43.9
Cranial dystonia	21	1033	55.7	55.0–56.4

Adapted from O'Riordan et al., 2004.[15]

and the average age at onset varies substantially according to the gene involved (Table 4.3).[9] These differences have been confirmed in other epidemiological studies.[13,23]

Dystonia is also more common in female individuals compared with male individuals. For most adult-onset focal dystonias, women substantially outnumber men in most studies (Figure 4.3). In one large study addressing sex differences for 3,222 individuals with predominantly adult-onset focal and segmental isolated dystonias, women outnumbered men for all types of dystonia (Figure 4.4).[7] Similar sex differences have been summarized in prior reviews of sex differences in primary dystonia (Table 4.4),[6,17] and they are evident in both meta-analyses.[13,23]

For early-onset monogenic dystonias, female individuals outnumber male individuals for some genes (*ANO3, GNAL, GCH1*) but not other genes (*TH, THAP1, TOR1A*).[7] In one study of nine families with dopa-responsive dystonia, affected girls outnumbered boys by four-fold.[4] Dopa-responsive dystonia is only partly penetrant, and overall penetrance was estimated to be 87% for girls and 38% for boys.[4]

Table 4.3 **Age at onset among monogenic dystonias**

Gene	Total cases	Median age at onset (yrs)	Interquartile range (yrs)
TOR1A	409	9	7–12
THAP1	211	15	9–26
ANO3	39	30	12–42
GNAL	74	38	25–46

Adapted from Lange et al., 2021.[9]

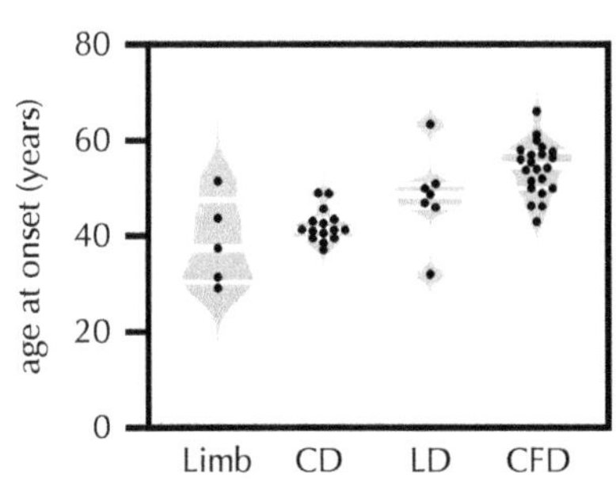

Figure 4.2. Age at onset for different types of isolated dystonia. This figure was created by pooling data across prior publications. Source data were obtained by reviewing the literature and including articles where age at onset was available for adult-onset focal dystonias with at least 100 cases (CD, cervical dystonia; CFD, craniofacial dystonia; LD, laryngeal dystonia; Limb, limb dystonia). Age at onset for monogenic dystonias was taken from cases with genes causing isolated dystonia that were listed in MDSgene (www.mdsgene.org). For this diagram, interventional clinical trials and surgical series were excluded because inclusion criteria often specify age limits

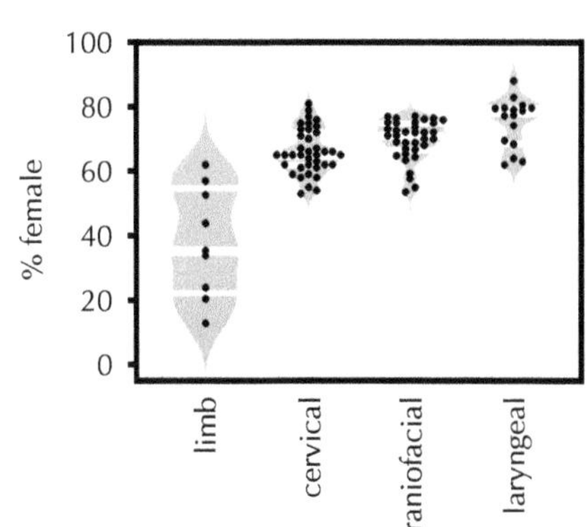

Figure 4.3. Sex differences in the literature for adult-onset isolated dystonias. This figure was created by pooling data across prior publications. Source data were obtained by reviewing the literature and including articles where sex was reported for adult-onset focal dystonias with at least 100 cases (CD, cervical dystonia; CFD, craniofacial dystonia; LD, laryngeal dystonia; Limb, limb dystonia).

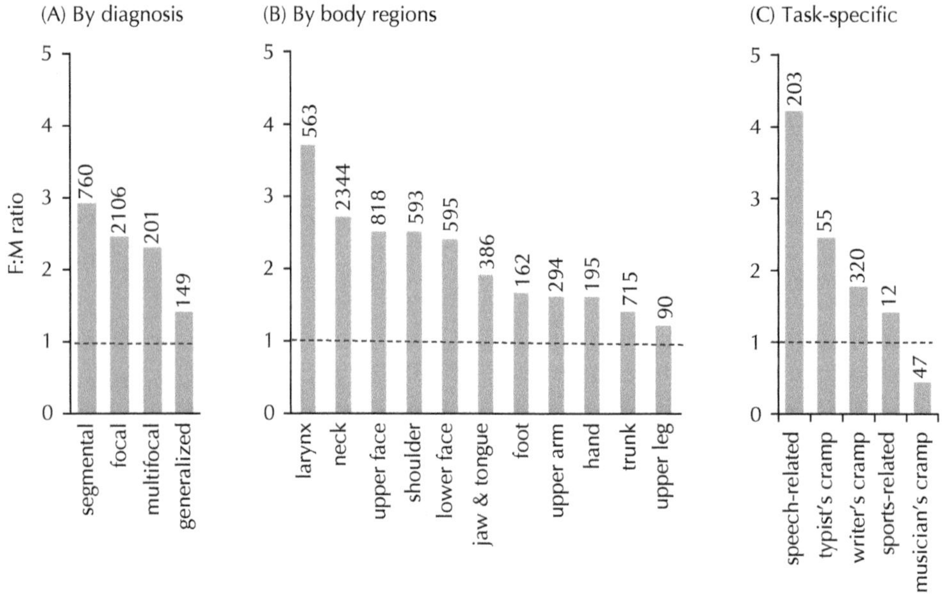

Figure 4.4. Sex differences in a single large study of isolated dystonias. This figure was adapted from a study of 3,222 individuals with all types of isolated dystonias.[7] Panel A shows the female-to-male (F:M) ratios for subgroups of individuals based on body distribution affected. Panel B shows the same ratios according to individual body regions affected. Panel C shows the same ratios for task-specific dystonias. The numbers at the top of the bar show total numbers of individuals in the group.

PREVALENCE OF COMBINED OR SECONDARY DYSTONIA

The epidemiology of combined and acquired dystonias has been less well studied than the isolated dystonias. However, it is likely that the overall prevalence of these types of dystonia exceeds that of the isolated dystonias. For example, dystonia is common in cerebral palsy, which has an estimated prevalence of 1–2 per 1,000 births.[14] Several subtypes are recognized. Dystonia is the predominant feature of the dyskinetic subtype, which comprises 15% of the total. Dystonia is also an accompanying feature of other subtypes of cerebral palsy, including the spastic and ataxic subtypes. The most methodical studies of all subtypes of cerebral palsy combined have suggested 80% of all individuals have at least some dystonic features (see Chapter 16, "Dystonia and Cerebral Palsy").[18]

Table 4.4 **Sex differences in adult-onset isolated focal dystonias**

Focal dystonia	Total cases	Female-to-male ratio
Cervical dystonia	2,634	1.5
Laryngeal dystonia	1,411	2.0
Blepharospasm	739	2.0
Upper limb dystonia	296	0.6
Oromandibular dystonia	37	3.1

Adapted from Jinnah et al., 2013.[6]

Dystonia is also common in Parkinson disease and related parkinsonian disorders,[22] where the prevalence is more than 100–200 cases per 100,000 population. Dystonia is the presenting feature for approximately 10–15% of all cases of Parkinson disease, particularly those with early-onset Parkinson disease. Dystonia may also occur later in the course of the disease, often as a side effect of levodopa treatment. Methodical studies addressing the prevalence of dystonia during the course of the disease are lacking, but it has been estimated that approximately 30–40% of all individuals with Parkinson disease have dystonia at some point. Dystonia may be even more common in the related Parkinsonian disorders, especially corticobasal degeneration, progressive supranuclear palsy, and multiple system atrophy (see Chapter 13, "Dystonia and Parkinsonism").

Dystonia is part of the spectrum of many additional acquired or genetically determined syndromes with more complex phenotypes.[3] For example, dystonia can be the most prominent feature of tardive dyskinesia, and the term *tardive dystonia* is sometimes used (see Chapter 19, "Dystonia Induced by Medications, Illicit Drugs, and Environmental Toxins").[21] Dystonia also is common in Huntington disease and often is the predominant feature in juvenile-onset cases (see Chapter 18, "Dystonias Combined with Other Features").[11] Dystonia also is common in some of the spinocerebellar ataxias and may occasionally be the presenting or dominant feature (see Chapter 14, "Dystonia and Ataxia").[20] Although all of these disorders are uncommon, the combined prevalence of dystonia is considerable.

Despite wide recognition of dystonia as a feature of many other neurological disorders, only two published studies address the overall prevalence of nonisolated dystonias. One community-based study of 706 randomly selected inhabitants from the Bruneck area of Northern Italy, aged 50–89, found the prevalence of secondary dystonia to be 1.07% (CI, 0.61–1.54).[26] The same study found the prevalence of primary dystonia to be 0.76% (CI, 0.38–1.14). This study implies that secondary dystonia is more common than primary dystonia. However, another study of residents in Kolkata estimated a crude prevalence of 11.45 (CI, 4.20–24.95)/100,000 for secondary dystonia compared with 43.91 (CI, 28.41–64.81)/100,000 for primary dystonia.[2] This second study may reflect an underestimate relating to methods of ascertainment, given that only six cases with secondary dystonia were identified from a population of 52,377.

PREVALENCE OF MONOGENIC DYSTONIAS

It is difficult to assess the relative prevalences of idiopathic and monogenic dystonias. For almost all large cohorts of adult-onset focal dystonias, candidate gene studies have revealed abnormalities for only a small fraction (usually <5%) of affected cases.[5,10,24]

On the other hand, more comprehensive studies involving broad dystonia gene panels or clinical exome sequencing often report higher frequencies of monogenic disorders. One study involving a panel with 94 dystonia genes in 61 individuals with dystonia revealed the overall prevalence of monogenic causes to be 15%.[25] Whole-exome studies have reported the overall prevalence of monogenic causes to be 20% in an American cohort of 189 individuals,[16] 19% in a European cohort of 764 individuals,[27] and 18% in a cohort of 65 individuals from China.[12] A whole-genome study of a cohort of 111 Australian cases found a genetic cause in 12%.[8] However, cohorts selected for these types of genetic studies are typically enriched for cases more likely to have a monogenic cause because of a family history, early onset, generalized rather than focal dystonia, or additional neurological or medical problems.

In the largest study of all types of dystonia, the percentage with a monogenic cause was low for isolated dystonias (4%), higher when dystonia was combined with another movement disorder (19%), and highest among those with additional neurological or medical problems (45%).[27] Therefore, most of the available genetic studies cannot be used to estimate the relative prevalences of idiopathic versus monogenic dystonias.

SYNOPSIS AND FUTURE PROSPECTS

Numerous epidemiological studies have documented the isolated dystonias to be rare disorders, with adult-onset focal dystonias being far more common than early-onset generalized dystonias. Monogenic causes for isolated dystonia appear to be even less common, although the exact prevalence is unknown because of the lack of methodical studies of large populations. Because of methodological issues associated with challenges of assessing rare disorders without widely accepted diagnostic criteria, all of the available studies very likely underestimate the numbers of affected individuals.

Perhaps more importantly, epidemiological studies focusing on isolated dystonias usually do not include other types of dystonia. There are very few large epidemiological studies of dystonia associated with cerebral palsy, tardive syndromes, or neurodegenerative disorders such as Parkinson or Huntington disease. Collectively, these types of dystonia are more common than the isolated dystonias. When these other forms of dystonia are considered, the dystonias are not so rare. Further studies of these other populations are needed for a fuller understanding of the true burden of dystonia in the community.

REFERENCES

1. Albanese A, Bhatia K, Bressman SB, DeLong MR, Fahn S, Fung VSC, et al. Phenomenology and classification of dystonia: A consensus update. Mov Disord 2013;28:863–873.
2. Das SK, Banerjee TK, Biswas A, Roy T, Raut DK, Chaudhuri A, Hazra A. Community survey of primary dystonia in the city of Kolkata, India. Mov Disord 2007;22:2031–2036.
3. Fung VS, Jinnah HA, Bhatia K, Vidailhet M. Assessment of the patient with dystonia: An update on dystonia syndromes. Mov Disord 2013;28:889–898.
4. Furukawa Y, Lang AE, Trugman JM, Bird TD, Hunter A, Sadeh M, et al. Gender-related penetrance and de novo GTP-cyclohydrolase I gene mutation in dopa-responsive dystonia. Neurology 1998;50:1015–1020.
5. Hammer M, Abravanel A, Peckham E, Mahloogi A, Majounie E, Hallett M, Singleton A. Blepharospasm: A genetic screening study in 132 patients. Parkinsonism Relat Disord 2019;64:315–318.
6. Jinnah HA, Berardelli A, Comella C, Defazio G, DeLong M, Factor S, et al. The focal dystonias: Current views and challenges for future research. Mov Disord 2013;7:926–943.
7. Kilic-Berkmen G, Scorr LM, McKay L, Donsante Y, Perlmutter JS, Norris SA, et al. Sex differences in dystonia. Mov Disord Clin Pract 2024;11:972–983.
8. Kumar KR, Davis RL, Tchan MC, Wali GM, Mahant N, Ng K, et al. Whole genome sequencing for the genetic diagnosis of heterogenous dystonia phenotypes. Parkinsonism Relat Disord 2019;69:111–118.
9. Lange LM, Junker J, Loens S, Baumann H, Olschewski L, Schaake S, et al. Genotype-phenotype relations for isolated dystonia genes: MDSGene systematic review. Mov Disord 2021;36:1086–1103.
10. LeDoux MS, Vemula SR, Xiao J, Thompson MM, Perlmutter JS, Wright LJ, et al. Clinical and genetic features of cervical dystonia in a large multicenter cohort. Neurol Genet 2016;2:e69.
11. Louis ED, Lee P, Quinn L, Marder K. Dystonia in Huntington's disease: Prevalence and clinical characteristics. Mov Disord 1999;14:95–101.
12. Ma J, Wang L, Yang YM, Wan XH. Targeted gene capture sequencing in diagnosis of dystonia patients. J Neurol Sci 2018;390:36–41.
13. Medina A, Nilles C, Martino D, Pelletier C, Pringsheim T. The prevalence of idiopathic or inherited isolated dystonia: A systematic review and meta-analysis. Mov Disord Clin Pract 2022;9:860–868.
14. Monbaliu E, Himmelmann K, Lin JP, Ortibus E, Bonouvrie L, Feys H, et al. Clinical presentation and management of dyskinetic cerebral palsy. Lancet Neurol 2017;16:741–749.
15. O'Riordan S, Raymond D, Lynch T, Saunders-Pullman R, Bressman SB, Daly L, Hutchinson M. Age at onset as a factor in determining the phenotype of primary torsion dystonia. Neurology 2004;63:1423–1426.
16. Powis Z, Towne MC, Hagman KDF, Blanco K, Palmaer E, Castro A, et al. Clinical diagnostic exome sequencing in dystonia: Genetic testing challenges for complex conditions. Clin Genet 2019;97:305–307.
17. Rafee S, O'Riordan S, Reilly R, Hutchinson M. We must talk about sex and focal dystonia. Mov Disord 2021;36:604–608.
18. Rice J, Skuza P, Baker F, Russo R, Fehlings D. Identification and measurement of dystonia in cerebral palsy. Dev Med Child Neurol 2017;59:1249–1255.
19. Richter T, Nestler-Parr S, Babela R, Khan ZM, Tesoro T, Molsen E, Hughes DA, International Society for P, Outcomes Research Rare Disease Special Interest G. Rare disease terminology and definitions—a systematic global review: Report of the ISPOR rare disease special interest group. Value Health 2015;18:906–914.
20. Rossi M, Balint B, Millar Vernetti P, Bhatia KP, Merello M. Genetic dystonia-ataxia syndromes: Clinical spectrum, diagnostic approach, and treatment options. Mov Disord Clin Pract 2018;5:373–382.
21. Savitt D, Jankovic J. Tardive syndromes. J Neurol Sci 2018;389:35–42.
22. Shetty AS, Bhatia KP, Lang AE. Dystonia and Parkinson's disease: What is the relationship? Neurobiol Dis 2019;132:104462.
23. Steeves TD, Day L, Dykeman J, Jette N, Pringsheim T. The prevalence of primary dystonia: A systematic review and meta-analysis. Mov Disord 2012;27:1789–1796.
24. Tian J, Vemula SR, Xiao J, Valente EM, Defazio G, Petrucci S, et al. Whole-exome sequencing for variant discovery in blepharospasm. Mol Genet Genomic Med 2018;57:1651–1654.
25. van Egmond ME, Lugtenberg CHA, Brouwer OF, Contarino MF, Fung VSC, Heiner-Fokkema MR, et al. A post hoc study on gene panel analysis for the diagnosis of dystonia. Mov Disord 2017;32:569–575.
26. Wenning GK, Kiechl S, Seppi K, Muller J, Hogl B, Saletu M, et al. Prevalence of movement disorders in men and women aged 50–89 years (Bruneck Study cohort): A population-based study. Lancet Neurol 2005;4:815–820.
27. Zech M, Jech R, Boesch S, Skorvanek M, Weber S, Wagner M, et al. Monogenic variants in dystonia: An exome-wide sequencing study. Lancet Neurol 2020;19:908–918.

SECTION II

The Isolated (Pure) Dystonia Syndromes

Chapter 5

Cervical Dystonias

INTRODUCTION

Cervical dystonia (CD) is characterized by excessive contraction of muscles connected to the upper spine, skull base, and shoulder.[2] Over the years, various terms have been used to describe CD, including spastic torticollis, spasmodic torticollis, and others. The term *wry neck* has also been used to describe a variety of causes of a painful and stiff neck. The term *cervical dystonia* was eventually adopted as a label that is both more accurate and more broadly inclusive of its different manifestations.[22] The term *spastic* was dropped because CD is not a disorder of spasticity, and the term *spasmodic* was dropped because many cases lack spasmodic jerking. The term *torticollis* refers now more specifically to rotation of the head to the right or left, while the term CD is more broadly inclusive of many abnormal movements of the head and neck.

In the majority of epidemiological studies, CD is the most common subtype of all of the isolated adult-onset dystonias. A meta-analysis of studies published from 1985 to 2010 revealed an overall prevalence of five cases of CD per 100,000.[133] Another meta-analysis of studies published from 2010 to 2022 revealed an overall prevalence of 10 per 100,000[93] (see Chapter 4, "Epidemiology of the Dystonias"). This apparent increase in prevalence probably is not due to a real increase, but to better recognition of CD. CD typically emerges in adults between 40 and 60 years of age (Table 5.1 and Figure 5.1), although children may be affected, too. In most large case series, females outnumber males (Figure 5.2).

The motor manifestations are quite heterogeneous, with different combinations of abnormal movements involving the neck, head, and/or shoulders. Abnormal movements vary among different individuals with CD, but each individual tends to maintain a relatively characteristic pattern of movements. Non-motor features are common, too, most notably pain or psychiatric comorbidities. These features are summarized below, along with the typical workup and treatment strategies.

MOTOR FEATURES

Abnormal Postures of the Head and Neck

Abnormal movements in CD may be relatively constant, or they may be more dynamic, with constant pulling or jerking of the head and neck toward the abnormal position. It is common for the head and neck to favor a relatively consistent abnormal posture, and CD is often

Table 5.1 **Large descriptive studies of cervical dystonia**

Study	Country	Cases	Female (%)	Age at onset	Main focus
Duane 1988[44]	USA	347	63.3	F: 42.8 M: 41.8	Detailed comparison of 3 cohorts with motor features and comorbid conditions
Chan 1991[22]	USA	226	65.0	41.3±8.2	Motor features, pain, and comorbid conditions
Rondot 1991[119]	Canada	220	62.0	NR	Motor features and psychosocial comorbidities
Heinen 1996[64]	Germany	256	59.3	49.1±13.3	Motor features and responses to oral and surgical therapies
Misra 2012[98]	MC	404	64.9	NR	Multicenter observational study of motor features and factors associated with poor response to BoNT
Ferreira 2014[52]	MC	201	61.2	NR	Multicenter observational study of motor features and factors associated with poor response to BoNT
Comella 2015[29]	ISS	1071	76.0	NR	Survey study of patient perspectives regarding diagnosis and treatment
Jankovic 2015[23,51,67]	MC	1046	74.4	49.0±16.7	Multicenter observational study of onabotulinumtoxin (CD-PROBE) with motor and non-motor features, injection patterns, and outcomes
Norris 2016[10,31,84,105,134]	MC	1477	74.6	45.8±14.2	Multicenter study (Dystonia Coalition) of clinical features relevant for spread of dystonia
Trosch 2017[139]	MC	347	75.2	48.9±15.6	Multicenter observational study of abobotulinumtoxin (ANCHOR-CD) with motor and non-motor features, injection patterns, and outcomes
Ortiz 2019[107]	Finland	937	73.1	NR	Evaluation of comorbid medical and psychiatric conditions as they relate to disability
Jost 2020[73]	MC	306	67.0	NR	Multicenter study of head and neck movements using the Col-Cap approach
Di Biasio 2020[40]	Italy	842	62.9	NR	Multicenter study of sensory and motor subtypes
Liang 2022[87]	China	333	64.6	40.6±13.3	Motor and non-motor features impacting quality of life

This table summarizes studies of cervical dystonia that included at least 200 subjects with detailed clinical descriptions. Treatment trials and surgical series were excluded because inclusion criteria bias in the cohorts. When cohorts were reported more than once for different reasons, only the largest or most complete is shown. Abbreviations: IS, international survey study; MC, multiple countries.

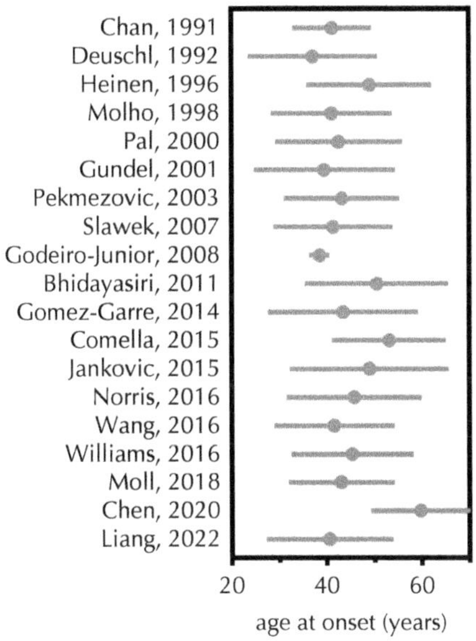

Figure 5.1. Age at onset for cervical dystonia. This figure was prepared by collecting data from studies that included at least 100 individuals with cervical dystonia and included age at onset.

described according to the predominant direction of movement. Historically, the directions of movement were described in four groups (Figure 5.3). The most common abnormality is *torticollis*, which refers to rotation of the head/neck in the yaw direction (turning the chin left or right). The second most common is *laterocollis*, which refers to lateral bending of the head/neck in the roll direction (tilting of an ear toward the ipsilateral shoulder). Abnormal movements in the pitch direction include *anterocollis* (flexion or forward bending of the head/neck) and *retrocollis* (extension or backward bending of the head/neck).

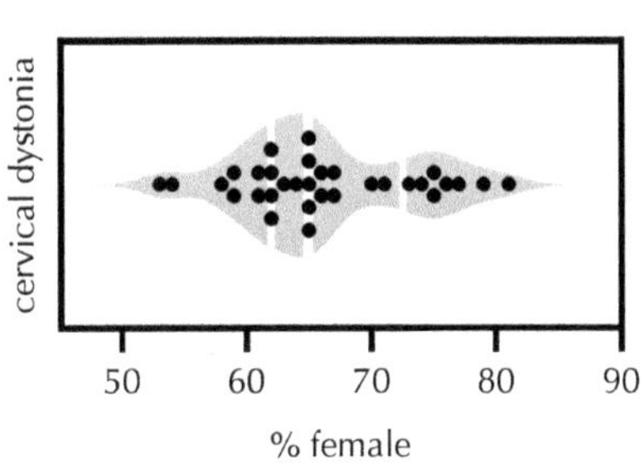

Figure 5.2. Sex distributions for cervical dystonia. This figure was prepared by collecting data from studies that included at least 100 individuals with cervical dystonia and included information on sex.

Although this approach for describing the main directions of abnormal movements is adequate for the majority of CD cases where the head and neck move in the same direction, it is not entirely suitable for some individuals who have more complex patterns of movement. Occasionally, the root of the neck may be shifted laterally, or forward or backward on the shoulders. In some cases, the head and neck move in opposing directions. The *col-cap* approach provides a more precise way of describing abnormal postures in these cases (Figure 5.4).[53] These more complex patterns occur because some muscles primarily move the neck (*collum*) by virtue of their connections with the cervical spine, while other muscles primarily move the head (*caput*) because they connect to the skull. For example, it is possible to have left latero-*collis* (neck tilting left) combined with right latero-*caput* (head tilting right, opposite to the neck direction). It is also possible to have antero-*collis* (forward bending of the neck) combined with either antero-*caput* (chin down) or retro-*caput* (chin up).[53] Most affected individuals have some combination of abnormal movements of the head and/or neck in different directions (Figure 5.5).

Other Abnormal Movements

Isolated focal CD is characterized chiefly by abnormal postures of the head and neck, but other abnormal movements also occur. The shoulder is often elevated because the cervical spine is connected to the shoulder by several muscles such as the trapezius and levator scapulae. When the shoulder is fixed, these muscles contribute to laterocollis. When the neck is fixed, the same muscles elevate the shoulder. Often there is some combination of laterocollis and shoulder elevation. Sometimes the shoulder is rotated anteriorly. This anterior rotation may also be caused by abnormal activity of the muscles moving the shoulder. However, anterior shoulder rotation may also reflect a behavioral compensation, when torticollis to one direction is compensated by rotation of the torso and shoulders in the opposite direction so the head can remain straight ahead. In view of these observations, the diagnosis of isolated *focal* CD may include involvement of the shoulder.[77] CD may also occur in segmental patterns that involve the head and neck (and sometimes shoulder) along with other areas such as an arm or the lower face

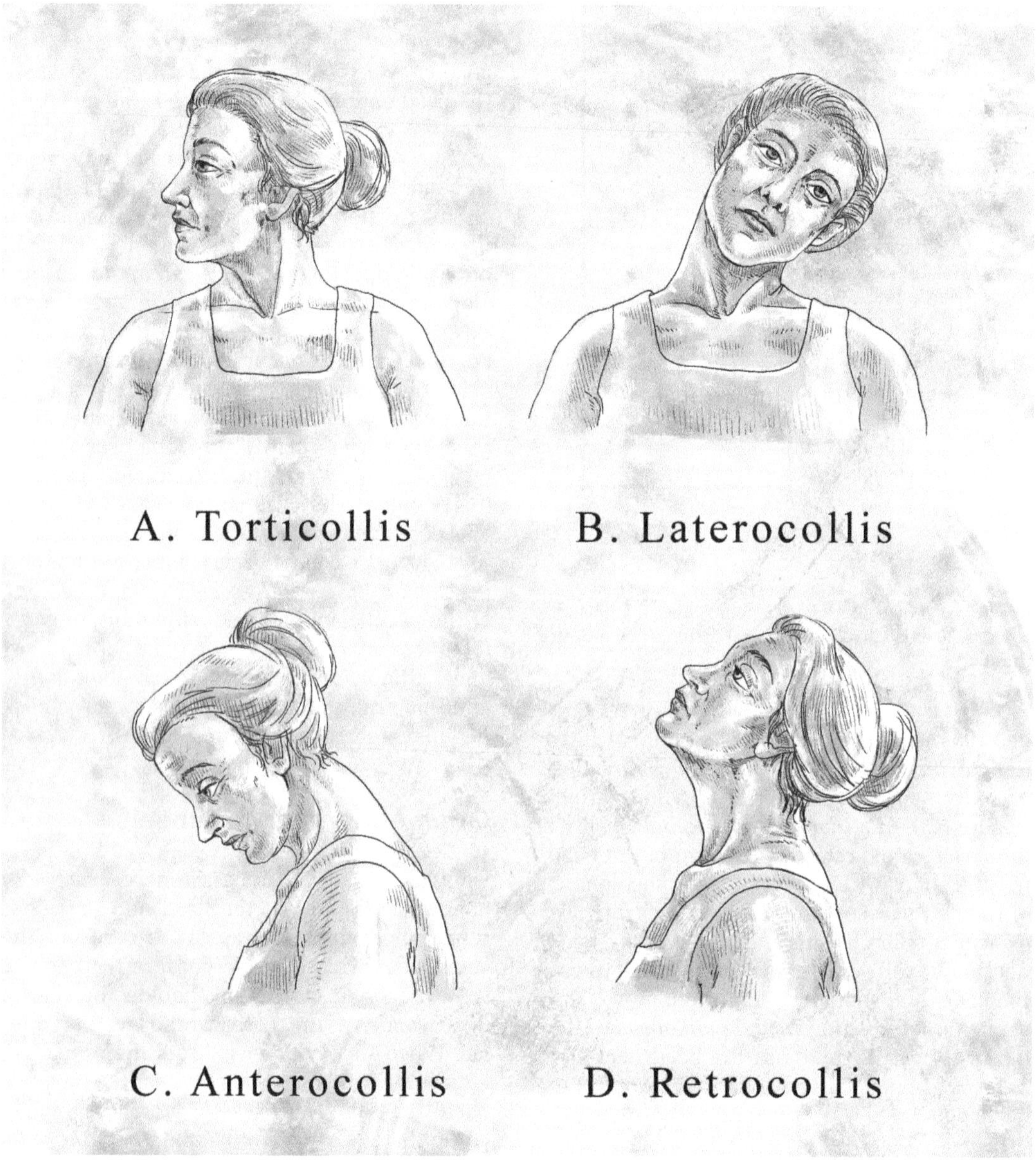

Figure 5.3. Classically recognized abnormal postures of cervical dystonia. The four main abnormalities include (A) torticollis, or rotation of the head/neck in the yaw direction marked by turning of the chin right or left; (B) laterocollis, or lateral bending of head/neck in the roll direction with tilting of the ear toward the ipsilateral shoulder; (C) anterocollis, or flexion with forward bending of the head/neck in the pitch direction; and (D) retrocollis, or extension with backward bending of the head/neck.

Illustration by Loren Bergantini.

and jaw.[77] Multifocal and generalized patterns of dystonia may also include CD.

In addition to postural abnormalities in CD, there are often faster intermittent movements. Some cases have sudden repetitive jerks of the head, often at a semi-regular frequency of 0.2 to 2 Hz.[127] These jerks often pull the head suddenly in one direction, although they can sometimes be multidirectional. This phenomenon is highly characteristic of CD, and it is the origin of the term *spasmodic torticollis*. However, these jerks only occur in 10–20% of individuals, usually

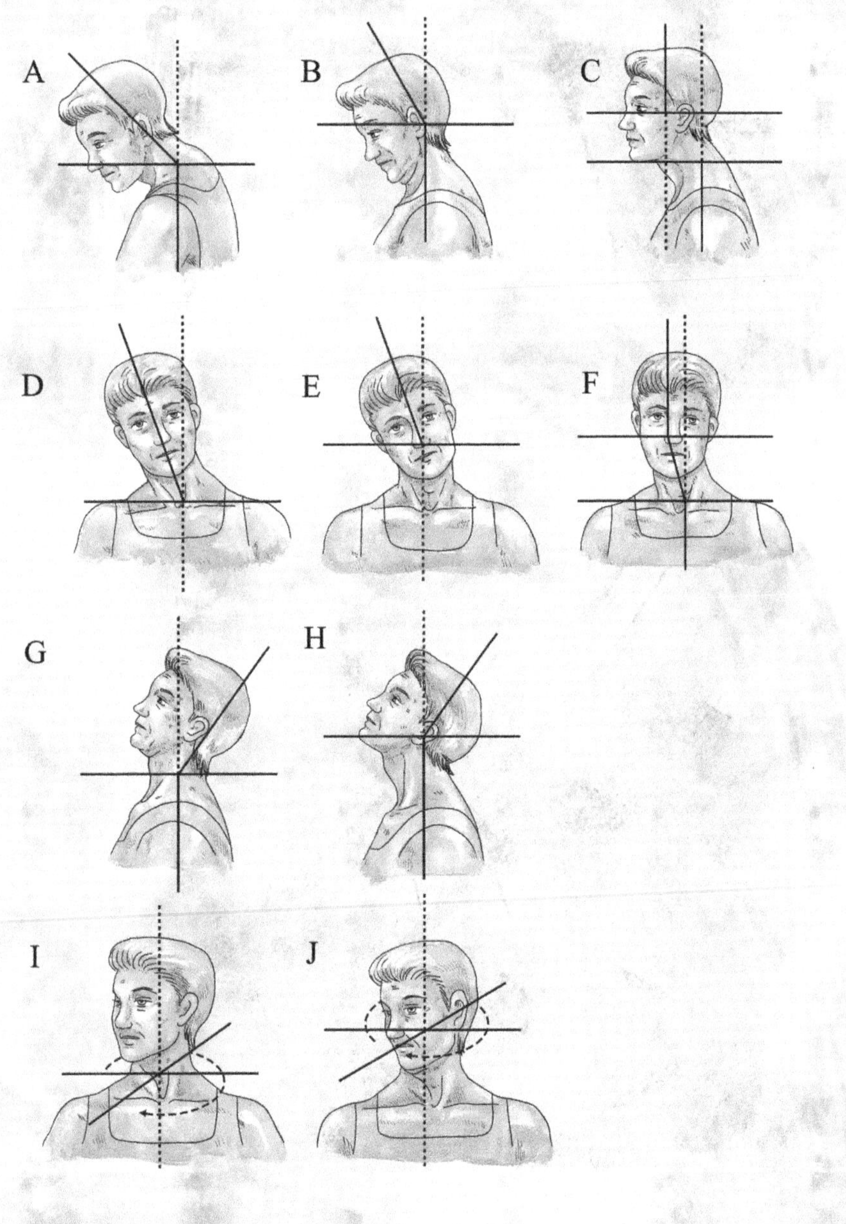

Figure 5.4. Collum-Caput concept for abnormal postures of cervical dystonia. This approach for describing abnormal postures in cervical dystonia acknowledges that some muscles control the head while others control the neck, leading to the possibility that the head and neck may move in the same or different directions. The examples show (A) anterocollis, (B) anterocaput, (C) anterocollis with retrocaput, (D) right laterocollis, (E) right laterocaput, (F) right laterocollis with left laterocaput, (G) retrocollis, (H) retrocaput, (I) torticollis, and (J) torticaput.

Illustration by Loren Bergantini.

early after onset, and they tend to diminish as the abnormal head position becomes more consistent with time. Rarely, these spasms can be the main presenting feature of CD, leading to diagnostic confusion with head tremor or neck tics.

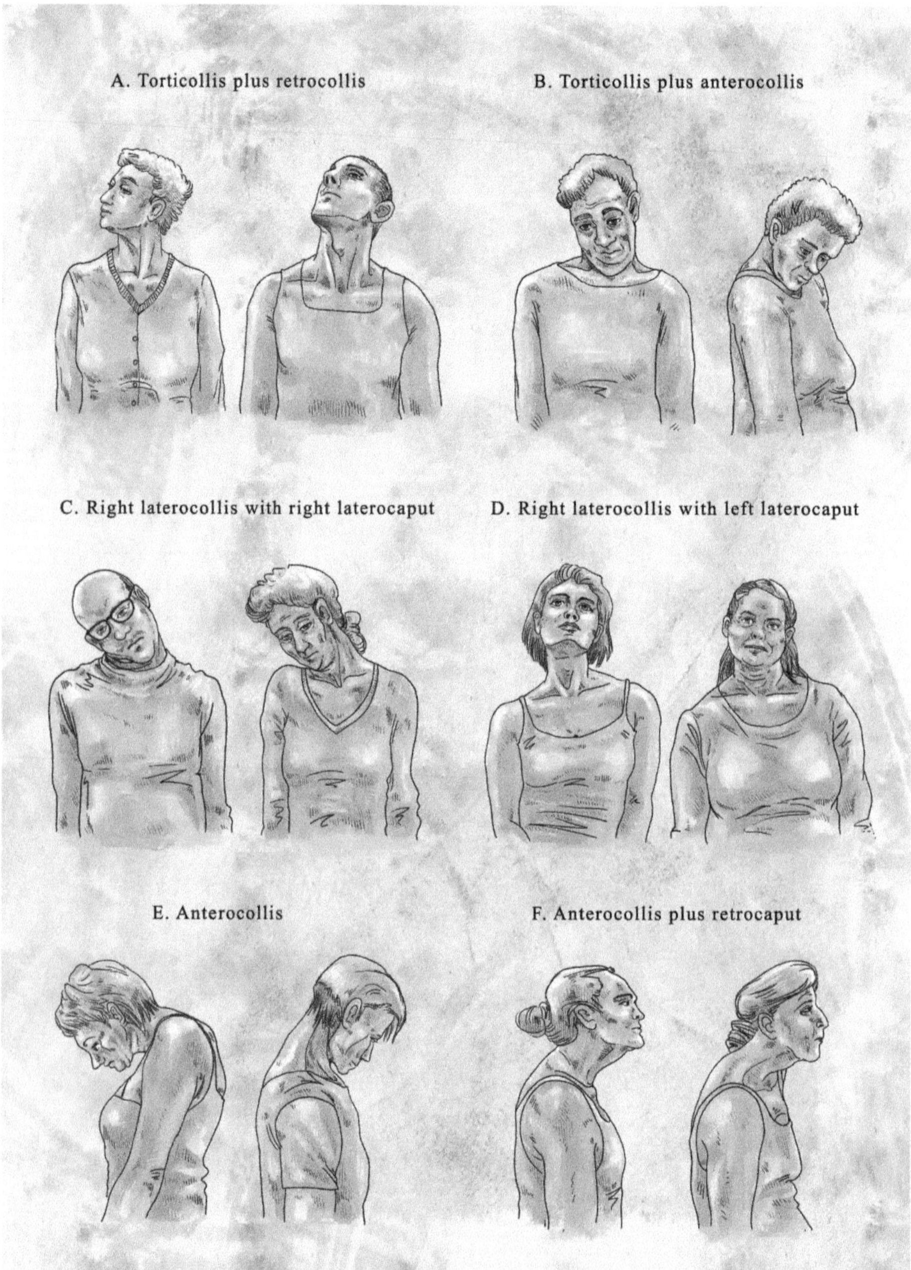

Figure 5.5. Examples of individuals with cervical dystonia. This schematic shows the varied combinations of abnormal postures that occur in actual individuals with cervical dystonia. Examples shown include (A) torticollis with retrocaput, (B) torticollis with anterocollis, (C) right laterocollis with right laterocaput, (D) right laterocollis with left laterocaput, (E) anterocollis with anterocaput, and (F) anterocollis with retrocaput.

Illustration by Loren Bergantini.

A tremor of the head occurs in approximately half of all individuals with CD.[126] This head tremor is more regular and occurs at a frequency of 4–6 Hz. The term *dystonic tremor* is sometimes used when this head tremor is combined with other abnormal dystonic movements of CD (see Chapter 12, " Dystonia and Tremor"). Many individuals also have hand tremor that resembles the tremor of essential tremor. This combination of dystonia in the neck with tremor in another region is sometimes called *tremor associated with dystonia*. Rare cases may have an isolated tremor of the head with little or no abnormal posturing of the head/neck. Some investigators favor the concept that isolated head tremor is a subtype of essential tremor, but others favor the concept that it is a subtype of dystonia instead (see Chapter 12).

Many patients with CD have a *null point*, a head position where abnormal muscle pulling and head tremor attenuate significantly or disappear.[126] As the head moves further from this point, muscle pulling and tremulous movement may worsen. Many individuals with CD also discover that they can attenuate the severity of muscle pulling with some action known as a *geste antagoniste*, sensory trick, or alleviating maneuver. In one methodical study of 154 individuals with CD, 90% reported a sensory trick that was at least partly effective in reducing abnormal movements.[109] Common examples include touching the side of the face or neck, or the back of the head.

Natural History

CD does not usually start suddenly. CD typically worsens over a period of weeks or months. Further progression may occur, but it is usually slower. Some cases continue to worsen over many years, or they may remain stable for a period and then undergo a subsequent phase of worsening.

The pattern of abnormal movements usually remains the same, but it may become more severe or it may spread to involve other body regions. In 5 years, approximately 20% of cases experience spread of dystonia from the neck to other areas. Spread usually affects a contiguous region such as the shoulder and arm, or the craniofacial region or larynx.[1,10,105,135,136,152] Remission occurs in 15% of cases, usually within the first few years of onset, but two-thirds of those who remit eventually relapse.[91]

ASSOCIATED FEATURES

Pain

Approximately 60–80% of cases with CD have pain in the neck or shoulders and/or recurrent headache.[2,23,120] There are several potential causes for pain. One obvious cause is excessive muscle pulling and spasms leading to muscle soreness. Long-standing abnormal postures and jerking movements of the head/neck can also lead to degenerative joint disease of the spine, with pain originating primarily from orthopedic causes. Finally, abnormal postures of the head/neck along with arthritic changes of the cervical spine can lead to cervical spondylotic myelopathy or radiculopathy.[80] In CD, these orthopedic changes often occur in the upper cervical spine (C2–4) instead of the more common age-related degenerative changes that usually affect lower joints.[26] In severe cases, CD can lead to atlantoaxial dislocation.

There is only a loose correlation between pain and abnormal movements.[120] Some patients have severely abnormal movements of the head/neck with no pain. Other patients have minimally abnormal movement with severe pain. Treatment may alleviate movement but not pain, or treatment may alleviate pain and not movement. This poor correlation between pain and movement is likely due to the different potential causes of pain combined with individual patient perceptions and reporting of pain.

Psychiatric Features

Psychiatric features are common in CD (see Chapter 11, "Non-Motor Features of Dystonia"). A meta-analysis of 34 studies of predominantly adult-onset focal dystonias showed a high frequency of anxiety-related disorders, including generalized anxiety disorder, panic attacks, and social phobia.[94] The frequency of any anxiety-related disorders in CD (33%) was similar to other focal dystonias including craniofacial dystonia (25%), limb dystonia (32%), laryngeal dystonia (26%), and mixed dystonias (40%). A separate meta-analysis of 54 studies of predominantly adult-onset focal dystonias also showed a high frequency of mood-related disorders including chronic dysthymia or major depression.[95] In this study, the frequency of any mood disorder in CD (32%) was similar to the frequencies in craniofacial dystonia (29%) and other mixed types of dystonia (31%).

These psychiatric features may reflect a reaction to the motor disorder. Alternatively, they may reflect an intrinsic feature of CD because the brain regions responsible for dystonia are also involved the regulation of psychiatric state.[11,158] Cluster analyses of large cohorts have implied that the combination of anxiety and mood disorders with poor quality of life identifies a subgroup of individuals with CD where intrinsic factors play an important role.[148] On the other hand, it seems likely there is also a subgroup where psychiatric features reflect a reaction to the movement disorder.

Quality of Life

CD has an enormous impact on quality of life.[58,74] Difficulty holding the head straight and still impacts many work-related activities, such as viewing a computer screen, interacting with clients, and driving. These problems also impact leisure activities such as hobbies that require good eye–hand skills, watching television, or reading. Several studies have shown that the pain and psychiatric comorbidities in CD have an even bigger impact on quality of life than do the motor features.[74]

DIFFERENTIAL DIAGNOSIS AND WORKUP

Diagnosis and Assessment

The diagnosis of CD is largely based on clinical recognition of its characteristic features and exclusion of potential mimics.[4,38] Cardinal features supporting the diagnosis include patterned abnormal movements and postures of the head and neck, often with tremor. Supportive features include a *geste antagonist*, pain in the neck and/or shoulders, and a null point. A diagnostic algorithm for adults has been suggested (Figure 5.6).[38]

There are many tools for assessing the severity of CD, including abnormal movements, pain, and quality of life.[3] In the clinical setting, simple tools can be used to estimate the severity of the motor disorder, such as a Likert-type scale or a visual analog scale that is rated by the affected individual, or a clinical global impression scale that is rated by the clinician. For example, treated individuals may be asked what percentage of improvement they experienced following treatment.[27,63] In the research setting, the Toronto Western Torticollis Rating Scale (TWSTRS) is most popular.[32] The original TWSTRS remains widely used, but a revised version (TWSTRS2) has improved clinometric properties and includes an item to score tremor.[30] Motor severity can also be rated using scales developed for dystonia in all body regions, such as the Global Dystonia Rating Scale or the Burke-Fahn-Marsden Dystonia Rating scale, although the latter has several limitations when it comes to CD.[14]

Pain in CD can also be assessed using simple tools such as Likert-like scales and visual analog

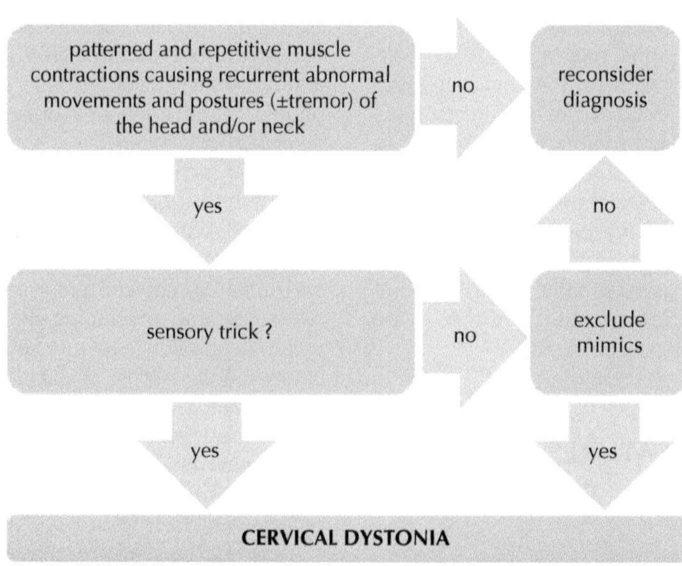

Figure 5.6. Diagnostic algorithm for cervical dystonia. Mimics may have fixed head postures from orthopedic problems, neck muscle weakness, head tilt from ocular misalignment, or others (see Chapter 26, "Pseudodystonia and Differential Diagnosis"). Adapted from a prior publication.[38]

scales. The TWSTRS also includes a subsection for rating pain. Two additional scales have been developed specifically for addressing pain in dystonia.[17,88] The best-studied scale for quality of life in CD is the Cervical Dystonia Impact Profile (CDIP-58), which has 58 questions divided into multiple domains of function.[19]

Adult-Onset Cases

Although the clinical features of CD may be similar across ages, the differential diagnosis and workup vary considerably for adults and children so they are considered separately. Most cases of adult-onset CD are idiopathic, and a cause is not usually found even with an extensive workup.[4,118] Many adults with CD report a potential trigger, such as trauma to the head or neck. However, epidemiological studies have suggested that these reports may reflect recall bias.[39,55,106]

For most cases, routine bloodwork is normal, so it is not usually conducted. Autoimmune thyroid disease is common in CD,[78] so some authorities recommend thyroid function tests.[144] Lesions disclosed by routine brain imaging studies are very uncommon causes for adult-onset CD. Lesions have been described in a number of different regions of the nervous system,[34,83] but lesion network mapping has suggested they connect to a common circuit involving the cerebellum and sensorimotor cortex.[35] Even when focal lesions are found, there is often a delay between the lesion and development of symptoms, making the relationship between the lesion and CD uncertain.[34] In view of the low frequency of responsible lesions, brain or spine imaging is not routinely required.

Isolated focal CD, or syndromes in which CD is the most prominent clinical feature, have been described for a number of genes, most notably *ANO3*.[25,131] CD may be the initial manifestation or the only feature associated with numerous genes usually associated with more complicated phenotypes (Table 5.2). Although 10–15% of individuals with CD have another family member affected with dystonia, several large genetic studies have shown that pathogenic variants in known genes account for only 2–4% of cases, even in familial cases, and even with large dystonia gene panels or whole-exome sequencing.[111,157]

Table 5.2 **Genes rarely associated with cervical dystonia**

Gene	Usual disease association
ANO3 [25,68,82,131]	Isolated segmental dystonia with frequent onset in the neck
ATM [24,89 121]	Ataxia-telangiectasia
ATXN2[13,92,150]	Spinocerebellar ataxia type 2 (SCA2)
ATXN3[92]	Spinocerebellar ataxia type 3 (SCA3)
C9orf72[50]	Frontotemporal dementia and/or motor neuron disease
CIZ1[154]	Adult-onset isolated cervical dystonia
COL6A3[72]	Early-onset cranio-cervical dystonia with frequent generalization
GBA[79]	Hereditary spastic paraplegia type 46 (SPG46)
GCH1[138,153]	Dopa-responsive dystonia ± parkinsonism
GNAL[20,41,46,81, 82, 84, 97,151]	Isolated segmental or generalized dystonia
HTT[5]	Huntington disease
KMT2B[18,28]	Early-onset generalized dystonia often with cognitive disability and/or seizures
PRKN[76]	Parkinson disease (PARK2)
SETX [16]	Progressive ataxia with oculomotor apraxia type 2
SGCE[6]	Early-onset segmental myoclonus-dystonia syndrome
THAP1[59,84,130,145]	Isolated early-onset segmental or generalized dystonia with frequent laryngeal and/or neck involvement
TGM6[137]	Spinocerebellar ataxia type 35 (SCA35)
TOR1A[42,82,84,86,143]	Isolated early-onset limb dystonia with subsequent spread to segmental or generalized dystonia
TTPA[9]	Progressive ataxia with vitamin E deficiency
TUBB4A[147]	Early-onset generalized dystonia with whispering dysphonia

This table summarizes representative reports in which a pathogenic or probably pathogenic gene variant was associated with a clinical phenotype in which cervical dystonia was the presenting or dominant movement disorder.

Therefore, genetic testing is not routinely conducted in adult-onset CD.

Although a detailed laboratory workup is not usually revealing for most adults who develop CD, there are some clinical features that provide useful clues for a discoverable underlying etiology. Idiopathic CD usually develops over several weeks or months, so sudden onset, such as overnight or in less than a day, is a useful clue for a potential cause. Sudden-onset CD can be seen with acute dystonic reactions from neuroleptics and with behavioral (psychogenic) etiologies.[48,124] The acute wry neck syndrome may also develop suddenly on awakening or sometimes after a sudden head movement. It is associated with neck pain and stiffness, sometimes with a relatively tonic abnormal posture lasting hours or days. The wry neck syndrome is probably musculoskeletal in origin.

The direction of posturing can also be helpful in pointing toward a cause. Movements dominated by retrocollis or anterocollis are not common in idiopathic CD. On the other hand, prominent retrocollis is characteristic of tardive dystonia,[102,123] so a medication history is important (see Chapter 19, "Dystonia Induced by Medications, Illicit Drugs, and Environmental Toxins"). Predominant retrocollis or anterocollis also occur Parkinson disease and related parkinsonian conditions, so a careful examination for parkinsonian features is valuable (see Chapter 13, "Dystonia and Parkinsonism").[60,108,117,155] CD may occur as an early manifestation of one of these disorders,[8] but it more often occurs during the course of the illness. Unlike idiopathic CD, the anterocollis in parkinsonian conditions sometimes develops rapidly, over a few days, often following a change in treatment.

CD must be distinguished from nondystonic causes of abnormal postures and movements of the head and neck (see Chapter 26, "Pseudodystonia and Differential Diagnosis"). For example, dystonic anterocollis must be distinguished from the dropped head syndrome due to neck extensor weakness associated with myasthenia gravis, motor neuron disease, and neck extensor myopathy.[117,122] Extensor spasms with retrocollis can occur with disorders affecting inhibitory neurons of the spine, such as stiff person syndrome, tetanus, or strychnine poisoning. Abnormal postures and movements of the head/neck may also result from orthopedic problems such as the Klippel-Flail anomaly, ankylosing spondylitis, vertebral compression fractures, and atlanto-axial dislocation. Behavioral compensations due to vestibular abnormalities or oculomotor weakness may also result in abnormal postures of the head/neck sometimes called *ocular torticollis*.

Early-Onset Cases

Isolated CD is uncommon in children and adults younger than 30 years. For these cases, there is a greater chance of discovering a cause, so a more extensive workup is warranted. Individuals with dyskinetic cerebral palsy often have generalized dystonia and other abnormal movements, and a very mobile form of CD is a common feature of this syndrome.[47,103] Imaging studies are valuable because they may reveal evidence for stroke or hypoxia-ischemia, or they may provide clues to a disorder that is degenerative, developmental, or metabolic.[100]

A genetic etiology is more likely for early-onset cases, so genetic testing is warranted, too. Many of the genes described above are associated with early-onset dystonia, most commonly starting in one limb and spreading to a segmental or generalized pattern. However, the initial or predominant syndrome in early-onset cases may occasionally resemble focal CD. Because of the many genes that may cause CD, exome sequencing is more useful than single-gene testing, unless there are other features that point to a specific syndrome (see Chapter 22, "Dystonia Genetics").

The label *benign paroxysmal torticollis of infancy* has been used to describe a rare syndrome of recurrent attacks of CD that begin in the first year of life.[61] The label is a misnomer for several reasons. The condition is not always benign since episodes of dystonia are often associated emesis, irritability, and lethargy. The condition is not limited to infancy because episodes may persist for several years. Many cases also evolve to have migraine, so the condition is sometimes considered an early-onset migraine equivalent. Finally, the predominant abnormal movement is head tilt (laterocollis), not torticollis. This syndrome may be linked with several genes, such as *CACNA1A* (see Chapter 14, "Dystonia and Ataxia").

Nondystonic postures and movements of the head and neck described above for adults must also be considered, along with some additional conditions that are more common in early-onset cases, such as congenital muscular torticollis,

Sandifer syndrome, retropharyngeal irritation, and others (see Chapter 26). Tic disorders may also present as repetitive jerking of the head. In addition, severe retrocollis, often combined with opisthotonic postures of the trunk, raises suspicion for neurodegeneration with brain iron accumulation (see Chapter 13, "Dystonia and Parkinsonism") and a number of other inherited metabolic disorders that usually begin very early in life.[71,132]

TREATMENT

Botulinum Toxins

The treatment of CD may involve botulinum toxin (BoNT), oral medications, physical therapy, and/or surgery. For most cases, BoNT is considered the first line of treatment because it is usually more effective with fewer side effects than other options (see Chapter 30, "Botulinum Toxin Treatment of Dystonia"). Several different BoNT preparations are available in different countries, and results from multiple double-blind, placebo-controlled trials have been summarized in prior reviews,[45,128] so only broadly relevant principles are described here.

For the majority of cases with CD, the BoNTs are effective for reducing abnormal movements and pain while improving disability and quality of life. Benefits usually emerge in 5–10 days, reach a peak at 4–6 weeks, and then start to wear off at 8–10 weeks.[99] Numerous longitudinal cohort studies have demonstrated sustained benefits following repeated treatment cycles over many years.[15,43,57,62,66,75,96,101,114,115,129] When applied by experienced injectors, side effects are uncommon and usually transient. The most common side effects include excessive muscle weakness (leading to head drop or difficulty raising the head from supine) and dysphagia (from spread of toxin into pharyngeal muscles). A systemic flu-like syndrome may occur as well.[7,56]

The longitudinal studies show a significant drop-out rate over time.[69,85] Within 3–5 years, approximately one-third of CD patients discontinue BoNT. Several studies have sought to delineate the reasons for discontinuing therapy.[15,57,62,66,70,75,104,129,141] They include insufficient efficacy, unrealistic expectations from treatment, the recurring waxing-waning effect associated with treatment cycles, frequent side effects, development of resistance, misdiagnosis, unusually complex patterns of movement, and practical issues such as repeated travel to the clinic and cost.[49] Patients who discontinue therapy because of poor initial response or a waning of response are often labeled has having primary or secondary resistance to therapy. However, true immune-mediated resistance to BoNT is uncommon. The two most common reasons for failure of BoNT are inadequate dose or improper muscle selection.[70,104,141] Therefore, failure of BoNT should lead to a reconsideration of the diagnosis and treatment plan or referral to an expert center.

It is also important to recognize that some subtypes of CD are more challenging to treat than others.[52,70] CD with severe anterocollis is more difficult to treat than torticollis, laterocollis, and retrocollis.[108,149] Some injectors have advocated injecting the deep anterior pre-vertebral muscles for anterocollis,[12] although methodical studies are lacking. CD with prominent head tremor can also be challenging to treat, especially if the tremor is multidirectional.[98] Some injectors have recommended specifically targeting the obliquus capitus inferior muscles for horizontal head tremor,[125] but methodical studies are again lacking. Some patients with particularly complex patterns of abnormal movements require careful consideration of the col-cap approach to achieve optimal results.[12,49,142] Poor responses are also seen in untreated CD with long-standing and severe abnormal postures. In these cases, there may be underlying muscle contractures or orthopedic changes in the spine that will not respond to BoNT.[26] Assessments of BoNT responses may also be clouded by psychiatric comorbidities,[36] which should be assessed and treated as needed.

Oral Medications

Many oral medications have been suggested for CD, often in combination with BoNT. They may be useful when BoNT benefits wane at the end of a treatment cycle, or they may be needed for pain that does not respond to BoNT. There are no rigorous large-scale studies that guide their application in CD, so choices are driven largely by experience. The most commonly used include benzodiazepines,[110,113] but numerous others are sometimes offered including anticholinergics, baclofen, levodopa, tizanidine, and muscle relaxants (see Chapter 28, "Symptom-Targeted Oral Medications for Dystonia").

Physical Therapy

Physical forms of therapy are an intuitively attractive approach for CD because of the abnormal postures, muscle spasms, and pain. Numerous strategies have been reported including stretching and strengthening exercises, various chiropractic techniques, sensori-motor retraining, massage, acupuncture and dry needling, yoga, and others (see Chapter 32, "Physiotherapy and Complementary Medicine for Dystonia").[37,54,112] Positive outcomes have been reported in many small and unblinded trials, but the largest and most rigorous trials have failed to show enduring benefits.

Although there is limited evidence supporting the use of these methods for CD, many patients ask for them, and some seem to benefit. As a result, these procedures may be offered according to individual preferences. Physiotherapy may be particularly useful in three circumstances. One involves individuals with severe CD who are starting BoNT therapy because grossly abnormal postures may challenging to correct with BoNT alone without stretching of the affected muscles or strengthening those that have become overextended and weak. Another situation where physical therapy is valuable involves individuals with short-duration BoNT responses, so that they have some methods they can apply when the benefits of BoNT wane. The third involves individuals with depression who get discouraged with chronic BoNT therapy.

Some traditionally used methods, such as repositioning procedures, may cause too much pain, so it is valuable to find a therapist who has experience with CD or to advise against certain procedures that may be counterproductive in CD. For example, rapid head and neck manipulations are best avoided because of their uncertain value in dystonia, tendency to increase pain, and small risk of arterial dissection.

Surgical Approaches

Several surgical therapies are available for CD, including deep brain stimulation (DBS), selective peripheral denervation, and sometimes pallidotomy. All are usually reserved for medically refractory cases. DBS is useful for many types of dystonia including CD (see Chapter 31, "Surgical Treatments for Dystonia"). Most studies of CD have targeted the pallidum, although some have targeted the subthalamic nucleus or other regions. One multicenter, double-blind study involving 62 cases of medically refractory CD were evaluated using the Toronto Western Torticollis Rating Scale. After 3 months of pallidal stimulation, there was an overall 21% decrease in motor severity, 36% decrease in disability, and 40% decrease in pain.[146] Numerous unblinded studies have also described positive outcomes for CD. A meta-analysis of 39 reports that included a total of 208 individuals with CD studied for an average duration of 2 years following pallidal or subthalamic stimulation described an overall 58% improvement in motor severity, 47% improvement in pain, and 61% improvement in disability.[140] Benefits vary significantly across cases, and many still require BoNT or oral therapy for optimal symptom relief. Several longitudinal studies have indicated that benefits from DBS are quite durable, lasting at least 10 years. The side effects are typical of those seen with DBS (see Chapter 31). For reasons that are not entirely clear, rare CD cases may also develop a hesitant gait or other parkinsonian features after DBS.[90]

Selective peripheral denervation may be useful for medically refractory CD when DBS is not an option, although it is offered at only a handful of centers worldwide. Denervation is most useful for specific patterns of abnormal movement, so cases must be carefully selected. With careful selection, the efficacy of selective peripheral denervation is similar to DBS.[33,116] Common side effects include focal muscle weakness and atrophy, sensory anomalies in the neck due to resection of local sensory nerves, and sometimes dysphagia.

Ablative procedures have also been evaluated in CD.[21,65] Relatively small numbers of cases have been reported, and there are no large, rigorous, blinded studies. The most common target has involved pallidotomy, either unilateral or bilateral. Benefits are similar to those reported for DBS, but with a higher risk for permanent side effects.

SYNOPSIS AND FUTURE PROSPECTS

Dystonia commonly affects the muscles of the head, neck, and shoulder. CD has numerous different clinical manifestations that include abnormal positions of the head/neck or shoulder, jerky or tremulous movements of the head/neck, and neck or shoulder pain. These problems are often associated with psychiatric comorbidities, and they have a strong impact on quality of life. Isolated CD is the most common of the adult-onset focal dystonias, but it is less common in children.

The diagnosis of CD is often delayed for many years. It may be initially misdiagnosed as more common musculoskeletal problems, sometimes leading to inappropriate treatments. The diagnosis is based chiefly on recognizing its characteristic clinical features and excluding potential mimics. CD is a chronic disorder for which there is no cure. However, it is important to recognize because effective treatments are available. These include botulinum toxins, physical therapy, oral medications, and surgery.

An etiology often cannot be established for most adult-onset cases, but an etiology is more likely to be found in early-onset cases. There are many known etiologies, both genetic and acquired. However, the pathogenesis of CD remains largely unknown. Further research into etiologies and pathogenesis is needed.

REFERENCES

1. Abbruzzese G, Berardelli A, Girlanda P, Marchese R, Martino D, Morgante F, et al. Long-term assessment of the risk of spread in primary late-onset focal dystonia. J Neurol Neurosurg Psychiatry 2008;79:392–396.
2. Albanese A, Bhatia KP, Cardoso F, Comella C, Defazio G, Fung VSC, et al. Isolated cervical dystonia: Diagnosis and classification. Mov Disord 2023;38:1367–1348.
3. Albanese A, Sorbo FD, Comella C, Jinnah HA, Mink JW, Post B, et al. Dystonia rating scales: Critique and recommendations. Mov Disord 2013;28:874–883.
4. Albanese A, Wissel J, Jost WH, Castagna A, Althaus M, Comes G, et al. Pain reduction in cervical dystonia following treatment with incobotulinumtoxinA: A pooled analysis. Toxins (Basel) 2023;15:333.
5. Ashizawa T, Jankovic J. Cervical dystonia as the initial presentation of Huntington's disease. Mov Disord 1996;11:457–459.
6. Asmus F, Zimprich A, Tezenas Du Montcel S, Kabus C, Deuschl G, et al. Myoclonus-dystonia syndrome: Epsilon-sarcoglycan mutations and phenotype. Ann Neurol 2002;52:489–492.
7. Baizabal-Carvallo JF, Jankovic J, Feld J. Flu-like symptoms and associated immunological response following therapy with botulinum toxins. Neurotox Res 2013;24:298–306.
8. Balint B, Mulroy E, Govert F, Latorre A, Di Lazarro G, Erro R, et al. Development of parkinsonism after long-standing cervical dystonia: A cohort. J Neurol Sci 2021;427:117477.
9. Becker AE, Vargas W, Pearson TS. Ataxia with vitamin E deficiency may present with cervical dystonia. Tremor Other Hyperkinet Mov 2016;6:374.
10. Berman BD, Groth CL, Sillau SH, Pirio Richardson S, Norris SA, Junker J, et al. Risk of spread in adult-onset isolated focal dystonia: A prospective international cohort study. J Neurol Neurosurg Psychiatry 2020;91:314–320.
11. Berman BD, Junker J, Shelton E, Sillau SH, Jinnah HA, Perlmutter JS, et al. Psychiatric associations of adult-onset focal dystonia phentypes. J Neurol Neurosurg Psychiat 2017;88:505–602.
12. Bhidayasiri R. Treatment of complex cervical dystonia with botulinum toxin: Involvement of deep-cervical muscles may contribute to suboptimal responses. Parkinsonism Relat Disord 2011;17 Suppl 1:S20–24.
13. Boesch SM, Muller J, Wenning GK, Poewe W. Cervical dystonia in spinocerebellar ataxia type 2: Clinical and polymyographic findings. J Neurol Neurosurg Psychiatry 2007;78:520–522.
14. Boz D, Kilic-Berkmen G, Perlmutter JS, Norris SA, Wright LJ, Klein C, et al. An empirical comparison of commonly universal rating scales for dystonia. Mov Disord Clin Pract 2023;10:1777–1786.
15. Brashear A, Bergan K, Wojcieszek J, Siemers ER, Ambrosius W. Patients' perception of stopping or continuing treatment of cervical dystonia with botulinum toxin type A. Mov Disord 2000;15:150–153.
16. Brugger F, Schupbach M, Koenig M, Muri R, Bohlhalter S, Kaelin-Lang A, et al. The clinical spectrum of ataxia with oculomotor apraxia type 2. Mov Disord Clin Pract 2014;1:106–109.
17. Bruno V, Achen B, Morgante F, Erro R, Fox SH, Edwards MJ, et al. The Pain in Dystonia Scale (PIDS): Development and validation in cervical dystonia. Mov Disord 2023;38:1175–1186.
18. Buzo EL, De la Casa-Fages B, Sanchez MG, Sanchez JRP, Carballal CF, Vidorreta JG, et al. Pallidal deep brain stimulation response in two siblings with atypical adult-onset dystonia related to a KMT2B variant. J Neurol Sci 2022;438:120295.
19. Cano SJ, Warner TT, Linacre JM, Bhatia KP, Thompson AJ, Fitzpatrick R, Hobart JC. Capturing the true burden of dystonia on patients: The Cervical Dystonia Impact Profile (CDIP-58). Neurology 2004;63:1629–1633.
20. Carecchio M, Panteghini C, Reale C, Barzaghi C, Monti V, Romito L, et al. Novel GNAL mutation with intra-familial clinical heterogeneity: Expanding the phenotype. Parkinsonism Relat Disord 2016;23:66–71.
21. Centen LM, Oterdoom DLM, Tijssen MAJ, Lesman-Leegte I, van Egmond ME, van Dijk JMC. Bilateral pallidotomy for dystonia: A systematic review. Mov Disord 2021;36:547–557.
22. Chan J, Brin MF, Fahn S. Idiopathic cervical dystonia: Clinical characteristics. Mov Disord 1991;6:119–126.
23. Charles PD, Adler CH, Stacy M, Comella C, Jankovic J, Manack Adams A, et al. Cervical dystonia and pain: Characteristics and treatment patterns from CD PROBE (Cervical Dystonia Patient Registry for Observation of OnabotulinumtoxinA Efficacy). J Neurol 2014.
24. Charlesworth G, Mohire MD, Schneider SA, Stamelou M, Wood NW, Bhatia KP. Ataxia telangiectasia presenting as dopa-responsive cervical dystonia. Neurology 2013;81:1148–1151.
25. Charlesworth G, Plagnol V, Holmstrom KM, Bras J, Sheerin UM, Preza E, et al. Mutations in ANO3

cause dominant craniocervical dystonia: Ion channel implicated in pathogenesis. Am J Hum Genet 2012;91:1041–1050.
26. Chawda SJ, Munchau A, Johnson D, Bhatia K, Quinn NP, Stevens J, et al. Pattern of premature degenerative changes of the cervical spine in patients with spasmodic torticollis and the impact on the outcome of selective peripheral denervation. J Neurol Neurosurg Psychiatry 2000;68:465–471.
27. Chueluecha C, Moore AP. LIVECHART Patient-Reported Outcome Tool for Botulinum Toxin Treatment in Cervical Dystonia. Mov Disord Clin Pract 2022;9:198–205.
28. Cif L, Demailly D, Lin JP, Barwick KE, Sa M, Abela L, et al. KMT2B-related disorders: Expansion of the phenotypic spectrum and long-term efficacy of deep brain stimulation. Brain 2020;143:3242–3261.
29. Comella C, Bhatia K. An international survey of patients with cervical dystonia. J Neurol 2015;262:837–848.
30. Comella CL, Fox SH, Bhatia KP, Perlmutter JS, Jinnah HA, Zurowski M, et al. Development of the comprehensive cervical dystonia rating scale: Methodology. Mov Disord Clin Pract 2014;2:135–141.
31. Comella CL, Perlmutter JS, Jinnah HA, Waliczek TA, Rosen AR, Galpern WR, et al. Clinimetric testing of the comprehensive cervical dystonia rating scale. Mov Disord 2016;31:563–569.
32. Comella CL, Stebbins GT, Goetz CG, Chmura TA, Bressman SB, Lang AE. Teaching tape for the motor section of the Toronto western spasmodic torticollis scale. Mov Disord 1997;12:570–575.
33. Contarino MF, Van Den Munckhof P, Tijssen MA, de Bie RM, Bosch DA, Schuurman PR, Speelman JD. Selective peripheral denervation: Comparison with pallidal stimulation and literature review. J Neurol 2014;261:300–308.
34. Corp DT, Greenwood C, Morrison-Ham J, Pullinen J, McDowall G, Younger E, et al. Clinical and structural findings in patients with lesion-induced dystonia: Descriptive and quantitative analysis of published cases. Neurology 2022;99:e1957–e1967.
35. Corp DT, Joutsa J, Darby RR, Delnooz CCS, van de Warrenburg BPC, Cooke D, et al. Network localization of cervical dystonia based on causal brain lesions. Brain 2019;2019:1660–1674.
36. Cotton AC, Scorr L, McDonald W, Comella C, Perlmutter JS, Goetz CG, et al. Assessing the severity of cervical dystonia: Ask the doctor or ask the patient. Mov Disord Clin Pract 2023;10:1399–1403.
37. De Pauw J, Van der Velden K, Meirte J, Van Daele U, Truijen S, Cras P, et al. The effectiveness of physiotherapy for cervical dystonia: A systematic literature review. J Neurol 2014;261:1857–1865.
38. Defazio G, Belvisi D, Comella C, Hallett M, Jinnah HA, Cimino P, et al. Validation of a guideline to reduce variability in diagnosing cervical dystonia. J Neurol 2023;270:2606–2612.
39. Defazio G, Fabbrini G, Erro R, Albanese A, Barone P, Zibetti M, et al. Does acute peripheral trauma contribute to idiopathic adult-onset dystonia? Parkinsonism Relat Disord 2020;71:40–43.
40. Di Biasio F, Marchese R, Abbruzzese G, Baldi O, Esposito M, Silvestre F, et al. Motor and sensory features of cervical dystonia subtypes: Data from the italian dystonia registry. Front Neurol 2020;11:906.
41. Dobricic V, Kresojevic N, Westenberger A, Svetel M, Tomic A, Ralic V, et al. De novo mutation in the GNAL gene causing seemingly sporadic dystonia in a Serbian patient. Mov Disord 2014;29:1190–1193.
42. Dobricic V, Kresojevic N, Zarkovic M, Tomic A, Marjanovic A, Westenberger A, et al. Phenotype of non-c.907_909delGAG mutations in TOR1A: DYT1 dystonia revisited. Parkinsonism Relat Disord 2015;21:1256–1259.
43. Dressler D, Paus S, Seitzinger A, Gebhardt B, Kupsch A. Long-term efficacy and safety of incobotulinumtoxinA injections in patients with cervical dystonia. J Neurol Neurosurg Psychiatry 2013;84:1014–1019.
44. Duane DD. Spasmodic torticollis: Clinical and biologic features and their implications for focal dystonia. Adv Neurol 1988;50:473–492.
45. Duarte GS, Rodrigues FB, Marques RE, Castelao M, Ferreira J, Sampaio C, et al. Botulinum toxin type A therapy for blepharospasm. Cochrane Database Syst Rev 2020;11:CD004900.
46. Dufke C, Sturm M, Schroeder C, Moll S, Ott T, Riess O, et al. Screening of mutations in GNAL in sporadic dystonia patients. Mov Disord 2014;29:1193–1196.
47. Ebara S, Harada T, Yamazaki Y. Unstable cervical spine in athetoid cerebral palsy. Spine 1989;14:1154–1159.
48. Ercoli T, Defazio G, Geroin C, Marcuzzo E, Fabbrini G, Bono F, et al. Sudden onset, fixed dystonia and acute peripheral trauma as diagnostic clues for functional dystonia. Mov Disord Clin Pract 2021;8:1107–1111.
49. Erro R, Picillo M, Pellecchia MT, Barone P. Improving the efficacy of botulinum toxin for cervical dystonia: A scoping review. Toxins 2023;15:391.
50. Estevez-Fraga C, Magrinelli F, Hensman Moss D, Mulroy E, Di Lazzaro G, Latorre A, et al. Expanding the spectrum of movement disorders associated with C9orf72 hexanucleotide expansions. Neurol Genet 2021;7:e575.
51. Evidente VG, Pappert EJ. Botulinum toxin therapy for cervical dystonia: The science of dosing. Tremor Other Hyperkinet Mov 2014;4:273.
52. Ferreira JJ, Colosimo C, Bhidayasiri R, Marti MJ, Maisonobe P, Om S. Factors influencing secondary non-response to botulinum toxin type A injections in cervical dystonia. Parkinsonism Relat Disord 2015;21:111–115.
53. Finsterer J, Maeztu C, Revuelta GJ, Reichel G, Truong D. Collum-caput (COL-CAP) concept for conceptual anterocollis, anterocaput, and forward sagittal shift. J Neurol Sci 2015;355:37–43.
54. Fleming BM, Schwab EL, Nouer SS, Wan JY, LeDoux MS. Prevalence, predictors, and perceived effectiveness of complementary, alternative and integrative medicine in adult-onset primary dystonia. Parkinsonism Relat Disord 2012;18:936–940.
55. Frei K. Posttraumatic dystonia. J Neurol Sci 2017;379: 183–191.
56. George EB, Cotton AC, Shneyder N, Jinnah HA. A strategy for managing flu-like symptoms after botulinum toxin injections. J Neurol 2018;265:1932–1933.
57. Gill CE, Manus ND, Pelster MW, Cook JA, Title W, Molinari AL, Charles D. Continuation of long-term care for cervical dystonia at an academic movement disorders clinic. Toxins (Basel) 2013;5:776–783.
58. Girach A, Vinagre Aragon A, Zis P. Quality of life in idiopathic dystonia: A systematic review. J Neurol 2019;266:2897–2906.
59. Giri S, Naiya T, Equbal Z, Sankhla CS, Das SK, Ray K, Ray J. Genetic screening of THAP1 in primary dystonia patients of India. Neurosci Lett 2017;637:31–37.

60. Godeiro-Junior C, Felicio AC, Barsottini OG, Aguiar PM, Silva SM, Borges V, Ferraz HB. Clinical features of dystonia in atypical parkinsonism. Arq Neuropsiquiatr 2008;66:800–804.
61. Greene KA, Lu V, Luciano MS, Qubty W, Irwin SL, Grimes B, Gelfand AA. Benign paroxysmal torticollis: Phenotype, natural history, and quality of life. Pediatr Res 2021;90:1044–1051.
62. Haussermann P, Marczoch S, Klinger C, Landgrebe M, Conrad B, Ceballos-Baumann A. Long-term follow-up of cervical dystonia patients treated with botulinum toxin A. Mov Disord 2004;19:303–308.
63. Hefter H, Urer B, Brauns R, Rosenthal D, Meuth SG, Lee JI, et al. The complex relationship between antibody titers and clinical outcome in botulinum toxin type A long-term treated patients with cervical dystonia. J Neurol 2022;269:5991–6002.
64. Heinen F, Scheidt CE, Nickel T, Rayki O, Wissel J, Poewe W, et al. Spasmodic torticollis: A multicentre study on behavioural aspects II: Signs, symptoms and course. Behav Neurol 1996;9:81–88.
65. Horisawa S, Fukui A, Kohara K, Kawamata T, Taira T. Unilateral pallidotomy in the treatment of cervical dystonia: A retrospective observational study. J Neurosurg 2019;134:216–222.
66. Hsiung GY, Das SK, Ranawaya R, Lafontaine AL, Suchowersky O. Long-term efficacy of botulinum toxin A in treatment of various movement disorders over a 10-year period. Mov Disord 2002;17:1288–1293.
67. Jankovic J, Adler CH, Charles D, Comella C, Stacy M, Schwartz M, et al. Primary results from the Cervical Dystonia Patient Registry for Observation of OnabotulinumtoxinA Efficacy (CD PROBE). J Neurol Sci 2015;349:84–93.
68. Jiang LT, Li LX, Liu Y, Zhang XL, Pan YG, Wang L, et al. The expanding clinical and genetic spectrum of ANO3 dystonia. Neurosci Lett 2021;746:135590.
69. Jinnah HA, Comella CL, Perlmutter J, Lungu C, Hallett M, Dystonia Coalition I. Longitudinal studies of botulinum toxin in cervical dystonia: Why do patients discontinue therapy? Toxicon 2018;147:89–95.
70. Jinnah HA, Goodmann E, Rosen AR, Evatt M, Freeman A, Factor S. Botulinum toxin treatment failures in cervical dystonia: Causes, management, and outcomes. J Neurol 2016;263:1188–1194.
71. Jinnah HA, Visser JE, Harris JC, Verdu A, Larovere L, Ceballos-Picot I, et al. Delineation of the motor disorder of Lesch-Nyhan disease. Brain 2006;129:1201–1217.
72. Jochim A, Zech M, Gora-Stahlberg G, Winkelmann J, Haslinger B. The clinical phenotype of early-onset isolated dystonia caused by recessive COL6A3 mutations (DYT27). Mov Disord 2016;31:747–750.
73. Jost WH, Tatu L, Pandey S, Slawek J, Druzdz A, Biering-Sorensen B, et al. Frequency of different subtypes of cervical dystonia: A prospective multicenter study according to Col-Cap concept. J Neural Transm 2020;127:45–50.
74. Junker J, Berman BD, Hall J, Wahba D, Brandt V, Permutter JS, et al. Quality of life in dystonia: Non-motor manifestations matter. J Neurol Neurosurg Psychiat 2021;92:622–628.
75. Kessler KR, Skutta M, Benecke R. Long-term treatment of cervical dystonia with botulinum toxin A: Efficacy, safety, and antibody frequency. German Dystonia Study Group. J Neurol 1999;246:265–274.
76. Khan NL, Graham E, Critchley P, Schrag AE, Wood NW, Lees AJ, et al. Parkin disease: A phenotypic study of a large case series. Brain 2003;126:1279–1292.
77. Kilic-Berkmen G, Pirio Richardson S, Perlmutter JS, Hallett M, Klein C, Wagle-Shukla A, et al. Current guidelines for classifying and diagnosing cervical dystonia: Empirical evidence and recommendations. Mov Disord Clin Pract 2021;9:183–190.
78. Kilic-Berkmen G, Scorr LM, Rosen A, Wu E, Freeman A, Silver M, et al. Thyroid disease in cervical dystonia. Parkinsonism Relat Disord 2023;107:10524.
79. Kloth K, Cozma C, Bester M, Gerloff C, Biskup S, Zittel S. Dystonia as initial presentation of compound heterozygous GBA2 mutations: Expanding the phenotypic spectrum of SPG46. Eur J Med Genet 2020;63:103992.
80. Konrad C, Vollmer-Haase J, Anneken K, Knecht S. Orthopedic and neurological complications of cervical dystonia: Review of the literature. Acta Neurol Scand 2004;109:369–373.
81. Kumar KR, Lohmann K, Masuho I, Miyamoto R, Ferbert A, Lohnau T, et al. Mutations in GNAL: A novel cause of craniocervical dystonia. JAMA Neurol 2014;71:490–494.
82. Lange LM, Junker J, Loens S, Baumann H, Olschewski L, Schaake S, et al. Genotype-phenotype relations for isolated dystonia genes: MDSGene systematic review. Mov Disord 2021;36:1086–1103.
83. LeDoux MS, Brady KA. Secondary cervical dystonia associated with structural lesions of the central nervous system. Mov Disord 2003;18:60–69.
84. LeDoux MS, Vemula SR, Xiao J, Thompson MM, Perlmutter JS, Wright LJ, et al. Clinical and genetic features of cervical dystonia in a large multicenter cohort. Neurol Genet 2016;2:e69.
85. Lee JI, Jansen A, Samadzadeh S, Kahlen U, Moll M, Ringelstein M, et al. Long-term adherence and response to botulinum toxin in different indications. Ann Clin Transl Neurol 2021;8:15–28.
86. Leube B, Kessler KR, Ferbert A, Ebke M, Schwendemann G, Erbguth F, et al. Phenotypic variability of the DYT1 mutation in German dystonia patients. Acta Neurol Scand 1999;99:248–251.
87. Liang Y, Lin J, Hou Y, Zhang L, Ou R, Li C, et al. Health-related quality of life in cervical dystonia using EQ-5D-5L: A large cross-sectional study in China. Front Neurol 2022;13:895272.
88. Listik C, Listik E, de Paiva Santos Rolim F, Meneses Cury Portela DM, Perez Lloret S, de Alves Araujo NR, et al. Development and validation of the Dystonia-Pain Classification System: A multicenter study. Mov Disord 2023;38:1163–1174.
89. Lohmann E, Kruger S, Hauser AK, Hanagasi H, Guven G, Erginel-Unaltuna N, et al. Clinical variability in ataxia-telangiectasia. J Neurol 2015;262:1724–1727.
90. Mahlknecht P, Georgiev D, Akram H, Brugger F, Vinke S, Zrinzo L, et al. Parkinsonian signs in patients with cervical dystonia treated with pallidal deep brain stimulation. Brain 2018;141:3023–3034.
91. Main ka T, Erro R, Rothwell J, Kuhn AA, Bhatia KP, Ganos C. Remission in dystonia: Systematic review of the literature and meta-analysis. Parkinsonism Relat Disord 2019;66:9–15.
92. Markovic V, Dragasevic-Miskovic NT, Stankovic I, Petrovic I, Svetel M, Kostic VS. Dystonia in patients with

spinocerebellar ataxia type 2. Mov Disord Clin Pract 2016;3:292–295.
93. Medina A, Nilles C, Martino D, Pelletier C, Pringsheim T. The prevalence of idiopathic or inherited isolated dystonia: A systematic review and meta-analysis. Mov Disord Clin Pract 2022;9:860–868.
94. Medina Escobar A, Martino D, Goodarzi Z. The prevalence of anxiety in adult-onset isolated dystonia: A systematic review and meta-analysis. Eur J Neurol 2021;28:4238–4250.
95. Medina Escobar A, Pringsheim T, Goodarzi Z, Martino D. The prevalence of depression in adult onset idiopathic dystonia: Systematic review and metaanalysis. Neurosci Biobehav Rev 2021;125:221–230.
96. Mejia NI, Vuong KD, Jankovic J. Long-term botulinum toxin efficacy, safety, and immunogenicity. Mov Disord 2005;20:592–597.
97. Miao J, Wan XH, Sun Y, Feng JC, Cheng FB. Mutation screening of GNAL gene in patients with primary dystonia from northeast China. Parkinsonism Relat Disord 2013;19:910–912.
98. Misra VP, Ehler E, Zakine B, Maisonobe P, Simonetta-Moreau M, Group IIC. Factors influencing response to Botulinum toxin type A in patients with idiopathic cervical dystonia: Results from an international observational study. BMJ Open 2012;2:e000881.
99. Mitsikostas DD, Dekundy A, Hanschmann A, Althaus M, Scheschonka A, Pagan F, Jankovic J. Duration and onset of effect of incobotulinumtoxinA for the treatment of blepharospasm in botulinum toxin-naive subjects. Curr Med Res Opin 2021:1–8.
100. Mohammad SS, Angiti RR, Biggin A, Morales-Briceno H, Goetti R, Perez-Duenas B, et al. Magnetic resonance imaging pattern recognition in childhood bilateral basal ganglia disorders. Brain Commun 2020;2:fcaa178.
101. Mohammadi B, Buhr N, Bigalke H, Krampfl K, Dengler R, Kollewe K. A long-term follow-up of botulinum toxin A in cervical dystonia. Neurol Res 2009;31:463–466.
102. Molho ES, Feustel PJ, Factor SA. Clinical comparison of tardive and idiopathic cervical dystonia. Mov Disord 1998;13:486–489.
103. Monbaliu E, Himmelmann K, Lin JP, Ortibus E, Bonouvrie L, Feys H, et al. Clinical presentation and management of dyskinetic cerebral palsy. Lancet Neurol 2017;16:741–749.
104. Nijmeijer SW, Koelman JH, Standaar TS, Postma M, Tijssen MA. Cervical dystonia: Improved treatment response to botulinum toxin after referral to a tertiary centre and the use of polymyography. Parkinsonism Relat Disord 2013;19:533–538.
105. Norris SA, Jinnah HA, Espay AJ, Klein C, Bruggemann N, Barbano RL, et al. Clinical and demographic characteristics related to onset site and spread of cervical dystonia. Mov Disord 2016;31:1874–1882.
106. O'Riordan S, Hutchinson M. Cervical dystonia following peripheral trauma: A case-control study. J Neurol 2004;251:150–155.
107. Ortiz R, Scheperjans F, Mertsalmi T, Pekkonen E. The prevalence of adult-onset isolated dystonia in Finland 2007-2016. PLoS One 2018;13:e0207729.
108. Papapetropoulos S, Tuchman A, Sengun C, Russell A, Mitsi G, Singer C. Anterocollis: Clinical features and treatment options. Med Sci Monit 2008;14:CR427–430.
109. Patel N, Hanfelt J, Marsh L, Jankovic J, Coalition on Motion Disorders. Alleviating manoeuvres (sensory tricks) in cervical dystonia. J Neurol Neurosurg Psychiatry 2014;85:882–884.
110. Pirio Richardson S, Wegele AR, Skipper B, Deligtisch A, Jinnah HA. Dystonia treatment: Patterns of medication use in an international cohort. Neurology 2017;88:1–8.
111. Powis Z, Towne MC, Hagman KDF, Blanco K, Palmaer E, Castro A, et al. Clinical diagnostic exome sequencing in dystonia: Genetic testing challenges for complex conditions. Clin Genet 2019;97:305–307.
112. Prudente CN, Zetterberg L, Bring A, Bradnam L, Kimberley TJ. Systematic review of rehabilitation in focal dystonias: Classification and recommendations. Mov Disord Clin Pract 2018;5:237–245.
113. Raluy-Callado M, Gabriel S, Dinet J, Wang M, Wasiak R. A retrospective study to assess resource utilization in patients with cervical dystonia in the United Kingdom. Neuropsychiatr Dis Treat 2015;11:647–655.
114. Ramirez-Castaneda J, Jankovic J. Long-term efficacy and safety of botulinum toxin injections in dystonia. Toxins (Basel) 2013;5:249–266.
115. Ramirez-Castaneda J, Jankovic J. Long-term efficacy, safety, and side effect profile of botulinum toxin in dystonia: A 20-year follow-up. Toxicon 2014;90:344–348.
116. Ravindran K, Kumar N, Englot DJ, Wilson TJ, Zuckerman SL. Deep brain stimulation versus peripheral denervation for cervical dystonia: A systematic review and meta-analysis. World Neurosurg 2018;122:e940–e946.
117. Revuelta GJ, Benatar M, Freeman A, Wichmann T, Jinnah HA, Delong MR, Factor SA. Clinical subtypes of anterocollis in parkinsonian syndromes. J Neurol Sci 2011;315:100–103.
118. Risvoll H, Kerty E. To test or not? The value of diagnostic tests in cervical dystonia. Mov Disord 2001;16:286–289.
119. Rondot P, Marchand MP, Dellatorlas G. Spasmodic torticollis-review of 220 patients. Can J Neurol Sci 1991;18:143–151.
120. Rosales RL, Cuffe L, Regnault B, Trosch RM. Pain in cervical dystonia: Mechanisms, assessment and treatment. Expert Rev Neurother 2021;21:1125–1134.
121. Saunders-Pullman R, Raymond D, Stoessl AJ, Hobson D, Nakamura T, Pullman S, et al. Variant ataxia-telangiectasia presenting as primary-appearing dystonia in Canadian Mennonites. Neurology 2012;78:649–657.
122. Savica R, Kumar N, Ahlskog JE, Josephs KA, Matsumoto JY, McKeon A. Parkinsonism and dropped head: Dystonia, myopathy or both? Parkinsonism Relat Disord 2012;18:30–34.
123. Savitt D, Jankovic J. Tardive syndromes. J Neurol Sci 2018;389:35–42.
124. Schrag A, Trimble M, Quinn N, Bhatia K. The syndrome of fixed dystonia: An evaluation of 103 patients. Brain 2004;127:2360–2372.
125. Schramm A, Huber D, Mobius C, Munchau A, Kohl Z, Baumer T. Involvement of obliquus capitis inferior muscle in dystonic head tremor. Parkinsonism Relat Disord 2017;44:119–123.
126. Shaikh AG, Beylergil SB, Scorr L, Kilic-Berkmen G, Freeman A, Klein C, et al. Dystonia & tremor: A cross-sectional study of the Dystonia Coalition cohort. Neurology 2021;96:e563–e574.
127. Shaikh AG, Wong AL, Zee DS, Jinnah HA. Keeping your head on target. J Neurosci 2013;33:11281–11295.
128. Simpson DM, Hallett M, Ashman EJ, Comella CL, Green MW, Gronseth GS, et al. Practice guideline update

summary: Botulinum neurotoxin for the treatment of blepharospasm, cervical dystonia, adult spasticity, and headache: Report of the Guideline Development Subcommittee of the American Academy of Neurology. Neurology 2016;86:1818–1826.
129. Skogseid IM, Kerty E. The course of cervical dystonia and patient satisfaction with long-term botulinum toxin A treatment. Eur J Neurol 2005;12:163–170.
130. Sohn AS, Glockle N, Doetzer AD, Deuschl G, Felbor U, Topka HR, et al. Prevalence of THAP1 sequence variants in German patients with primary dystonia. Mov Disord 2010;25:1982–1986.
131. Stamelou M, Charlesworth G, Cordivari C, Schneider SA, Kagi G, Sheerin UM, et al. The phenotypic spectrum of DYT24 due to ANO3 mutations. Mov Disord 2014;29:928–934.
132. Stamelou M, Lai SC, Aggarwal A, Schneider SA, Houlden H, Yeh TH, et al. Dystonic opisthotonus: A "red flag" for neurodegeneration with brain iron accumulation syndromes? Mov Disord 2013;28:1325–1329.
133. Steeves TD, Day L, Dykeman J, Jette N, Pringsheim T. The prevalence of primary dystonia: A systematic review and meta-analysis. Mov Disord 2012;27:1789–1796.
134. Sun YV, Li C, Hui Q, Huang Y, Barbano R, Rodriguez R, Malaty IA, et al. A multi-center genome-wide association study of cervical dystonia. Mov Disord 2021;36:2795–2801.
135. Svetel M, Pekmezovic T, Jovic J, Ivanovic N, Dragasevic N, Maric J, Kostic VS. Spread of primary dystonia in relation to initially affected region. J Neurol 2007;254:879–883.
136. Svetel M, Pekmezovic T, Tomic A, Kresojevic N, Kostic VS. The spread of primary late-onset focal dystonia in a long-term follow up study. Clin Neurol Neurosurg 2015;132:41–43.
137. Thirumurugesan SL, Delhikumar CG, Karunakar P, Sugumaran R, Biswal N, Kalatheeswaran S. Cervical dystonia - A rare presentation of spinocerebellar ataxia type 35. Indian J Pediatr 2022;89:626.
138. Trender-Gerhard I, Sweeney MG, Schwingenschuh P, Mir P, Edwards MJ, Gerhard A, et al. Autosomal-dominant GTPCH1-deficient DRD: Clinical characteristics and long-term outcome of 34 patients. J Neurol Neurosurg Psychiatry 2009;80:839–845.
139. Trosch RM, Espay AJ, Truong D, Gil R, Singer C, LeWitt PA, et al. Multicenter oberservational study of abobotulinumtoxinA neurotoxin in cervical dystonia: The ANCHOR-CD registry. J Neurol Sci 2017;376:84–90.
140. Tsuboi T, Wong JK, Almeida L, Hess CW, Wagle Shukla A, Foote KD, et al. A pooled meta-analysis of GPi and STN deep brain stimulation outcomes for cervical dystonia. J Neurol 2020;267:1278–1290.
141. Tucker H, Osei-Poku F, Ashton D, Lally R, Jesuthasan A, Latorre A, et al. Management of secondary poor response to botulinum toxin in cervical dystonia: A multicenter audit. Mov Disord Clin Pract 2021;8:541–545.
142. Tyslerowicz M, Kiedrzynska W, Adamkiewicz B, Jost WH, Slawek J. Cervical dystonia - improving the effectiveness of botulinum toxin therapy. Neurol Neurochir Pol 2020;54:1–11.
143. Van Coller R, Schutte CM, Lubbe E, Ngele B. TOR1A mutation-related isolated childhood-onset generalised dystonia in South Africa. S Afr Med J 2021;111:946–949.
144. van Egmond ME, Lagrand TJ, Lizaitiene G, Smit M, Tijssen MAJ. A novel diagnostic approach for patients with adult-onset dystonia. J Neurol Neurosurg Psychiatry 2022;93:1039–1048.
145. Vemula SR, Xiao J, Zhao Y, Bastian RW, Perlmutter JS, Racette BA, et al. A rare sequence variant in intron 1 of THAP1 is associated with primary dystonia. Mol Genet Genomic Med 2014;2:261–272.
146. Volkmann J, Mueller J, Deuschl G, Kuhn AA, Krauss JK, Poewe W, et al. Pallidal neurostimulation in patients with medication-refractory cervical dystonia: A randomised, sham-controlled trial. Lancet Neurol 2014;13:875–884.
147. Vulinovic F, Schaake S, Domingo A, Kumar KR, Defazio G, Mir P, et al. Screening study of TUBB4A in isolated dystonia. Parkinsonism Relat Disord 2017;41:118–120.
148. Wadon ME, Bailey GA, Yilmaz Z, Hubbard E, AlSaeed M, Robinson A, et al. Non-motor phenotypic subgroups in adult-onset idiopathic, isolated, focal cervical dystonia. Brain Behav 2021;11:e2292.
149. Waln O, Ledoux MS. Blepharospasm plus cervical dystonia with predominant anterocollis: A distinctive subphenotype of segmental craniocervical dystonia? Tremor Other Hyperkinet Mov 2011;tre-01-33-140-2.
150. Walsh R, O'Dwyer JP, O'Riordan S, Bradley D, Moroney J, Hutchinson M. Cervical dystonia presenting as a phenocopy in an Irish SCA2 family. Mov Disord 2009;24:466–467.
151. Wang X, Mei S, Tian Z, Wang L, Hao G, Zhu X, et al. Case report: Clinical outcome from pallidal stimulation in a patient with levodopa-resistant dopa-responsive dystonia. Front Neurol 2022;13:921577.
152. Weiss EM, Hershey T, Karimi M, Racette B, Tabbal SD, Mink JW, et al. Relative risk of spread of symptoms among the focal onset primary dystonias. Mov Disord 2006;21:1175–1181.
153. Weissbach A, Pauly MG, Herzog R, Hahn L, Halmans S, Hamami F, et al. Relationship of genotype, phenotype, and treatment in dopa-responsive dystonia: MDSGene review. Mov Disord 2021;2022:237–252.
154. Xiao J, Uitti RJ, Zhao Y, Vemula SR, Perlmutter JS, Wszolek ZK, et al. Mutations in CIZ1 cause adult onset primary cervical dystonia. Ann Neurol 2012;71:458–469.
155. Yoon WT. Comparison of dystonia between Parkinson's disease and atypical parkinsonism: The clinical usefulness of dystonia distribution and characteristics in the differential diagnosis of parkinsonism. Neurol Neurochir Pol 2018;52:48–53.
156. Yoon WT, Chung EJ, Lee SH, Kim BJ, Lee WY. Clinical analysis of blepharospasm and apraxia of eyelid opening in patients with parkinsonism. J Clin Neurol 2005;1:159–165.
157. Zech M, Jech R, Boesch S, Skorvanek M, Weber S, Wagner M, et al. Monogenic variants in dystonia: An exome-wide sequencing study. Lancet Neurol 2020;19:908–918.
158. Zurowski M, Marsh L, McDonald W. Psychiatric comorbidities in dystonia: Emerging concepts. Mov Disord 2013;28:914–920.

Chapter 6

Craniofacial Dystonias

INTRODUCTION

Dystonia commonly affects the muscles of the face and other cranial regions. Blepharospasm (BSP) is characterized by involvement of the muscles around the eyes, particularly the orbicularis oculi and nearby muscles of the upper face.[22] Oromandibular dystonia (OMD) is characterized by involvement of muscles of the mouth including the lower face, jaw, and tongue. However, BSP and OMD are frequently combined (Table 6.1). Approximately half of all individuals who start with BSP experience spread of dystonia over 5 years, and the most common area for spread is the oromandibular region.[1,9,69,93,94,105] Conversely, subjects who start with OMD often experience spread to the upper face.[88] Since BSP and OMD often occur simultaneously as segmental craniofacial dystonia, they are considered together in this chapter.

In most epidemiological studies, BSP is the second most common of all dystonia syndromes, with cervical dystonia being the most common. However, BSP is sometimes more common than cervical dystonia in epidemiological studies from Asia. A meta-analysis of studies published from 1985 to 2010 revealed an overall prevalence of 4.2 cases of BSP per 100,000,[91] while another meta-analysis of studies published from 2010 to 2022 revealed an overall prevalence of 2.4 cases per 100,000[71] (see Chapter 4, "Epidemiology of the Dystonias"). Meta-analyses for OMD have placed the prevalence at 0.5–0.6 cases per 100,000.[71,91] These results imply that OMD is quite rare. However, this figure reflects cases with pure OMD and does not include many cases where BSP coexists. Both CFD and OMD typically emerge in adults between 50 and 60 years of age (Figure 6.1), although they may instead arise in children. In most large case series, females substantially outnumber males (Figure 6.2).

The combination of BSP with OMD is sufficiently common to have its own eponym, *Meige syndrome*.[98] However, the use of this eponym has been discouraged.[63] Henri Meige was not the first to describe the combination of BSP with OMD. This combination was first described by Horatio Wood. In fact, the original focus of Meige was not to describe BSP with OMD. Instead, his intent was to discriminate *spasm facial median* from other facial spasms that involved muscles more laterally in the face.[98] However, he described involvement of some muscles that are not midline (orbicularis oculi and jaw), and the value of discriminating medial from lateral facial spasms in the cranial dystonias has never been clear. In view of this history, it is not clear that the combination of BSP and OMD should be called *Meige syndrome*. Another reason this eponym has been discouraged is that it has been variably applied

Table 6.1 **Large descriptive studies of craniofacial dystonias**

Study	Country	Cases	Female (%)	Age at onset	Main focus	Additional regions with dystonia	Additional symptoms
Jankovic 1984[51]	USA	250	75.0	NR	BSP	32% OMD, 29% LD, 20% CD, 14% limb	Initial symptom was blinking in 78%, other symptoms NR
Grandas 1988[42]	UK	264	64.4	56±12	BSP	OMD 71%, CD 23%, LD 17%, RD 15%	Initial symptoms included photophobia 25, dry eyes 16%, eye pain 12%
Mauriello 1996[70]	USA	239	57.7	NR	BSP	7% OMD	NR
Anderson 1998[3]	USA	1653	73.0	55±NR	BSP	OMD 25%, CD 24%, RD 20%	Initial symptoms included blinking 77%, eye spasms 66%, eye irritation 55%, dry eye 49%
Peckham, 2011[77]	USA	240	73.8	NR	BSP	OMD 31%, 8% CD, 1% LD	Initial symptoms included photophobia 25% and eye irritation 22%
Martino, 2012[69]	Italy	281	73.7	57±10	BSP	43% OMD, 17% CD	NR
Slaim, 2018[90]	France	240	240	52±19	OMD	BSP 39%, CD 27%, SD 20%, Gen 11%, limb 6%	NR
Wakakura, 2018[103]	Japan	1116	72.8	66±17	BSP	NR	Chief complaints included difficulty opening eyes, photophobia, eye pain, eye irritation, blinking
Fang, 2020[31]	China	338	71.0	50±12	BSP	NR	Coexisting symptoms including blinking 92%, photophobia 82%, blurry vision 80%, eye strain 76%, dry eye 58%
Scorr, 2021[88]	Intl	727	70.0	50±16	OMD	Seg 43%, Multi 6%, Gen 11%	NR
	USA	116	70.0	54±15	OMD	Seg 49%, Gen 5%	NR
	USA	56	70.0	50±14	OMD	Seg 16%, Gen 2%	NR
Scorr, 2022[87]	Intl	884	66.9	49±14	BSP	CD 60%, OMD 56%, LD 19%	Coexisting symptoms included photophobia 82%, dry eyes 78%, eye irritation 70%
Balal, 2023[6]	Turkey	82	53.6	43±18	OMD	Other CFD 28%, CD 6%, LD 2%	NR

This table summarizes studies of craniofacial dystonia that included more than 200 research participants and provided detailed clinical information on coexisting features. Although many articles focused on BSP or OMD, many articles included overlapping cases.

Abbreviations: BSP, blepharospasm; CD, cervical dystonia; Gen, generalized dystonia; Int, international; LD, laryngeal dystonia; limb, arm or leg dystonia; NR, not reported; RD, respiratory dystonia; Seg, segmental dystonia.

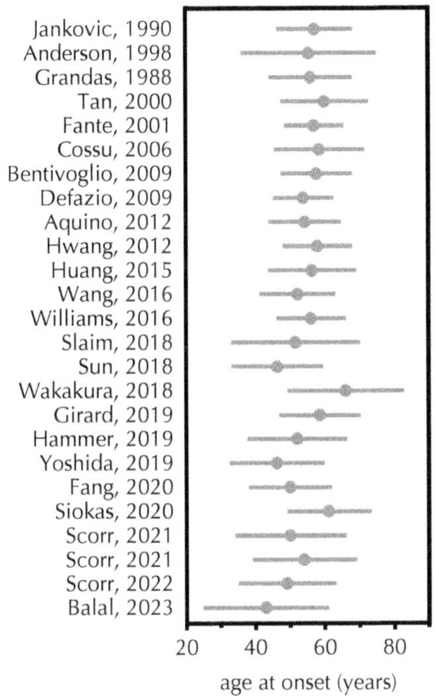

Figure 6.1. Age at onset for blepharospasm and oromandibular dystonia. This figure was prepared by collecting data from studies that included at least 100 individuals with craniofacial dystonia and included age at onset.

in the literature to isolated BSP, isolated OMD, the combination of BSP and OMD, and occasionally BSP with laryngeal or cervical dystonia. As a result, the eponym lacks a broadly accepted meaning. Finally, medical errors may result from confusion of *Meige syndrome* with *Meig syndrome*, which refers to the combination of an ovarian tumor with ascites and hydrothorax. In view of these observations and in keeping with the Council of Science Editors recommendations

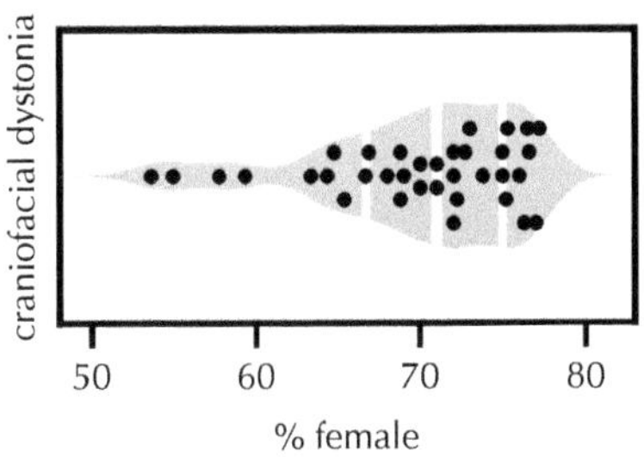

Figure 6.2. Sex distributions for blepharospasm and oromandibular dystonia. This violin plot was prepared by collecting data from studies that included at least 100 individuals with craniofacial dystonia and included information on sex.

discouraging the use of possessive eponyms in science and medicine, the term *craniofacial segmental dystonia* is used to refer to the combination of BSP and OMD in this chapter, rather than Meige syndrome.[58]

BLEPHAROSPASM: CLINICAL FEATURES

Motor Features

The most characteristic feature of BSP is excess activity of the orbicularis oculi muscles. The orbicularis oculi muscle has multiple distinct portions, with different functions (Figure 6.3). The orbital portion of the muscle surrounds the eye and contributes to downward movement of the eyebrow and/or upward movement of the upper cheek area. The palpebral portion of the muscle is part of the upper and lower eyelids, and it is divided into pretarsal and preseptal segments. Riolan's muscle is a very thin portion of the pretarsal orbicularis oculi in the vermillion border of the eyelid; it is responsible for keeping the eyelid closed.

Each portion of the orbicularis oculus muscle has a different action, and overactivity results in different types of abnormal movements. Excess activity of the orbital portion of the orbicularis oculi produces a squeezing appearance around the eyes (Figure 6.4A). Spasms are usually bilateral, symmetric, and synchronous. However, spasms sometimes begin on one side, or they may remain asymmetric for many years. Spasms may be brief, lasting less than a second. They may also be much longer, leading to lengthy periods of eye closure that may produce functional blindness.

Excess activity of the palpebral portion of the orbicularis oculi contributes to excessive blinking. In one detailed study, normal individuals averaged 17 blinks/min, with substantial modulation by activities such as reading (4 blinks/min) or speaking (26 blinks/min).[7] Individuals with BSP may have more than 100 blinks/min.[8] The blink rate in BSP also varies under different conditions. The blink rate may be normal at rest, but it may increase substantially with bright lights or stress. Sometimes there are rapid trains of 3–5 blinks or more with only partial opening between blinks, a phenomenon called *eyelid fluttering*.

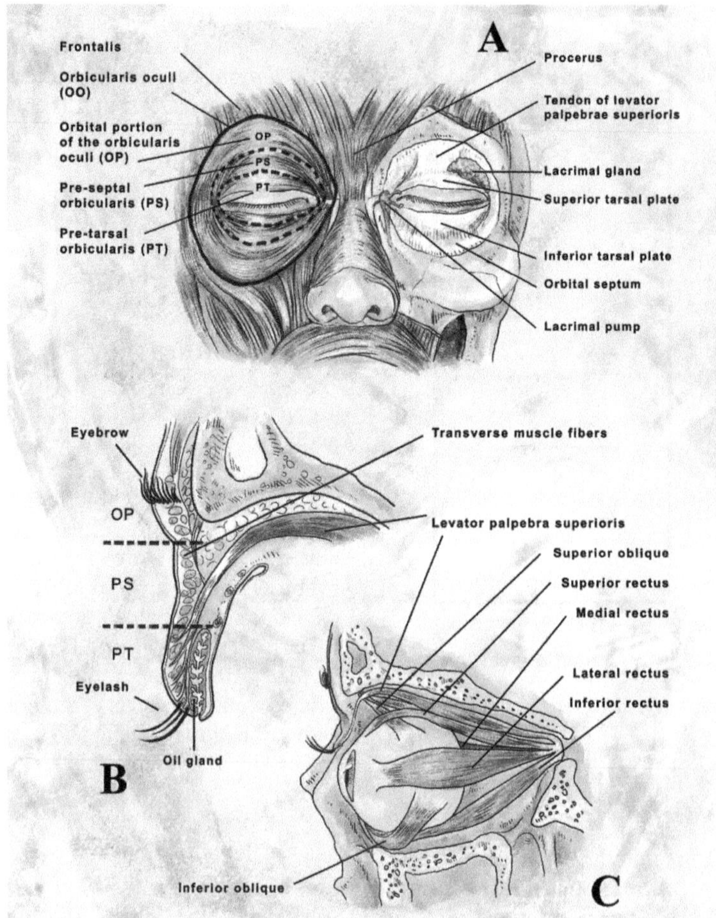

Figure 6.3. Facial muscles responsible for the craniofacial dystonias. Understanding the abnormal movements and treatment of blepharospasm is greatly aided by a detailed understanding of the muscles involved. A key muscle is the orbicularis oculus (OO), a complex muscle with distinct parts. These parts have different functions, and they may be differentially affected in blepharospasm. The orbital portion of the OO is a ring-like muscle that surrounds the eye, with two separate parts that include an upper half and a lower half. The upper half draws the eyebrow down while the lower half draws the tissue under the eyes upward. Simultaneous contraction of both halves gives a squeezing appearance around the eyes. The palpebral portion of the OO is in the eyelid itself, also with upper and lower portions. The upper half is further subdivided into two parts, pretarsal (contained within the most mobile portion of the upper eyelid) and preseptal (between the moving part of the upper eyelid and the superior orbital rim). Blinking involves contraction of the palpebral OO along with simultaneous relaxation of the levator palpebrae muscle. Contraction of the palpebral OO can often be seen in eyelid fluttering. A fine strip of the pretarsal OO muscle just above the eyelid rim is known as Riolan's muscle, which contracts to keep the eyelid closed. For eye opening, Riolan's muscle must relax to allow the eyelid stretching that is required to travel over the globe of the eye. Failure of relaxation in this portion of the OO may be responsible for pretarsal blepharospasm.

Illustration by Loren Bergantini.

Fluttering may reflect a more persistent spasm of the palpebral portions of the orbicularis oculi muscles.

Another feature of BSP has been labeled *apraxia of eyelid opening* or *pretarsal BSP*.[28,95] It is defined as nonparalytic difficulty in initiating eyelid opening in the absence of clinically apparent contraction of the orbicularis oculi. Its frequency depends on how it is defined. In its mildest form, there is a slight delay in opening the eyelids, a phenomenon that is common in BSP. In its more severe form, there is a marked delay in eyelid opening, or the eyelids will not open without using the fingers. Sometimes contraction of the frontalis is used as a compensatory tactic to open the eyes (Figure 6.4B). These phenomena are thought to be caused by excessive activity of the pretarsal orbicularis

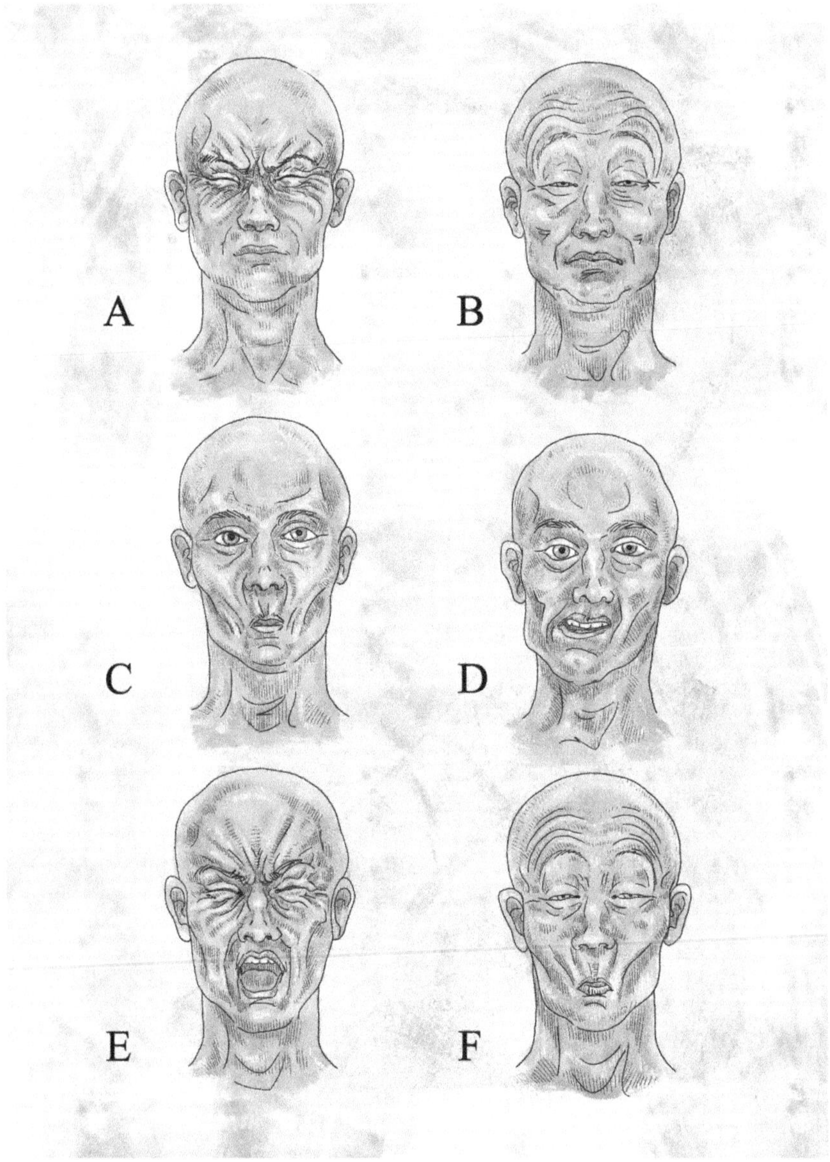

Figure 6.4. Typical appearances of craniofacial dystonias. Panel A shows the typical spasms of blepharospasm involving the orbital orbicularis oculi. There is downward movement of the eyebrow, upward movement of the face below the eyes, and a squeezing appearance around the eyes. Panel B shows pretarsal BSP, where the eyes remain closed with no obvious spasm. Instead, there is compensatory contraction of the frontalis in an attempt to open the eyes. Oromandibular dystonia may appear as taught lips (Panel C) or deviation of the jaw (Panel D). Combinations are common, including typical blepharospasm with jaw opening dystonia (Panel E) or pretarsal BSP with lower facial contortions (Panel F).

Illustration by Loren Bergantini.

oculi and Riolan's muscle in particular, rendering the eyelid rim unable to relax so that it can stretch as is moves over the globe of the eye.[43,95] Therefore, these eyelid phenomena in BSP are not truly apraxia, and the term *pretarsal BSP* is preferable. Indeed, true apraxia of eyelid opening may also occur because of nonparalytic failure of the levator palpebrae to pull the eyelid open.[95]

Most individuals with BSP have some combination of orbital orbicularis oculi spasm, excessive blinking or fluttering, and sometimes delayed eyelid opening without apparent spasm. In one multicenter study of 131 cases, 98% had excessive blinking, 93% had periocular spasms, and 29% had pretarsal BSP.[88] In some cases, one of these problems may dominate the clinical picture. Some individuals with BSP may have prominent orbital spasms with a normal or reduced blink rate. Others may have extreme blinking and fluttering but few spasms. Excessive blinking and fluttering may precede the development of spasms of the orbital portion of the orbicularis oculi.[15] Pretarsal BSP may occur in isolation but more often occurs among individuals who have more obvious periocular spasms and excessive blinking for many years.

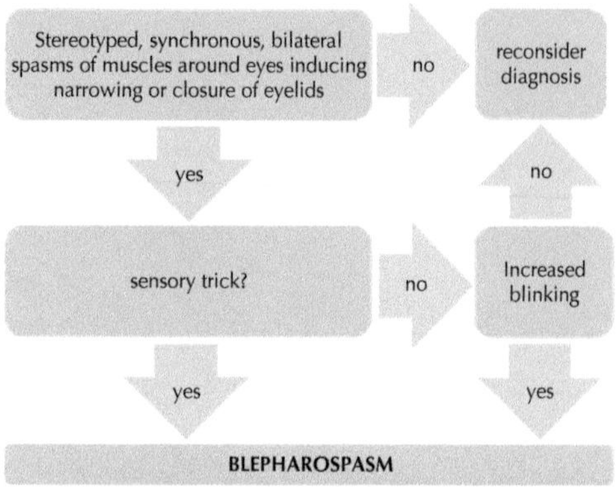

Figure 6.5. Diagnostic algorithm for blepharospasm.

Adapted from previous publications.[21,23]

Non-Motor features

Although BSP is defined by its motor features, non-motor features are common. Sensory symptoms relating to the eyes are very common and may precede the development of motor symptoms.[41,47,48,64,76,77,92,103] In the multicenter study of 131 cases described above, 82% endorsed symptoms of photophobia, 78% reported dry eyes, and 70% noted irritating sensations such as feelings of sand or grit in the eyes, or a burning feeling in the eyes.[88]

Psychiatric features are also common, most notably the anxiety spectrum disorders, and particularly social anxiety, which refers to anxiousness in social settings.[10] Depressed mood also is common, with approximately a quarter meeting criteria for clinical depression.

Differential Diagnosis

The diagnosis of BSP rests on clinical recognition of its characteristic features and exclusion of potential mimics.[17,21,23] A diagnostic algorithm has been proposed (Figure 6.5).[18,21] Although the symptoms and signs of BSP are sufficiently characteristic to suggest an almost immediate diagnosis, multiple studies have revealed that the time from symptom onset to diagnosis averages from 3 to 6 years.[41,47,53,68,78] Misdiagnosis of initial presentations is common.[47,48,103] Sensory symptoms in the eyes often suggest more common problems such as dry eyes, allergies, conjunctivitis, or keratitis. Inability to open the eyes may be confused with myasthenia gravis. Coexisting psychiatric symptoms may also lead to incorrect initial psychiatric diagnoses.

When there are obvious eye spasms, common alternative diagnoses to consider include eye tics, hemifacial spasm, and psychogenic disorders (Table 6.2).[30] Tics can often be identified because they typically affect a younger age group, they may be accompanied by a premonitory urge, they are often suppressible, and there may be additional tics producing other body movements. Hemifacial spasm is not considered a subtype of dystonia because it is thought to be caused by irritation of the seventh cranial nerve with ephaptic transmission. Hemifacial spasm is characterized by sudden irregular jerks of the facial muscles sometimes combined with more tonic muscle contraction. Hemifacial spasm frequently affects the upper face, but usually only on one side. BSP more commonly affects both eyes, although it can be asymmetric, especially at onset. Bilateral hemifacial spasm is rare.[35] It can be discriminated from BSP because spasms of each eye are usually asynchronous, unlike spasms of BSP, where both eyes spasm together. Eye spasms may also be a manifestation of a tardive syndrome resulting from exposure to drugs that block dopamine receptors.

Excessive eyelid blinking may also be caused by irritation from dry eyes, inflammatory conditions, and others. Pretarsal BSP can be difficult to distinguish from disorders of eyelid weakness, such as myasthenia gravis. In pretarsal BSP, the main problem is opening the eyes after a blink because of failure of the palpebral orbicularis oculi to relax. Once the eyelids are open, they can usually stay open until there is another blink that closes them. In myasthenia gravis, the main problem is levator weakness leading to progressive

Table 6.2 **Differential diagnosis of blepharospasm**

Diagnosis	Discriminating features
Dry eye syndrome	Dry eye syndrome may be associated with behavioral compensations such as excessive blinking or forced eye closures, but the motor features are typically under voluntary control
Inflammatory disorders of the eye	Irritation from keratitis or conjunctivitis may also be associated with blinking and forced eye closures that are under voluntary control, and they may be associated with visible signs of inflammation
Eye tics	Tics are often associated with a premonitory urge and voluntary suppressibility, and they may be combined with tics in other regions of the body
Eyelid myokymia	Subtle irregular contractions of the eyelids that do not typically provoke eyelid closure.
Hemi-facial spasm	Hemifacial spasm usually affects only one half the face, usually the first (upper) division of cranial nerve VII
Myasthenia gravis	Myasthenia gravis is associated with eyelid weakness and drooping; spasms are not common
Psychogenic facial movements	Suggestive findings include unilateral tonic unilateral eye closure, convergence spasms of the eyes, and sudden onset.
Ptosis	Ptosis refers to eyelid drooping due to muscle weakness or structural defects of the skin or connective tissues of the eyes; spasms are not common

drooping of the eyelid until it closes. A diagnosis of BSP is more likely if there are associated eye spasms. A diagnosis of myasthenia is more likely if there other symptoms of muscle weakness such as diplopia. While it may be possible to discriminate pretarsal BSP from myasthenia gravis on clinical grounds, diagnostic testing may be needed. Rarely, blepharospasm and myasthenia gravis may occur in the same case.[33,52,62] Eyelid myokymia, a subtle irregular and often asynchronous contraction of small muscles of the eyelid might be confused with BSP. However, eyelid myokymia does not typically provoke eyelid closure, and it is often limited to the lower preseptal region.

Psychogenic (functional) movements of the face are common,[34,55] and are perhaps the most difficult to discriminate from BSP. Psychogenic movements may closely resemble typical BSP or OMD. Features that favor a psychogenic diagnosis include tonic unilateral contraction of the lower face (often with ipsilateral jaw deviation), prominent involvement of the platysma, inconsistent facial movements, movement patterns that are suggestible, reduction in abnormal movements with distraction, abrupt onset of symptoms, and coexisting convergence eye spasms. Some of these characteristics are described in more detail in Chapter 25, "Psychogenic (Functional) Dystonia." Sensory tricks occur in about half of individuals with BSP and a third of individuals with hemifacial spasm, but they are uncommon in tics and psychogenic disorders.

OROMANDIBULAR DYSTONIA: CLINICAL FEATURES

Motor Features

The motor features of OMD are quite varied.[6,67,88,97] Involvement of the orbicularis oris and nearby muscles of the lower face produces tightening of the lips over the mouth, puckering or protrusion of the lips, grimacing or a taut smile, tremor-like movements, and other facial contortions (Figure 6.4C). Involvement of the jaw is often characterized according to the most prominent abnormality. Jaw closing dystonia appears as excessive clenching or inability to open the mouth and is caused by overactivity of the masseters, medial pterygoids, or temporalis muscles. Jaw opening dystonia appears as unwanted opening of the mouth or inability to close the mouth and is caused by overactivity of the lateral pterygoids, with occasional contributions from the anterior digastric muscles or platysma. Jaw deviation is produced by excessive activity of the lateral pterygoid contralateral to the direction of deviation (Figure 6.4D), and jaw retraction can be caused by overactivity of the temporalis muscles.

Excessive activity of the lingual muscles can produce unwanted protrusion of the tongue, retraction, or lateral movements.

OMD often combines various movements of the perioral muscles, jaw, and tongue (Figure 6.4E–F). Although quite varied among different individuals, abnormal movements tend to be relatively stereotyped within one individual. The movements may occur at rest, but they are often triggered by speaking or chewing. For example, chewing can trigger involuntary jaw opening with food falling out of the mouth, or the tongue may push food out of the mouth. Task-specific OMD can also be seen in musicians, such those who play a flute or trumpet. In these musicians, dystonia may involve the facial muscles, jaw, or tongue (see Chapter 10, "Musician's and Other Task-Specific Dystonias."

Non-Motor Features

Jaw involvement in OMD is often associated with pain in the affected muscles or in the temporomandibular joint (TMJ). Individuals with severe jaw dystonia may break teeth or bite their tongue. Lower facial and tongue involvement in OMD may be associated with sialorrhea. All regions may contribute to difficulty in speaking or eating. Like BSP, psychiatric features of depression and anxiety are common in OMD.

Differential Diagnosis

OMD in adults is often idiopathic, with several related conditions that must be considered (Table 6.3). Tardive syndromes due to dopamine receptor antagonists may cause OMD (see Chapter 19, "Dystonia Induced by Medications, Illicit Drugs, and Environmental Exposures"). Tardive dystonia often affects the lower face, jaw, and/or tongue.[86] Edentulous dyskinesias occur spontaneously in older individuals who have had their teeth removed. This disorder most closely resembles typical tardive dyskinesias with repetitive and stereotypical movements of the lips and tongue, but there is no history of exposure to relevant drugs.[60] Tics also may involve the lower face, jaw, or tongue. Hemi-masticatory spasm is analogous to hemifacial spasm, except that it is caused by irritation of the fifth cranial nerve.[79] It is characterized by sudden jerking of the jaw, sometimes combined with more tonic contractions. Trismus or "lockjaw" caused by tetanus may resemble jaw-closing OMD. Occasionally OMD may be confused with bulbar amyotrophic lateral sclerosis (motor neuron disease).

A number of diagnostic terms describe clinical syndromes with multiple potential etiologies. *Bruxism* refers to grinding of the teeth. Jaw dystonia may cause bruxism. However, unlike most other forms of dystonia that remit during sleep, most cases of bruxism occur during sleep so the relationship to dystonia is not clear.[26] Stuttering is another common disorder that may result from OMD.[59] However, stuttering has many causes, and dystonia is probably not the cause in most cases. OMD is often confused with the temporomandibular joint (TMJ) syndrome, a diagnosis that encompasses a number of different disorders associated with discomfort during jaw movement.[82] OMD may cause the TMJ syndrome,

Table 6.3 **Differential diagnosis of oromandibular dystonia**

Diagnosis	Discriminating features
Bruxism	Bruxism refers to grinding of the teeth while sleeping; OMD usually resolves during sleep
Edentulous dyskinesias	Repetitive and stereotyped movements of the lips and tongue that occur in elderly individuals who had their teeth removed; spasms are uncommon
Hemi-masticatory spasm	Analogous to hemifacial spasm, but caused by cranial nerve V and associated with sudden jaw movements
Mouth tics	Tics are often associated with a premonitory urge and voluntary suppressibility, and they may be combined with tics in other regions of the body
Psychogenic facial movements	Suggestive findings include unilateral tonic deviation of the lower face and/or jaw, prominent platysma involvement, and sudden onset.
Temporomandibular joint syndrome	An umbrella term that refers to pain during jaw movements, usually at the articulation point between the mandible and the cranium
Trismus	Forced and often prolonged jaw spasms due to tetanus

including frank dislocation of the joint, but not all causes of the TMJ syndrome result from dystonia. The TMJ syndrome may result instead from arthritis of the jaw joints, trauma, bruxism, autoimmune disorders, and others.

ETIOLOGY AND WORKUP

For the majority of adults with isolated BSP, a cause cannot usually be found despite extensive testing. A careful medication history is useful because isolated BSP can sometimes occur as a tardive syndrome following exposure to dopamine receptor antagonists.[86] BSP rarely may be linked with a genetic cause, or with focal lesions of the nervous system.[40,57] BSP may also be combined with other neurological or medical problems, most notably Parkinson disease and the related parkinsonian syndromes.[80] Eye spasms and excessive blinking may occur early in these diseases or later in response to treatment. Pretarsal BSP has also been reported in these conditions, particularly progressive supranuclear palsy. Because BSP in adults is usually idiopathic, it is not mandatory to conduct neuroimaging studies, routine bloodwork, or genetic testing. However, such studies are required in children because a cause is more likely to be found.

Similar to BSP, OMD in adults is usually idiopathic. A careful history of drug exposure is important to exclude tardive syndromes affecting the oromandibular regions. Focal lesions that cause OMD are rare, so routine brain imaging studies are not warranted in adults. Genetic causes are uncommon among older adults, but more common in children and young adults. Some genes appear to predispose to prominent OMD including those associated with neuroacanthocytosis (e.g., *VPS13A*), rapid-onset dystonia-parkinsonism (e.g., *ATP1A3*), neurodegeneration with brain iron accumulation (e.g., *PANK2*), pathogenic variants in *YY1*,[37] and others.[38]

TREATMENT

Botulinum Toxins

The treatment of first choice for the motor features of BSP is botulinum toxin (BoNT). Several different formulations of BoNT are available in different parts of the world, and results from many studies have been described in numerous prior reviews,[25,89] so only general principles are summarized here. In most cases, the BoNTs are very effective for reducing eye spasms and excessive blinking. Benefits typically emerge in 5–10 days, peak at 4–6 weeks, and begin to wane after 8–10 weeks.[61,73] Most cases show sustained improvements with repeated treatment over many years, although worsening symptoms or spread of dystonia beyond the upper face may require changes in dose patterns over time.[27,36,49,50,99,101] In experienced hands, side effects are uncommon. The most common side effects when treating BSP include ptosis, lagophthalmos, dry eye, epiphoria, and diplopia.

There are no widely accepted guidelines regarding dilution, doses, dosing interval, and injection locations. Many studies describe injection of a standard dose pattern around the eyes in all cases, with a fixed interval of 12 weeks. Standardized treatment algorithms have been proposed,[83] although there has been increasing recognition that dose patterns and intervals need to be customized for each individual based on the nature of the problems observed.[4,31,47,61,73]

The pattern of treatments around the eyes has received considerable attention. Individuals with squeezing spasms around the eyes may need more BoNT directed to the orbital portion of the orbicularis oculi muscles, whereas those with excessive blinking or fluttering of the eyelids may need more directed to the palpebral portions of the muscle (Figure 6.3). Several studies have compared pretarsal with preseptal injections, with the most common conclusion that pretarsal injections are more effective with fewer side effects.[12,66,83–85,96] Cases with prominent pretarsal BSP may need high doses in the pretarsal portion of the muscle and especially Riolan's muscle, while avoiding the upper portion of the orbital orbicularis oculi because affected individuals often contract the nearby frontalis as a behavioral compensation to open the eyes (Figures 6.3 and 6.4).[2,5,29,81]

Discomfort from dry eyes is common in BSP. These cases may benefit from treating the lower medial eyelid region, a strategy that reduces the effectiveness by which the lacrimal pump removes tear liquid from the eyes (Figure 6.3).[46] In these cases, it may also be useful to avoid treating the upper outer preseptal eyelid region to avoid impacting the lacrimal gland and the eyelid margin where the Meibomian oil glands reside and contribute to tear quality. Usually, treatment of some combination of the orbital and palpebral portions of the orbicularis oculi yields best outcomes.

OMD can also be treated with BoNT, although good responses are not as reliable as those obtained in BSP.[14,16,45,88,106] For involvement of the lower face, the orbicularis oris may be targeted. Low doses must be used to avoid sialorrhea, slurred speech, or undesirable cosmetic effects such as facial asymmetry or loss of smiling. When the jaw is involved, BoNT must be targeted to muscles most responsible for the dominant abnormal movement pattern.[107] BoNT can also be used for lingual dystonia,[106] but satisfactory results can be challenging because of the complex anatomy of tongue muscles and movement and the risk for side effects such as dysphagia and dysarthria.

Other Medical Treatments

Symptoms of dry eyes are common in BSP, and BoNT often makes these symptoms worse. As a result, treatments directed to dry eyes are also important. These include artificial tears or other lubricants that can be added to the eyes as needed. Photophobia can be addressed with tinted eyeglasses, especially those that have tinted FL-41 lenses.[11]

Oral medications may be used for the craniofacial dystonias, either alone or in combination with BoNT. Most reports are anecdotal, and there are no large-scale studies to guide selection of oral agents. Options include anticholinergics, baclofen, levodopa, methylphenidate, tizanidine, and zolpidem (see Chapter 28, "Symptom-Targeted Oral Medications for Dystonia"). Anticholinergics are often not well tolerated in older individuals, and they may exaggerate dry eye symptoms. One double-blind placebo-controlled trial with only three patients in each group suggested some value of cannabis oil, but larger studies are needed to verify any benefits.[72]

Surgical Treatments

For individuals with medically refractory craniofacial dystonia, there are several surgical options. Most of these procedures are offered by specialized centers and are not widely available. None has been subject to rigorous blinded clinical trials, but they may be helpful for cases who do not respond to BoNT.

Deep brain stimulation (DBS) can be effective for many types of dystonia, including the craniofacial dystonias (see Chapter 31, "Surgical Treatments for Dystonia"). There are no rigorous blinded trials of DBS for BSP or OMD, with most information coming from case reports and small series from specialized centers. These types of studies are known to be influenced by a publication bias favoring positive outcomes.[74] With these caveats in mind, a meta-analysis of 23 studies including a total of 115 cases with craniofacial dystonia suggested significant improvement on the Burke-Fahn-Marsden dystonia rating scale following DBS.[104] However, results vary considerably among cases, and DBS may worsen or trigger BSP in certain cases.[65,100]

Orbital myectomy may also be offered to individuals with BSP, especially those with pretarsal BSP that is more difficult to treat satisfactorily with BoNT.[75] This procedure involves partial or complete stripping of the muscles responsible for closing the eyes. Again, there are no rigorous blinded trials of this type of surgery, and most reports come from specialized centers. However, encouraging results have been published from many independent centers.[13,39,44,56]

The frontalis suspension or frontalis sling procedure was originally developed for the treatment of ptosis, but it has also been used in BSP. In this procedure, an artificial surgical connection is made subcutaneously between the frontalis muscle and the upper eyelid, making it possible for contraction of the frontalis to aid eye opening. Once again, there are no rigorous blinded trials for this procedure, but encouraging results have been reported from several centers.[24,44,54,102]

Differential section of the seventh cranial nerve was offered for BSP prior to availability of BoNT, and its use has since been described for cases refractory to BoNT.[32] Initial success rates of approximately 50% have been reported, although reoperation and permanent side effects are not uncommon. This procedure is now only rarely offered because other surgical options are preferable.

SYNOPSIS AND FUTURE PROSPECTS

Dystonia commonly affects cranial muscles in various combinations. The craniofacial dystonias are often misdiagnosed as other disorders, but they are important to recognize because good treatments are available. The treatment of choice for the motor features involves BoNT. Successful application of BoNT requires a careful clinical examination to assess the many different clinical manifestations that may occur and precise targeting of muscles responsible for these manifestations on a case-by-case basis.

Additional oral medications may be useful, too. Non-motor features such as dry eyes or psychiatric issues are common and may also require treatment. Affected individuals who have inadequate responses to more conservative therapies may proceed to surgical interventions such as DBS, orbital myectomy, frontalis suspension, or others. There are no studies comparing these surgical options, and recommendations for the type of surgical procedure are often driven by factors such as local expertise.

The pathogenesis of BSP and OMD remains largely unknown, and studies addressing the underlying causes and biology are an important need for future research efforts.[22] Whether or not there are subtypes of BSP with differing biologies also needs further attention.[19,20] Considering the time it takes to reach a diagnosis, studies addressing strategies to reduce the time to diagnosis would also be valuable. Of course, the development of additional therapies that do not require repeated injections in the eyelids or surgery would be very welcome, too.

REFERENCES

1. Abbruzzese G, Berardelli A, Girlanda P, Marchese R, Martino D, Morgante F, et al. Long-term assessment of the risk of spread in primary late-onset focal dystonia. J Neurol Neurosurg Psychiatry 2008;79:392–396.
2. Albanese A, Bentivoglio AR, Colosimo C, Galardi G, Maderna L, Tonali P. Pretarsal injections of botulinum toxin improve blepharospasm in previously unresponsive patients. J Neurol Neurosurg Psychiatry 1996;60:693–694.
3. Anderson RL, Patel BC, Holds JB, Jordan DR. Blepharospasm: Past, present, and future. Ophthalmic Plast Reconstr Surg 1998;14:305–317.
4. Aquino CC, Felicio AC, Castro PC, Oliveira RA, Silva SM, Borges V, Ferraz HB. Clinical features and treatment with botulinum toxin in blepharospasm: A 17-year experience. Arq Neuropsiquiatr 2012;70:662–666.
5. Aramideh M, Ongerboer de Visser BW, Brans JW, Koelman JH, Speelman JD. Pretarsal application of botulinum toxin for treatment of blepharospasm. J Neurol Neurosurg Psychiatry 1995;59:309–311.
6. Balal M, Demirkiran M. Oromandibular dystonia: Clinical and demographic data from eight-two patients. Tremor Other Hyperkinet Mov (N Y) 2023;13;3.
7. Bentivoglio AR, Bressman SB, Cassetta E, Carretta D, Tonali P, Albanese A. Analysis of blink rate patterns in normal subjects. Mov Disord 1997;12:1028–1034.
8. Bentivoglio AR, Daniele A, Albanese A, Tonali PA, Fasano A. Analysis of blink rate in patients with blepharospasm. Mov Disord 2006;21:1225–1229.
9. Berman BD, Groth CL, Sillau SH, Pirio Richardson S, Norris SA, Junker J, et al. Risk of spread in adult-onset isolated focal dystonia: A prospective international cohort study. J Neurol Neurosurg Psychiatry 2020;91:314–320.
10. Berman BD, Junker J, Shelton E, Sillau SH, Jinnah HA, Perlmutter JS, et al. Psychiatric associations of adult-onset focal dystonia phentypes. J Neurol Neurosurg Psychiat 2017;88:505–602.
11. Blackburn MK, Lamb RD, Digre KB, Smith AG, Warner JE, et al. FL-41 tint improves blink frequency, light sensitivity, and functional limitations in patients with benign essential blepharospasm. Ophthalmology 2009;116:997–1001.
12. Cakmur R, Ozturk V, Uzunel F, Donmez B, Idiman F. Comparison of preseptal and pretarsal injections of botulinum toxin in the treatment of blepharospasm and hemifacial spasm. J Neurol 2002;249:64–68.
13. Chapman KL, Bartley GB, Waller RR, Hodge DO. Follow-up of patients with essential blepharospasm who underwent eyelid protractor myectomy at the Mayo Clinic from 1980 through 1995. Ophthalmic Plast Reconstr Surg 1999;15:106–110.
14. Comella CL. Systematic review of botulinum toxin treatment for oromandibular dystonia. Toxicon 2018;147:96–99.
15. Conte A, Ferrazzano G, Defazio G, Fabbrini G, Hallett M, Berardelli A. Increased blinking may be a precursor of blepharospasm: A longitudinal study. Mov Disord Clin Pract 2017;4:733–736.
16. Dadgardoust PD, Rosales RL, Asuncion RM, Dressler D. Botulinum neurotoxin a therapy efficacy and safety for oromandibular dystonia: A meta-analysis. J Neural Transm (Vienna) 2019;126:141–148.
17. Defazio G, Albanese A, Pellicciari R, Scaglione CL, Esposito M, Morgante F, et al. Expert recommendations for diagnosing cervical, oromandibular, and limb dystonia. Neurol Sci 2019;40:89–95.
18. Defazio G, Belvisi D, Comella C, Hallett M, Jinnah HA, Cimino P, et al. Validation of a guideline to reduce variability in diagnosing cervical dystonia. J Neurol 2023;270:2606–2612.
19. Defazio G, Conte A, Gigante AF, Ferrazzano G, Pellicciari R, Dagostino S, Fabbrini G, Berardelli A. Clinical heterogeneity in patients with idiopathic blepharospasm: A cluster analysis. Parkinsonism Relat Disord 2017;40:64–68.
20. Defazio G, Gigante AF, Hallett M, Berardelli A, Perlmutter JS, Berman BD, et al. Motor and psychiatric features in idiopathic blepharospasm: A data-driven cluster analysis. Parkinsonism Relat Disord 2022;104:94–98.
21. Defazio G, Hallett M, Jinnah HA, Berardelli A. Development and validation of a clinical guideline for diagnosing blepharospasm. Neurology 2013;81:236–240.
22. Defazio G, Hallett M, Jinnah HA, Conte A, Berardelli A. Blepharospasm 40 years later. Mov Disord 2017;32:498–509.

23. Defazio G, Jinnah HA, Berardelli A, Perlmutter JS, Berkmen GK, Berman BD, et al. Diagnostic criteria for blepharospasm: A multicenter international study. Parkinsonism Relat Disord 2021;91:109–114.
24. Dressler D, Karapantzou C, Rohrbach S, Schneider S, Laskawi R. Frontalis suspension surgery to treat patients with blepharospasm and eyelid opening apraxia: Long-term results. J Neural Transm (Vienna) 2017;124:253–257.
25. Duarte GS, Rodrigues FB, Marques RE, Castelao M, Ferreira J, Sampaio C, et al. Botulinum toxin type A therapy for blepharospasm. Cochrane Database Syst Rev 2020;11:CD004900.
26. Ella B, Ghorayeb I, Burbaud P, Guehl D. Bruxism in movement disorders: A comprehensive review. J Prosthodont 2017;26:599–605.
27. Elston JS. Long-term results of treatment of idiopathic blepharospasm with botulinum toxin injections. Br J Ophthalmol 1987;71:664–668.
28. Elston JS. A new variant of blepharospasm. J Neurol Neurosurg Psychiatry 1992;55:369–371.
29. Esposito M, Fasano A, Crisci C, Dubbioso R, Iodice R, Santoro L. The combined treatment with orbital and pretarsal botulinum toxin injections in the management of poorly responsive blepharospasm. Neurol Sci 2013;35:397–400.
30. Fabbrini G, Defazio G, Colosimo C, Thompson PD, Berardelli A. Cranial movement disorders: Clinical features, pathophysiology, differential diagnosis and treatment. Nat Clin Pract Neurol 2009;5:93–105.
31. Fang XB, Xie MS, Song ZB, Zhong ZG, Wang Y, Ou ZL, et al. Long-term treatment of blepharospasm with botulinum toxin A: A service-based study over a 16-year follow-up in southern China. Neurol Sci 2020;41:645–652.
32. Fante RG, Frueh BR. Differential section of the seventh nerve as a tertiary procedure for the treatment of benign essential blepharospasm. Ophthalmic Plast Reconstr Surg 2001;17:276–280.
33. Fasano A, Bentivoglio AR, Ialongo T, Soleti F, Evoli A. Treatment with botulinum toxin in a patient with myasthenia gravis and cervical dystonia. Neurology 2005;64:2155–2156.
34. Fasano A, Valadas A, Bhatia KP, Prashanth LK, Lang AE, Munhoz RP, et al. Psychogenic facial movement disorders: Clinical features and associated conditions. Mov Disord 2012;27:1544–1551.
35. Felicio AC, Godeiro-Junior Cde O, Borges V, Silva SM, Ferraz HB. Bilateral hemifacial spasm: A series of 10 patients with literature review. Parkinsonism Relat Disord 2008;14:154–156.
36. Fernandez HH, Pagan F, Danisi F, Greeley D, Jankovic J, Verma A, et al. Prospective study evaluating incobotulinumtoxinA for cervical dystonia or blepharospasm: Interim results from the first 145 subjects with cervical dystonia. Tremor Other Hyperkinet Mov 2013;3:tre-03-139-2924-1.
37. Ferng A, Thulin P, Walsh E, Weissbrod PA, Friedman J. YY1: A new gene for childhood onset dystonia with prominent oromandibular-laryngeal involvement? Mov Disord 2022;37:227–228.
38. Fujioka S, Strongosky AJ, Hassan A, Rademakers R, Dickson DW, Wszolek ZK. Clinical presentation of a patient with SLC20A2 and THAP1 deletions: Differential diagnosis of oromandibular dystonia. Parkinsonism Relat Disord 2015;21:329–331.
39. Georgescu D, Vagefi MR, McMullan TF, McCann JD, Anderson RL. Upper eyelid myectomy in blepharospasm with associated apraxia of lid opening. Am J Ophthalmol 2008;145:541–547.
40. Girard B, Davoudi O, Tatry M, Tassart M. Secondary blepharospasm, analysis and pathophysiology of blepharospasm. J Fr Ophtalmol 2021;44:e1–e12.
41. Girard BC, Levy P. Dry eye syndrome in benign essential blepharospasm. J Fr Ophtalmol 2019;42:1062–1067.
42. Grandas F, Elston J, Quinn N, Marsden CD. Blepharospasm: A review of 264 patients. J Neurol Neurosurg Psychiatry 1988;51:767–772.
43. Grandas F, Traba A, Perez-Sanchez JR, Esteban A. Pretarsal blepharospasm: Clinical and electromyographic characteristics. Clin Neurophysiol 2020;131:1678–1685.
44. Grivet D, Robert PY, Thuret G, De Feligonde OP, Gain P, Maugery J, Adenis JP. Assessment of blepharospasm surgery using an improved disability scale: Study of 138 patients. Ophthal Plast Reconstr Surg 2005;21:230–234.
45. Hassell TJW, Charles D. Treatment of blepharospasm and oromandibular dystonia with botulinum toxins. Toxins (Basel) 2020;12:269.
46. Ho RW, Fang PC, Chang CH, Liu YP, Kuo MT. A review of periocular botulinum neurotoxin on the tear film homeostasis and the ocular surface change. Toxins (Basel) 2019;11:66.
47. Huang XF, Wang KY, Liang ZH, Du RR, Zhou LN. Clinical analysis of patients with primary blepharospasm: A report of 100 cases in China. Eur Neurol 2015;73:337–341.
48. Hwang WJ. Demographic and clinical features of patients with blepharospasm in southern Taiwan: A university hospital-based study. Acta Neurol Taiwan 2012;21:108–114.
49. Jankovic J, Comella C, Hanschmann A, Grafe S. Efficacy and safety of incobotulinumtoxinA (NT 201, Xeomin) in the treatment of blepharospasm-a randomized trial. Mov Disord 2011;26:1521–1528.
50. Jankovic J, Kenney C, Grafe S, Goertelmeyer R, Comes G. Relationship between various clinical outcome assessments in patients with blepharospasm. Mov Disord 2009;24:407–413.
51. Jankovic J, Orman J. Blepharospasm: Demographic and clinical survey of 250 patients. Ann Ophthalmol 1984;16:371–376.
52. Jankovic J, Patten BM. Blepharospasm and autoimmune disease. Mov Disord 1987;2:159–163.
53. Jog M, Chouinard S, Hobson D, Grimes D, Chen R, Bhogal M, Simonyi S. Causes for treatment delays in dystonia and hemifacial spasm: A Canadian survey. Can J Neurol Sci 2011;38:704–711.
54. Karapantzou C, Dressler D, Rohrbach S, Laskawi R. Frontalis suspension surgery to treat patients with essential blepharospasm and apraxia of eyelid opening-technique and results. Head Face Med 2014;10:44.
55. Kaski D, Bronstein AM, Edwards MJ, Stone J. Cranial functional (psychogenic) movement disorders. Lancet Neurol 2015;14:1196–1205.
56. Kent TL, Petris CK, Holds JB. Effect of upper eyelid myectomy on subsequent chemodenervation in the management of benign essential blepharospasm. Ophthalmic Plast Reconstr Surg 2015;31:222–226.
57. Khooshnoodi MA, Factor SA, Jinnah HA. Secondary blepharospasm associated with structural lesions of the brain. J Neurol Sci 2013;331:98–101.

58. Kilic-Berkmen G, Defazio G, Hallett M, Berardelli A, Ferrazzano G, Belvisi D, et al. Diagnosis and classification of blepharospasm: Recommendations based on empirical evidence. J Neurol Sci 2022;439:120319.
59. Kiziltan G, Akalin MA. Stuttering may be a type of action dystonia. Mov Disord 1996;11:278–282.
60. Kolle WC. Edentulous orodyskinesia. Ann Neurol 1983;13:97–99.
61. Kollewe K, Mohammadi B, Kohler S, Pickenbrock H, Dengler R, Dressler D. Blepharospasm: Long-term treatment with either Botox(R), Xeomin(R) or Dysport(R). J Neural Transm 2015;122:427–431.
62. Kurlan R, Jankovic J, Rubin A, Patten B, Griggs R, Shoulson I. Coexistent Meige's syndrome and myasthenia gravis. A relationship between blinking and extraocular muscle fatigue? Arch Neurol 1987;44:1057–1060.
63. LeDoux MS. Meige syndrome: What's in a name? Parkinsonism Relat Disord 2009;15:483–489.
64. Lee JM, Baek JS, Choi HS, Kim SJ, Jang JW. Clinical features of benign essential blepharospasm in Korean patients. Korean J Ophthalmol 2018;32:339–343.
65. Limotai N, Go C, Oyama G, Hwynn N, Zesiewicz T, Foote K, et al. Mixed results for GPi-DBS in the treatment of cranio-facial and cranio-cervical dystonia symptoms. J Neurol 2011;258:2069–2074.
66. Lolekha P, Choolam A, Kulkantrakorn K. A comparative crossover study on the treatment of hemifacial spasm and blepharospasm: Preseptal and pretarsal botulinum toxin injection techniques. Neurol Sci 2017;38:2031–2036.
67. Ma H, Qu J, Ye L, Shu Y, Qu Q. Blepharospasm, oromandibular dystonia, and Meige syndrome: Clinical and genetic update. Front Neurol 2021;12:630221.
68. Macerollo A, Superbo M, Gigante AF, Livrea P, Defazio G. Diagnostic delay in adult-onset dystonia: Data from an Italian movement disorder center. J Clin Neurosci 2015;22:608–610.
69. Martino D, Berardelli A, Abbruzzese G, Bentivoglio AR, Esposito M, Fabbrini G, et al. Age at onset and symptom spread in primary adult-onset blepharospasm and cervical dystonia. Mov Disord 2012;27:1447–1450.
70. Mauriello JA, Jr., Dhillon S, Leone T, Pakeman B, Mostafavi R, Yepez MC. Treatment selections of 239 patients with blepharospasm and Meige syndrome over 11 years. Br J Ophthalmol 1996;80:1073–1076.
71. Medina A, Nilles C, Martino D, Pelletier C, Pringsheim T. The prevalence of idiopathic or inherited isolated dystonia: A systematic review and meta-analysis. Mov Disord Clin Pract 2022;9:860–868.
72. Millman N, van der Woerd B, Sund LT, Johns M. Cannabinoid use in the treatment of laryngeal dystonia and vocal tremor: A pilot investigation. J Voice 2023;in press.
73. Mitsikostas DD, Dekundy A, Hanschmann A, Althaus M, Scheschonka A, Pagan F, Jankovic J. Duration and onset of effect of incobotulinumtoxinA for the treatment of blepharospasm in botulinum toxin-naive subjects. Curr Med Res Opin 2021;37:1761–1768.
74. Nissen T, Wynn R. The clinical case report: A review of its merits and limitations. BMC Res Notes 2014;7:264.
75. Pariseau B, Worley MW, Anderson RL. Myectomy for blepharospasm 2013. Curr Opin Ophthalmol 2013;24:488–493.
76. Patel N, Jankovic J, Hallett M. Sensory aspects of movement disorders. Lancet Neurol 2014;13:100–112.
77. Peckham EL, Lopez G, Shamim EA, Richardson SP, Sanku S, Malkani R, et al. Clinical features of patients with blepharospasm: A report of 240 patients. Eur J Neurol 2011;18:382–386.
78. Powell AT, Bidewell JW, Walker AC. Diagnosing idiopathic dystonia: Must it take so long? Aust Health Rev 1995;18:120–131.
79. Radhakrishnan DM, Goyal V, Shukla G, Singh MB, Ramam M. Hemi masticatory spasm: Series of 7 cases and review of literature. Mov Disord Clin Pract 2019;6:316–319.
80. Rana AQ, Kabir A, Dogu O, Patel A, Khondker S. Prevalence of blepharospasm and apraxia of eyelid opening in patients with parkinsonism, cervical dystonia and essential tremor. Eur Neurol 2012;68:318–321.
81. Rana AQ, Shah R. Combination of blepharospasm and apraxia of eyelid opening: A condition resistant to treatment. Acta Neurol Belg 2012;112:95–96.
82. Raudino F. Is temporomandibular dysfunction a cranial dystonia? An electrophysiological study. Headache 1994;34:471–475.
83. Rayess YA, Awaida CJ, Jabbour SF, Ballan AS, Sleilati FH, Abou Zeid SM, Nasr MW. Botulinum toxin for benign essential blepharospasm: A systematic review and an algorithmic approach. Rev Neurol 2021;177:107–114.
84. Sacramento DRC, Lima A, Maia DP, Cunningham M, Maciel RH, Camargos ST, Cardoso F. Comparison of techniques of botulinum toxin injections for blepharospasm and hemifacial spasm. Mov Disord 2019;34:1401–1403.
85. Sanguandikul L, Apinyawasisuk S, Jariyakosol S, Hirunwiwatkul P, Chongpison Y. Complications of preseptal versus pretarsal botulinum roxin injection in eenign essential blepharospasm: A randomized controlled trial. Am J Ophthalmol 2021;232:9–16.
86. Savitt D, Jankovic J. Tardive syndromes. J Neurol Sci 2018;389:35–42.
87. Scorr L, Cho HJ, Kilic-Berkmen G, McKay JL, Hallett M, Klein C, et al. Clinical features and evolution of blepharospasm: A multicenter international cohort and systematic literature review. Dystonia 2022;1:10359.
88. Scorr LM, Factor SA, Perez-Parra S, Kaye R, Paniello RC, Norris SA, et al. Oromandibular dystonia: A clinical examination of 2,020 cases. Front Neurol 2021;12:700714.
89. Simpson DM, Hallett M, Ashman EJ, Comella CL, Green MW, Gronseth GS, et al. Practice guideline update summary: Botulinum neurotoxin for the treatment of blepharospasm, cervical dystonia, adult spasticity, and headache: Report of the Guideline Development Subcommittee of the American Academy of Neurology. Neurology 2016;86:1818–1826.
90. Slaim L, Cohen M, Klap P, Vidailhet M, Perrin A, Brasnu D, et al. Oromandibular dystonia: Demographics and clinical data from 240 patients. J Mov Disord 2018;11:78–81.
91. Steeves TD, Day L, Dykeman J, Jette N, Pringsheim T. The prevalence of primary dystonia: A systematic review and meta-analysis. Mov Disord 2012;27:1789–1796.
92. Sun Y, Tsai PJ, Chu CL, Huang WC, Bee YS. Epidemiology of benign essential blepharospasm: A nationwide population-based retrospective study in Taiwan. PLoS One 2018;13:e0209558.
93. Svetel M, Pekmezovic T, Jovic J, Ivanovic N, Dragasevic N, Maric J, Kostic VS. Spread of primary

dystonia in relation to initially affected region. J Neurol 2007;254:879–883.
94. Svetel M, Pekmezovic T, Tomic A, Kresojevic N, Kostic VS. The spread of primary late-onset focal dystonia in a long-term follow up study. Clin Neurol Neurosurg 2015;132:41–43.
95. Tawfik HA, Dutton JJ. Debunking the puzzle of eyelid apraxia: The muscle of Riolan hypothesis. Ophthalmic Plast Reconstr Surg 2023;39:211–220.
96. Teekaput C, Teekaput K, Thiankhaw K. Preseptal and pretarsal botulinum toxin injection in hemifacial spasm and blepharospasm: A 10-year comparative study. Ther Clin Risk Manag 2023;19:35–42.
97. Termsarasab P, Tanenbaum DR, Frucht SJ. The phenomenology and natural history of idiopathic lower cranial dystonia. J Clin Mov Disord 2014;1:3.
98. Tolosa ES, Klawans HL. Meiges disease: A clinical form of facial convulsion, bilateral and medial. Arch Neurol 1979;36:635–637.
99. Truong DD, Gollomp SM, Jankovic J, LeWitt PA, Marx M, Hanschmann A, et al. Sustained efficacy and safety of repeated incobotulinumtoxinA (Xeomin((R))) injections in blepharospasm. J Neural Transm (Vienna) 2013;120:1345–1353.
100. Vagefi MR, Lin CC, McCann JD, Anderson RL. Exacerbation of blepharospasm associated with craniocervical dystonia after placement of bilateral globus pallidus internus deep brain stimulator. Mov Disord 2008;23:454–456.
101. Vivancos-Matellano F, Rodriguez-Sanz A, Herrero-Infante Y, Mascias-Cadavid J. Efficacy and safety of long-term therapy with type A Botulinum toxin in patients with blepharospasm. Neuroophthalmology 2019;43:277–283.
102. Wabbels B, Roggenkamper P. Long-term follow-up of patients with frontalis sling operation in the treatment of essential blepharospasm unresponsive to botulinum toxin therapy. Graefes Arch Clin Exp Ophthalmol 2007;245:45–50.
103. Wakakura M, Yamagami A, Iwasa M. Blepharospasm in Japan: A clinical observational study from a large referral hospital in Tokyo. Neuroophthalmology 2018;42:275–283.
104. Wang X, Zhang Z, Mao Z, Yu X. Deep brain stimulation for Meige syndrome: A meta-analysis with individual patient data. J Neurol 2019;266:2646–2656.
105. Weiss EM, Hershey T, Karimi M, Racette B, Tabbal SD, Mink JW, Paniello RC, Perlmutter JS. Relative risk of spread of symptoms among the focal onset primary dystonias. Mov Disord 2006;21:1175–1181.
106. Yoshida K. Botulinum neurotoxin therapy for lingual dystonia using an individualized injection method based on clinical features. Toxins (Basel) 2019;11:51.
107. Yu GLT, Rosales RL. Treatment of oromandibular dystonia using botulinum toxin: Case series and illustrative muscle targeting. Basal Ganglia 2018;13:7–16.

Chapter 7

Laryngeal Dystonias

INTRODUCTION

Dystonia may affect the muscles of the larynx, resulting in abnormalities of vocalization or breathing. Laryngeal dystonia (LD) is traditionally divided into two subgroups, adductor spasmodic dysphonia (AdSD) and abductor spasmodic dysphonia (AbSD), although both may occasionally occur together. LD involves only a few very small muscles, but there is an enormous impact on quality of life because it affects the ability to communicate with others.[44]

In addition to these classic presentations, there are several related conditions. Rarely, LD may occur only when singing or breathing rather than speaking. Other conditions include dystonia of nearby pharyngeal or respiratory muscles, vocal tremor (VT), and muscular tension dysphonia (MTD). These other conditions may occur in isolation, or they may coexist with LD.

The prevalence of laryngeal dystonia (LD) ranges between 7 and 70 cases per million (see Chapter 4, "Epidemiology of Dystonia").[39] In most epidemiological studies, LD is less common than cervical dystonia or blepharospasm. However, its manifestations and subtypes are poorly recognized, with long delays between symptom onset and diagnosis,[18,24,39,74,88] so it may be more common than epidemiological studies indicate. LD typically emerges in adults between 40 and 60 years of age (Figure 7.1), although children are rarely affected as well. In virtually all studies, female individuals outnumber male individuals (Figure 7.2).

The nomenclature of this group of disorders has evolved over the years. It was first described in 1871 by Traube as *spastic dysphonia*.[95] Other terms were occasionally used as well. Recognizing that spasticity was not the underlying problem, Aronson and colleagues recommended the name *spasmodic dysphonia* in 1968.[4] Once the relationship of these disorders with other focal dystonias was recognized in the early 1980s, the term *laryngeal dystonia*

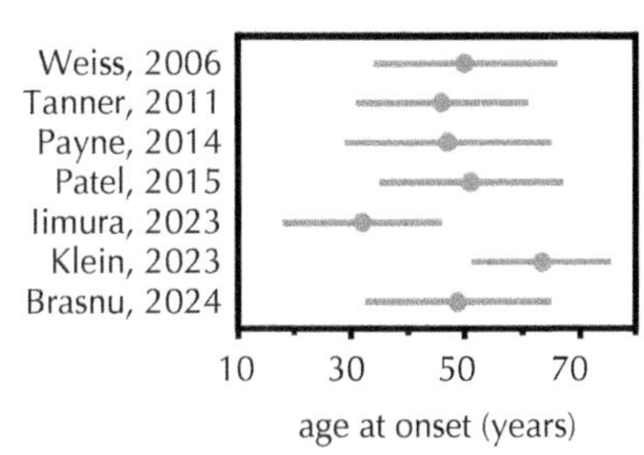

Figure 7.1. Age at onset for laryngeal dystonia. This figure shows the average (±SD) age at onset for studies in the literature that included more than 100 cases of laryngeal dystonia. When the same center had multiple reports over the years, only the largest series was included.

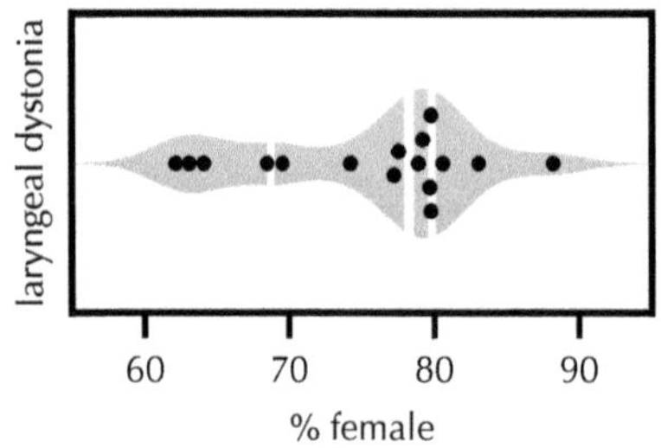

Figure 7.2. Sex distribution in laryngeal dystonia. This violin plot shows the distribution of female and male individuals for studies in the literature that included more than 100 cases of laryngeal dystonia. When the same center had multiple reports over the years, only the largest series was included.

was introduced. Although the term *spasmodic dysphonia* is still widely used, the term *laryngeal dystonia* is a more inclusive and accurate label.

CHARACTERISTIC PHENOTYPES

Adductor Spasmodic Dysphonia

AdSD is the most common form of LD, accounting for 80–90% of all cases (Table 7.1). It is characterized by a strained and strangled voice that is very effortful (Table 7.2). It is a task-specific dystonia, emerging predominantly during articulation of normal speech.[56] It is absent or less prominent when making other types of sounds such as singing, yelling, crying, laughing, or whispering.[36] Sometimes individuals find they can speak better when they change the task such as use a higher pitch, speak in a false accent, or even speak in a different language.

The characteristic feature is intermittent breaks in the voice, expressed as sudden brief hesitations in vocalization. Voice breaks in AdSD are most prominent with voiced vowels. When a vowel occurs at the start of a word (e.g., *eat*), there is strain to get the word started (*e-e—eeat*). When a vowel occurs in the middle of a word (e.g., *lawn*), the word comes out broken (*la—aawn*). When a vowel occurs at the end of word (e.g., *heavily*), the word is cut off at the end (*heavilll—*).

The adductor subtype of LD is caused by excessive activity of muscles responsible for adducting the vocal cords, most notably the thyroarytenoid.[48] The strained-strangled quality with voice breaks is caused by persistent adduction of the vocal cords restricting the exit of air. The voice breaks are caused by superimposed spasms that transiently block airflow.

Abductor Spasmodic Dysphonia

The abductor subtype of LD (AbSD) is less common than AdSD, accounting for 5–10% of all LD (Table 7.1). It is characterized by an airy or hoarse voice that is very effortful, often with voice breaks (Table 7.2). Like AdSD, AbSD is task-specific, occurring mostly during normal speaking, and less common with other types of vocalizations. Unlike AdSD, voice breaks in AbSD are most prominent with voiceless consonants (p, t, k, h, s, f) before vowels. Usually, the voice cuts out just after the start of the voiceless constant, so *funny* becomes *f—uunny*.

The abductor subtype of LD is caused by excessive activity of muscles responsible for abducting the vocal cords, most notably the posterior cricoarytenoid.[48] The airy and hoarse quality with voice breaks results from persistent of abduction of the vocal cords required during vocalization.

Vocal Tremor

Vocal tremor is characterized by rhythmical oscillations of voice strength, with a frequency of 6–8 Hz.[73,86,94,105] The tremor is best elicited with prolonged vocalization of vowels such as "E" and "A" to permit recognition of rhythmicity (Table 7.2). Oscillations in VT can be difficult to discriminate from LD because they may be somewhat irregular or they may be sufficiently prominent that they produce voice breaks resembling LD. Vocal tremor may occur in isolation, or it may be combined with LD or with tremor of another body region, most often the upper limbs.

Whether isolated VT should be considered an unusual manifestation of essential tremor or a manifestation of dystonia is not clear (see Chapter 12, "Dystonia and Tremor").[6] The tremor is caused by rhythmical oscillations of many laryngeal muscles,[48] and often additional muscles outside of the larynx.

Muscular Tension Dysphonia

The concept of MTD was introduced to describe a voice disorder distinct from LD or VT. It is thought to be primarily behavioral.[67] This voice

Table 7.1 **Large descriptive studies of laryngeal dystonia (LD)**

Study	Country	Cases	Female (%)	Age at onset	AdLD (%)	AbLD (%)	AdLD+ AbLD (%)	VT (%)	Extra-laryngeal symptoms
Izdebski, 1984[42]	USA	200	69.5	43	NR	NR	NR	NR	
Schweinfurth, 2002[83]	USA	168	79.8	NR	NR	NR	NR	NR	Tremor 26% Dystonia 11%
Tish, 2003[91]	Australia	169	62.1	51±NR	89.4	1.8	4.7	32.0	Tremor 7.7% Dystonia 13%
Klotz, 2004[48]	USA	214	74.3	NR	61.7	7.4	9.8	21.0	
Weiss, 2006[102]	USA	117	NR	50±16	81.1	11.1	7.7	NR	Dystonia 9%
Tanner, 2011[88]	USA	150	64.0	46±15	96.7	1.3	2.0	27.3	
White, 2011[104]	USA	128	78.9	NR	95.3	3.9	NR	25.8	
Patel, 2015[72]	USA	718	77.6	51±16	91.8	8.2	NR	52.6	Dystonia 5.7%
Payne, 2014[74]	Australia	193	68.4	47±18	86.0	4.7	2.1	NR	
Blitzer, 2018[9,10,11]	USA	1400	63.0	NR	82.0	17.0	0.4	25.0	Dystonia 5.3%
Guiry, 2019[36]	USA	178	79.8	NR	56.7	43.3	NR	29.8	
Valenzuela, 2019[98]	Canada	101	79.2	NR	98.0	2.0	1.0	NR	
Hyodo, 2021[39]	Japan	1534	80.6	31±NR	93.2	5.7	1.0	NR	
Lagos-Villaseca, 2023[50]	USA	255	88.2	NR	78.0	4.3	2.4	5.1	
Iimura, 2023[41]	Japan	834	83.1	32±14.7	96.2	2.8	1.1	NR	
Dupuch, 2023[24]	France	516	77.3	48.8±16.2	61.0	26.4	2.3	13.2	Dystonia 9.1%
Ghanouni, 2023[33]	USA	143	79.7	49.4±12.1	NR	NR	NR	39.9	Dystonia 22.3%

This table summarizes studies of laryngeal dystonia that included more than 100 research participants and provided clinical information regarding at least 2 of 3 variables (sex, age at onset, type of LD).

Abbreviations: AbSD, abductor spasmodic dysphonia; AdSD, adductor spasmodic dysphonia; NR, not reported; VT, vocal tremor (in some reports combined with spasmodic dysphonia).

Table 7.2 **Comparison of voice disorders**

Feature	AdSD	AbSD	VT	MTD
Voice quality	Strained, strangled, tight	Airy, hoarse	Rhythmic change in voice pitch or strength	Constant strain and tightness
Voice breaks	Common	Common	Occasional	Uncommon
Most apparent condition	Voiced vowels	Voiceless consonants before vowels	Sustained vowels	All aspects of voicing
Underlying cause	Excessive vocal cord adduction	Excessive vocal cord abduction	Oscillation of laryngeal and pharyngeal muscles	Tensing of many laryngeal and pharyngeal muscles
Main muscles involved	Thyroarytenoid	Posterior cricoarytenoid	Laryngeal, pharyngeal, sometimes tongue and others	Laryngeal, pharyngeal
Treatment	BoNT to thyroarytenoids	BoNT to posterior cricoarytenoid	BoNT to multiple muscles or anti-tremor medications	Voice therapy

Abbreviations: AbSD, abductor spasmodic dysphonia; AdSD, adductor spasmodic dysphonia; BoNT, botulinum toxin; MTD, muscular tension dysphonia; VT, vocal tremor.

disorder sometimes emerges after a period of excessive shouting or loud singing and may reflect an unconscious behavioral adaptation to vocal cord strain or injury, laryngeal pain, or vocal weakness.[2,21] Unlike LD, where vocal problems are task-specific, MTD is characterized by a more constant strain or hoarseness of the voice across many types of vocalizations (Table 7.2).[57,80] Voice breaks are uncommon in MTD. It may occur in isolation, but it may also occur in association with LD or VT. When it occurs with LD or VT, MTD may again reflect behavioral compensation for impaired vocalization.

Mixed Phenotypes

Although the voice disorders outlined above are often described as distinct entities, mixed phenotypes are common. LD is combined with VT in 21–52% of cases, especially AdSD but less commonly AbSD as well (Table 7.1). The syndrome of LD with VT is sometimes called *dystonic tremor* of the voice,[75] although most experts consider this to be a combination of two different movements. LD is frequently combined with MTD, too. The frequency of combined LD and MTD is unclear because of differences in the criteria used by experts for defining and discriminating these disorders.[57]

Even AdSD and AbSD may be combined in 1–5% of individuals (Table 7.1). There are reports of patients who have voice characteristics of AdSD and AbSD simultaneously, and others who had adductor or abductor SD and later evolved into the other. Some have suggested that all individuals with LD have both adductor and abductor muscle overactivity, and the net voice outcome reflects the predominance of one subtype.[14] In fact, detailed laryngeal muscle electromyography (EMG) studies have confirmed widespread laryngeal muscle involvement in both subtypes of LD and in VT, with more involvement of specific muscles in specific subtypes (Table 7.3).[48]

The term *whispering dysphonia* refers to speaking in a whisper with a very airy voice. It may reflect AbSD with full vocal cord abduction. Alternatively, it may reflect a combination of LD with behavioral compensation to avoid spasms.

Related Phenotypes

There are a number of less common phenotypes related to LD. Symptoms of LD are worse with normal speaking and may disappear with singing. In rare cases, LD may be triggered by singing rather than speaking.[16] Some individuals with singing-specific LD later progress to LD with other vocal tasks.

Dystonia may affect both laryngeal and pharyngeal muscles, or rarely may affect the pharyngeal muscles in isolation. Pharyngeal dystonia is described by a nasal or strained voice, sometimes with voice breaks resembling LD.[1,46,69,71,84] The nasal voice and dysphagia in pharyngeal dystonia are often mistaken for pharyngeal muscle weakness such as that which may occur in myasthenia gravis or motor neuron disease. Different pharyngeal muscles may be involved, alone or in various combinations. Pharyngeal dystonia is often associated with dysphagia.

Table 7.3 **Muscles affected in laryngeal dystonia**

	AdSD (n = 100)		AbSD (n = 16)		Mixed (n = 21)		VT (n = 77)	
Muscle	**Number**	**%**	**Number**	**%**	**Number**	**%**	**Number**	**%**
Thyroarytenoid	68/92	74	2/13	15	13/18	72	42/73	58
Lateral cricoarytenoid	30/68	44	0/4	0	2/5	40	32/60	53
Interarytenoid	16/49	33	NT	NT	0/2	0	6/42	14
Posterior cricoarytenoid	NT	NT	12/14	86	6/18	33	NT	NT

This table was adapted from a comprehensive electromyography study of 214 individuals with various types of LD or VT.[14] Columns indicating "number" reflect the number of cases tested among the total number of cases. All muscles were not tested in every case.

Abbreviations: AbSD, abductor spasmodic dysphonia, AdSD, adductor spasmodic dysphonia; VT, vocal tremor (with or without SD).

Dystonia may also affect respiration by interrupting the normal coordination between the diaphragm and the larynx. During normal breathing, laryngeal muscles usually open the vocal cords to allow passage of air. Active closure of the vocal cords (or failure to open them) disrupts the passage of air during inspiration or expiration. This phenomenon has been given many labels in the literature including *respiratory dystonia*, *breathing dystonia*, *laryngeal breathing dystonia*, *laryngeal dyspnea*, *respiratory dyskinesia*, and others.

This phenomenon may occur in isolation but more commonly occurs in combination with dystonia affecting another region of the body.[34,59,74,90,91,108] Affected individuals may have inspiratory or expiratory stridor and irregular breathing, and they may develop anxiety related to the sensation of air hunger. This problem is often mistaken for vocal cord weakness, structural restriction of airflow due to asthma or bronchitis, or hysteria. Breathing dystonia also accounts for stridor in some cases of multiple system atrophy.[49,63,92] It may also occur as a tardive syndrome following neuroleptic exposure.[82] In these cases, difficulties with breathing can develop suddenly, leading to emergency intubation and tracheostomy. Although rare, breathing dystonia is important to recognize because withholding neuroleptics or use of botulinum toxins may avoid more invasive interventions such as tracheostomy.

Dystonia may also affect the diaphragm, either in isolation or in combination with dystonia in another region of the body. It, too, has been given many labels, most commonly *respiratory dyskinesia* or *diaphragmatic dystonia*. The clinical appearance is an irregular breathing tempo. Alternatively, regular breathing may be interrupted by short inspirations or expirations. It was particularly common following post-encephalitic parkinsonism in the 1920s,[70] but now is more commonly seen as a tardive syndrome following neuroleptic exposure or as a consequence of levodopa treatment in Parkinson disease.[82] It is often mistakenly diagnosed as cardiorespiratory disease, anxiety, or even hysteria.

Dystonia of the laryngeal and related muscles may also manifest as recurrent sniffing sounds, coughing, or paroxysmal coughing.[19,74] Such cases are often initially misdiagnosed with tics or a pulmonary problem such as asthma or irritable larynx.

ASSOCIATED FEATURES

Extra-Laryngeal Movement Disorders

Individuals with LD may have dystonia in other body regions, most notably the neck, shoulders, or upper limbs. The frequency of extra-laryngeal dystonia has been reported to range from 0% to 32% (Table 7.1).[7,15,27,72,73,83,91,102] Differences in the frequency of extra-laryngeal dystonia are likely due to several factors including how individuals were evaluated, whether assessments came otolaryngology or neurology clinics, referral biases to these clinics, whether assessments were based on examination or history, and other issues. Longitudinal studies assessing spread of dystonia have indicated that dystonia may begin in the larynx and spread elsewhere, or it may begin elsewhere and spread to the larynx.[7,10,24,27,33] The overall risk of spread for focal LD is 15–20% over 5 years.

Individuals with LD, with or without VT, often have tremor of other body regions, most notably the upper limbs (see Chapter 12). Once again, the frequency of extra-laryngeal tremor varies among different studies due to methodological differences.[33,83,91,104] Some studies have indicated that subclinical tremor may be detectable by EMG even when there is no audibly perceptible voice tremor.[48]

Non-Motor Features

Non-motor features, particularly anxiety and depression, are common among individuals with all types of dystonia. The impact of these problems should not be underestimated because they have a disproportionate effect on quality of life, even more so than the motor features (see Chapter 11, "Non-Motor Features of Dystonia").[44]

A meta-analysis of 34 independent studies of various types of dystonia revealed that a substantial proportion of individuals with all types of dystonias had an anxiety-related disorder such as generalized anxiety disorder, panic attacks, or social phobia.[60] In these studies, the frequency of any anxiety-related disorder in LD (26%) was similar to other focal dystonias, such as cervical dystonia (33%), craniofacial dystonia (25%), limb dystonia (32%), or mixed dystonias (40%). *Social phobia* refers to emotional discomfort that is provoked by interacting with others, such as speaking in public or speaking to strangers. It is therefore not surprising that many individuals with LD meet diagnostic criteria for social phobia.

Another meta-analysis of 54 studies revealed that a substantial proportion of individuals with all type of dystonias had a mood-related disorder such as major depression or dysthymia.[61] The overall frequencies of any mood disorder were 32% for cervical dystonia and 29% for craniofacial dystonia. There were no studies of LD large enough to be evaluated separately, so they were combined into a group of mixed dystonias, where the overall frequency of any mood disorder was 31%. These studies imply a high frequency of psychiatric disorders in LD, although one case-control study suggested that psychiatric disorders were no more common in 128 individuals compared with 146 individuals with other voice disorders.[103]

DIFFERENTIAL DIAGNOSIS AND WORKUP

The main route to diagnosis is clinical recognition of the characteristic vocal features and exclusion of potential mimics. Even experts in voice disorders do not always agree on key diagnostic features. The source of the disagreement is that perceiving the key voice abnormalities requires a high level of training and it is subjective. Furthermore, many of the key voice abnormalities overlap among the different conditions, and the borders between them are sometimes hard to define. However, some consensus-based approaches for diagnosis have been published for the more common problems such as AbSD and VT.[57,94]

Many individuals report a history of some triggering event, such as an upper respiratory illness, stress, or trauma.[15,20,42,83,89] However, recall bias makes establishing a true causal relationship between these events and dystonia unclear. A medication history is important because LD and its related conditions can occur as a tardive syndrome with use of dopamine receptor antagonists (see Chapter 19, "Dystonia Induced by Medications, Illicit Drugs, and Environmental Toxins").[82]

A careful otolaryngology evaluation including laryngoscopy is recommended to rule out structural abnormalities that might mimic LD, such as weakness of one or both vocal cords, vocal cord polyps or other mass lesions, or vocal fold tears. A neurological exam can be useful because some individuals may have dystonia outside the larynx.[7,15,27,72,73,83,91,102] Features suggestive of Parkinson disease or another parkinsonian condition should be sought because these individuals may have abnormalities of the voice such as hypophonia or stuttering, which could mimic LD.[58] Individuals with related parkinsonian conditions, most notably multiple system atrophy, often have a hoarse and airy voice that can resemble AbSD (see Chapter 13, "Dystonia and Parkinsonism").[49] Some individuals with multiple system atrophy or anti-IgLON5 antibodies develop prominent stridor, during both waking hours and sleep. This problem has been attributed to LD, but it may also result from weakness of laryngeal muscles.[51,92]

Beyond laryngoscopy, further laboratory workup in adults is not usually revealing and often not conducted. Brain imaging studies only rarely disclose a potential cause, so they are not always necessary. Bloodwork does not usually provide an explanation for LD. A family history of LD or a related condition such as dystonia or tremor is reported for 2–16% of cases.[10,72,74] However, discoverable genetic etiologies are uncommon in adult-onset LD.

An etiology is more likely to be found in early-onset cases of LD. In some early-onset cases, the severity of laryngeal spasms reaches a point where individuals become aphonic and/or anarthric.[32] In children, brain MRI and genetic testing are more useful. In most cases with a genetic etiology, LD is part of a broader spectrum of segmental or generalized dystonia. However, the same genes may occasionally be associated with isolated focal LD, or LD may be the initial manifestation before other problems develop. LD has most frequently been associated with *KMT2B*,[17] *THAP1*,[22,35,52,101,107] and *TUBB4A*.[5,55] *TUBB4A* has been linked with a characteristic *whispering dysphonia* which is not typical of idiopathic LD and may partly reflect a behavioral compensation for laryngeal spasms.[5,55] LD has also been described less commonly for a number of other genes including *ANO3*,[85] *GCH1*,[96] *GNAL*,[23,76] *KCTD17*,[93] *TOR1A*,[106] and *YY1*.[30]

LD along with other manifestations of dystonia has also been linked with genes more often associated with ataxia such as ataxia telangiectasia (*ATM*),[3] Friedreich ataxia (*FXN*),[79] and spinocerebellar ataxia type 12 (*PPP2R2*). In fact, "ataxia" genes may sometimes cause a prominent dystonic phenotype instead.[25] The relationships between ataxia and dystonia are summarized further in Chapter 14, "Dystonia and Ataxia."[78]

TREATMENT

Botulinum Toxins

The treatment of LD and related voice disorders may include oral medications, botulinum toxin (BoNT), voice therapy, and/or surgery. BoNT is probably the most commonly used treatment (see Chapter 30, "Botulinum Toxin Treatment of Dystonia"). There are two small, randomized, double-blind, placebo-controlled trials of BoNT for LD. One of these controlled trials had 13 individuals (all AdSD),[97] and the other had 24 individuals (22 with AdSD and 2 with AbSD).[37,40] Despite the small size of these trials, both showed significant improvements in clinician-rated vocal measures, patient impressions of voice improvement, objective measures of voice quality, and quality of life.

In addition to these controlled trials, there are numerous unblinded studies, some of which included hundreds of individuals followed for many years. Systematic reviews of the most rigorous of these unblinded studies[47,100] and one large post-marketing surveillance study[41] revealed some common trends. The AdSD subtype responds most consistently to BoNT, with satisfactory results in more than 80% of individuals. There is a less consistent response to BoNT in AbSD and pure VT, with satisfactory results in less than 50%. For AdSD, doses range from 1 to 3 units per side, and some advocate unilateral injections, alternating the side with each treatment.[26,31,53] For AdSD, benefits of BoNT typically emerge in 2–10 days, peak at 4–10 weeks, and begin to wane after 6–16 weeks. Dose intervals range widely from 6 weeks to 6 months. A common side effect when treating AdSD is a period of breathiness or hoarseness of the voice with vocal weakness lasting a few days to a few weeks. Other less common side effects include dysphagia or local bleeding.

Most cases show sustained improvements with repeated treatment over many years. With long-term therapy, true functional resistance is rare; one large study estimated a frequency of true resistance at only 8/1,400 cases (0.6%).[65] Unlike other focal dystonias, where there is evidence for increased doses over time, longitudinal studies in LD have suggested the need for smaller doses with repeated treatments over time.[8,12,53,68,87] A systematic review and meta-analysis that included 474 individuals with LD spanning 17 articles revealed BoNT to produce very consistent improvements quality of life.[29]

Surgical Approaches

Numerous surgical approaches have been developed for LD, although they are offered only by a handful of specialized centers across the world. A systematic review of the most common procedures found no large, randomized, double-blinded, controlled trials.[100] There are many uncontrolled reports of positive outcomes, but negative outcomes are rarely reported, and those that report positive outcomes sometimes claim no adverse events (a finding that is unusual for a surgical procedure), or they do not address the outcomes of the sometimes high frequency of cases lost to follow-up (many of whom may have had poor outcomes). Despite these limitations, the positive outcomes reported from multiple centers in different parts of the world suggest they may be useful in expert hands. Some have argued that surgical approaches may be preferable to BoNT because surgery provides a sustainable effect and eliminates the need for repeated injections, associated swings in vocal function, and sometimes high costs and associated travel.[62]

The most common surgeries for LD include myectomy, denervation, and thyroplasty. AdSD is caused by excessive activity of vocal cord adductor muscles, so one approach involves myectomy or myoneurotomy targeting the thyroarytenoid muscles, the main vocal cord adductors. The goal is to destroy 50–80% of the muscle and weaken vocal fold adduction. Good long-term results have been reported from several centers using objective acoustic or aerodynamic measures of vocal function, clinician-rated measures of voice, patient-rated measures, and quality of life.[100] Side effects are common and include a weak voice or a breathy-husky voice, which may last for several months. There is also a smaller risk of aspiration.

A related approach to treating AdSD involves sectioning the adductor branch of the recurrent laryngeal nerve, leaving the posterior branch to the abductor muscles intact. The goal is to selectively weaken the adductors. To prevent the re-establishment of its original connections, the severed branch is connected to a branch of the ansa cervicalis. Once again, there are several reports of good long-term outcomes, with side effects similar to myectomy.[100] A very different approach to AdSD involves permanently widening the gap between the vocal cords to reduce the strength of vocal cord closure. This procedure is called *lateralization thyroplasty*, or *thyroplasty type 2*. Side effects include weak glottal closure in 10–15% of individuals.[100]

Deep brain stimulation is useful for many different types of dystonia (see Chapter 31, "Surgical Treatments for Dystonia"). One randomized, double-blind, controlled trial of six individuals with AdSD reported positive outcomes following stimulation of the ventral intermediate nucleus of the thalamus.[38] Positive outcomes with similar surgical strategies have also been reported for nine additional patients in unblinded reports.[28] Additional information regarding the potential value of this approach comes from case reports or series where LD is more often part of a broader pattern of dystonia that is segmental or generalized, such as genetic dystonias associated with *KMT2B*[17] or *TUBB4A*.[5] These studies often describe substantially less improvement in LD compared to dystonia of the neck or limbs, although the target in these cases is usually the internal segment of the globus pallidus. Whether the poorer responses of LD in these reports reflects differences in the target stimulated remains to be determined. Broader application of deep brain stimulation in LD has been limited by the sometimes unpredictable outcomes and observations that it can sometimes worsen the ability to communicate by causing dysarthria, hypophonia, or stuttering.[66,77]

Other Treatment Options

Oral medications have a relatively limited role in treating LD. None is entirely effective, and all have side effects.[43] The benzodiazepines can sometimes be helpful when stress and anxiety contribute to worsening symptoms. Propranolol and other beta-blockers may be at least partly helpful for VT.[45] Sodium oxybate has been suggested as well, but it is habit-forming and has numerous cognitive side effects, so it is not widely used.[81] Cannabinoids may be helpful, too, but rigorous studies assessing risk-benefit ratios are lacking.[64]

There also has been considerable attention to behavioral strategies to improve the voice in LD and related conditions,[54] and some centers advocate a combination of BoNT and voice therapy for all cases. Individuals with pure MTD do not need BoNT because good results can be achieved with voice therapy alone.[67]

SYNOPSIS AND FUTURE PROSPECTS

Dystonia may affect the muscles of the larynx as well as muscles in the pharynx or diaphragm. Dystonia in these regions can have several different manifestations that include a strained-strangled voice, an airy or hoarse voice, and vocal tremor. There may also be related problems that affect airflow such as dyspnea, respiratory irregularities, or recurrent coughing or sneezing.

The laryngeal dystonias and related conditions are often misdiagnosed, even among experts. Recent studies have suggested that diagnosis might be achieved by applying artificial intelligence to acoustic recordings,[13] or even certain characteristics from brain MRI.[99] Further development of these methods may ultimately provide valuable tools for diagnosis. Very little is known about the pathogenesis of these disorders, so further work is needed in this arena, too.

Despite the difficulties in diagnosis, recognition is important because treatments are available. The most commonly offered treatments include BoNT, voice therapy, and/or various surgical options. There are no studies comparing BoNT with surgery, and the ideal approach may depend on patient preferences and local expertise.

REFERENCES

1. Alappan N, Shyam Sundar A, Varghese ST. Neuroleptic induced laryngo-pharyngeal dystonia. J Neuropsychiatry Clin Neurosci 2008;20:241–242.
2. Altman KW, Atkinson C, Lazarus C. Current and emerging concepts in muscle tension dysphonia: A 30-month review. J Voice 2005;19:261–267.
3. Arican P, Dundar NO, Kirbiyik O, Cavusoglu D, Yilmaz SB, Gencpinar P. Variant ataxia-telangiectasia in a child presenting with laryngeal dystonia. Turk J Pediatr 2020;62:491–494.
4. Aronson AE, Brown JR, Litin EM, Pearson JS. Spastic dysphonia. II. Comparison with essential (voice) tremor and

other neurologic and psychogenic dysphonias. J Speech Hear Disord 1968;33:219–231.

5. Bally JF, Kern DS, Fearon C, Camargos S, Pereira da Silva-Junior F, Barbosa ER, et al. DYT-TUBB4A (DYT4 dystonia): Clinical anthology of 11 cases and systematized review. Mov Disord Clin Pract 2022;9:659–675.
6. Barkmeier-Kraemer JM. Isolated voice tremor: A clinical variant of essential tremor or a distinct clinical phenotype? Tremor Other Hyperkinet Mov (N Y) 2020;10. doi:10.7916/tohm.v0.738.
7. Berman BD, Groth CL, Sillau SH, Pirio Richardson S, Norris SA, Junker J, et al. Risk of spread in adult-onset isolated focal dystonia: A prospective international cohort study. J Neurol Neurosurg Psychiatry 2020;91:314–320.
8. Birkent H, Maronian N, Waugh P, Merati AL, Perkel D, Hillel AD. Dosage changes in patients with long-term botulinum toxin use for laryngeal dystonia. Otolaryngol Head Neck Surg 2009;140:43–47.
9. Blitzer A. Spasmodic dysphonia and botulinum toxin: Experience from the largest treatment series. Eur J Neurol 2010;17 Suppl 1:28–30.
10. Blitzer A, Brin MF, Simonyan K, Ozelius LJ, Frucht SJ. Phenomenology, genetics, and CNS network abnormalities in laryngeal dystonia: A 30-year experience. Laryngoscope 2018;128 Suppl 1:S1–S9.
11. Blitzer A, Brin MF, Stewart CF. Botulinum toxin management of spasmodic dysphonia (laryngeal dystonia): A 12-year experience in more than 900 patients. Laryngoscope 1998;108:1435–1441.
12. Bradley JP, Barrow EM, Hapner ER, Klein AM, Johns MM, 3rd. Botulinum toxin-A dosing trends for adductor spasmodic dysphonia at a single institution over 10 years. J Voice 2017;31:363–365.
13. Cala F, Frassineti L, Manfredi C, Dejonckere P, Messina F, Barbieri S, et al. Machine learning assessment of spasmodic dysphonia based on acoustical and perceptual parameters. Bioengineering 2023;10.
14. Cannito MP, Johnson JP. Spastic dysphonia: A continuum disorder. J Commun Disord 1981;14:215–233.
15. Childs L, Rickert S, Murry T, Blitzer A, Sulica L. Patient perceptions of factors leading to spasmodic dysphonia: A combined clinical experience of 350 patients. Laryngoscope 2011;121:2195–2198.
16. Chitkara A, Meyer T, Keidar A, Blitzer A. Singer's dystonia: First report of a variant of spasmodic dysphonia. Ann Otol Rhinol Laryngol 2006;115:89–92.
17. Cif L, Demailly D, Lin JP, Barwick KE, Sa M, Abela L, et al. KMT2B-related disorders: Expansion of the phenotypic spectrum and long-term efficacy of deep brain stimulation. Brain 2020;143:3242–3261.
18. Creighton FXJ, Hapner ER, Klein AM, Rosen A, Jinnah HA. Diagnostic delays in spasmodic dysphonia: A call for clinician education. J Voice 2015;29:592–594.
19. Crone NE, Jinnah HA, Reich SG. Wilson disease presenting with an unusual cough. Mov Disord 2005;20:891–893.
20. de Lima Xavier L, Simonyan K. The extrinsic risk and its association with neural alterations in spasmodic dysphonia. Parkinsonism Relat Disord 2019;65:117–123.
21. Desjardins M, Apfelbach C, Rubino M, Verdolini Abbott K. Integrative review and framework of suggested mechanisms in primary muscle tension dysphonia. J Speech Lang Hear Res 2022;65:1867–1893.
22. Djarmati A, Schneider SA, Lohmann K, Winkler S, Pawlack H, Hagenah J, et al. Mutations in THAP1 (DYT6) and generalised dystonia with prominent spasmodic dysphonia: A genetic screening study. Lancet Neurol 2009;8:447–452.
23. Dos Santos CO, Masuho I, da Silva-Junior FP, Barbosa ER, Silva SM, Borges V, et al. Screening of GNAL variants in Brazilian patients with isolated dystonia reveals a novel mutation with partial loss of function. J Neurol 2016;263:665–668.
24. Dupuch G, Mailly M, Guillaume J, Daval M, Ayache D, Brasnu D. Incidence and risk factors for secondary extralaryngeal dystonia in patients with laryngeal dystonia. Am J Otolaryngol 2023;45:104090.
25. Dzinovic I, Boesch S, Skorvanek M, Necpal J, Svantnerova J, Pavelekova P, et al. Genetic overlap between dystonia and other neurologic disorders: A study of 1,100 exomes. Parkinsonism Relat Disord 2022;102:1–6.
26. Elmiyeh B, Prasad VM, Upile T, Saunders N, Youl BD, Epstein R, Rubin JS. A single-centre retrospective review of unilateral and bilateral Dysport injections in adductor spasmodic dysphonia. Logoped Phoniatr Vocol 2010;35:39–44.
27. Esposito M, Fabbrini G, Ferrazzano G, Berardelli A, Peluso S, Cesari U, et al. Spread of dystonia in patients with idiopathic adult-onset laryngeal dystonia. Eur J Neurol 2018;25:1341–1344.
28. Evidente VGH, Ponce FA, Evidente MH, Lambert M, Garrett R, Sugumaran M, Lott DG. Adductor spasmodic dysphonia improves with bilateral thalamic deep brain stimulation: Report of 3 cases done asleep and review of literature. Tremor Other Hyperkinet Mov 2020;10:60.
29. Faham M, Ahmadi A, Silverman E, Harouni GG, Dabirmoghaddam P. Quality of life after botulinum toxin injection in patients with adductor spasmodic dysphonia; a systematic review and meta-analysis. J Voice 2021;35:271–283.
30. Ferng A, Thulin P, Walsh E, Weissbrod PA, Friedman J. YY1: A new gene for childhood onset dystonia with prominent oromandibular-laryngeal involvement? Mov Disord 2022;37:227–228.
31. French G, Bosch JD, Randall DR. Retrospective review of dosing trends in botulinum toxin injections for the treatment of adductor spasmodic dysphonia in a long-term cohort. J Otolaryngol Head Neck Surg 2020;49:4.
32. Ganos C, Crowe B, Stamelou M, Kresojevic N, Lukic MJ, Bras J, et al. The clinical syndrome of dystonia with anarthria/aphonia. Parkinsonism Relat Disord 2016;24:20–27.
33. Ghanouni A, Jona N, Jinnah HA, Kilic-Berkmen G, Shelly S, Klein AM. Demographics and clinical characteristics associated with the spread of new-onset laryngeal dystonia. Laryngoscope 2024;134:2295–2299.
34. Grillone GA, Blitzer A, Brin MF, Annino DJ, Saint-Hilaire MH. Treatment of adductor laryngeal breathing dystonia with botulinum toxin type A. Laryngoscope 1994;104:30–32.
35. Groen JL, Ritz K, Contarino MF, van de Warrenburg BP, Aramideh M, Foncke EM, et al. DYT6 dystonia: Mutation screening, phenotype, and response to deep brain stimulation. Mov Disord 2010;25:2420–2427.
36. Guiry S, Worthley A, Simonyan K. A separation of innate and learned vocal behaviors defines the symptomatology of spasmodic dysphonia. Laryngoscope 2019;129:1627–1633.
37. Hirose K, Asano K, Sakaguchi M, Nagao A, Nakahira M, Doi N, et al. Post-treatment clinical course following botulinum toxin injection therapy for adductor spasmodic dysphonia: Analysis of data from a placebo-controlled,

randomized, double-blinded clinical trial in Japan. Laryngoscope Investig Otolaryngol 2021;6:1088–1095.
38. Honey CR, Kruger MT, Almeida T, Rammage LA, Tamber MS, Morrison MD, et al. Thalamic deep brain stimulation for spasmodic dysphonia: A phase I prospective randomized double-blind crossover trial. Neurosurgery 2021;89:45–52.
39. Hyodo M, Hisa Y, Nishizawa N, Omori K, Shiromoto O, Yumoto E, et al. The prevalence and clinical features of spasmodic dysphonia: A review of epidemiological surveys conducted in Japan. Auris Nasus Larynx 2021;48:179–184.
40. Hyodo M, Nagao A, Asano K, Sakaguchi M, Mizoguchi K, Omori K, et al. Botulinum toxin injection into the intrinsic laryngeal muscles to treat spasmodic dysphonia: A multicenter, placebo-controlled, randomized, double-blinded, parallel-group comparison/open-label clinical trial. Eur J Neurol 2021;28:1548–1556.
41. Iimura S, Nose Y, Tabata K, Oda K, Yamashita Y, Takahashi N, Kawano Y. Safety and effectiveness of onabotulinumtoxinA in patients with laryngeal dystonia: Final report of a 52-week, multicenter postmarketing surveillance study. Toxins 2023;15:553.
42. Izdebski K, Dedo HH, Boles L. Spastic dysphonia: A patient profile of 200 cases. Am J Otolaryngol 1984;5:7–14.
43. Jinnah HA. Medical and surgical treatments for dystonia. Neurol Clin 2020;38:325–348.
44. Junker J, Berman BD, Hall J, Wahba D, Brandt V, Perlmutter JS, et al. Quality of life in dystonia: Non-motor manifestations matter. J Neurol Neurosurg Psychiat 2021;92:622–628.
45. Justicz N, Hapner ER, Josephs JS, Boone BC, Jinnah HA, Johns MM, 3rd. Comparative effectiveness of propranolol and botulinum for the treatment of essential voice tremor. Laryngoscope 2015;126:113–117.
46. Kahn L, Jordaan H. The swallowing and voicing characteristics of pharyngeal dystonia: A single case report. S Afr J Commun Disord 2001;48:21–31.
47. Khan HA. Use of botulinum toxin in spasmodic dysphonia: A review of recent studies. Cureus 2023;15:e33486.
48. Klotz DA, Maronian NC, Waugh PF, Shahinfar A, Robinson L, Hillel AD. Findings of multiple muscle involvement in a study of 214 patients with laryngeal dystonia using fine-wire electromyography. Ann Otol Rhinol Laryngol 2004;113:602–612.
49. Kollensperger M, Geser F, Seppi K, Stampfer-Kountchev M, Sawires M, Scherfler C, et al. Red flags for multiple system atrophy. Mov Disord 2008;23:1093–1099.
50. Lagos-Villaseca A, Bhatt NK, Abdolhosseini P, Quinonez L, Paoletti MF, Gochman G, et al. Assessment of patients receiving short-interval botulinum toxin chemodenervation treatment for laryngeal dystonia and essential tremor of the vocal tract. JAMA Otolaryngol Head Neck Surg 2023;149:615.
51. Lalich IJ, Ekbom DC, Starkman SJ, Orbelo DM, Morgenthaler TI. Vocal fold motion impairment in multiple system atrophy. Laryngoscope 2014;124:730–735.
52. LeDoux MS, Xiao J, Rudzinska M, Bastian RW, Wszolek ZK, Van Gerpen JA, et al. Genotype-phenotype correlations in THAP1 dystonia: Molecular foundations and description of new cases. Parkinsonism Relat Disord 2012;18:414–425.
53. Lee SJ, Kang MS, Choi HS, Lim JY. Alternating unilateral versus bilateral injections of botulinum toxin for the treatment of adductor spasmodic dysphonia. Otolaryngol Head Neck Surg 2021;164:815–820.
54. Lester-Smith RA, Miller CH, Cherney LR. Behavioral therapy for temor or dystonia affecting voice in speakers with hyperkinetic dysarthria: A systematic review. J Voice 2023;37:561–573.
55. Lohmann K, Wilcox RA, Winkler S, Ramirez A, Rakovic A, Park JS, et al. Whispering dysphonia (DYT4 dystonia) is caused by a mutation in the TUBB4 gene. Ann Neurol 2012;73:537–545.
56. Ludlow CL. Spasmodic dysphonia: A laryngeal control disorder specific to speech. J Neurosci 2011;31:793–797.
57. Ludlow CL, Domangue R, Sharma D, Jinnah HA, Perlmutter JS, Berke G, et al. Consensus-based attributes for identifying patients with spasmodic dysphonia and other voice disorders. JAMA Otolaryngol Head Neck Surg 2018;144:657–665.
58. Ma A, Lau KK, Thyagarajan D. Voice changes in Parkinson's disease: What are they telling us? J Clin Neurosci 2020;72:1–7.
59. Marion MH, Klap P, Perrin A, Cohen M. Stridor and focal laryngeal dystonia. Lancet 1992;339:457–458.
60. Medina Escobar A, Martino D, Goodarzi Z. The prevalence of anxiety in adult-onset isolated dystonia: A systematic review and meta-analysis. Eur J Neurol 2021;28:4238–4250.
61. Medina Escobar A, Pringsheim T, Goodarzi Z, Martino D. The prevalence of depression in adult onset idiopathic dystonia: Systematic review and metaanalysis. Neurosci Biobehav Rev 2021;125:221–230.
62. Mendelsohn AH, Berke GS. Surgery or botulinum toxin for adductor spasmodic dysphonia: A comparative study. Ann Otol Rhinol Laryngol 2012;121:231–238.
63. Merlo IM, Occhini A, Pacchetti C, Alfonsi E. Not paralysis, but dystonia causes stridor in multiple system atrophy. Neurology 2002;58:649–652.
64. Millman N, van der Woerd B, Sund LT, Johns M. Cannabinoid use in the treatment of laryngeal dystonia and vocal tremor: A pilot investigation. J Voice 2023;in press.
65. Mor N, Tang C, Blitzer A. Botulinum toxin in secondarily nonresponsive patients with spasmodic dysphonia. Otolaryngol Head Neck Surg 2016;155:458–461.
66. Moro E, LeReun C, Krauss JK, Albanese A, Lin JP, Walleser Autiero S, et al. Efficacy of pallidal stimulation in isolated dystonia: A systematic review and meta-analysis. Eur J Neurol 2017;24:552–560.
67. Morrison MD, Rammage LA, Belisle GM, Pullan CB, Nichol H. Muscular tension dysphonia. J Otolaryngol 1983;12:302–306.
68. Namin AW, Christopher KM, Eisenbeis JF. Botulinum toxin dosing trends in spasmodic dysphonia over a 20-year period. J Voice 2017;31:107–110.
69. Norby E, Orbelo D, Strand E, Duffy J, Ekbom D, Bower J, Matsumoto J. Hyoid muscle dystonia: A distinct focal dystonia syndrome. Parkinsonism Relat Disord 2015;21:1210–1213.
70. Parker HL. Epidemic encephalitis: Respiratory syndrome. Med Clin North Am 1930;13:1347–1362.
71. Patel A, Sulica L, Frucht S. Velopharyngeal dystonia: An unusual focal task-specific dystonia. Tremor Other Hyperkinetic Mov 2017;7:365. doi:10.7916/d8611961.
72. Patel AB, Bansberg SF, Adler CH, Lott DG, Crujido L. The Mayo Clinic Arizona spasmodic dysphonia experience: A demographic analysis of 718 patients. Ann Otol Rhinol Laryngol 2015;124:859–863.

73. Patel PN, Kabagambe EK, Starkweather JC, Keller M, Ahmed ZA, Gruber SC, et al. Defining differences in patient characteristics between spasmodic dysphonia and laryngeal tremor. Laryngoscope 2019;129:170–176.
74. Payne S, Tisch S, Cole I, Brake H, Rough J, Darveniza P. The clinical spectrum of laryngeal dystonia includes dystonic cough: Observations of a large series. Mov Disord 2014;29:729–735.
75. Pinto JV, Perez SS, Garcia-Lopez I. Laryngeal dystonia, dystonic tremor and vocal tremor: Three different entities. J Voice 2023. doi:10.1016/j.jvoice.2023.11.017.
76. Putzel GG, Fuchs T, Battistella G, Rubien-Thomas E, Frucht SJ, Blitzer A, et al. GNAL mutation in isolated laryngeal dystonia. Mov Disord 2016;31:750–755.
77. Rodrigues FB, Duarte GS, Prescott D, Ferreira J, Costa J. Deep brain stimulation for dystonia. Cochrane Database Syst Rev 2019;1:CD012405.
78. Rossi J, Cavallieri F, Giovannini G, Budriesi C, Gessani A, Carecchio M, et al. Spasmodic dysphonia as a presenting symptom of spinocerebellar ataxia type 12. Neurogenetics 2019;20:161–164.
79. Rota S, Marchina E, Todeschini A, Nanetti L, Rinaldi F. Very late onset Friedreich ataxia with laryngeal dystonia. Case Rep Neurol 2014;6:287–290.
80. Roy N, Gouse M, Mauszycki SC, Merrill RM, Smith ME. Task specificity in adductor spasmodic dysphonia versus muscle tension dysphonia. Laryngoscope 2005;115:311–316.
81. Rumbach AF, Blitzer A, Frucht SJ, Simonyan K. An open-label study of sodium oxybate in spasmodic dysphonia. Laryngoscope 2017;127:1402–1407.
82. Savitt D, Jankovic J. Tardive syndromes. J Neurol Sci 2018;389:35–42.
83. Schweinfurth JM, Billante M, Courey MS. Risk factors and demographics in patients with spasmodic dysphonia. Laryngoscope 2002;112:220–223.
84. Shi LL, Simpson CB, Hapner ER, Jinnah HA, Johns MM, 3rd. Pharyngeal dystonia mimicking spasmodic dysphonia. J Voice 2018;32:234–238.
85. Stamelou M, Charlesworth G, Cordivari C, Schneider SA, Kagi G, Sheerin UM, et al. The phenotypic spectrum of DYT24 due to ANO3 mutations. Mov Disord 2014;29:928–934.
86. Sulica L, Louis ED. Clinical characteristics of essential voice tremor: A study of 34 cases. Laryngoscope 2010;120:516–528.
87. Tang CG, Novakovic D, Mor N, Blitzer A. Onabotulinum toxin A dosage trends over time for adductor spasmodic dysphonia: A 15-year experience. Laryngoscope 2016;126:678–681.
88. Tanner K, Roy N, Merrill RM, Sauder C, Houtz DR, Smith ME. Spasmodic dysphonia: Onset, course, socioemotional effects, and treatment response. Ann Otol Rhinol Laryngol 2011;120:465–473.
89. Tanner K, Roy N, Merrill RM, Sauder C, Houtz DR, Smith ME. Case-control study of risk factors for spasmodic dysphonia: A comparison with other voice disorders. Laryngoscope 2012;122:1082–1092.
90. Tierney WS, Bryson PC, Nelson R, Kaplan SE, Benninger MS, Milstein CF. Respiratory laryngeal dystonia: Characterization and diagnosis of a rare neurogenic disorder. Laryngoscope 2020;130:2843–2846.
91. Tisch SH, Brake HM, Law M, cole IE, Darveniza P. Spasmodic dysphonia: Clinical features and effects of botulinum toxin therapy in 169 patients - an Australian experience. J Clin Neurosci 2003;10:434–438.
92. Todisco M, Alfonsi E, Isaias IU, Zangaglia R, Minafra B, Cosentino G, et al. Vocal cord electromyographic correlates of stridor in multiple system atrophy phenotypes. Parkinsonism Relat Disord 2020;70:31–35.
93. Todisco M, Gana S, Cosentino G, Errichiello E, Arceri S, Avenali M, et al. KCTD17-related myoclonus-dystonia syndrome: Clinical and electrophysiological findings of a patient with atypical late onset. Parkinsonism Relat Disord 2020;78:129–133.
94. Torrecillas V, Dwenger K, Barkmeier-Kraemer JM. Classification of vocal tremor using updated consensus-based tremor classification criteria. Laryngoscope Investig Otolaryngol 2021;6:261–276.
95. Traube L. *Gesammelte Beitrage zur Pathologie und Physiologie*, 2 ed. Verlag von August Hirshwald; 1871.
96. Trender-Gerhard I, Sweeney MG, Schwingenschuh P, Mir P, Edwards MJ, Gerhard A, et al. Autosomal-dominant GTPCH1-deficient DRD: Clinical characteristics and long-term outcome of 34 patients. J Neurol Neurosurg Psychiatry 2009;80:839–845.
97. Truong DD, Rontal M, Rolnick M, Aronson AE, Mistura K. Double-blind controlled study of botulinum toxin in adductor spasmodic dysphonia. Laryngoscope 1991;101:630–634.
98. Valenzuela D, Singer J, Lee T, Hu A. The impact of socioeconomic status on voice outcomes in patients with spasmodic dysphonia treated with botulinum Toxin injections. Ann Otol Rhinol Laryngol 2019;128:316–322.
99. Valeriani D, Simonyan K. A microstructural neural network biomarker for dystonia diagnosis identified by a DystoniaNet deep learning platform. Proc Natl Acad Sci 2020;117:26398–26405.
100. van Esch BF, Wegner I, Stegeman I, Grolman W. Effect of botulinum toxin and surgery among spasmodic dysphonia patients. Otolaryngol Head Neck Surg 2017;156:238–254.
101. Vemula SR, Xiao J, Zhao Y, Bastian RW, Perlmutter JS, Racette BA, et al. A rare sequence variant in intron 1 of THAP1 is associated with primary dystonia. Mol Genet Genomic Med 2014;2:261–272.
102. Weiss EM, Hershey T, Karimi M, Racette B, Tabbal SD, Mink JW, et al. Relative risk of spread of symptoms among the focal onset primary dystonias. Mov Disord 2006;21:1175–1181.
103. White LJ, Hapner ER, Klein AM, Delgaudio JM, Hanfelt JJ, Jinnah HA, Johns MM, 3rd. Coprevalence of anxiety and depression with spasmodic dysphonia: A case-control study. J Voice 2012;26:667 e661–666.
104. White LJ, Klein AM, Hapner ER, Delgaudio JM, Hanfelt JJ, Jinnah HA, Johns MM, 3rd. Coprevalence of tremor with spasmodic dysphonia: A case-control study. Laryngoscope 2011;121:1752–1755.
105. Wolraich D, Vasile Marchis-Crisan C, Redding N, Khella SL, Mirza N. Laryngeal tremor: Co-occurrence with other movement disorders. ORL J Otorhinolaryngol Relat Spec 2010;72:291–294.
106. Xiao J, Bastian RW, Perlmutter JS, Racette BA, Tabbal SD, Karimi M, et al. High-throughput mutational analysis of TOR1A in primary dystonia. BMC Med Genet 2009;10:24.
107. Xiromerisiou G, Houlden H, Scarmeas N, Stamelou M, Kara E, Hardy J, et al. THAP1 mutations and dystonia phenotypes: Genotype phenotype correlations. Mov Disord 2012;27:1290–1294.
108. Zwirner P, Dressler D, Kruse E. Spasmodic laryngeal dyspnea: A rare manifestation of laryngeal dystonia. Eur Arch Otorhinolaryngol 1997;254:242–245.

Chapter 8

Limb Dystonias

INTRODUCTION

Dystonia may affect any region of the body, either alone or in combinations with other regions. Sometimes, a single limb may be affected, either upper or lower. Occasionally, only one part of an upper limb may be affected, such as one finger, the whole hand, wrist, upper arm, or shoulder. The same is true for the lower limb, with occasional involvement of only one toe, multiple toes, the foot, lower or upper leg, or hip and pelvis.

This chapter focuses on focal limb dystonias.[46] In children, dystonia of one limb is a relatively common initial sign for several monogenic disorders. In these cases, limb dystonia often spreads to a generalized pattern. Childhood-onset limb dystonias are covered only briefly here, with more details in Chapter 9, "Isolated Generalized Dystonias," and Chapter 22 "Dystonia Genetics." Therefore, this chapter mostly addresses adult-onset limb dystonias. Task-specific dystonias affecting the upper limbs and upper limb dystonic syndromes that resemble tremor have unique characteristics that differentiate them from more typical isolated focal upper limb dystonia. They are therefore addressed in separate Chapter 10, "Musician's and Other Task-Specific Dystonias," and Chapter 12, "Dystonia and Tremor."

Upper and lower limb dystonias have distinct clinical, etiological, and therapeutic implications. Large descriptive studies have suggested the average age of onset for upper limb dystonias is 30–50 years of age, while the age of onset for the lower limb tends to be older (Figure 8.1). Walking-induced dystonia tends to be much more common in female individuals compared to male individuals, while studies of writer's

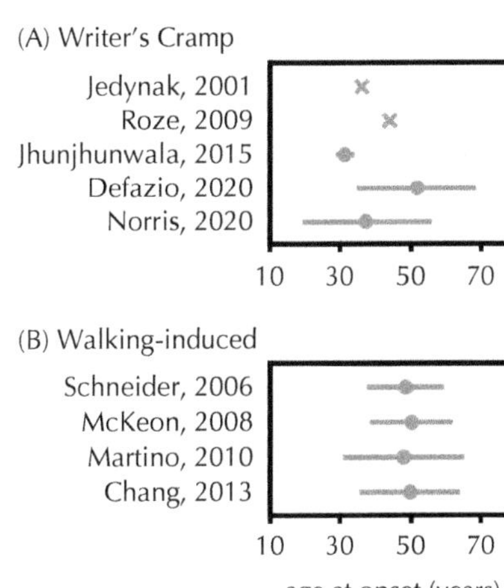

Figure 8.1. Age at onset for upper and lower limb dystonias. This figure shows the average (±SD) age at onset for studies in the literature that included at least 50 cases of writer's cramp or 10 cases of walking dystonia. When the same center had multiple reports over the years, only the largest series was included.

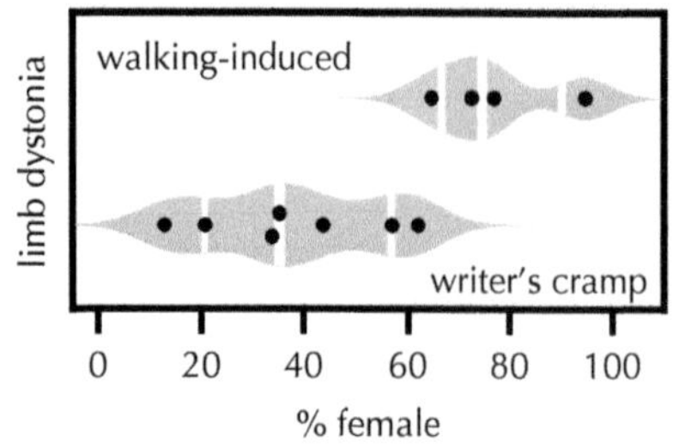

Figure 8.2. Sex distribution for task-specific limb dystonias. This violin plot shows the distribution of female and male individuals for studies in the literature that included that included at least 50 cases of writer's cramp or 10 cases of walking-induced dystonia. When the same center had multiple reports over the years, only the largest series was included.

cramp do not always show a female preponderance (Figure 8.2). As a result of the differences between the upper and lower limb dystonias, they are addressed separately.

ISOLATED FOCAL UPPER LIMB DYSTONIA

Epidemiology

In children, upper limb dystonia is uncommon but often an early sign of a monogenic dystonia. By contrast, most cases that emerge in adults are idiopathic. Isolated focal limb dystonia is less common than focal isolated dystonia of the neck or cranial muscles (see Chapter 4, "Epidemiology of Dystonia"). In most epidemiological studies, isolated limb dystonia is one of the least common forms of dystonia among adults, although it is more commonly a part of segmental or generalized dystonia (see Chapter 4). Among the limb dystonias, the upper limb is far more commonly affected than the lower limb.

In two different meta-analyses of published epidemiological studies, the prevalence of isolated focal upper limb dystonia was estimated at 1.3–2.2 per 100,000 individuals, compared with 5–10 per 100,000 for cervical dystonia and 2.8–4.2 per 100,000 for blepharospasm.[38,58] The majority of upper limb dystonias are task-specific, most notably writer's cramp. Upper limb dystonias that are not task-specific are less common, with several differences from task-specific dystonias that imply a different etiopathogenesis.

The most common presentations of isolated focal upper limb dystonia is either writer's cramp or jerky dystonic movements sometimes called dystonic tremor or primary writer's tremor (see Chapter 12). Probably the next most common manifestation of isolated focal upper limb dystonia is also a task-specific dystonia, musician's dystonia. Other than these task-specific syndromes, isolated focal upper limb dystonias are uncommon. As task-specific dystonias are addressed in Chapter 10, the remainder of this chapter focuses mainly on non–task-specific upper limb dystonia.

Clinical Characteristics and Evolution

Several large descriptive studies of cases with upper limb dystonia have been published, although most focus on writer's cramp.[13,23,24,51] Only two large series of cases with upper limb dystonia that are not task-specific have been published. The Italian Dystonia Registry, comprised of 1,522 consecutively recruited clinic patients with idiopathic adult-onset dystonia from 37 centers, included 182 individuals (12%) with upper limb dystonia, either focal or as part of a segmental/multifocal dystonia.[14] In this study 70 individuals had writer's cramp, and 80% of them had focal onset. In contrast, the same study included 112 individuals with non–task-specific upper limb dystonia, and onset was focal in 46%, with the remainder split evenly between those who had upper limb involvement as part of segmental dystonia at onset and those who had upper limb dystonia that developed after onset of dystonia elsewhere. In 107 individuals with focal upper limb onset from both groups, there was subsequent spread of dystonia in only 18% of the writer's cramp group versus 49% in the non–task-specific group. Those with writer's cramp had a mean age at onset of 44 years, while those with non–task-specific dystonia had mean age of onset of 52 years. Those with writer's cramp were less likely to have associated action tremor (26%) compared with those with no task-specificity (48%). These differences may imply that the mechanisms responsible for task-specific versus non–task-specific upper limb dystonia differ.[14] No data were given about the proportion of individuals with writer's cramp in whom dystonia subsequently became non–task-specific, although the loss of specificity is known to occur in some individuals over time.

Another large series came from the Dystonia Coalition, comprised of 3,320 cases of mostly adult-onset dystonias from 38 centers across North America, Europe, and Australia.[42] A total of 367 cases (11%) had upper limb dystonia at onset. Onset was focal in 292 (80%) and non-focal in 75 (20%). Dystonia was task-specific in 67% of the whole group, 70% of the focal onset group, and 55% of the non–focal onset groups. It started in the dominant limb in approximately 80% of both groups. In the focal onset group, spread of dystonia occurred in approximately one-third, who were more likely to be younger (mean age of onset 29.5 vs. 38.9 years), have had dystonia for longer (24.1 vs. 14.5 years), have non–task-specific dystonia (54% vs. 18%), and have a sensory trick (52% vs. 29%). There were important differences in those with young adult-onset (<21 years) versus older adult-onset (≥21 years), with the younger-onset group being less likely to have task-specificity (45% vs. 73%) and more likely to have spread after onset (49% vs. 19%). Overall, onset was task-specific in 246/367, and the majority (194) had writer's cramp. Those with pure musician's cramp of an upper limb were least likely to become non–task-specific (3/30). These differences again imply etiological heterogeneity among isolated upper limb dystonias.[42]

History

Individuals with isolated focal upper limb dystonias that are not task-specific usually present with difficulty using the limb or involuntary posturing of the limb. Common tasks affected, in addition to writing which is the most common task-specific complaint, are using eating utensils or drinking. However, use of any tool or object may be affected. Resting dystonia is uncommon. However occasionally the complaint will be of the upper limb adopting an abnormal posture when performing another task, for example becoming flexed or pulled behind the body when walking. There may be accompanying tremor-like movements, which may dominate the picture, rather than abnormal posturing (see Chapter 12). Patients rarely lose the ability to use the limb altogether, but the performance becomes slow and clumsy. With prolonged attempts to perform a task, pain may occur. The main problem may be in the hand, upper arm, shoulder, or neck. Other sensory symptoms (loss of sensation or paraesthesia, pain at rest beyond that triggered by limb use) should not be present and suggest added pathology. However, the term *numbness* is sometimes used to explain various sensations in a limb, including altered motor function, and clarification should be sought before accepting it as a true red flag. Sensory tricks are present in approximately half of all individuals.

Examination

The key finding on examination is abnormal posturing of the fingers or wrist and sometimes the arm (Figure 8.3A–B). This posturing may only be observable during specific tasks. The most common abnormal posture is flexion of the wrist and/or fingers with varying degrees of radial or ulnar deviation of the hand and splaying of the fingers, although wrist extension can occur instead of flexion. A classic posture is described as "spooning," characterized by slight wrist flexion with metacarpophalangeal hyperextension (Figure 8.3C).[30] The specificity of this sign for dystonia is not clear since it can be seen in other neurological disorders and even in otherwise normal children. Elbow flexion is more common than extension, and the shoulder is often elevated and anteriorly rotated rather than depressed or pulled backward. Both adduction and abduction of the shoulder can be present. Some degree of abnormal posturing when holding the arms in posture, either outstretched or in the targeting nose position, is seen in the majority. Abnormal upper limb posturing during walking is common, although usually less than when using the upper limb. Frequently, abnormal upper limb posturing worsens or emerges when the gait is stressed, such as toe-walking or heel-walking.

Superimposed action tremor is present in approximately half[14,54] and may be dependent on limb position. When performing a task affected by upper limb dystonia, such as writing, there is often overflow of muscle activity to more proximal segments of the limb, leading to abnormal posturing of the upper limb, shoulder, or neck. When the affected limb is relaxed, dystonic posturing can frequently be elicited when a task is performed by the contralateral, unaffected limb. This posturing is similar to that when the limb is used, but it is usually less severe. This phenomenon is termed *mirror dystonia*.[34,56]

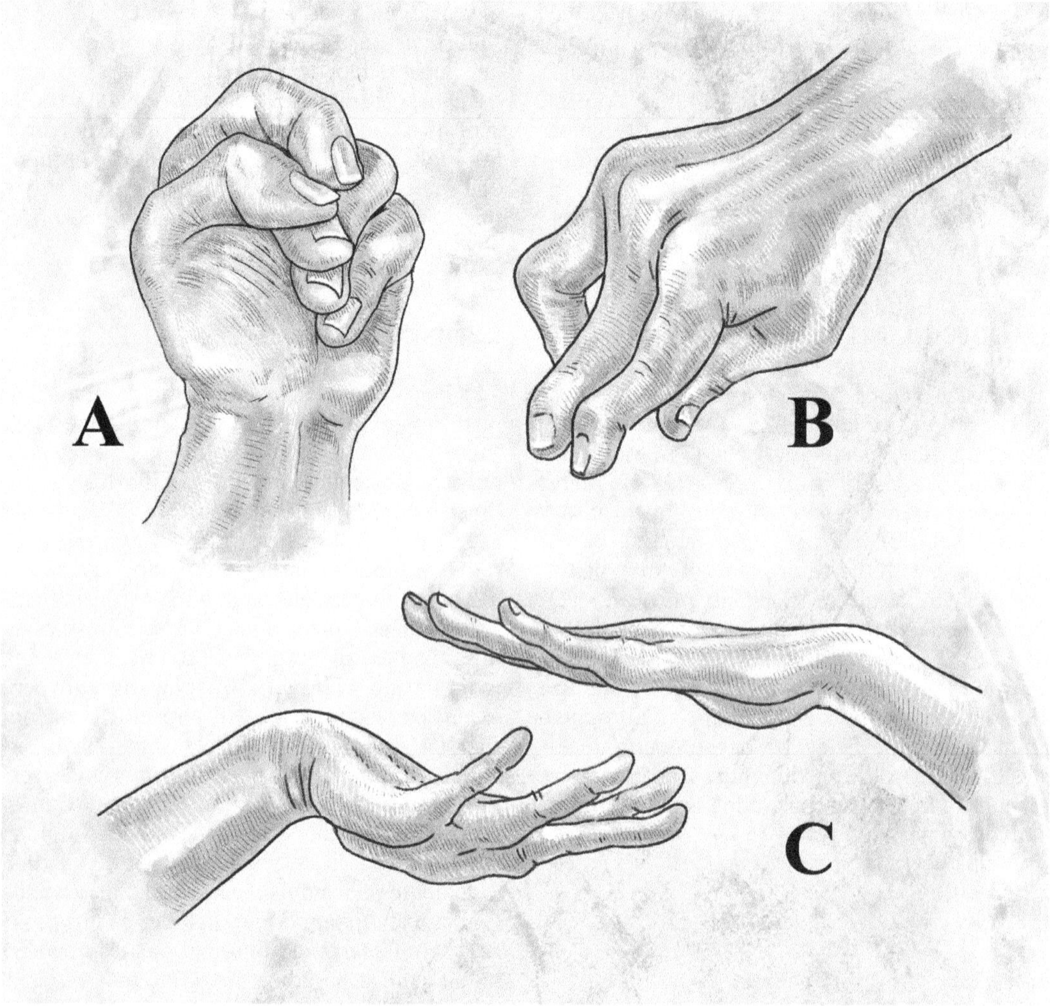

Figure 8.3. Dystonic upper limb postures. Panel A shows excessive flexion of the fingers and thumb. Panel B shows a more complex pattern with abnormal finger postures that have extension at the proximal interphalangeal joints but flexion at the distal interphalangeal and metacarpophalangeal joints. Panel C shows dystonic spooning of the right hand with a relatively normal left hand.

Illustration by Loren Bergantini.

Weakness or sensory impairment should not be present and suggests a different pathology. However repetitive finger tapping may be clumsy, slow, or variable in amplitude. These abnormalities are presumably caused by superimposed dystonic muscle contractions, and they can be difficult to differentiate from parkinsonism or ataxia.[3] In contrast, the ability to fractionate finger movements and perform tasks requiring fine motor control, even in the presence of moderate-severe dystonic posturing, can be remarkably preserved, presumably because corticospinal motor control is intact.

Causes and Investigation

The differential diagnosis of upper limb dystonia includes several problems that produce abnormal posturing (Table 8.1). Because isolated non–task-specific focal upper limb dystonia is relatively uncommon, an underlying lesion should be excluded with neuroimaging (Table 8.2). A systematic review of single, localized lesions reported to cause focal upper limb dystonia in 72 cases revealed that the pathology could potentially arise from multiple regions.[35] The thalamus was the site for the majority

Table 8.1 **Differential diagnosis of movements suggestive of limb dystonias**

Cause	Notes
Parkinson disease	May occur in upper or lower limb before other parkinsonian features emerge, sometimes by many years
Parkinsonian syndromes	May occur with corticobasal syndrome or progressive supranuclear palsy
Stiff limb syndrome	Variant of stiff-syndrome person, which often affects the trunk and proximal limbs, but may occasionally affect the distal part of one limb
Spastic paraparesis	Can be unilateral and occasionally mimics isolated dystonia
Spinal claudication	Usually exercise-induced and often associated with pain
Radiculopathy	May be associated with foot drop or leg pain
Neuromuscular	Focal involvement of specific muscles may result in abnormal posturing resembling dystonia
Orthopedic	Joint abnormalities may result in abnormal postures resembling dystonia

(n = 39), but there were also lesions in the basal ganglia (n = 17), cortex (n = 4), brainstem (n = 4), cerebellum (n = 1), and cervical spine (n = 7). A second systematic study of published reports of lesion-induced dystonia confirmed limb dystonia could result from lesions in many regions.[11] This second study suggested that focal hand dystonia more likely resulted from thalamic lesions, while involvement of the whole upper limb was more likely to result from basal ganglia lesions.

Younger individuals with isolated focal upper limb onset of dystonia are more likely to generalize and also more likely to have an underlying genetic etiology (Table 8.2). No large studies of childhood-onset focal upper limb onset dystonia are available. However, in a recent systematic review of genotype-phenotype correlations in seven monogenic causes of mostly isolated dystonia (*TOR1A, THAP1, GNAL, ANO3, PRKRA, KMT2B*, and *HPCA*), the upper limb was the most common site of onset for *TOR1A, THAP1*, and *PRKRA*. For all of these genes, onset is most commonly in childhood or adolescence and less commonly in adults.[32]

Genetic variants in *GNAL* and *ANO3* are more common monogenic causes of adult-onset isolated dystonia.[32] The upper limbs are the second most common site of onset in *ANO3*-related dystonia, whereas *GNAL* presents uncommonly in the upper limbs. Dystonia associated with *ANO3* is often accompanied by tremor. Isolated upper limb onset has also been described as the initial manifestation of biallelic *AOPEP* (*C9orf3*) mutations with onset of symptoms in young adulthood, whereas lower limb or generalized dystonia is the more common presenting feature in childhood.[67] *SGCE*-related myoclonus-dystonia usually presents with myoclonic jerks in the upper limbs, sometimes also with upper limb dystonia, but the dystonia tends to be cervical or manifest as writer's cramp (see Chapter 15, "Dystonia and Myoclonus").[1,40,48]

In addition to lesions and genetic causes of focal upper limb dystonia, there may be other causes (Table 8.2). Focal upper limb dystonia can occasionally be the presenting feature of neurodegenerative disease that is not associated with overt focal brain pathology. The most common neurodegenerative disorders presenting with focal upper limb dystonia include sporadic and monogenic Parkinson disease.[27,28,33,49,60] Upper limb dystonia also occurs in atypical parkinsonisms,[7,9,17,49,63,66] and rapid-onset dystonia parkinsonism due to genetic variants in *ATP1A3*.[6] Although dystonia can occur in isolation, most cases have

Table 8.2 **Potential causes for isolated focal limb dystonia**

Causes	Notes
Idiopathic	Upper limb is far more common than lower limb in adults
Monogenic	Common in children and adolescents, but may occasionally occur in adults
Parkinson disease	May occur in upper or lower limb before other parkinsonian features emerge, sometimes by many years
Focal brain lesions	Lesions may occur in different regions, and upper limb more common than lower limb
Tardive syndromes	Uncommon, but upper limb more frequent than lower limb
Post-traumatic	May involve either upper or lower limb, often fixed and painful

additional features of parkinsonism (see Chapter 13, "Dystonia and Parkinsonism"). Isolated upper limb dystonia may also occur in the spinocerebellar ataxias before other cerebellar features become obvious (see Chapter 14, "Dystonia and Ataxia").[50]

Some Specific Upper Limb Dystonia Syndromes

In its early stages and even after many years of progression, dystonia almost always remains mobile, with worsening of abnormal postures during action and less prominent dystonia at rest. In contrast, individuals with the syndrome of fixed dystonia develop abnormal postures that escalate over days to weeks and become completely or near-completely immobile.[53] An upper limb is affected most commonly, followed by a lower limb, then the jaw. Pain is often prominent, and some individuals fulfill criteria for complex regional pain syndrome.[61] A history of onset following injury is present in the majority, compared with a minority in classical idiopathic focal dystonia. The injury may be minor, including a history of immobilization in a cast. Clinical evidence of a psychogenic etiology or somatization disorder is present in many. Many affected patients do not respond to botulinum toxins, although a minority exhibit a non-physiologic immediate response, which may be useful diagnostically or therapeutically.[15] However, in a minority of patients, no evidence to support a psychological contribution can be found, and the differential diagnosis includes post-immobilization dystonia in Parkinson disease,[55] corticobasal syndrome,[57] or stiff-limb syndrome,[5] as well as musculoskeletal causes (see Chapter 26, "Pseudodystonia and Differential Diagnosis").

Dystonia of the shoulder commonly coexists with dystonia of the upper limb[42] or neck.[29] Isolated involvement of the shoulder, without involvement of the upper limb or neck, may also occur as a distinct syndrome.[59,64] The typical manifestation is tonic elevation or anterior displacement, and it is often fixed. The syndrome often occurs after trauma, with atypical features such as rapid onset within hours or days, a relatively fixed nature of shoulder elevation, prominent pain, and a lack of a torsional component. These characteristics share some similarities with the syndrome of fixed limb dystonia and psychogenic dystonia. However, a case arising from accessory nerve injury with neurogenic hypertrophy has been reported.[12]

Individuals with a tremor that resembles *essential tremor* often have dystonia, and the tremor typically involves an upper limb (see Chapter 12).[54] Some individuals have subtle abnormal postures of unclear clinical significance, and the term *essential tremor plus* may be applied.[8,45,47] It remains to be determined whether these postures in essential tremor plus reflect a very mild form of dystonia, a behavioral compensation for tremor, or a soft neurological sign with low specificity.

Isolated involuntary thumb flexion has been reported as a peculiar form of focal dystonia among inhabitants of the Faroe Islands.[31] It remains to be determined if this is a dystonic phenomenon unique to this population, a dystonic phenomenon that has been overlooked in other populations, or another movement disorder that mimics dystonia.

ISOLATED LOWER LIMB DYSTONIA

Epidemiology

The lower limbs are almost universally affected in cerebral palsy, a relatively common problem in children (see Chapter 16, "Dystonia and Cerebral Palsy"). However, there is often a relevant history or additional corticospinal signs that point to the diagnosis, and isolated lower limb dystonia is uncommon for cerebral palsy. Monogenic dystonias often present with involvement of a lower limb, although as a group they are all quite rare and, again, most commonly occur in children.[32]

For adults, isolated focal lower limb dystonia is among the least common of the focal isolated dystonias. Many epidemiology studies do not address focal lower limb dystonia, but one study from Finland placed the crude prevalence at 1 per 1,000,000[44] and another study focusing specifically on the lower limb found that it accounted for only 0.7% of subjects in 579 consecutive clinic patients from nine Italian university centers for movement disorders.[36] There are only a few prior case series of focal lower limb dystonia, and most are relatively small.[37,52] Most of these cases had lower limb dystonia induced by walking, so they are addressed in Chapter 10.

History

Isolated focal lower limb dystonia is most commonly task-specific, presenting as a gait disturbance.[36] It is usually present when walking but commonly worsens with prolonged walking. When it is occasionally not task-specific, it still often gets worse with walking. It is more commonly unilateral but can spread to the opposite side while remaining asymmetrical.

Affected individuals may have a relatively nonspecific complaint when walking, such as the leg "not doing what it should do," "kicking out," or the foot "dragging" or "turning in." Sometimes there is associated pain, which may be due to the involuntary muscle spasm or secondary musculoskeletal problems that may have developed if the diagnosis has been delayed. Complaints of abnormal postures are relatively uncommon. Affected individuals often complain that hard, shiny floor surfaces worsen their gait (e.g., walking in smooth-tiled shopping malls), whereas walking on uneven surfaces such as sand or grass may be easier. This phenomenon is the opposite in ataxia, where irregular surfaces are more difficult.

Delay in diagnosis is frequent, with initial suspicions of an underlying orthopedic problem, which can sometimes develop secondary to the disordered gait mechanics. Neurological referral may not occur until the gait disturbance fails to resolve after orthopedic treatment. Structural pathology should always be excluded with imaging of the brain and spinal cord. Once this is performed, in addition to orthopedic misdiagnosis, spondylotic spinal canal narrowing causing cord flattening may lead to a mistaken diagnosis of myelopathy. These misdiagnoses may lead to inappropriate surgery.[52]

Examination

The key finding on examination is abnormal posturing of the foot and leg (Figure 8.4A).[36] Posturing may sometimes occur when seated as rest with the dangling foot displaying intorsion. However, abnormal posturing may only be observable during the affected task (e.g., walking). It may be necessary to observe the individual walking long distances, such as doing repeated laps of a room

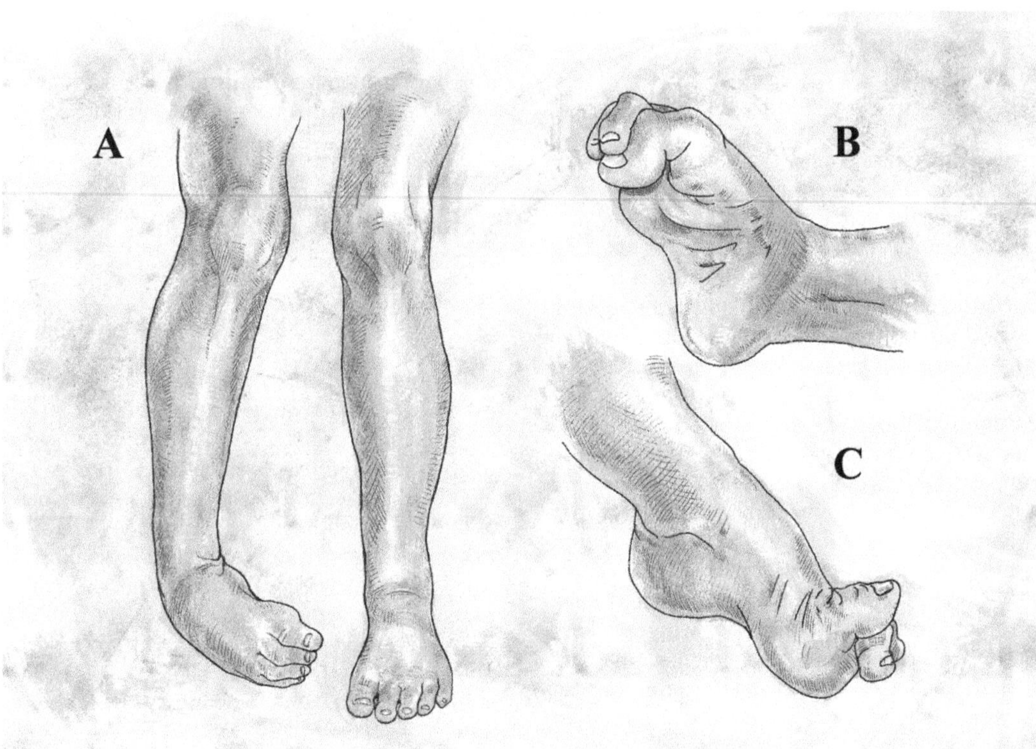

Figure 8.4. Dystonic lower limb postures. Panel A shows a typical dystonic posture with intorsion and plantar flexion of the foot combined with some flexion of the toes. Panel B shows more extreme flexion of the toes, which sometimes cross over each other. Panel C shows the striatal dystonic toe, which resembles the Babinski extensor plantar reflex.

Illustration by Loren Bergantini.

if it is small, in order for the abnormal posture to become obvious. Classic gaits (ataxic, parkinsonian, spastic, weak, fearful, psychogenic, antalgic, or orthopedic) have fairly consistent features and are therefore often easy to recognize.[4,16] In contrast, dystonic gaits are quite varied and often difficult to classify.

The most common abnormality is downward curling of the toes with plantar flexion and intorsion of the foot (Figure 8.4A–B).[52] The abnormal posture should be stereotyped (patterned) at any particular phase of the gait cycle (i.e., heel strike or swing phase) but the posture may vary according to the gait cycle. For example, the ankle may invert and plantar flex during the swing phase, then dorsiflex and evert just before heel strike, only to invert and plantar flex again during the next swing phase. Abnormalities in position of the knee or hips may be subtle, for example a reduction in knee bend during the swing phase, or premature or rapid extension before heel strike, or, in the case of the hip, delay in relaxation of hip flexion during the swing phase so that the leg appears slightly "hung up" due to a delay in heel strike compared with the opposite leg. Sometimes, with dystonic plantar extension of the foot, there is increased flexion of the hip with a high stepping gait as a behavioral compensation to avoid scuffing the ball of the foot. The pelvis may rotate excessively or inappropriately during a phase of the gait cycle, often leading to the mistaken diagnosis of hip pathology.

Task-specific gait dystonia is often normalized or improved significantly during walking backward and sometimes also during running[65] or tandem gait, although persistence during any of these tasks may also occur. There may be reduced arm swing on the same side, but this is non-specific and can occur with any problem of the ipsilateral leg present when walking (e.g., painful osteoarthritis of the knee). It is quite common for affected individuals to be aware that their gait is significantly better, or worse, when wearing certain footwear. The gait should be examined both with and without such footwear. Rarely, there may be more restricted task-specificity, such as dystonia only when walking stairs.[39] In one series of 17 individuals with lower limb dystonia restricted to walking stairs, dystonia when walking down was more common than dystonia walking up.[2] In these cases, the examination needs to be carried out while performing this specific task.

Causes and Investigation

The investigation of isolated lower limb dystonia is informed by its potential causes and the knowledge that idiopathic lower limb dystonia is an uncommon syndrome (Tables 8.1 and 8.2). In most if not all cases, neuroimaging is indicated to exclude both cerebral and spinal pathology. When focal lower limb dystonia occurs in a child or adolescent, a monogenic dystonia is the most commonly identifiable cause. The lower limb is the most common site of dystonia onset associated with *KMT2B*, a close second most common site of onset is associated with *TOR1A*, and it is relatively common also with *PRKRA*.[32] Dystonia of the foot or leg is the most common presenting feature of dopa-responsive dystonia due to genetic variants in *GCH1* (Segawa syndrome).[62]

In adults, focal lower limb dystonia should raise concern for Parkinson disease or, less likely, another parkinsonian syndrome. Some such cases present with isolated focal lower limb dystonia before the other parkinsonian features emerge, and they may account for up to 40–50% of cases.[37,52] A good response to levodopa increases the likelihood of the leg dystonia being the initial manifestation of Parkinson disease, although an apparent clinical response may be seen with other disorders.[10] Imaging dopamine transporters can be of assistance in this setting.

Some Specific Lower Limb Dystonia Syndromes

Lower limb dystonia that is exercise-induced is a particular category of task-specific gait dystonia that implies that the dystonia is not present at rest and does not always occur when walking but instead emerges only after more prolonged walking or running, for example after 5–10 minutes. Often, the greater the walking or running speed or effort, the shorter the latency. In contrast, task-specific gait dystonia as described above is usually present with walking any distance, even though it may worsen with prolonged walking. Also unlike task-specific gait dystonia, exercise-induced leg dystonia can persist for seconds or minutes even after walking stops. Exercise-induced gait dystonia is less likely to be idiopathic. The possibilities of an initial presentation of early-onset Parkinson disease, as well as—especially in childhood or adolescence—glucose transporter deficiency and dopa-responsive dystonia, should also be considered. The differential diagnosis of leg dysfunction that worsens with exercise includes transient neurological deficits from spinal claudication due to lumbar spinal canal stenosis; rarely, steal phenomena due to spinal arteriovenous malformation; and musculoskeletal problems involving the hip or ankle joints.

Another well-characterized lower limb dystonia is the *striatal toe* or *dystonic toe*. These terms refer to prominent dorsal extension of the great toe (Figure 8.4C). The sign may occur spontaneously, or it may be triggered by walking. It can also be triggered by sensory stimulation of the foot, and it can closely resemble the extensor plantar reflex (Babinksi sign) of corticospinal injury.[20] However, it is common in Parkinson disease[22,41] and many types of dystonia[21,43] where its pathogenesis is thought to involve striatal dysfunction (thus *striatal toe*). As a result, the value of the upgoing toe sign as a localizing sign in movement disorders is sometimes unclear.

TREATMENT

Oral medications used for upper and lower limb dystonias include levodopa, anticholinergics, baclofen, benzodiazepines, and others. Some patients may benefit, although the degree of improvement tends to be mild or moderate rather than marked (see Chapter 28, "Symptom-Targeted Oral Medications for Dystonia").

A trial of levodopa is often given for upper and lower limb dystonias because of the possibility of late-onset dopa-responsive dystonia or an early dystonic sign of Parkinson disease. In adults, a proper trial of levodopa requires escalating the dose to approximately 1,000 mg/d in divided doses for at least 1 month. In children, the dose should be titrated to 20 mg/kg/d for at least 1 month. Many individuals will respond to lower doses in a shorter duration of time, especially those with early-onset Parkinson disease or dopa-responsive dystonia, but a small number of cases require higher doses or longer durations to see any effect.

There are few randomized controlled studies of any therapies for limb dystonias. A recent review of published literature for the upper limb concluded that the best evidence of efficacy is with botulinum toxin injections, with 20–90% of patients experiencing improvement (see Chapter 30, "Botulinum Toxin Treatment for Dystonia").[18] However, many treated individuals eventually discontinue this treatment, presumably because of the complex muscle patterns often involved in limb dystonias and the challenge associated with delivering exactly the right dose to the right muscles.[26] Individuals with simple patterns of dystonia, such as those with involvement of one finger or isolated wrist flexion, do better than those with more complex movements.

Functional neurosurgery including deep brain stimulation, and ablative methods, have all been reported to be effective in selected individuals (see Chapter 31, "Surgical Treatments for Dystonia").[19] Behavioral techniques, sensorimotor training, and neuromodulation have all been reported to provide good outcomes in small series, but larger confirmatory studies are required (see Chapter 32, "Physiotherapy and Complementary Medicine for Dystonia").

SUMMARY AND FUTURE PROSPECTS

Dystonia may affect a single limb. Although focal dystonia of an upper or lower limb is a common presentation among children, it is an uncommon presentation among adults. Among adults, the upper limb is far more frequently affected than the lower limb. Adult-onset upper limb dystonias are most commonly task-specific, such as writer's cramp or musician's dystonia. Adult-onset lower limb dystonias are also often task-specific, occurring with walking, running, or sometimes only going down stairs. Upper and lower limb dystonias that are not task-specific also occur and often raise concern for a structural lesion or a neurodegenerative disorder such as Parkinson disease.

Dystonia of a limb should prompt an evaluation for its cause. Among children, apart from cerebral palsy, monogenic causes are common, so neuroimaging and genetic testing are both required. Among adults, a genetic cause may be found, but a focal lesion or neurodegenerative cause is more likely. Therefore, neuroimaging is important for adults, but the value of genetic testing is lower. For both children and adults, a levodopa trial is essential because it has implications for potential causes. If levodopa fails, other oral agents or functional neurosurgery may be useful.

The pathogenesis of limb dystonias seems to be a bit different from other more common dystonias such as cervical dystonia or blepharospasm.[25] Among children, limb dystonias are more common than cervical dystonia or blepharospasm. Yet among adults, the converse is true. Among adults, limb dystonias are far more likely to be task-specific, whereas cervical dystonia and blepharospasm are not. These observations imply etiological heterogeneity among the adult-onset focal dystonias.

REFERENCES

1. Asmus F, Zimprich A, Tezenas Du Montcel S, Kabus C, Deuschl G, et al. Myoclonus-dystonia syndrome: Epsilon-sarcoglycan mutations and phenotype. Ann Neurol 2002;52:489–492.
2. Baik JS, Ma HI, Lee PH, Taira T. Focal task-specific lower limb dystonia only when walking stairs: Is it a new disease entity? Front Neurol 2019;10:1081.
3. Bajaj NP, Gontu V, Birchall J, Patterson J, Grosset DG, Lees AJ. Accuracy of clinical diagnosis in tremulous parkinsonian patients: A blinded video study. J Neurol Neurosurg Psychiatry 2010;81:1223–1228.
4. Baker JM. Gait disorders. Am J Med 2018;131:602–607.
5. Balint B, Mahant N, Meinck HM, Fung V. Stiff limb syndrome mimicking corticobasal syndrome. Mov Disord Clin Pract 2014;1:354–356.
6. Balint B, Stephen CD, Udani V, Sankhla CS, Barad NH, Lang AE, Bhatia KP. Paroxysmal asymmetric dystonic arm posturing: A less recognized but characteristic manifestation of ATP1A3-related disease. Mov Disord Clin Pract 2019;6:312–315.
7. Barclay CL, Lang AE. Dystonia in progressive supranuclear palsy. J Neurol Neurosurg Psychiatry 1997;62:352–356.
8. Bellows ST, Jankovic J. Phenotypic features of isolated essential tremor, essential tremor plus, and essential tremor-Parkinson's disease in a movement disorders clinic. Tremor Other Hyperkinet Mov (N Y) 2021;11:12.
9. Boesch SM, Wenning GK, Ransmayr G, Poewe W. Dystonia in multiple system atrophy. J Neurol Neurosurg Psychiatry 2002;72:300–303.
10. Chang FC, Josephs KA. Levodopa responsiveness in adult-onset lower limb dystonia is associated with the development of Parkinson's disease. Tremor Other Hyperkinet Mov 2013;tre-03-150-3598-2.
11. Corp DT, Greenwood C, Morrison-Ham J, Pullinen J, McDowall G, Younger E, et al. Clinical and structural findings in patients with lesion-induced dystonia: Descriptive and quantitative analysis of published cases. Neurology 2022;99:e1957–e1967.
12. Cossu G, Melis M, Melis G, Ferrigno P, Molari A. Persistent abnormal shoulder elevation after accessory nerve injury and differential diagnosis with post-traumatic focal shoulder-elevation dystonia: Report of a case and literature review. Mov Disord 2004;19:1109–1111.
13. Das CP, Prabhakar S, Truong D. Clinical profile of various sub-types of writer's cramp. Parkinsonism Relat Disord 2007;13:421–424.
14. Defazio G, Ercoli T, Erro R, Pellicciari R, Mascia MM, Fabbrini G, et al. Idiopathic non-task-specific upper limb dystonia, a neglected form of dystonia. Mov Disord 2020;35:2038–2045.
15. Edwards MJ, Bhatia KP, Cordivari C. Immediate response to botulinum toxin injections in patients with fixed dystonia. Mov Disord 2011;26:917–918.
16. Fasano A, Bloem BR. Gait disorders. Continuum 2013;19:1344–1382.
17. Godeiro-Junior C, Felicio AC, Barsottini OG, Aguiar PM, Silva SM, Borges V, Ferraz HB. Clinical features of dystonia in atypical parkinsonism. Arq Neuropsiquiatr 2008;66:800–804.
18. Gupta N, Pandey S. Treatment of focal hand dystonia: Current status. Neurol Sci 2021;42:3561–3584.
19. Horisawa S, Ochiai T, Goto S, Nakajima T, Takeda N, Fukui A, et al. Safety and long-term efficacy of ventro-oral thalamotomy for focal hand dystonia: A retrospective study of 171 patients. Neurology 2019;92:e371–e377.
20. Horstink MW, Haaxma C, Bloem BR, Duysens J. Babinski, pseudo-Babinski, and dystonia. Arch Neurol 2007;64:1207–1209.
21. Jan MMS. Misdiagnoses in children with dopa-responsive dystonia. Pediatr Neurol 2004;31:298–303.
22. Jankovic J. Dystonia and other deformities in Parkinson's disease. J Neurol Sci 2005;229:1–3.
23. Jedynak PC, Tranchant C, de Beyl DZ. Prospective clinical study of writer's cramp. Mov Disord 2001;16:494–499.
24. Jhunjhunwala K, Lenka A, Pal PK. A clinical profile of 125 patients with writer's cramp. Eur Neurol 2015;73:316–320.
25. Jinnah HA, DeFazio G. Adult-onset focal dystonias: To lump or split. Int Rev Neurobiol 2023;169:317–327.
26. Karp BI, Cole RA, Cohen LG, Grill S, Lou JS, Hallett M. Long-term botulinum toxin treatment of focal hand dystonia. Neurology 1994;44:70–76.
27. Khan NL, Graham E, Critchley P, Schrag AE, Wood NW, Lees AJ, et al. Parkin disease: A phenotypic study of a large case series. Brain 2003;126:1279–1292.
28. Kidron D, Melamed E. Forms of dystonia in patients with Parkinson's disease. Neurology 1987;37:1009–1011.
29. Kilic-Berkmen G, Pirio Richardson S, Perlmutter JS, Hallett M, Klein C, et al. Current guidelines for classifying and diagnosing cervical dystonia: Empirical evidence and recommendations. Mov Disord Clin Pract 2021;9:183–190.
30. Kim CY, Louis ED. "Spooning": A subtle sign of limb dystonia. Tremor Other Hyperkinet Mov (N Y) 2018;8:607.
31. Kim CY, Petersen MS, Eliasen EH, Defazio G, Greene P, Jinnah HA, et al. Involuntary thumb flexion on neurological examination: An unusual form of upper limb dystonia in the Faroe islands. Tremor Other Hyperkinet Mov (N Y) 2019;9. doi:10.7916/tohm.v0.686.
32. Lange LM, Junker J, Loens S, Baumann H, Olschewski L, Schaake S, et al. Genotype-phenotype relations for isolated dystonia genes: MDSGene systematic review. Mov Disord 2021;36:1086–1103.
33. LeWitt PA, Burns RS, Newman RP. Dystonia in untreated Parkinsonism. Clinical Neuropharmacology 1986;9:293–297.

34. Liu P, Yuan Y, Zhang N, Liu X, Yu L, Luo B. Mirror movements in acquired neurological disorders: A mini-review. Front Neurol 2021;12:736115.
35. Liuzzi D, Gigante AF, Leo A, Defazio G. The anatomical basis of upper limb dystonia: Lesson from secondary cases. Neurol Sci 2016;37:1393–1398.
36. Martino D, Macerollo A, Abbruzzese G, Bentivoglio AR, Berardelli A, Esposito M, et al. Lower limb involvement in adult-onset primary dystonia: Frequency and clinical features. Eur J Neurol 2010;17:242–246.
37. McKeon A, Matsumoto JY, Bower JH, Ahlskog JE. The spectrum of disorders presenting as adult-onset focal lower extremity dystonia. Parkinsonism Relat Disord 2008;14:613–619.
38. Medina A, Nilles C, Martino D, Pelletier C, Pringsheim T. The prevalence of idiopathic or inherited isolated dystonia: A systematic review and meta-analysis. Mov Disord Clin Pract 2022;9:860–868.
39. Menon S, Muglan JA, Shimon L, Stewart D, Snow B, Hayes M, et al. Down the stairs dystonia: A novel task-specific focal isolated syndrome. Mov Disord Clin Pract 2017;4:121–124.
40. Nardocci N, Zorzi G, Barzaghi C, Zibordi F, Ciano C, Ghezzi D, Garavaglia B. Myoclonus-dystonia syndrome: Clinical presentation, disease course, and genetic features in 11 families. Mov Disord 2008;23:28–34.
41. Nausieda PA, Weiner WJ, Klawans HL. Dystonic foot response of Parkinsonism. Arch Neurol 1980;37:132–136.
42. Norris SA, Jinnah HA, Klein C, Jankovic J, Berman BD, Roze E, et al. Clinical and demographic characteristics of upper limb dystonia. Mov Disord 2020;35:2086–2090.
43. Nygaard TG, Marsden CD, Fahn S. Dopa-responsive dystonia: Long-term treatment response and prognosis. Neurology 1991;41:174–181.
44. Ortiz R, Scheperjans F, Mertsalmi T, Pekkonen E. The prevalence of adult-onset isolated dystonia in Finland 2007–2016. PLoS One 2018;13:e0207729.
45. Pandey S, Bhattad S. Questionable dystonia in essential tremor plus: A video-based assessment of 19 patients. Mov Disord Clin Pract 2019;6:722–723.
46. Pirio Richardson S, Altenmuller E, Alter K, Alterman RL, Chen R, Frucht S, et al. Research priorities in limb and task-specific dystonias. Front Neurol 2017;8:170.
47. Rajalingam R, Breen DP, Lang AE, Fasano A. Essential tremor plus is more common than essential tremor: Insights from the reclassification of a cohort of patients with lower limb tremor. Parkinsonism Relat Disord 2018;56:109–110.
48. Raymond D, Saunders-Pullman R, de Carvalho Aguiar P, Schule B, Kock N, Friedman J, et al. Phenotypic spectrum and sex effects in eleven myoclonus-dystonia families with epsilon-sarcoglycan mutations. Mov Disord 2008;23:588–592.
49. Rivest J, Quinn N, Marsden CD. Dystonia in Parkinson's disease, multiple system atrophy, and progressive supranuclear palsy. Neurology 1990;40:1571–1578.
50. Rossi M, Balint B, Millar Vernetti P, Bhatia KP, Merello M. Genetic dystonia-ataxia syndromes: Clinical spectrum, diagnostic approach, and treatment options. Mov Disord Clin Pract 2018;5:373–382.
51. Roze E, Soumare A, Pironneau I, Sangla S, de Cock VC, Teixeira A, et al. Case-control study of writer's cramp. Brain 2009;132:756–764.
52. Schneider SA, Edwards MJ, Grill SE, Goldstein S, Kanchana S, Quinn NP, et al. Adult-onset primary lower limb dystonia. Mov Disord 2006;21:767–771.
53. Schrag A, Trimble M, Quinn N, Bhatia K. The syndrome of fixed dystonia: An evaluation of 103 patients. Brain 2004;127:2360–2372.
54. Shaikh AG, Beylergil SB, Scorr L, Kilic-Berkmen G, Freeman A, Klein C, et al. Dystonia & tremor: A cross-sectional study of the Dystonia Coalition cohort. Neurology 2021;96:e563–e574.
55. Singer C, Papapetropoulos S. Lower limb post-immobilization dystonia in Parkinson's disease. J Neurol Sci 2005;239:111–114.
56. Sitburana O, Wu LJ, Sheffield JK, Davidson A, Jankovic J. Motor overflow and mirror dystonia. Parkinsonism Relat Disord 2009;15:758–761.
57. Stamelou M, Alonso-Canovas A, Bhatia KP. Dystonia in corticobasal degeneration: A review of the literature on 404 pathologically proven cases. Mov Disord 2012;27:696–702.
58. Steeves TD, Day L, Dykeman J, Jette N, Pringsheim T. The prevalence of primary dystonia: A systematic review and meta-analysis. Mov Disord 2012;27:1789–1796.
59. Thyagarajan D, Kompoliti K, Ford B. Post-traumatic shoulder dystonia: Persistent abnormal postures of the shoulder after minor trauma. Neurology 1998;51:1205–1207.
60. Tolosa E, Compta Y. Dystonia in Parkinson's disease. J Neurol 2006;253 Suppl. 7:7–13.
61. Verdugo RJ, Ochoa JL. Abnormal movements in complex regional pain syndrome: Assessment of their nature. Muscle Nerve 2000;23:198–205.
62. Weissbach A, Pauly MG, Herzog R, Hahn L, Halmans S, Hamami F, et al. Relationship of genotype, phenotype, and treatment in dopa-responsive dystonia: MDSGene review. Mov Disord 2021;2022:237–252.
63. Wenning GK, Tison F, Ben Shlomo Y, Daniel SE, Quinn NP. Multiple system atrophy: A review of 203 pathologically proven cases. Mov Disord 1997;12:133–147.
64. Wright RA, Ahlskog JE. Focal shoulder-elevation dystonia. Mov Disord 2000;15:709–713.
65. Wu LJ, Jankovic J. Runner's dystonia. J Neurol Sci 2006;251:73–76.
66. Yoon WT. Comparison of dystonia between Parkinson's disease and atypical parkinsonism: The clinical usefulness of dystonia distribution and characteristics in the differential diagnosis of parkinsonism. Neurol Neurochir Pol 2018;52:48–53.
67. Zech M, Kumar KR, Reining S, Reunert J, Tchan M, Riley LG, et al. Biallelic AOPEP loss-of-function variants cause progressive dystonia with prominent limb involvement. Mov Disord 2022;37:137–147.

Chapter 9

Isolated Generalized Dystonias

INTRODUCTION

A key aspect for classifying the many different types of dystonia involves the affected body distribution.[1] *Focal dystonia* refers to involvement of a single body region, *segmental dystonia* refers to involvement of two or more contiguous body regions, *multifocal dystonia* refers to involvement of two or more non-contiguous body regions, and *generalized dystonia* refers to a relatively broader distribution of affected body regions (see Chapter 3, "Classification of the Dystonias").

Another key aspect for classifying the dystonias is based on whether dystonia is an isolated problem or whether it is combined with other movement disorders or additional neurological or systemic problems (see Chapter 18, "Dystonias Combined with Other Features").[1] Individuals with isolated dystonia may have tremor, because tremor is frequently associated with dystonia (see Chapter 13, "Dystonia and Tremor"). However, individuals with isolated dystonia do not have other movement disorders such as parkinsonism or ataxia. They also do not have other neurological or medical problems unless these other problems are only coincidental and etiologically unrelated to their dystonia syndrome.

This chapter addresses the isolated generalized dystonias as well as their relationship to segmental and multifocal dystonias. The common isolated focal dystonias are described in dedicated chapters. Dystonia syndromes that are combined with other problems are addressed in chapters that focus on the main problem dystonia is combined with. Epidemiological studies have indicated that generalized dystonia is the least common subtype of the isolated dystonias, constituting fewer than 1% of all cases (see Chapter 4, "Epidemiology of the Dystonias").

A NOTE ABOUT NOMENCLATURE

Classification Based on Body Distribution

Exactly which body regions and how many regions must be affected to define *generalized* dystonia is bit arbitrary, and criteria have changed over the years (see Chapter 3). Historically, generalized dystonia was defined by involvement of both legs and at least one other body region.[2–6] This definition derived from observations that individuals with early-onset dystonia often had leg involvement before it spread to other regions. *Bicrural dystonia* may be relatively common in children with generalized dystonia, but it is uncommon in adults.

The 2013 Dystonia Consensus group suggested that generalized dystonia should be defined instead by involvement of the trunk and at least two additional regions.[1] A limitation of this approach is that truncal dystonia is often underreported. Truncal dystonia is easily overlooked in individuals with more obvious dystonia in other body regions. In addition, truncal dystonia has many manifestations, some of which have specific labels that are not readily recognized as dystonic. Truncal dystonia can include forward flexion, as in the dromedary gait of individuals with dystonia associated with the *TOR1A* gene or parkinsonism, where it is often called *camptocormia*.[3,52] Truncal dystonia can be manifested also as backward arching or spasms, often seen in tardive dystonias or metabolic dystonias, where it is called opisthotonos.[47] Bending of the trunk may be labeled *scoliosis*, and more obvious bending at the hip is called *Pisa* syndrome.[10,16,43,54] Some individuals may have only truncal jerking or wobbling. Concerns about poor recognition of the many manifestations of truncal dystonia have been confirmed in studies that it is reported for fewer than 5% of cases with genetic disorders typically linked with generalized dystonia.[32]

Because it remains unclear if core defining features of generalized dystonia should include both legs or the trunk, terms referring to the distribution of dystonia in the body should be viewed as guidelines rather than rules. Accordingly, the 2025 Dystonia Consensus group suggested that the definition of generalized dystonia should be more flexible, for example including three limbs even without the trunk.[2] Regardless of how generalized dystonias are defined, there can be many different combinations of body regions affected. These combinations tend to cluster into syndromic patterns defined by the underlying etiology, although there is considerable overlap among these syndromes.

The precise definition of "segmental" dystonia also is a bit arbitrary (see Chapter 3). Historically there were no guidelines for defining *single* body regions, leading to variations of opinion regarding how to discriminate focal from segmental dystonia. For example, some movement disorder specialists consider the upper and lower face to be separate regions, while others consider them to be one region, leading to disagreement regarding whether the combination is a segmental or focal dystonia.[29] A similar arbitrary division occurs when considering the hand versus the arm. There also were no guidelines defining contiguous body regions, resulting also in some variations of opinion regarding *segmental* versus *multifocal* dystonia. An example here involves the neck and larynx, which are often affected together.[30] There also remains some uncertainty regarding how many body regions may be combined in *segmental* or *multifocal* dystonia before it should be classified as *generalized*. Specific guidelines now exist for common focal and segmental patterns, such as cervical dystonia or blepharospasm,[29,30] but similar guidelines are lacking for most body regions. This chapter focuses on generalized dystonias, but it includes patterns that may also be considered segmental or multifocal.

Classification as Isolated Versus Combined Dystonia

Criteria that distinguish relatively pure forms of dystonia from disorders where dystonia is combined with other problems are also a bit arbitrary, leading again to different opinions regarding what disorders to include among the *isolated* generalized dystonias. It is important to remember that characteristics of isolated dystonia are defined by clinical phenomenology only (Axis I of the classification system) not etiology or pathogenesis (Axis II of the classification system). Axis I and Axis II are not tightly correlated (see Chapter 3), so an individual may present with a clinical picture of isolated dystonia, but the etiology may be more often associated with combined dystonia.

A well-known example of this imperfect correlation between Axis I and Axis II is dopa-responsive dystonia caused by pathogenic variants in *GCH1*.[51] This gene is normally considered among the combined dystonias because a significant portion of individuals also have some parkinsonism, and, in some cases, the parkinsonian features predominate (see Chapter 13). However, many individuals may have isolated dystonia without parkinsonism. Another good example is the myoclonus dystonia syndrome associated with genetic variants in *SGCE*.[53] Some individuals present with a clinical phenotype of isolated dystonia, some present with myoclonus alone (essential myoclonus), and many present with both dystonia and myoclonus (see Chapter 15, "Dystonia and Myoclonus"). As a result, *SGCE* also is normally considered among the combined dystonias, although it can cause the syndrome of isolated dystonia.

The frequency with which a second phenomenology must occur to link a gene with isolated versus combined dystonia is a bit arbitrary, leading to some differences of opinion regarding this distinction, too. For example, the *PRKRA* gene may be associated with isolated generalized dystonia, but a significant proportion of cases have developmental delay or parkinsonism. Similarly, *KMT2B* and *HPCA* can be associated with isolated dystonia, but many cases also have intellectual disability.[7,12,46] *TUBB4A* provides another example where the phenotype is varied. Pathogenic variants in this gene are most commonly associated with the syndrome of *hypomyelination and atrophy of the basal ganglia and cerebellum* (H-ABC syndrome), but a small number of cases (<50 total) have been described with an isolated dystonia syndrome that combines laryngeal dystonia often with additional involvement of the trunk and limbs.[8] In view of observations that these genes are commonly associated with dystonia that is combined with other features (*PRKRA, HPCA, KMT2B*), or even syndromes without dystonia (*TUBB4A*), some experts discuss these genes along with genes causing isolated segmental or generalized dystonias, while other experts discuss these genes with those genes that are more typically associated with combined dystonias. There is an imperfect correlation between clinical phenomenology and many other genes. The isolated dystonia phenotype may sometimes occur with almost all genes usually associated with more complicated phenotypes.

Evolution over Time

Most isolated generalized dystonias first present with involvement of one body region, followed by spread over several months or years to a generalized pattern.[35,56] In other words, focal dystonia may evolve to segmental or multifocal dystonia and later to generalized dystonia. Most such cases begin in childhood, and most have a genetic etiology. Adult-onset focal or segmental dystonia may also evolve to isolated generalized dystonia, but adult-onset cases that evolve to generalized dystonia are uncommon.

Just as a focal dystonia may evolve over time into a generalized distribution, an isolated dystonia may change to a combined dystonia. For the majority of genes typically associated with more complex phenotypes, the initial clinical impression of the phenomenology may be isolated dystonia. Associated features may be missed on initial evaluation because they are relatively mild. A good example is the mild intellectual disability often associated with *KMT2B* or *HPCA*, which is easy to miss during the routine neurological exam unless neuropsychological testing is conducted.[7,12,46]

Alternatively, associated clinical features may emerge over time. Examples include Wilson disease or Niemann-Pick type C, where the initial clinical impression may be isolated focal dystonia but progression of the neurodegenerative process eventually produces generalized dystonia and makes other features, such as dementia, more obvious. This potential evolution over time is important to keep in mind during the workup because the most appropriate way to classify an individual may change with time.

GENETIC SYNDROMES OF ISOLATED GENERALIZED DYSTONIA

Overview

Hundreds of genes can cause generalized dystonia (see Chapter 22, "Dystonia Genetics"). Most of these genes typically cause dystonia combined with other neurological or systemic features, although most can rarely present with the syndrome of isolated generalized dystonia. Only a few genes are consistently associated with isolated generalized dystonia without accompanying neurological or systemic features (Table 9.1). Most of these genes can sometimes also cause dystonia with a more limited focal or segmental pattern, too.

TOR1A

The *TOR1A* gene was the first gene to be linked with isolated generalized dystonia.[41] The associated disorder is most often called *DYT1 dystonia*, although alternative names such as *Oppenheim dystonia* or DYT-*TOR1A* have also been used. Early studies described a relatively characteristic phenotype,[9] but later studies revealed additional less-common phenotypes.[32] The typical age at onset is in a child or young teen. In one

Table 9.1 **Most common genes linked with isolated dystonia syndromes**

Gene	Inheritance	Gene product	Usual age at onset	Typical body distribution	Evolution to generalized
ANO3	Autosomal dominant	Anoctamin-3	Adulthood	Focal or segmental, with prominent neck involvement and tremor	Uncommon
COL6A3	Autosomal recessive	Alpha-3 subunit of type VI collagen	Early childhood	Segmental involving neck, arms	Common
GNAL	Autosomal dominant	G-protein subunit alpha-l	Adulthood	Segmental involving head, neck, arms	Uncommon
THAP1	Autosomal dominant	Thanatos-associated domain-containing apoptosis protein 1	Adolescence	Segmental involving head, neck, arms	Common
TOR1A	Autosomal dominant	TorsinA	Childhood	Segmental starting with limbs	Very common

meta-analysis of 694 cases, the median age at onset was 9 years with an interquartile range of 7–12 years. The complete range of onset was broad, from 1 to 70 years, but only 5% of individuals had onset after age 30 years. Males and females were nearly equally affected. The typical and most common evolution involved insidious onset of dystonia in one arm or leg, followed by spread over many months or years to other body regions into a broader pattern. Involvement of the face and larynx may occur, but they are uncommon. Less common variant phenotypes include limited spread that remains focal or segmental, or spread to generalized pattern following onset in the neck, larynx, or craniofacial region. In some cases, the phenotype is dominated by what appears to be an action or resting tremor, or repetitive jerking that resembles myoclonus.

The vast majority of cases (98%) with DYT1 dystonia harbor a genetic variant that consists of deletion of three bases (CAG) in *TOR1A*, although a handful of other genetic variants have also been reported.[15,22] The disorder is usually dominantly inherited, but penetrance among carriers is only 30%. Biallelic variants have been associated with congenital arthrogryposis multiplex type 5, with a spectrum of severity that varies from motor delay with mild gait disturbance to more severe global delay, severe flexion contractions, and early death.[44]

The common deletion can be explained by a founder effect in some populations, such as the Ashkenazi Jews. However, it appears to have arisen spontaneously in many other populations as well. The common deletion is in-frame, so it leads to deletion of a single amino acid (glutamate) in an otherwise intact protein. The exact functions of the normal protein (torsinA) have not been fully delineated.[22] The normal torsinA protein is found predominantly in the endoplasmic reticulum of most cells of the body, while the mutant protein tends to accumulate in the nuclear envelope. The consequences of this redistribution of the protein may have many effects, including mislocalization of partner proteins in the nucleus, endoplasmic reticulum, and downstream destinations of these other proteins, such as the Golgi apparatus or synapse. Routine clinical brain imaging is usually normal, but advanced imaging methods reveal abnormalities in all major nodes of the motor network responsible for dystonia, including the basal ganglia, cerebellum, and sensorimotor cortex. The precise mechanisms responsible for causing dystonia remain to be determined.

THAP1

Syndromes associated with variants in the *THAP1* gene have most often been called DYT6 dystonia or *THAP1*-related dystonia, but DYT-*THAP1* has also been used. Similar to *TOR1A* dystonia, *THAP1* dystonia has been associated with a relatively characteristic phenotype, but also with many variations. The typical age at onset is in a teen or young adult. In one early review, the mean age at onset was 16.8 years.[33] In a survey of 100 cases from the United Kingdom, the mean age at onset was 24.4 years of age.[53] In an aggregate analysis of 241 reports with case-level data, the median age at onset was 15 years with an interquartile range of 9–29 years. Onset ranged from 2 to 69 years.[32] In many studies, there was a slight preponderance of females compared to males. Unlike DYT1 dystonia, the typical body distributions for DYT6 dystonia include prominent involvement of the neck, upper limbs, and larynx. However, any region of the body can be affected, and patterns that remain focal or segmental are common. Coexisting tremor-like or jerking movements resembling myoclonus are common and may be the most prominent feature in some cases.

THAP1 encodes Thanatos-associated protein 1, which is a DNA transcription factor. This function means that it controls the synthesis of mRNAs responsible for other proteins. Genetic variants in *THAP1* dystonia are quite varied and include missense, nonsense, splice site defects, insertions and deletions, and others.[32] The disorder is dominantly inherited, with a penetrance of 48%. The precise proteins and mechanisms involved in the pathogenesis of dystonia remain to be determined. Routine clinical neuroimaging studies are usually normal, but advanced imaging methods reveal an impact on all nodes of the motor network responsible for dystonia, most notably the cerebellum.

GNAL

Syndromes associated with variants in the *GNAL* gene have been given a number of different labels including *GNAL*-associated dystonia, DYT25, and DYT-*GNAL*. This disorder has been associated with a relatively characteristic phenotype, along with many variations. The typical age at onset is in a young or middle-aged adult. In a meta-analysis of 76 cases, the median age at onset was 38 years with an interquartile range of 25–47 years.[32] Rarely, onset was as early as 2 years of age. Females accounted for approximately two-thirds of affected individuals. The typical body distributions involve the neck with segmental spread to the larynx and/or craniofacial regions. Involvement of the limbs and spread to more generalized patterns occurs less commonly. Phenotypes with prominent tremor or jerking movements resembling myoclonus may also occur,[11,20,40] and some cases may also have ataxia.[17]

GNAL encodes guanine nucleotide binding protein, alpha-activating L-subunit. This protein is sometimes referred to as G-olf or Golf, because it is a G-protein (guanine-nucleotide binding protein) first associated with neurons of the olfactory bulb. It is expressed in many brain regions, with high expression in the basal ganglia and particularly in synaptic terminals. It stimulates the activity of adenylate cyclase, a membrane-bound enzyme that converts adenosine triphosphate (ATP) to cyclic adenosine monophosphate (cAMP) during the process of neurotransmitter signal transduction. Therefore, the initial molecular mechanism of pathogenesis involves distortion of synaptic transmission, but how this distortion results in dystonia remains to be determined. Like *THAP1*, genetic variants of *GNAL* linked with dystonia are quite varied.[21,32] Inheritance is usually dominant, with insufficient cases reported to estimate penetrance. Biallelic variants were reported for two siblings from a consanguineous family.[36] The phenotype was more severe, with mild intellectual disability combined with hypertonia in the first year of age and subsequent evolution to generalized dystonia. Routine clinical brain imaging studies are normal.

ANO3

Syndromes associated with variants in the *ANO3* gene have been given a number of different labels including *ANO3*-associated dystonia, DYT24, and DYT-*ANO3*. The typical age at onset is in a young or middle-aged adult. In a meta-analysis of 53 cases, the median age at onset was 23 years with an interquartile range of 9–42 years.[32] Rarely, onset was in the first year of life or as late as 69 years of age. Females accounted for approximately 60% of affected individuals. The typical body distributions involve the neck, with prominent head tremor and head jerking. Presentations with head tremor alone were not uncommon. Spread to the shoulder and upper limbs was most common, spread to the craniofacial regions may also occur, but spread to more generalized patterns was less common.

ANO3 encodes the protein anoctamin-3. Like *THAP1* and *GNAL*, genetic variants are heterogeneous for *ANO3*.[21,32] Pathogenic *ANO3* variants are dominantly inherited, with too few cases reported to estimate penetrance. The protein is homologous with several other anoctamin proteins, which function as chloride channels. However, anoctamin-3 does not possess ion channel function and may instead be a regulatory subunit for these channels. Clinical brain imaging is normal, and the mechanisms leading to dystonia remain to be determined.

COL6A3

The *COL6A3* gene has been linked with isolated dystonia, with very few cases so far reported.[42] This gene is currently classified among the isolated dystonias, but this designation may change as more cases with broader phenotypes may be found. Onset is usually in late childhood or adolescence, starting as a focal dystonia involving the arms or neck, and then spreading to a segmental or generalized pattern.

The disorder is inherited in an autosomal recessive manner. The same gene has been associated with Ulrich congenital muscular dystrophy and Bethlehem myopathy. The gene encodes one of the subunits of type VI collagen, but the mechanisms responsible for causing dystonia remain to be determined.

OTHER SYNDROMES OF ISOLATED GENERALIZED DYSTONIA

Idiopathic

For both early-onset and late-onset cases, a genetic etiology cannot be established for some cases, even after extensive testing. These cases may be caused by known dystonia genes with genetic variants that are not detected by existing methods. Examples include genetic variants in non-coding regions of introns or upstream regulatory regions, which are not usually evaluated by routine clinical diagnostic tests. Alternatively, these cases may have variants in other dystonia genes that have yet to be discovered. It also is possible that some cases do not have a genetic etiology.

Acquired

There are relatively few acquired etiologies for isolated generalized dystonias. Medications that block dopamine receptors can cause both acute dystonic reactions and tardive dystonia. In both cases, there is often prominent involvement of extensor muscles of the neck and trunk, leading to retrocollis and opisthotonus. The face or limbs are sometimes affected, too, producing a clinical picture of isolated generalized dystonia, although many have some parkinsonian features as well (see Chapter 19, "Dystonia Induced by Medications, Illicit Drugs, and Environmental Exposures").

The syndrome of acute striatal necrosis is characterized by sudden and severe encephalopathy, usually in a child, with obvious bilateral abnormalities in the basal ganglia on MRI, followed by a recovery period during which many individuals develop generalized dystonia. Most of them also have some parkinsonism or cognitive impairment, so the syndrome is only rarely isolated dystonia. It can be caused by a number of different genes,[37,50] but it has also been reported following exposure to certain toxins found as food contaminants (3-nitropropionic acid)[24] or infection with mycoplasma[5,23,31] or *Streptococcus*.[13]

DIFFERENTIAL DIAGNOSIS AND WORKUP

Differential Diagnosis

Isolated generalized dystonia is usually readily recognizable because its phenomenology is unique. Nevertheless, there are a few mimics that should be considered, most notably cerebral palsy.[27,38] Historically, this diagnosis was given to young children with known or presumed perinatal brain injury. The clinical picture is quite varied, usually with some combination of corticospinal signs, dystonia, and ataxia. However, there are cerebral palsy subtypes dominated by only one of these problems, and some cases may have isolated generalized dystonia (see Chapter 16, "Dystonia and Cerebral Palsy"). In recent years, the diagnosis of cerebral palsy has become a descriptive label with many potential etiologies, and approximately a third have a genetic etiology.[18,34,39,55] Many young children are given this descriptive diagnosis before an etiological diagnosis is found, including children who have genetic isolated generalized dystonia.

For adults, the most frequent conditions referred for assessment of possible isolated generalized dystonia are neuromuscular disorders associated with the common problem of recurrent idiopathic cramping. Cramping may be quite severe, and it may involve many muscles throughout the body, occasionally raising concern for isolated generalized dystonia.[28,48] Many are idiopathic, but some may have myotonia. These neuromuscular disorders can usually be discriminated from dystonia by several features. They are often associated with a random and changing distribution of muscle involvement, rather than the more patterned muscle involvement of dystonia. The neuromuscular disorders are often associated with brief and very painful cramps, in contrast to the often longer and less painful movements more typical of dystonia. Finally, many cramp and myotonic disorders have characteristic features on electromyography (EMG) (see Chapter 26, "Pseudodystonia and Differential Diagnosis").[25]

Perhaps the second most common group of mimics to consider are the behavioral disorders. They are called *conversion disorder* or *somatoform disorder* in the psychiatry literature, and *functional* or *psychogenic dystonia* in the neurological literature as summarized in Chapter 25, "Psychogenic (Functional) Dystonia." Individuals with behavioral movement disorders may closely mimic isolated generalized dystonia. However, they can usually be identified by a number of features. Behavioral disorders are often associated with patterns of muscle involvement that are different from typical dystonias. Muscle involvement in typical dystonia is usually patterned, while involvement in behavioral disorders often changes over time. Sudden onset may occur in behavioral disorders, while most typical dystonias usually have a more insidious onset.

Finally, *stiff person syndrome* is an autoimmune disorder affecting inhibitory neurons of the spine and may involve spasms or abnormal postures of many regions of the body in a manner that could resemble isolated generalized dystonia.[6,45] Stiff person syndrome can usually be recognized by its proclivity for extensor muscles of the trunk and legs, frequent coexistence of startle reactions and diabetes mellitus, and abnormal serological testing for antibodies to glutamic acid decarboxylase or amphiphysin (see Chapter 21, "Dystonia and Autoimmunity").

Workup

Unlike the majority of isolated focal dystonias where an etiology cannot be found despite extensive workup, a cause can be found for many individuals with isolated generalized dystonia. Workup starts with a careful clinical evaluation aimed to delineate a potentially recognizable syndromic pattern (see Chapter 27, "Workup of Dystonia").[19]

The history should focus on age at onset and manner of progression because this information can help narrow the list of potential causes. For example, the usual age at onset varies considerably for many genes associated with isolated generalized dystonia (Figure 9.1), a diurnal pattern with worsening in the evening is suggestive of dopa-responsive dystonia, and sudden onset might point to a behavioral disorder. The exam should focus on which body regions are most affected (Figure 9.2) and whether there are any other clinical features that point to a more specific syndromic pattern. This information can also provide clues toward specific etiologies. For example, each gene associated with isolated generalized dystonia is associated with a relatively characteristic pattern of body involvement. Brain MRI is also useful because it is usually normal for genetic disorders typically associated with isolated generalized dystonias, and any detectable abnormality might point instead toward an acquired disorder.

When it comes to genetic testing, a family history is helpful, although some cases are sporadic. Partial penetrance combined with a predilection for females to be affected more than males for some genes (Figure 9.3) can make recognition of

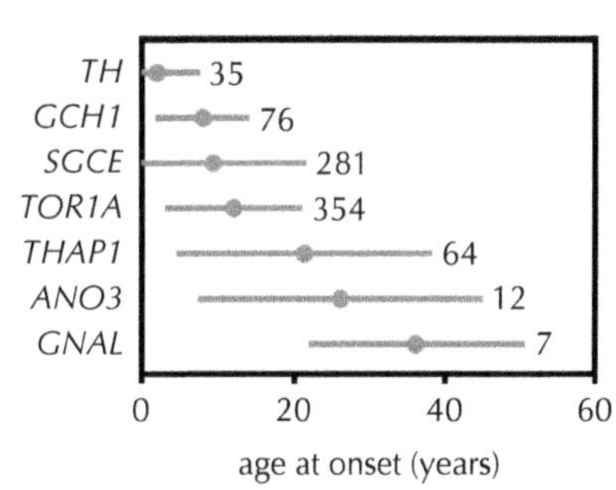

Figure 9.1. Age at onset for dystonia according to gene. This schematic shows the average age at onset (circular symbol) and standard deviation (bars) for select genes causing dystonia. Data were compiled from MDSgene (www.mdsgene.org).

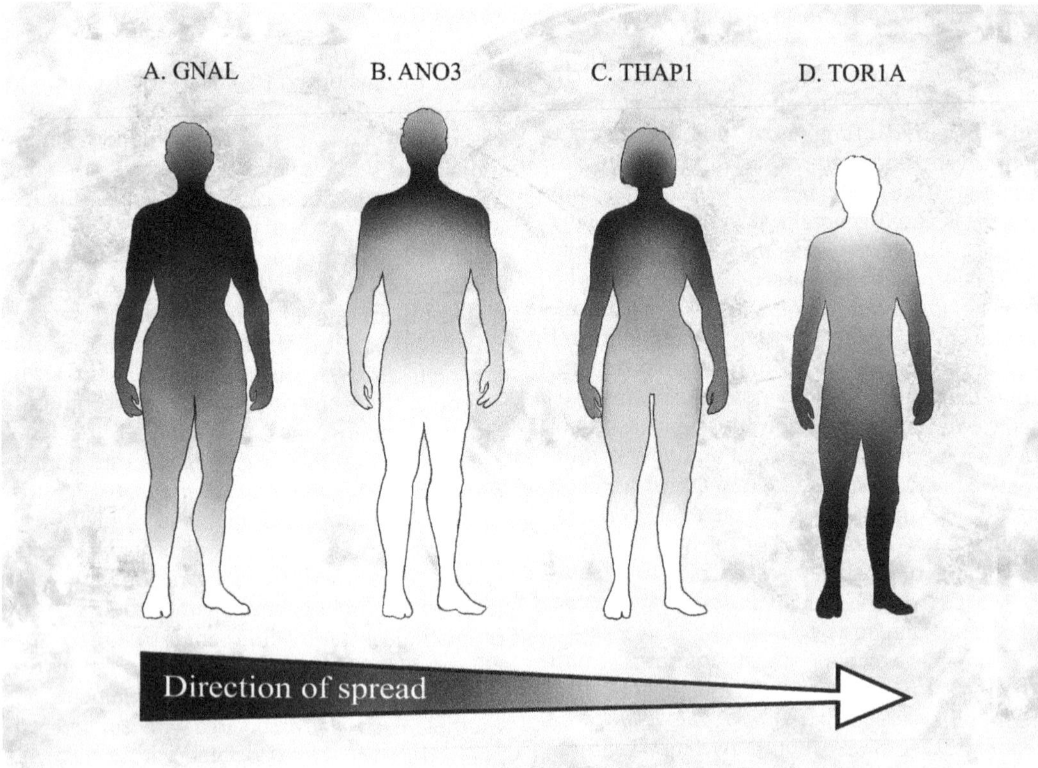

Figure 9.2. Body distributions for dystonia according to gene. This schematic shows how specific genes tend to impact different regions of the body. The arrows depict where dystonia initially starts and the direction of spread over time. Darker shading indicates regions most frequently affected, and lighter shading indicates less frequently affected. This diagram provides a general guideline only as many exceptions exist.

Illustration by Loren Bergantini.

family patterns difficult. It is sometimes tempting to use the phenotype to try to predict the most likely gene for testing. This strategy should be avoided because there is considerable overlap among the ages at onset and body distributions

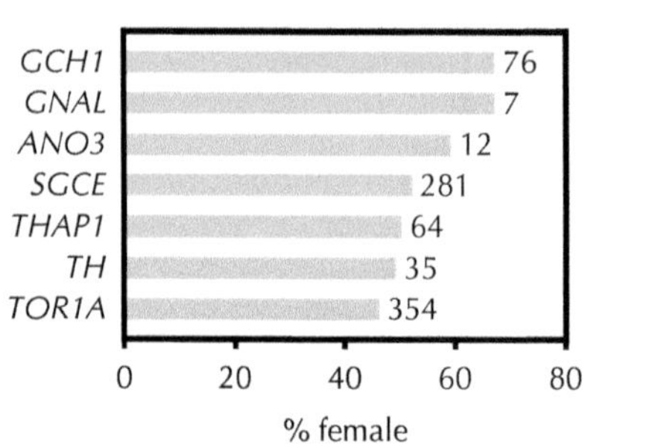

Figure 9.3. Sex distributions for dystonia according to gene. This schematic shows the percentage of females for select genes causing dystonia. Data were compiled from MDSgene (www.mdsgene.org).

for genes associated with generalized dystonia. A broader strategy such as exome sequencing is preferable to avoid the hassle and cost of sequential genetic testing. It is also tempting to focus testing only on a small panel of genes that cause isolated generalized dystonias. This strategy will miss many genes commonly linked with dystonia combined with other features because they may sometimes present with isolated dystonia before other features develop (see Chapter 22).

TREATMENT

The management of most generalized dystonias is largely symptom-based since there are few disease-specific treatments. Symptom-based oral medications can be at least partly helpful for many cases (see Chapter 28, “Symptom-Targeted

Oral Medications for Dystonia"). Targeted therapies are available for only a few disorders where the cause is better characterized (see Chapter 29, "Special Interventions for Certain Types of Dystonia"). Physical therapy may be useful to maintain function and prevent contractures (see Chapter 32, "Physiotherapy and Complementary Medicine for Dystonia"). The botulinum toxins can be useful for those in whom specific regions of the body are most problematic, such as individuals with prominent involvement of the neck, larynx, or an upper limb (see Chapter 30, "Botulinum Toxin Treatment for Dystonia").

Because oral therapies often produce only partial benefits and botulinum toxins address a limited number of muscles, surgical therapies often play a larger role in the treatment of generalized dystonia (see Chapter 31, "Surgical Treatments for Dystonia"). The value of deep brain stimulation depends on the etiology.[4,49] For *TOR1A*, consistently good outcomes for deep brain stimulation have been reported for relatively large numbers of cases. Poor outcomes are uncommon for *TOR1A* and should prompt reconsideration of surgical technique, stimulator settings, or equipment failure. For *THAP1*, responses are variable. While there are many reports of good outcomes, there are also reports of partial or poor outcomes. The reasons for this variability are not clear, but they may reflect differences in body regions affected in relation to the usual targets of stimulation. For *ANO3* and *GNAL*, progression to generalized dystonia is less common, and relatively small numbers of cases have been reported following surgery. The majority of reports describe favorable outcomes, but partial responses may also occur, and the risk of a publication bias favoring positive outcomes has to be considered.

SUMMARY AND FUTURE PROSPECTS

The isolated generalized dystonias are among the least common of all dystonias. They more commonly arise in childhood but may also arise in adults. Focal dystonias may spread over time, but precisely how much of the body must be affected to merit designations of segmental or generalized dystonia are a bit arbitrary.

Although they are the least common, they are the most disabling because the involvement of multiple body regions creates more serious disability and a greater impact on quality of life. A careful clinical and etiological evaluation is important because there are both acquired and genetic causes, often with implications for prognosis, risk for affecting other family members, and response to certain forms of treatment.

The mechanisms by which most genes cause isolated generalized dystonias are not well characterized. A variety of apparently unrelated biological mechanisms have been delineated,[55] and it is likely that they all impinge on the same sensorimotor network that causes dystonia. Because mechanisms are only partly understood, treatments are largely symptom-based. However, more specific targeted therapies exist for some of these disorders. As mechanisms for the genetic and acquired dystonias become better understood, it is likely that additional targeted therapies will be developed.

REFERENCES

1. Albanese A, Bhatia K, Bressman SB, DeLong MR, Fahn S, Fung VSC, et al. Phenomenology and classification of dystonia: A consensus update. Mov Disord 2013;28:863–873.
2. Albanese A, Bhatia K, Fung V, Hallett M, Jankovic J, et al. Definition and Classification of Dystonia, 2025 (first presented at the International Dystonia Symposium in 2023).
3. Ali F, Matsumoto JY, Hassan A. Camptocormia: Etiology, diagnosis, and treatment response. Neurol Clin Pract 2018;8:240–248.
4. Artusi CA, Dwivedi A, Romagnolo A, Bortolani S, Marsili L, Imbalzano G, et al. Differential response to pallidal deep brain stimulation among monogenic dystonias: Systematic review and meta-analysis. J Neurol Neurosurg Psychiatry 2020;91:426–433.
5. Ashtekar CS, Jaspan T, Thomas D, Weston V, Gayatri NA, Whitehouse WP. Acute bilateral thalamic necrosis in a child with Mycoplasma pneumoniae. Dev Med Child Neurol 2003;45:634–637.
6. Balint B, Charlesworth G, Erro R, Wood NW, Bhatia KP. Delineating the phenotype of autosomal-recessive HPCA mutations: Not only isolated dystonia! Mov Disord 2019;34:589–592.
7. Balint B, Vincent A, Meinck HM, Irani SR, Bhatia KP. Movement disorders with neuronal antibodies: Syndromic approach, genetic parallels and pathophysiology. Brain 2018;141:13–36.
8. Bally JF, Kern DS, Fearon C, Camargos S, Pereira da Silva-Junior F, Barbosa ER, et al. DYT-TUBB4A (DYT4 dystonia): Clinical anthology of 11 cases and systematized review. Mov Disord Clin Pract 2022;9:659–675.
9. Bressman SB, Sabatti C, Raymond D, de Leon D, Klein C, Kramer PL, et al. The DYT1 phenotype and guidelines for diagnostic testing. Neurology 2000;54:1746–1752.
10. Cannas A, Solla P, Floris G, Tacconi P, Serra A, Piga M, et al. Reversible Pisa syndrome in patients with

Parkinson's disease on dopaminergic therapy. J Neurol 2009;256:390–395.
11. Carecchio M, Panteghini C, Reale C, Barzaghi C, Monti V, Romito L, et al. Novel GNAL mutation with intra-familial clinical heterogeneity: Expanding the phenotype. Parkinsonism Relat Disord 2016;23:66–71.
12. Cif L, Demailly D, Lin JP, Barwick KE, Sa M, Abela L, et al. KMT2B-related disorders: Expansion of the phenotypic spectrum and long-term efficacy of deep brain stimulation. Brain 2020;143:3242–3261.
13. Dale RC, Church AJ, Benton S, Surtees RA, Lees A, Thompson EJ, et al. Post-streptococcal autoimmune dystonia with isolated bilateral striatal necrosis. Dev Med Child Neurol 2002;44:485–489.
14. Di Fonzo A, Albanese A, Jinnah HA. The apparent paradox of phenotypic diversity and shared mechanisms across dystonia syndromes. Curr Opin Neurol 2022;35:502–509.
15. Dobricic V, Kresojevic N, Zarkovic M, Tomic A, Marjanovic A, Westenberger A, et al. Phenotype of non-c.907_909delGAG mutations in TOR1A: DYT1 dystonia revisited. Parkinsonism Relat Disord 2015;21:1256–1259.
16. Doherty KM, van de Warrenburg BP, Peralta MC, Silveira-Moriyama L, Azulay JP, Gershanik OS, Bloem BR. Postural deformities in Parkinson's disease. Lancet Neurol 2011;10:538–549.
17. Erro R, Di Fonzo A, Percetti M, Monfrini E, Scannapieco S, Picillo M, Barone P. Childhood-onset dystonia with cerebellar signs: Expanding the spectrum of GNAL mutations. Eur J Neurol 2020;27:e66–e67.
18. Fahey MC, Maclennan AH, Kretzschmar D, Gecz J, Kruer MC. The genetic basis of cerebral palsy. Dev Med Child Neurol 2017;59:462–469.
19. Fung VS, Jinnah HA, Bhatia K, Vidailhet M. Assessment of the patient with dystonia: An update on dystonia syndromes. Mov Disord 2013;28:889–898.
20. Geoghegan AR, Al Hussona M, Beauchamp NJ, Hutchinson M, Sean O'Riordan MB, Lynch T, Webb D. A novel GNAL mutation in familial dystonia presenting with childhood tremor and myoclonus. Mov Disord 2019;34:923–924.
21. Gomez-Garre P, Jesus S, Perinan MT, Adarmes A, Alonso-Canovas A, Blanco-Ollero A, et al. Mutational spectrum of GNAL, THAP1 and TOR1A genes in isolated dystonia: Study in a population from Spain and systematic literature review. Eur J Neurol 2021;28:1188–1197.
22. Gonzalez-Alegre P. Advances in molecular and cell biology of dystonia: Focus on torsinA. Neurobiol Dis 2019;127:233–241.
23. Green C, Riley DE. Treatment of dystonia in striatal necrosis caused by Mycoplasma pneumoniae. Pediatr Neurol 2002;26:318–320.
24. He F, Zhang S, Qian G, Zhang C. Delayed dystonia with striatal CT lucencies induced by a mycotoxin (3-nitropropionic acid). Neurology 1995;45:2178–2183.
25. Hutto SK, Harrison TB. Electrodiagnostic assessment of hyperexcitable nerve disorders. Neurol Clin 2021;39:1083–1096.
26. Jinnah HA, Albanese A. The new classification for the dystonias: Why was it needed and how was it accomplished? Mov Disord Clin Pract 2014;1:280–284.
27. Jonsson U, Eek MN, Sunnerhagen KS, Himmelmann K. Cerebral palsy prevalence, subtypes, and associated impairments: A population-based comparison study of adults and children. Dev Med Child Neurol 2019;61:1162–1167.
28. Katzberg HD. Case studies in management of muscle cramps. Neurol Clin 2020;38:679–696.
29. Kilic-Berkmen G, Defazio G, Hallett M, Berardelli A, Ferrazzano G, Belvisi D, et al. Diagnosis and classification of blepharospasm: Recommendations based on empirical evidence. J Neurol Sci 2022;439:120319.
30. Kilic-Berkmen G, Pirio Richardson S, Perlmutter JS, Hallett M, Klein C, Wagle-Shukla A, et al. Current guidelines for classifying and diagnosing cervical dystonia: Empirical evidence and recommendations. Mov Disord Clin Pract 2021;9:183–190.
31. Kim JS, Choi IS, Lee MC. Reversible parkinsonism and dystonia following probable mycoplasma pneumoniae infection. Mov Disord 1995;10:510–512.
32. Lange LM, Junker J, Loens S, Baumann H, Olschewski L, Schaake S, et al. Genotype-phenotype relations for isolated dystonia genes: MDSGene systematic review. Mov Disord 2021;36:1086–1103.
33. LeDoux MS, Xiao J, Rudzinska M, Bastian RW, Wszolek ZK, Van Gerpen JA, et al. Genotype-phenotype correlations in THAP1 dystonia: Molecular foundations and description of new cases. Parkinsonism Relat Disord 2012;18:414–425.
34. MacLennan AH, Thompson SC, Gecz J. Cerebral palsy: Causes, pathways, and the role of genetic variants. Am J Obstet Gynecol 2015;213:779–788.
35. Marsden CD, Harrison MJ, Bundey S. Natural history of idiopathic torsion dystonia. Adv Neurol 1976;14:177–187.
36. Masuho I, Fang M, Geng C, Zhang J, Jiang H, Ozgul RK, et al. Homozygous GNAL mutation associated with familial childhood-onset generalized dystonia. Neurol Genet 2016;2:e78.
37. Mohammad SS, Angiti RR, Biggin A, Morales-Briceno H, Goetti R, Perez-Duenas B, et al. Magnetic resonance imaging pattern recognition in childhood bilateral basal ganglia disorders. Brain Commun 2020;2:fcaa178.
38. Monbaliu E, Himmelmann K, Lin JP, Ortibus E, Bonouvrie L, Feys H, et al. Clinical presentation and management of dyskinetic cerebral palsy. Lancet Neurol 2017;16:741–749.
39. Moreno-De-Luca A, Millan F, Pesacreta DR, Elloumi HZ, Oetjens MT, Teigen C, et al. Molecular diagnostic yield of exome sequencing in patients with cerebral palsy. JAMA 2021;325:467–475.
40. O'Connor A, Buckley M, O'Sullivan SS. Teenage onset head tremor due to novel mutation in GNAL gene. Mov Disord Clin Pract 2017;4:903–904.
41. Ozelius LJ, Hewett JW, Page CE, Bressman SB, Kramer PL, Shalish C, et al. The early-onset torsion dystonia gene (DYT1) encodes an ATP-binding protein. Nature Genet 1997;17:40–48.
42. Panda PK, Sharawat IK. COL6A3 mutation associated early-onset isolated dystonia (DYT)-27: Report of a new case and review of published literature. Brain Dev 2020;42:329–335.
43. Pellene A, Saenz-Farret M, Micheli F. Recurrent and alternating Pisa syndrome. Clin Neuropharmacol 2015;38:252–254.
44. Saffari A, Lau T, Tajsharghi H, Karimiani EG, Kariminejad A, Efthymiou S, et al. The clinical and genetic spectrum of autosomal-recessive TOR1A-related disorders. Brain 2023;146:3273–3288.

45. Sarva H, Deik A, Ullah A, Severt WL. Clinical spectrum of stiff person syndrome: A Review of recent reports. Tremor Other Hyperkinet Mov 2016;6:340.
46. Siegert S, Schmidt WM, Pletschko T, Bittner RE, Gobara S, Freilinger M. Specific cognitive changes due to hippocalcin alterations? A aovel familial homozygous hippocalcin variant associated with inherited dystonia and altered cognition. Neuropediatrics 2021;52: 377–382.
47. Stamelou M, Lai SC, Aggarwal A, Schneider SA, Houlden H, Yeh TH, et al. Dystonic opisthotonus: A "red flag" for neurodegeneration with brain iron accumulation syndromes? Mov Disord 2013;28:1325–1329.
48. Swash M, Czesnik D, de Carvalho M. Muscular cramp: Causes and management. Eur J Neurol 2019;26: 214–221.
49. Tisch S, Kumar KR. Pallidal deep brain stimulation for monogenic dystonia: The effect of gene on outcome. Front Neurol 2021;11:630391.
50. Tonduti D, Chiapparini L, Moroni I, Ardissone A, Zorzi G, Zibordi F, et al. Neurological disorders associated with striatal lesions: Classification and diagnostic approach. Curr Neurol Neurosci Rep 2016;16:54.
51. Weissbach A, Pauly MG, Herzog R, Hahn L, Halmans S, Hamami F, et al. Relationship of genotype, phenotype, and treatment in dopa-responsive dystonia: MDSGene review. Mov Disord 2021;2022:237–252.
52. Wijemanne S, Jankovic J. Hand, foot, and spine deformities in parkinsonian disorders. J Neural Transm 2019;126:253–264.
53. Xiromerisiou G, Houlden H, Scarmeas N, Stamelou M, Kara E, Hardy J, et al. THAP1 mutations and dystonia phenotypes: Genotype phenotype correlations. Mov Disord 2012;27:1290–1294.
54. Yokochi F. Lateral flexion in Parkinson's disease and Pisa syndrome. J Neurol 2006;253 Suppl 7:17–20.
55. Zech M, Jech R, Boesch S, Skorvanek M, Weber S, Wagner M, et al. Monogenic variants in dystonia: An exome-wide sequencing study. Lancet Neurol 2020;19:908–918.
56. Zilber N, Inzelberg R, Kahana E, Korczyn AD. Natural course of idiopathic torsion dystonia among Jews. Neuroepidemiology 1994;13:195–201.

Chapter 10

Musician's and Other Task-Specific Dystonias

INTRODUCTION

The task-specific dystonias (TSDs) are a unique subgroup of focal dystonias. As suggested by the term, TSDs emerge only when performing a specific task and not when performing other actions.[21,65,78,84] Although a single task triggers dystonia in any one individual, the types of tasks vary among individuals. The problem may remain task-specific, but sometimes a second task may also begin to trigger dystonia over time, and occasionally the task-specificity is lost and dystonia occurs with any activity.

The first detailed description of task-specific dystonia was *writer's cramp*. According to William Gowers,[23] writer's cramp was first recognised by Charles Bell in 1830, in British civil service clerks who were afflicted by abnormal hand movements when attempting to write, yet they had no neuromuscular deficit, nor impairment of other actions. Following Bell's description of writer's cramp, Solly coined the term *scrivener's palsy* or the *paralysis of writers*, recognizing the problem as a rare condition where the "muscles cease to obey the mandates of the will" when writing.[77] He described "a set of muscles being cramped and paralysed by long-continued exertion," and noted that Virchow had also earlier described "shoemakers' cramp, cow milking cramp, musicians' cramp, compositors' cramp, and sempstresses' cramp."[85] Hammond used the term *writer's spasm* in the first edition of his textbook of neurology, linking it to individuals in professions "who are required by any employment to perform delicate, complex, or uniform actions with the fingers for many hours each day."[26] He cited additional examples of cramps in violinists, pianists, watch-makers, jewelers and seamstresses. Hammond later coined the term *anapeiratic paralysis* (meaning "to do or attempt again") to emphasize the "habitual use of a particular class of muscles in the same way for a long time" as a potential cause. In his text *Diseases of the Nervous System*, Gowers entitled a chapter "Occupation Neuroses," adopting it from the German *Beschaftigungsneurosen* (meaning "employment neurosis") and added additional occupational cramps in telegraphists, metalsmiths, painters, harpists, artificial flowermakers, turners, knitters, engravers, masons, enamelers, cigarette makers, shoemakers, milkers, money counters, and even zither players.[23] He also recognized that TSDs could affect more than a single skill (e.g., piano playing as well as writing), yet other activities using the same limb were spared. Although these cramps were considered neurological conditions by these early authors, there ensued a debate over the next century about whether they were neurological or psychiatric in origin.[19,21]

Sheehy and Marsden were the first to propose that writer's cramp was a manifestation of focal dystonia, noting that it could be purely task-specific (simple writer's cramp), affect other tasks as well (dystonic writer's cramp), or it could be the initial or an accompanying manifestation of more widespread segmental or generalized dystonia.[69] Afflictions among athletes, including "the yips" in golfers, were described soon after.[45] Many TSDs in other regions have been described, for example the oromandibular region in musicians,[34] lower limbs in runners,[87] and the neck.[6,37,67] This chapter describes the key features of the more common types of TSD.

EPIDEMIOLOGY

The epidemiology of TSD is partly addressed in Chapter 8, "Limb Dystonias" and Chapter 4, "Epidemiology of Dystonia." In most epidemiological studies, TSDs are relatively rare or they are not specifically distinguished from other types of dystonia. However, they are likely to be more common than reported because mild manifestations are often not recognized or reported.

One epidemiological study from North America suggested writer's cramp to be a relatively uncommon subtype of dystonia, with an estimated prevalence of approximately 1:15,000 individuals.[51] However, another epidemiological study from India suggested that focal hand dystonia, and particularly writer's cramp, was the most common of all types of dystonia.[12] These differences likely reflect how writer's cramp was ascertained and additional cultural issues that may influence self-reporting of various ailments.

Unlike most other focal dystonias that are more common in female individuals, some studies have suggested writer's cramp to be more common in male individuals.[2,29,69,82] However, many of these studies were relatively small, and some of the largest studies have suggested more female than male individuals with writer's cramp.[64,76] In addition, the sex distribution seems to depend on task, with a more obvious prevalence of females for walking-induced dystonia and laryngeal dystonia (Figure 10.1). The age at onset also seems to vary across task-specific dystonias (Figure 10.2).

One key risk factor for TSD involves very frequent repetition of an activity in a susceptible individual. As a result, the prevalence of a TSD will be influenced by both the proportion of the population who are vulnerable and the number of people who repetitively engage in a particular task. For example, telegraphist's cramp affected 14% of employees in an Australian study from 1970, but has disappeared alongside the telegram.[17] An epidemic of writer's cramp was first recognized in Britain at a time when many in the civil service were required to write copiously as part of their profession, possibly exacerbated by the introduction of a new steel writing nib.[57,77] Writer's cramp may now be less common, being replaced by TSDs related to computer use, such as typist's cramp or mouser's cramp.[10,69,80]

In comparison to the changing needs for the telegraph and handwriting, amateur and professional musicians have always existed, and many practice extensively to perfect their technique. The prevalence of musician's dystonia has been estimated to be approximately 1% of all musicians.[1] In musicians who use their hands to play an instrument, the more dextrous limb tends to be affected. In brass or woodwind players, the oromandibular region can be affected and sometimes other craniofacial regions. Unlike other focal dystonias among adults, there is a clear male preponderance for musician's dystonia, although this may reflect the greater number of professional male muscians.[19]

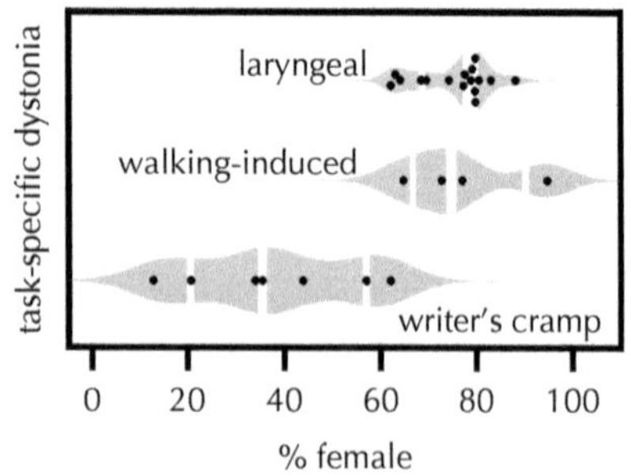

Figure 10.1. Sex distribution for task-specific dystonias. This figure shows the distribution of female and male individuals for studies in the literature that included at least 50 cases of writer's cramp, 10 cases of walking dystonia, or 100 cases of laryngeal dystonia. When the same center had multiple reports over the years, only the largest series was included.

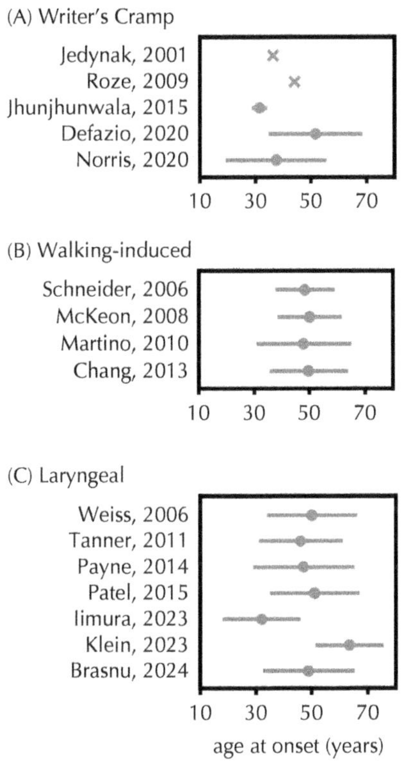

Figure 10.2. Age at onset for task-specific dystonia. This figure shows the average (±SD) age at onset for studies in the literature that included at least 50 cases of writer's cramp, 10 cases of walking dystonia, or 100 cases of laryngeal dystonia. When the same center had multiple reports over the years, only the largest series was included.

CLINICAL FEATURES

History

The diagnosis of TSD should be suspected in any person who presents with a history of progressive difficulty performing a single action, with preservation of the ability to perform other actions normally with the same body part. Sometimes more than one task may be affected, but the affected body region can do other tasks normally. The difficulty in performing the task may be described as inability to perform a task, loss of dexterity or skill, an unnatural feeling to the action, cramping, or pain. The task affected may be unusually specific at first before more obvious features become apparent. For example, there are individuals whose complaint was being unable to write a single number or a single letter for several years before writing other numbers and letters became more generally affected.[68] There are similar reports of task-specific laryngeal dystonia in individuals who began with difficulty only with very specific words or sounds before affecting other aspects of speech (see Chapter 7, "Laryngeal Dystonias").

The upper limbs are most commonly affected, presumably because they are most commonly used for highly trained and repetitive tasks, but almost any body part can be affected including the mouth, neck, trunk, and lower limbs. The evolution of disability is usually slow, typically over many months or even years, starting with minor difficulties only after sustained performance of the task for long periods. Later there is gradual progression so that difficulties are more severe and appear after a shorter interval of performance, typically minutes. Later still, abnormal postures may begin immediately upon starting the task. However, even when severe, symptoms still worsen with ongoing task performance rather than being maximal from the start.

The earliest reported symptoms of TSD affecting the upper limbs are often sensory, such as fatigue, or nonspecific tension or pain when performing the offending action. Individuals may complain of dysesthesia but not true loss of sensation. In writer's cramp, discomfort may be due to spasm or cramping during writing and therefore localized over the forearm or intrinsic hand muscles, but it can sometimes be localized instead over the joints or more proximal upper limb or neck. A TSD involving walking may be associated with painful leg cramps. For TSD of the upper and lower limbs, there usually is relief from discomfort when the task stops. Except for the limbs where pain or soreness are common with TSD, individuals with TSD in other body parts do not usually experience pain, although they may report other sensory symptoms. The affected individual may know of one or more *gestes antagonistes* (sensory tricks) that they can use to counteract the problem.

Major sensory or motor symptoms outside of performing the task should be absent. However, some individuals may complain of loss of sense of the position of the affected body part when performing an action, for example not knowing exactly where the hand and fingers of the affected hand are in a guitarist or loss of a sense of where the lips are in a wind instrument player with embouchure dystonia. Others report an unnatural feeling of the limb when performing the task. Some individuals may use the term *weakness*, where they are likely describing difficulty in wilfully moving the fingers and not true weakness. True weakness is usually absent. Occasionally the main complaint may be that the skilled movement is interrupted by jerking, spasm, tremor, or other abnormal movement. Although abnormal postures are a defining feature of dystonia, few individuals with TSD complain of abnormal posturing.

Eventually, the dominant complaint among individuals with TSD is difficulty or loss of skill in performing the affected action. Although most individuals will volunteer that the difficulty is restricted to a specific action, sometimes the significance of the task for diagnosis and a history of task-specificity must be explicitly ascertained.

Examination

The neurological examination in TSD should be normal when the individual is not performing the task. Since the dystonia is only present during a specific task, it follows that the affected individual should be examined performing the triggering action. The examination may require use of a particular tool, such as a pen or musical instrument. Instructions should be given to bring the tool if required, even if it is a large musical instrument. When the precise environment cannot be reproduced, it is sometimes feasible to review a video of the problem.

The key findings that allow a diagnosis of TSD are the presence of abnormal motor signs when performing the task but not other actions using the same body region. When not performing the offending task, there usually are no abnormal movements. A key element is the emergence of patterned (stereotyped) abnormal posturing with the task. The abnormal postures or movements are usually in the body part performing the main movement but occasionally may occur in muscles used for postural support to allow the action to be performed. For example, an individual with writer's cramp may experience involuntary excessive curling or extension of one or more fingers holding a pen. Alternatively, there may be overflow to the arm, with excessive flexion of the elbow or abduction of the shoulder. Another common finding is jerking or tremor of the affected body region when performing the task. These movements may occur in isolation, or they may be combined with abnormal postures.

Despite sensory complaints, sensation is usually normal when tested at the bedside. Similarly, even if the individual complains of weakness, power and reflexes are usually normal. It is important to consider whether the abnormal movements observed are pathological or compensatory. Many individuals can describe compensatory movements as volitional strategies to compensate for abnormal movements, such as an unusual manner of holding a pen or musical instrument. Others may be unaware that some abnormal movements reflect behavioral compensations that were unconsciously learned.

SOME EXAMPLES

The Spectrum

A huge number of different TSDs have been reported, so it is not practical to list every task and its variations. Novel forms of TSD continue to be reported in the modern literature. To give an indication of the breadth of the clinical spectrum, the most recently reported TSD include running-induced cervical dystonia,[37] weaver's dystonia,[4] vada maker's dystonia,[8] billiard player's dystonia,[20,75] axial dystonia when sitting in the lotus position,[43] leg dystonia when walking down stairs,[3,47] dystonic tremulous movements triggered by stepping on the brakes,[88] "club-cutting" hair,[63] pharyngeal or palatal dystonia when speaking,[56,71,72] and dystonia when using a computer mouse.[80]

The most well-characterized TSDs involve writing and playing musical instruments. The section below describes a few of the classic TSDs to provide some examples of what can be observed.

Writer's Cramp

Several large descriptive series of writer's cramp have been published, dividing individuals into various subgroups for comparisons (Table 10.1). One large early study divided cases into simple writer's cramp (only writing was affected) or complex writer's cramp (at least one additional task was affected).[30] Subsequent studies addressed whether flexion or extension movements were the main problem.[11,64] A later study addressed flexion or extension abnormalities according to

Table 10.1 **Descriptive studies of writer's cramp**

Study	Cases	Female (%)	Age at onset	Notes
Soland 1996[76]	186	33.9	NR	Few clinical details were provided other than sex distribution
Jedynak 2001[30]	65	35.4	36.3±NR	Subjects were classified as simple (WC only, *N* = 32) or complex (other tasks also affected, *N* = 33)
Das 2007[11]	141	20.6	NR	Subjects were classified as mainly flexion (*N* = 81) extension (*N* = 27), or dystonic tremor (*N* = 15)
Roze 2009[64]	104	62	44*	Subjects were classified as mainly flexion (*N* = 57), extension (*N* = 23), or pronation-supination (*N* = 9)
Jhunjhunwala 2015[31]	125	12.8	31.5±2.7	Subjects were classified according to region affected as wrist (*N* = 125), thumb (*N* = 104), fingers (*N* = 71), or upper arm (*N* = 12)
Defazio 2020[13]	70	43.9	43.8±15.9	Subjects were classified as focal or segmental patterns, or cases with or without spread
	112	52.7	51.6±16.7	These subjects did not have task-specificity, and had a greater tendency to spread than those with WC
Norris 2020[50]	367	57	37.5±18.1	All types of upper limb dystonia were included and classified into those with task-specificity (*N* = 246) vs no task-specificity; and those with spread to other regions (*N* = 195) vs no spread

This table summarizes studies that included at least 50 participants with writer's cramp (WC) where there was also additional clinical information on coexisting features. Age at onset is given usually in years ± standard deviation and sometimes as median (*).

Abbreviations: NR, not reported; WC, writer's cramp.

which region of the upper limb was affected.[31] The most recent studies focused on comparing writer's cramp with upper limb dystonias that are not task-specific or on risk factors for spread to another body region.[13,50]

Early in the illness, affected individuals may not experience overtly abnormal postures or movement but rather only feel tension or spasm of forearm muscles, which may be palpable. Involuntary flexion of the fingers is more common than extension (Figures 10.3 and 10.4).[11,31,64] Excessive flexion leads to progressive tightness of finger grip, with or without flexion of the wrist. Sometimes this finger flexion will lead to the affected fingers slipping off the shaft of the pen. In contrast, in extensor writer's cramp, typically the index finger (or less commonly the thumb) lifts off the pen with writing. This may lead to loss of pen grip and the pen slipping from the hand. Some affected individuals will attempt to overcome the tendency for the digits to lift off the pen by increasing activation of the finger flexors. Thus, with both flexor and extensor writer's cramp, the most obvious finding, at least initially when attempting to write, may be excessively forceful grip on the pen leading to the fingertips going pale due to reduced circulation, or intermittent stopping after writing a few words or sentences to rest or re-grip the pen.

In addition to abnormal flexion or extension of the fingers, dystonic posturing may also affect the wrist, leading to excessive flexion or

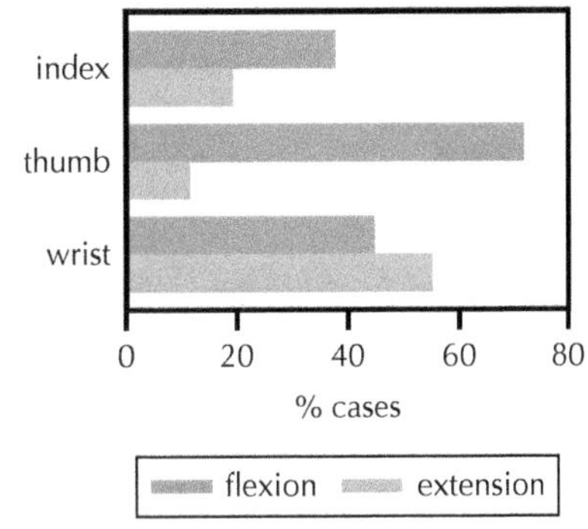

Figure 10.3. Hand involvement among 125 cases with writer's cramp focussing on the most common regions including the index finger, thumb, and wrist. Generated from results presented in a prior publication.[43]

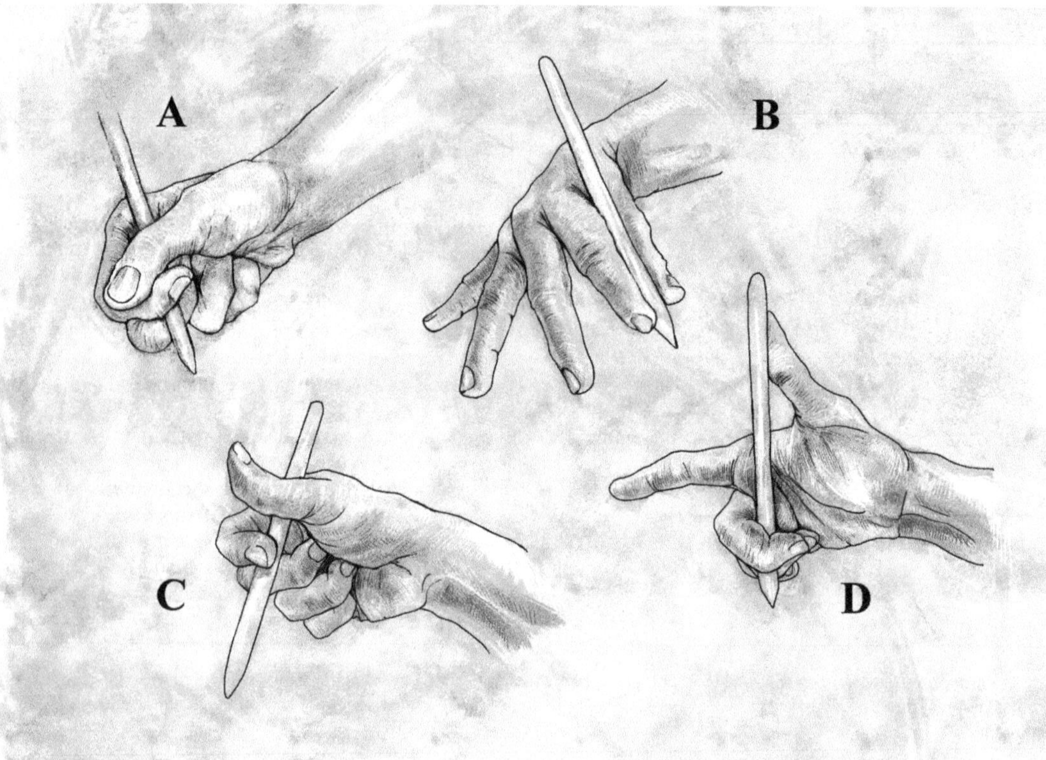

Figure 10.4. Examples of writer's cramp. These drawings show various abnormal postures in writer's cramp. Panel A shows excessive flexion of multiple digits, while Panel B shows excessive wrist flexion with splaying of the hand due to excessive extension of the digits. Panel C show a more complex combination of excessive flexion of digits 3–5 with extension of the thumb, and Panel D shows another complex combination of flexion with excessive extension of the thumb and forefinger and flexion of digits 3–5.

Illustration by Loren Bergantini.

extension, ulnar or radial deviation, or pronation or supination. The elbow is affected relatively less commonly, but more often the shoulder with progressive elevation during writing that can be accompanied by neck flexion. When the wrist extends, there may be compensatory elevation of the arm as a behavioral compensation to keep the pen in contact with the paper. Shoulder elevation can lead to compensatory elbow extension or a hunched posture with the elbow flexed and pushing against the table to keep the pen on the page.

In addition to abnormal posturing, approximately 50% of individuals will develop additional involuntary movements, either tremor or jerks, when attempting to write.[11,31,64] Sometimes jerking will be the dominant abnormality rather than abnormal posturing. Some individuals with tremor that is limited to the task of writing will have no observable abnormal posturing, raising the question of whether they have primary writing tremor. It is still debated whether primary writing tremor is a *forme fruste* of dystonia, a variant of essential tremor, or an independent entity, with evidence for and against each of these possibilities (see Chapter 12, "Dystonia and Tremor").[14,33,52,54,59]

Approximately 30–50% of affected individuals will exhibit *mirror dystonia*.[11,74] Mirror dystonia can be elicited by instructing the individual to write with the unaffected hand, leaving the affected hand at rest. The hypothenar eminence of the affected hand is relaxed in mid supination/pronation on a desk, or the forearm is rested on an elevated platform such as a pile of books or box with their pronated hand hanging passively over the edge. Writing with the unaffected hand will evoke dystonic posturing in the affected hand. Usually the mirror dystonia is not as severe as when using the affected limb for the task. This phenomenon can be useful in confirming the diagnosis and in clarifying what is the pathological dystonic posturing as opposed to any compensatory movements or postures.[55,73]

Musician's Dystonia

Oromandibular dystonia may also be a TSD in musicians (Figure 10.5A).[81] The term *embouchure* refers to the way a musician applies the lips, mouth, and tongue to the mouthpiece of a wind instrument. The formation of the embouchure differs according to whether it is a brass instrument, single- or double-reed instrument, or a flute. In brass instruments, pitch and airflow are controlled by adjusting the mouth aperture, especially the upper lip in higher register instruments. In single-reed instruments, such as the clarinet and saxophone, upper lip control dominates. In comparison, in double-reed instruments, such as the oboe and bassoon, the upper and lower lips contribute equally. Flautists control the direction and velocity of airflow using mainly the upper lip.[81] Embouchure dystonia typically affects the perioral region or tongue.

In a cross-sectional study of 585 professional players of brass wind instruments, 59% reported self-perceived embouchure problems, with 30% reporting embouchure fatigue and 26% embouchure cramping.[79] Given such a high rate of self-reported problems and variations in normal technique, it may be challenging to differentiate what is a true embouchure dystonia as opposed to a non-dystonic embouchure problem such as poor technique. Diagnostic criteria have been suggested.[86] Six characteristic patterns of embouchure dystonia have been recognized: tremor and lip-pulling (more common in high-register brass players), lip-locking (more common in low register brass players), jaw or tongue dystonia (wind players), and craniofacial dystonia (a smaller percentage of musicians).[18] The differential diagnosis includes neuromuscular disease such as infraorbital neuropathy or musculoskeletal issues such as muscle tear or temporomandibular joint disease.

Individuals with embouchure dystonia often report initial difficulties when playing a specific register or with specific techniques employed to switch notes. They may also lose ability to sustain trains of notes in terms of timing, pitch, or volume. Problems initially are more likely to occur with more difficult passages. Some individuals will develop stereotyped involuntary movements affecting components of the facial musculature, especially tremulous movements, or inappropriate movements ("lip pulling") which break the seal of their embouchure leading to air escape. In these cases, the diagnosis of dystonia is relatively easy. Others may clamp down too tightly onto the mouthpiece ("lip-lock" or "jaw-lock"). In subtle cases where individuals simply complain of fatigue or loss of coordination (e.g., "losing my lips" or "losing my buzz") without obvious involuntary movements, the diagnosis can be more difficult. A complaint of cramping supports the diagnosis,[79] whereas frank pain and discomfort are more supportive of a non-dystonic problem.[81] Affected individuals may not be aware of the precise nature of their impairment. They may even describe difficulty sensing the relationship between their mouth and mouthpiece, but there should be no evidence of sensory abnormality on formal testing.

Musicians can also develop hand dystonia (Figure 10.5B–C).[1,58,65,78] The hand with more demand (e.g., the right hand in pianists, the left hand in violinists, or the right hand in guitarists) is more commonly affected. Initially there may be only loss of dexterity. Eventually focal abnormal posturing occurs. Like writer's cramp, abnormal movements involve finger flexion more than extension. In a pianist, typical findings include slowness or difficulty lifting one or more (usually adjacent) fingers off the keys after playing a note, or progressive curling of the fingers due to excessive flexion at the distal or proximal interphalangeal or metacarpophalangeal joints in the readiness position. Excessive finger flexion may cause the finger to slip from its correct position with the musical instrument, a finding more common with wind instruments than keyboards, perhaps because piano keys are larger than wind instrument keys. Compensatory postures may be adopted. Other involuntary movements, both tremor and jerks, can be present. Pain is usually not a feature and should lead to the suspicion of a musculoskeletal or overuse syndrome or peripheral nerve entrapment. Commencing instruction before the age of 10 years old may be a protective factor.[58] Almost half of all individuals with musician's dystonia will have another affected task, such as writing or computer keyboarding, although the second task is usually not as severely affected.

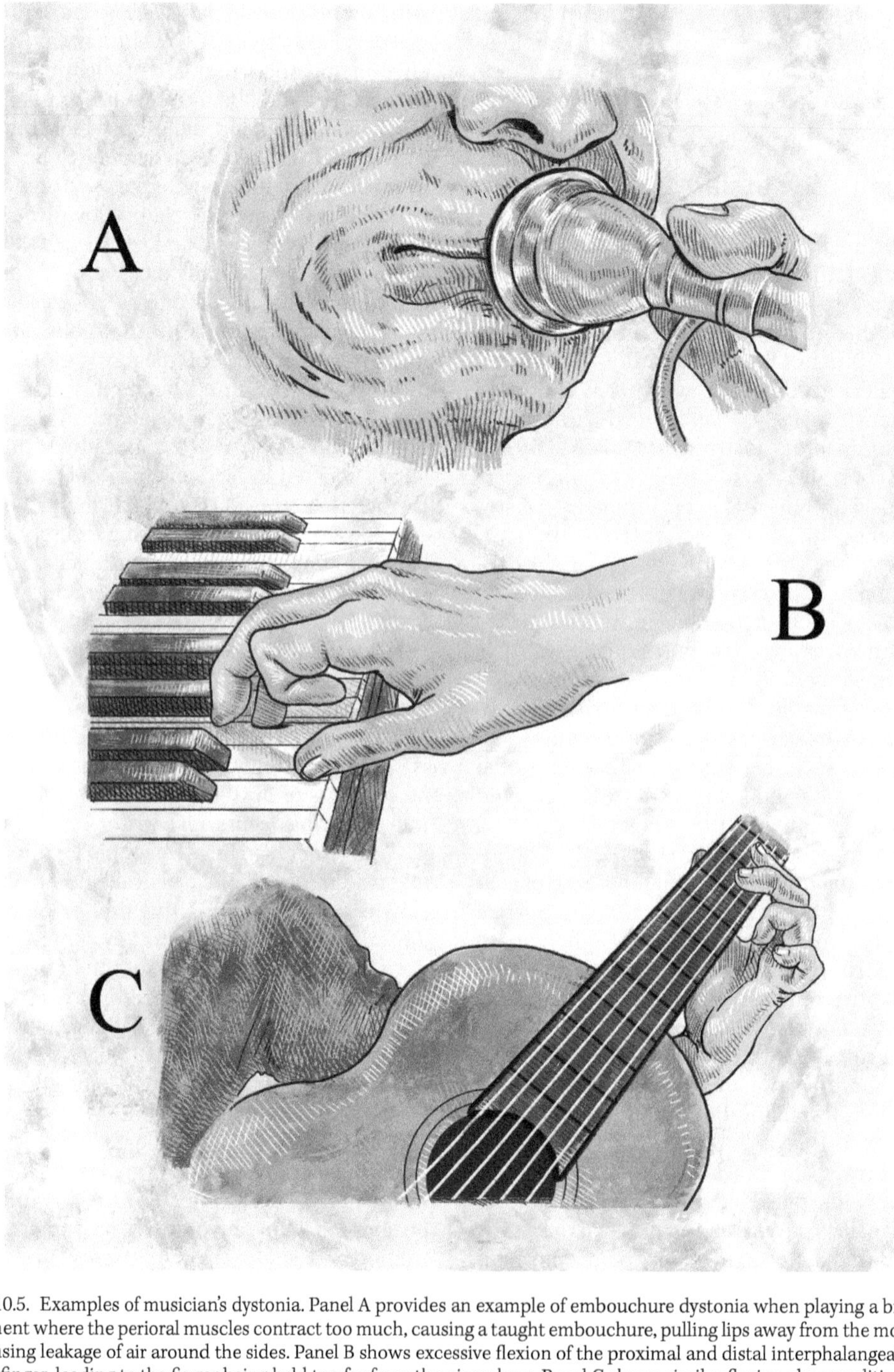

Figure 10.5. Examples of musician's dystonia. Panel A provides an example of embouchure dystonia when playing a brass wind instrument where the perioral muscles contract too much, causing a taught embouchure, pulling lips away from the mouthpiece and causing leakage of air around the sides. Panel B shows excessive flexion of the proximal and distal interphalangeal joints of the forefinger, leading to the finger being held too far from the piano keys. Panel C shows similar flexion abnormalities of digits 4–5 in a guitar player.

Illustration by Loren Bergantini.

Task-Specific Lower Limb Dystonia

Although a TSD of a lower limb may be a relatively common manifestation of childhood-onset dystonias that later generalize, focal isolated lower limb dystonia is one of the rarest dystonias of adults, whether task-specific or not. There are only a few prior case series of focal lower limb dystonia, and most are relatively small (Table 10.2).

The most common pattern among adult cases with walking-induced dystonia involves inversion of the ankle with toe flexion, but there are many variations.[61] When walking for an extended period, individuals with Parkinson disease may develop downward curling of the toes, cramping of the calf, or plantar flexion with intorsion of one foot (see Chapter 13, "Dystonia and Parkinsonism").[48,70] The same phenomenon may be seen in certain early-onset monogenic disorders, where the syndrome may resemble paroxysmal exertional dyskinesia (see Chapter 17, "Dystonia and Paroxysmal Dyskinesias").[49] Less common examples of task-specific lower limb dystonia include dystonia only with running,[32,37,87] going down stairs (but not up stairs),[3,47] cycling,[32] foot drumming,[32,35] using car brakes,[88] or dancing.[22]

Given the rarity of lower limb dystonias, the initial diagnosis is often some orthopedic problem. An incorrect orthopedic diagnosis is often further compounded by the high frequency of non-specific musculoskeletal abnormalities found with MRI of lower limb joints. Diagnosis rests on the observation of stereotyped abnormal posturing when performing a specific task but not other tasks. Normalization or marked improvement when walking backward can be helpful. A *geste antagoniste* is present only in a minority.

Laryngeal Dystonia

Laryngeal dystonia, also known as spasmodic dysphonia, may also be considered among the TSD because spasms of laryngeal muscles occur only with certain types of vocalizations.[24,41] Affected individuals may have great difficulty talking normally, but vocalization is normal when singing, shouting, whispering, or even speaking in an alternative language or accent. In adductor laryngeal dystonia, spasms are relatively specific to voiced vowels. In abductor laryngeal dystonia, spasms occur instead with voiceless consonants. In rare cases of singer's dystonia, vocalization is abnormal with singing but not when talking normally.[9] These conditions are covered in more detail in the Chapter 13, "Laryngeal Dystonias."

DIFFERENTIAL DIAGNOSIS AND INVESTIGATION

The main differential diagnoses of TSDs of the hand are neuromuscular and orthopedic issues. Examples include nerve entrapment syndromes, tendonitis and other musculoskeletal problems, or non-specific overuse syndromes (see Chapter 8, "Limb Dystonias"). Non-specific overuse syndromes are characterized by pain and discomfort

Table 10.2 **Descriptive studies of walking-induced dystonia**

Study	Cases	Female (%)	Age at onset	Notes
Schneider 2006[66]	17	64.7	48.4±10.7	Dystonia affected the toes (N = 13), foot (N = 10), and/or upper leg (N = 2); dystonia also occurred in the upper limb N = 2) or neck (N = 2)
McKeon 2008[46]	19	94.7	50.1±11.5	Dystonia affected the foot (N = 19), toes (N = 7) and/or upper leg (N = 2); Parkinson disease was eventually diagnosed in N = 3.
Martino 2010[44]	11	72.7	47.9±17.0	Dystonia affected the toes (N = 10), foot (N = 7) and/or upper leg (N = 2); dystonia also occurred in upper limb (N = 6) or larynx (N = 2)
Chang 2013[7]	22	77	49.7±14.0	Parkinson disease was eventually diagnosed in N = 8; and corticobasal syndrome in N = 2

This table summarizes studies that included at least 10 participants with lower limb dystonia where there was also additional clinical information on coexisting features. Age at onset is given in years ± standard deviation.

in the absence of clear explanatory findings on examination or objective measurement.

All of these diagnoses are especially relevant for individuals who perform highly repetitive tasks such as writers, musicians, or people who play sports.[39] The prevalence of performance-related musculoskeletal disorders is more than 70% among professional musicians.[36] In the case of neurological injury or nerve entrapment syndromes, focal sensory symptoms or signs and weakness are the major clues. Neurophysiological tests such as electromyography/nerve conduction velocity (EMG/NCV) testing or imaging can be useful for limb involvement. However, the high prevalence of non-specific abnormalities reported with both physiological and imaging tests can lead to overdiagnosis, and corroboration with clinical findings is crucial.[53] Neurophysiological and imaging tests are more difficult to apply and interpret for other conditions, such as cranial or axial TSD.

PATHOGENESIS

The pathogenesis of most forms of dystonia is summarized in Chapter 22, "Dystonia Genetics"; Chapter 24, "Dystonia Physiology"; and Chapter 23, "The Neuroanatomical Substrates of Dystonia." Early-onset monogenic dystonias may first present with TSD before evolving into more generalized dystonia that is not task-specific. Similarly, focal brain lesions may sometimes cause TSD. In this regard, TSD shares certain aspects of pathogenesis with other dystonias that are not task-specific. However, there also is some evidence that the pathogenesis of TSD may be different from dystonia that is not task-specific.[13,50,58,78] For example, many studies have indicated a strong predominance of women for most adult-onset focal dystonias such as cervical dystonia and craniofacial dystonias that are not task-specific. However, several studies have indicated that most TSDs, and particularly musician's dystonia, are more common in men. Other studies have indicated that the risk of spread in TSD seems to be lower than the risk of spread for other adult-onset focal dystonias.[13,50]

The most striking difference between TSD and non–task-specific dystonia is the association with extensive repetition of an action, usually over many years. This suggests that repeated activation of specific sensorimotor networks or pathways can lead to dystonia. This observation also implies that dystonia is not always purely an endogenously driven output of nervous system dysfunction but instead partially driven by repetitive activity. In some cases, an underlying predisposition might be playing a relatively minor role (i.e., an individual would never have developed dystonia had they not performed a highly repetitive activity). This observation further suggests the possibility that dystonia might potentially arise in an otherwise normal brain.

Epilepsy provides an example where seizures are usually associated with an underlying genetic predisposition or focal brain abnormality yet sometimes occur in an otherwise normal brain exposed to a biological stress. Other individuals, even if suffering from TSD in one body part such as writer's cramp, also manifest dystonia elsewhere, which might indicate a more important role for an underlying diathesis (e.g., in individuals with *SGCE* pathogenic variants).

Another point of difference among individuals with different TSDs relates to the type of task triggering dystonia. Some may develop TSD following an acquired, non-physiological, and highly skilled activity involving object use (e.g., playing a musical instrument). Others may develop TDS following performance of a relatively normal function, such as walking, running, or speaking. There might also be differences in motor activities that involve movements or body parts with differing levels of complexity (e.g., writing vs. violinist's dystonia affecting the bowing arm). Comparing the characteristics of individuals with task-specific dystonia divided according to these and other criteria may give insights into the nature of dystonia in general.

Several studies have compared neuroanatomical and neurophysiological findings in TSD versus non–task-specific dystonia. Structural and functional MRI techniques have found TSD and non–task-specific dystonia have differences in deep gray and white matter regions, as well as in sensorimotor, limbic, temporal, and occipital cortices. However, many of these studies have been quite small, and what constitutes an ideal comparison group is not always clear.[5,62,83] Fewer studies have specifically explored neurophysiological differences in TSD compared with other forms of dystonia. One study found pathological coherence in wrist flexors and extensors in both dystonia and writer's cramp patients but not controls. However, there were differences in the neurophysiological characteristics of co-contraction in the two groups.[16] Another study found differences in tactile and auditory perception of sequential sensory stimuli in musician's dystonia but not writer's cramp compared with controls, but concluded that the abnormalities in musicians were more likely to be secondary to dystonia rather than causal.[40]

TREATMENT

Many treatment strategies have been explored for individuals with TSD. Most of these treatments are similar to those used for other forms of dystonia, with some notable differences. Affected individuals may respond at least in part to oral medications used for other types of dystonia such as anticholinergics, benzodiazepines, and muscle relaxants (see Chapter 28, "Symptom-Targeted Oral Medications for Dystonia"). As a group, oral therapies have limited efficacy but may be used as adjunctive agents.[15]

Individuals with TSD of the hand may also respond to botulinum toxin injections (see Chapter 30, "Botulinum Toxin Treatment for Dystonia"). However, treating dystonia of the hand is more challenging than treating cervical dystonia or blepharospasm for several reasons. First, the large number of muscles controlling the fingers and hand can make it difficult to select the best combination of muscles for the best response. Second, these muscles are small, so precise targeting often requires EMG or ultrasound. Third, the dosing window is sometimes small, especially for wrist and finger extensors, making side effects from overtreatment common. Finally, it can be very difficult to discriminate pathological dystonic movements from intentional or unintentional behavioral compensations. Despite these challenges, experienced providers can achieve good outcomes for some individuals.[25] A systematic review of six controlled trials including a total of 139 individuals (most of whom had writer's cramp) suggested at least some improvement in 73%.[89] However, longitudinal studies have suggested that many patients discontinue therapy.[38,42]

For professional musicians with TSD of the hand, satisfactory responses are hard to achieve with botulinum toxins because the degree of motor control needed for top-level performance often cannot be restored. Satisfactory responses are only rarely achieved in musicians with embouchure dystonia because the sensitive muscles of the lower face have a low therapeutic margin, and restoring the degree of motor control required to play at a high level cannot usually be achieved. Satisfactory responses can sometimes be achieved with TSD of the hand, especially if the abnormal movement is relatively simple.

Neurosurgical methods can also provide relief from TSD of the hand. Deep brain stimulation is usually reserved for dystonia that is medically refractory and relatively severe, so it is not often offered to individuals with writer's cramp or other occupational TSDs. However, TSD of the hand appears to respond very well to small thalamic lesions.[28]

Rehabilitation medicine may also have a role in treating TSD. Many different types of studies have been reported. Two systematic reviews of these methods have grouped the many interventional trials into six categories: (1) movement practice, (2) training with constraint, (3) sensory reorganization, (4) biofeedback training, (5) neuromodulation with training, and (6) compensatory strategies.[27,60] Although many trials have reported positive outcomes, definitive recommendations are lacking due to the lack of rigorous experimental designs (see Chapter 32, "Physiotherapy and Complementary Medicine for Dystonia").

SYNOPSIS AND FUTURE PERSPECTIVES

A characteristic feature of most forms of dystonia is that abnormal movements are worsened or triggered by voluntary action. In some cases, the action that triggers dystonia may be highly specific. In these cases, dystonia is triggered only by a specific type of activity but not by other similar activities. Many types of activity can cause such a TSD, the most common being writing for writer's cramp or playing a musical instrument. The types of activities that trigger a task-specific dystonia tend to be highly repetitive, often requiring a high level of skill to perfect. These disorders are chiefly diagnosed by recognizing their characteristic features on history and examination.

The workup and treatment of these task-specific dystonias are similar to those for other forms of dystonia. However, it can be challenging to obtain satisfactory treatment, especially for professionals like musicians who need a very precise level of motor control to perform. Additional strategies for treatment clearly need to be developed.

Both task-specific and non–task-specific dystonias share some common clinical features. Although they also share some features of pathogenesis, there are some notable differences, with some evidence pointing to a distinct pathogenesis. Further studies are needed to understand how a highly repetitive activity can trigger dystonia because this may lead to insights into how to reverse TSD and possibly other types of dystonia.

REFERENCES

1. Altenmuller E, Jabusch HC. Focal dystonia in musicians: Phenomenology, pathophysiology and triggering factors. Eur J Neurol 2010;17 Suppl 1:31–36.
2. Amouzandeh A, Grossbach M, Hermsdorfer J, Altenmuller E. Pathophysiology of writer's cramp: An exploratory study on task-specificity and non-motor symptoms using an extended fine-motor testing battery. J Clin Mov Disord 2017;4:13.
3. Baik JS, Ma HI, Lee PH, Taira T. Focal task-specific lower limb dystonia only when walking stairs: Is it a new disease entity? Front Neurol 2019;10:1081.
4. Barad N. Weaver's dystonia: A novel form of focal task-specific dystonia. Mov Disord Clin Pract 2020;7:847–848.
5. Bianchi S, Fuertinger S, Huddleston H, Frucht SJ, Simonyan K. Functional and structural neural bases of task specificity in isolated focal dystonia. Mov Disord 2019;34:555–563.
6. Bouchard M, Furtado S. Speech-induced cervical dystonia. Can J Neurol Sci 2011;38:929–930.
7. Chang FC, Josephs KA. Levodopa responsiveness in adult-onset lower limb dystonia is associated with the development of Parkinson's disease. Tremor Other Hyperkinet Mov 2013:tre-03-150-3598-2.
8. Cherian A, Divya KP. Vada maker's dystonia: A new task-specific focal dystonia. Parkinsonism Relat Disord 2020;77:85–86.
9. Chitkara A, Meyer T, Keidar A, Blitzer A. Singer's dystonia: First report of a variant of spasmodic dysphonia. Ann Otol Rhinol Laryngol 2006;115:89–92.
10. Cohen LG, Hallett M. Hand cramps: Clinical features and electromyographic patterns in a focal dystonia. Neurology 1988;38:1005–1012.
11. Das CP, Prabhakar S, Truong D. Clinical profile of various sub-types of writer's cramp. Parkinsonism Relat Disord 2007;13:421–424.
12. Das SK, Banerjee TK, Biswas A, Roy T, Raut DK, Chaudhuri A, Hazra A. Community survey of primary dystonia in the city of Kolkata, India. Mov Disord 2007;22:2031–2036.
13. Defazio G, Ercoli T, Erro R, Pellicciari R, Mascia MM, Fabbrini G, et al. Idiopathic non-task-specific upper limb dystonia, a neglected form of dystonia. Mov Disord 2020;35:2038–2045.
14. Erro R, Ciocca M, Hirschbichler ST, Rothwell JC, Bhatia KP. Primary writing tremor is a dystonic trait: Evidence from an instructive family. J Neurol Sci 2015;356:210–211.
15. Faccioli S, Pagliano E, Ferrari A, Maghini C, Siani MF, Sgherri G, et al. Evidence-based management and motor rehabilitation of cerebral palsy children and adolescents: A systematic review. Front Neurol 2023;14:1171224.
16. Farmer SF, Sheean GL, Mayston MJ, Rothwell JC, Marsden CD, Conway BA, et al. Abnormal motor unit synchronization of antagonist muscles underlies pathological co-contraction in upper limb dystonia. Brain 1998;121:801–814.
17. Ferguson D. An Australian study of telegraphists' cramp. Br J Ind Med 1971;28:280–285.
18. Frucht SJ. Embouchure dystonia: Portrait of a task-specific cranial dystonia. Mov Disord 2009;24:1752–1762.
19. Frucht SJ. Focal task-specific dystonia: From early descriptions to a new, modern formulation. Tremor Other Hyperkinet Mov (N Y) 2014;4:230.
20. Frucht SJ. Billiards-related dystonia: A new task-specific dystonia. Parkinsonism Relat Disord 2019;60:12–13.
21. Garcia-Ruiz PJ. Task-specific dystonias: Historical review—a new look at the classics. J Neurol 2013;260:750–753.
22. García-Ruiz PJ, del Val J, Losada M, Campos JM. Task-specific dystonia of the lower limb in a flamenco dancer. Parkinsonism Relat Disord 2011;17:221–222.
23. Gowers WR. *A Manual of Diseases of the Nervous System*. Churchill; 1888.
24. Guiry S, Worthley A, Simonyan K. A separation of innate and learned vocal behaviors defines the symptomatology of spasmodic dysphonia. Laryngoscope 2019;129:1627–1633.
25. Gupta N, Pandey S. Treatment of focal hand dystonia: Current status. Neurol Sci 2021;42:3561–3584.
26. Hammond WA. *A Treatise on Diseases of the Nervous System*. D. Appleton; 1871.
27. Hautekiet A, Raes K, Geers S, Santens P, Oostra K. Evidence of rehabilitation therapy in task-specific focal dystonia: A systematic review. Eur J Phys Rehabil Med 2021;57:710–719.
28. Horisawa S, Ochiai T, Goto S, Nakajima T, Takeda N, Fukui A, et al. Safety and long-term efficacy of ventro-oral thalamotomy for focal hand dystonia: A retrospective study of 171 patients. Neurology 2019;92:e371–e377.
29. Jackman M, Delrobaei M, Rahimi F, Atashzar SF, Shahbazi M, Patel R, Jog M. Predicting improvement in writer's cramp symptoms following botulinum neurotoxin injection therapy. Tremor Other Hyperkinet Mov 2016;6:410.
30. Jedynak PC, Tranchant C, de Beyl DZ. Prospective clinical study of writer's cramp. Mov Disord 2001;16:494–499.
31. Jhunjhunwala K, Lenka A, Pal PK. A clinical profile of 125 patients with writer's cramp. Eur Neurol 2015;73:316–320.
32. Katz M, Byl NN, San Luciano M, Ostrem JL. Focal task-specific lower extremity dystonia associated with intense repetitive exercise: A case series. Parkinsonism Relat Disord 2013;19:1033–1038.
33. Latorre A, Rocchi L, Batla A, Berardelli A, Rothwell JC, Bhatia KP. The signature of primary writing tremor is dystonic. Mov Disord 2021;36:1715–1720.
34. Lederman RJ. Occupational cramp in instrumental musicians. Med Probl Perform Art 1988;3:45–51.

35. Lee A, Altenmüller E. Heavy metal curse: A task-specific dystonia in the proximal lower limb of a professional percussionist. Med Probl Perform Art 2014;29:174–176.
36. Lee HS, Park HY, Yoon JO, Kim JS, Chun JM, Aminata IW, et al. Musicians' medicine: Musculoskeletal problems in string players. Clin Orthop Surg 2013;5:155–160.
37. Lee JH, Kim HJ, Park DG, Yoon JH. A novel task-specific dystonia: Running-induced cervical dystonia in a triathlete. Neurol Sci 2021;42:3051–3052.
38. Lee JI, Jansen A, Samadzadeh S, Kahlen U, Moll M, Ringelstein M, et al. Long-term adherence and response to botulinum toxin in different indications. Ann Clin Transl Neurol 2021;8:15–28.
39. Lenka A, Jankovic J. Sports-related dystonia. Tremor Other Hyperkinet Mov (N Y) 2021;11:54.
40. Lim VK, Bradshaw JL, Nicholls ME, Altenmuller E. Perceptual differences in sequential stimuli across patients with musician's and writer's cramp. Mov Disord 2003;18:1286–1293.
41. Ludlow CL. Spasmodic dysphonia: A laryngeal control disorder specific to speech. J Neurosci 2011;31:793–797.
42. Lungu C, Karp BI, Alter K, Zolbrod R, Hallett M. Long-term follow-up of botulinum toxin therapy for focal hand dystonia: Outcome at 10 years or more. Mov Disord 2011;26:750–753.
43. Martin AJ, McGrath R, Fung VSC. A wilted flower: Lotus position dystonia. Mov Disord Clin Pract 2020;7:206–207.
44. Martino D, Macerollo A, Abbruzzese G, Bentivoglio AR, Berardelli A, Esposito M, et al. Lower limb involvement in adult-onset primary dystonia: Frequency and clinical features. Eur J Neurol 2010;17:242–246.
45. McDaniel KD, Cummings JL, Shain S. The "yips": A focal dystonia of golfers. Neurology 1989;39:192–195.
46. McKeon A, Matsumoto JY, Bower JH, Ahlskog JE. The spectrum of disorders presenting as adult-onset focal lower extremity dystonia. Parkinsonism Relat Disord 2008;14:613–619.
47. Menon S, Muglan JA, Shimon L, Stewart D, Snow B, Hayes M, et al. Down the stairs dystonia: A novel task-specific focal isolated syndrome. Mov Disord Clin Pract 2017;4:121–124.
48. Morales-Briceno H, Fung VSC, Bhatia KP, Balint B. Parkinsonism and dystonia: Clinical spectrum and diagnostic clues. J Neurol Sci 2022;433:120016.
49. Mulroy E, Magrinelli F, Mohd Fauzi NA, Kutty SK, Latorre A, Bhatia KP. Paroxysmal, exercise-induced, diurnally fluctuating dystonia: Expanding the phenotype of SPG8. Parkinsonism Relat Disord 2021;85:26–28.
50. Norris SA, Jinnah HA, Klein C, Jankovic J, Berman BD, Roze E, et al. Clinical and demographic characteristics of upper limb dystonia. Mov Disord 2020;35:2086–2090.
51. Nutt JG, Muenter MD, Aronson A, Kurland LT, Melton LJ. Epidemiology of focal and generalized dystonia in Rochester, Minnesota. Mov Disord 1988;3:188–194.
52. Ondo WG, Satija P. Task-specific writing tremor: Clinical phenotypes, progression, treatment outcomes, and proposed nomenclature. Int J Neurosci 2012;122:88–91.
53. Overton M, Du Plessis H, Sole G. Electromyography of neck and shoulder muscles in instrumental musicians with musculoskeletal pain compared to asymptomatic controls: A systematic review and meta-analysis. Musculoskelet Sci Pract 2018;36:32–42.
54. Pandey S, Datta A. A primary writing tremor is a form of dystonic tremor: Is the debate settled? Mov Disord 2021;36:1995–1996.
55. Papapetropoulos S, Singer C. Treatment of primary writing tremor with botulinum toxin type a injections: Report of a case series. Clin Neuropharmacol 2006;29:364–367.
56. Patel AS, Sulica L, Frucht SJ. Velopharyngeal dystonia: An unusual focal task-specific dystonia? Tremor Other Hyperkinet Mov (N Y) 2017;7:365.
57. Pearce JM. A note on scrivener's palsy. J Neurol Neurosurg Psychiatry 2005;76:513.
58. Pirio Richardson S, Altenmuller E, Alter K, Alterman RL, Chen R, Frucht S, et al. Research priorities in limb and task-specific dystonias. Front Neurol 2017;8:170.
59. Pita Lobo P, Quattrocchi G, Jutras MF, Sangla S, Apartis E, Vidailhet M, Grabli D. Primary writing tremor and writer's cramp: Two faces of a same coin? Mov Disord 2013;28:1306–1307.
60. Prudente CN, Zetterberg L, Bring A, Bradnam L, Kimberley TJ. Systematic review of rehabilitation in focal dystonias: Classification and recommendations. Mov Disord Clin Pract 2018;5:237–245.
61. Ramdhani RA, Frucht SJ. Adult-onset idiopathic focal lower extremity dystonia: A rare task-specific dystonia. Tremor Other Hyperkinet Mov (N Y) 2013;3:tre-03-142-2990-1.
62. Ramdhani RA, Kumar V, Velickovic M, Frucht SJ, Tagliati M, Simonyan K. What's special about task in dystonia? A voxel-based morphometry and diffusion weighted imaging study. Mov Disord 2014;29:1141–1150.
63. Roberts K, Mahon B, O'Rourke K, Lynch T. "Club-cutting" dystonic tremor: A case report. Tremor Other Hyperkinet Mov (N Y) 2013;3:tre-03-158-4183-1.
64. Roze E, Soumare A, Pironneau I, Sangla S, de Cock VC, Teixeira A, et al. Case-control study of writer's cramp. Brain 2009;132:756–764.
65. Sadnicka A, Kassavetis P, Parees I, Meppelink AM, Butler K, Edwards M. Task-specific dystonia: Pathophysiology and management. J Neurol Neurosurg Psychiatry 2016;87:968–974.
66. Schneider SA, Edwards MJ, Grill SE, Goldstein S, Kanchana S, Quinn NP, et al. Adult-onset primary lower limb dystonia. Mov Disord 2006;21:767–771.
67. Schramm A, Naumann M, Reiners K, Classen J. Task-specific craniocervical dystonia. Mov Disord 2008;23:1041–1043.
68. Shamim EA, Chu J, Scheider LH, Savitt J, Jinnah HA, Hallett M. Extreme task specificity in writer's cramp. Mov Disord 2011;26:2107–2109.
69. Sheehy MP, Marsden CD. Writers' cramp-a focal dystonia. Brain 1982;105:461–480.
70. Shetty AS, Bhatia KP, Lang AE. Dystonia and Parkinson's disease: What is the relationship? Neurobiol Dis 2019;132:104462.
71. Shi LL, Simpson CB, Hapner ER, Jinnah HA, Johns MM, 3rd. Pharyngeal dystonia mimicking spasmodic dysphonia. J Voice 2018;32:234–238.
72. Sinclair CF, Simonyan K, Brin MF, Blitzer A. Negative dystonia of the palate: A novel entity and diagnostic consideration in hypernasal speech. Laryngoscope 2015;125:1426–1432.
73. Singer C, Papapetropoulos S, Spielholz NI. Primary writing tremor: Report of a case successfully treated with botulinum toxin A injections and discussion of underlying mechanism. Mov Disord 2005;20:1387–1388.
74. Sitburana O, Wu LJ, Sheffield JK, Davidson A, Jankovic J. Motor overflow and mirror dystonia. Parkinsonism Relat Disord 2009;15:758–761.

75. Smilowska K, Domingos J, Pasman JW, van Wamelen DJ, van de Warrenburg BP, Bloem BR. Billiards-related dystonia: A new task-specific dystonia. Parkinsonism Relat Disord 2019;60:10–11.
76. Soland VL, Bhatia KP, Marsden CD. Sex prevalence of focal dystonias. J Neurol Neurosurg Psychiat 1996;60:204–205.
77. Solly S. Clinical lectures on scriveners' palsy, or the paralysis of writers. The Lancet 1864;84:709–711.
78. Stahl CM, Frucht SJ. Focal task specific dystonia: A review and update. J Neurol 2017;264:1536–1541.
79. Steinmetz A, Stang A, Kornhuber M, Rollinghoff M, Delank KS, Altenmuller E. From embouchure problems to embouchure dystonia? A survey of self-reported embouchure disorders in 585 professional orchestra brass players. Int Arch Occup Environ Health 2014;87:783–792.
80. Suzuki K, Takano M, Hashimoto K, Numao A, Nakamura T, Sakuta H, Hirata K. Computer mouse-related dystonia: A novel presentation of task-specific dystonia. J Neurol 2012;259:2221–2222.
81. Termsarasab P, Frucht SJ. Evaluation of embouchure dysfunction: Experience of 139 patients at a single center. Laryngoscope 2016;126:1327–1333.
82. Todt I, Baumann A, Knutzen A, Granert O, Tzvi E, Lindert J, et al. Abnormal effective connectivity in the sensory network in writer's cramp. Neuroimage Clin 2021;31:102761.
83. Tomic A, Agosta F, Sarasso E, Svetel M, Kresojevic N, Fontana A, et al. Brain structural changes in focal dystonia: What about task specificity? A multimodal MRI study. Mov Disord 2021;36:196–205.
84. Torres-Russotto D, Perlmutter JS. Task-specific dystonias: A review. Ann N Y Acad Sci 2008;1142: 179–199.
85. Virchow R. *Handbuch der speciellen Pathologie und Therapie*. Enke; 1854.
86. Woldendorp KH, Boschma H, Boonstra AM, Arendzen HJ, Reneman MF. Fundamentals of embouchure in brass players: Towards a definition and clinical assessment. Med Probl Perform Art 2016;31:232–243.
87. Wu LJ, Jankovic J. Runner's dystonia. J Neurol Sci 2006;251:73–76.
88. Yoo SW, Lee M, Kim JS. "Stepping on the brakes" dystonic tremor: A new type of task-specific dystonic tremor of the lower extremity. Neurol Sci 2020;41:477–479.
89. Zakin E, Simpson DM. Botulinum toxin therapy in writer's cramp and musician's dystonia. Toxins (Basel) 2021;13:899.

Chapter 11

Non-Motor Features of Dystonia

INTRODUCTION

Historically, dystonia was considered a psychiatric disorder, as described in Chapter 1, "A Brief History of the Concept of Dystonia and Its Evolution," and in Chapter 25, "Psychogenic (Functional) Dystonia." It is now widely accepted that dystonia is an organic disorder arising from structural or physiological changes in specific neural networks. However, it is also now well-recognized that psychiatric problems commonly coexist with dystonia. These psychiatric problems are important to recognize because they can have a greater impact on quality of life (QoL) than the movement disorder itself.

There has been a long debate regarding whether these psychiatric comorbidities are secondary to dystonia, play a causal role in triggering dystonia, or reflect an innate biology (endophenotype) that predisposes to both dystonia and psychiatric problems.[120] There is evidence to support each of these different ideas, and it is feasible that each is valid for certain subgroups of individuals with dystonia.

In addition to psychiatric comorbidities, a number of additional non-motor comorbidities can occur among individuals with dystonia. They include pain, impaired quality of sleep, cognitive features, and others. These other non-motor features can also have a profound impact on QoL, and they tend to co-occur along with psychiatric comorbidities for a substantial subgroup of individuals. Non-motor symptoms do not always correlate with motor severity, so they must be addressed separately.[26,108,115] This chapter addresses the main psychiatric and other non-motor problems in individuals with dystonia.

PSYCHIATRIC COMORBIDITIES

The Spectrum of Psychiatric Problems

Numerous studies have documented an increase in the prevalence of psychiatric problems among individuals with dystonia. Some studies address all types of psychiatric concerns across mixed populations of dystonia subtypes, while others address only specific dystonia subtypes or specific psychiatric problems.

One large study of a Welsh population health database spanning 1994–2017 compared 52,589 individuals with mostly idiopathic adult-onset dystonias with 216,754 controls.[8] Compared to the controls, those with dystonia had higher rates of psychiatric diagnoses (43% vs. 31%) and psychiatric medication prescriptions (45% vs. 38%). The most common problems were depression

(31%) and anxiety (28%). However, individuals with dystonia also had an increased risk for other problems including substance use disorder, eating disorders, attention-deficit/hyperactivity disorder, autism spectrum disorder, and conduct disorder. On the other hand, individuals with dystonia had a reduced risk of severe mental illness such as schizophrenia, schizotypal and delusional disorders, and bipolar disorder. Psychiatric diagnoses usually predated dystonia diagnoses, particularly in the 12 months prior to diagnosis, and especially for anxiety disorders. However, there also was an elevated rate of receiving a psychiatric diagnosis in the dystonia group throughout the illness, especially in the 12 months after dystonia diagnosis.[8]

The character of psychiatric manifestations in idiopathic dystonia may be influenced by the site of dystonia onset. Among 478 individuals with mostly adult-onset focal dystonias recruited by the Dystonia Coalition, psychiatric problems (depression and anxiety) occurred in all groups but varied according to the site of dystonia onset.[11] Individuals with onset in the cervical and laryngeal region had higher anxiety, whereas onset in the face was associated with relatively lower anxiety. Individuals with laryngeal onset had higher social anxiety. Higher pain levels were associated with worse neuropsychiatric symptoms in all groups.

Another detailed case-control study assessed individuals with the Structured Clinical Interview for Diagnostic and Statistical Manual disorders, Yale-Brown Obsessive-Compulsive Scale, Hamilton Rating Scale for Anxiety, and the Beck Depression Inventory.[34] It included 62 healthy controls, 26 disease controls with hemifacial spasm, and 89 consecutive individuals with various isolated focal dystonias (34 cervical dystonia, 28 blepharospasm, 16 laryngeal dystonia, and 11 upper limb dystonia). The prevalence of psychiatric disorders in the dystonia group was 57.3% compared with 24.1% of healthy controls and 34.6% of the disease controls. Individuals with cervical dystonia and blepharospasm had higher rates of depressive disorders than did healthy controls, but they did not have higher rates of anxiety disorders, obsessive-compulsive disorder, or adjustment disorders. The laryngeal and upper limb dystonia groups did not have higher rates of psychiatric illness, although this finding may have reflected the relatively small numbers of individuals with these diagnoses. Psychiatric symptoms developed before the diagnosis of dystonia in 69% of individuals with dystonia and after the onset of dystonia in 31%.[34]

Another thorough study compared psychiatric profiles as well as personality traits of 86 individuals who had focal dystonias with a population-based sample of 3,943 healthy controls.[58] The dystonia group had a lifetime prevalence for any psychiatric or personality disorder of 70.9% with an increased odds ratio (OR) of 4.5 compared to the control group. The highest ORs were found for social phobia (OR 21.6), agoraphobia (OR 16.7) and panic disorder (OR 11.5). The dystonia group also had an increased prevalence of 32.6% for anxious personality disorders comprising obsessive-compulsive (22.1%) and avoidant personality disorders (16.3%). Except for social phobia, psychiatric disorders often manifested prior to dystonia. In self-rated personality traits, individuals with dystonia showed greater agreeableness and conscientiousness, but reduced openness.[58]

Psychiatric Problems in Specific Dystonia Populations

Most of the prior studies addressed different types of psychiatric illness in mixed populations of dystonias. Most addressed the adult-onset focal dystonias, since they are the most common. A smaller number of studies have focused on more specific dystonia populations or children.

A longitudinal study assessed 53 individuals with cervical dystonia 2 years apart with several rating scales such as the Cervical Dystonia Impact Profile-58 and the Toronto Western Spasmodic Torticollis Rating Pain subscale.[74] It showed relatively stable scores for anxiety and depression as well as QoL. Mood disorders were associated with an earlier age of onset of dystonia. Mood disorders were also associated with an earlier age of onset in women in a cross-sectional study of 193 patients (128 female), although men had an earlier average age at onset. A history of a mood disorder was reported in 53/128 (41%) women, of whom a mood disorder occurred prior to dystonia in 33. Mood disorders were more common in women (41%) than men (31%).[77]

Other studies focusing on specific types of adult-onset focal dystonia noted an increased prevalence of anxiety and depression in blepharospasm,[26] writer's cramp,[116] and generalized dystonia.[60] Another study focusing on blepharospasm included a review of 10,324 previously published cases from 41 different reports, as well as 884 new cases from the Dystonia Coalition.[95] In this study, anxiety (34–40%) and depression (21–24%) were common. A similar analysis focused on oromandibular dystonia with 1,121 previously published cases and 727 new cases from the Dystonia Coalition found social anxiety more common than depression, with impaired QoL independent of dystonia severity.[96]

A systematic review did not find obsessive-compulsive disorder to be increased in generalized dystonia,[55] but some studies have reported positive findings for other types of dystonia. Using specific rating scales, at least four studies have found an increased prevalence of obsessive-compulsive disorder in focal dystonia,[27,75,107] with similar rates to hemifacial spasm in one[17] and higher than Parkinson disease in another.[27]

Most studies have addressed adults with dystonia, but some have also addressed children. Children with non-tic movement disorders (n = 102, 66 with dystonia) had an increased rate of psychiatric diagnoses using criteria from the Diagnostic and Statistical Manual of Mental Disorders (DSM-5) (39.2%) that was similar to children with tic disorder (41.8%) and neurology controls with peripheral neuropathy or epilepsy (29.7%).[64] All groups had significantly higher rates of psychiatric diagnoses than community controls (9.5%) or controls evaluated in emergency departments (18%). Another study of 50 children aged 7–17 with dystonia from all causes found higher levels of prosocial difficulties, with 48% experiencing clinically significant anxiety.[9] However, they experienced significantly lower levels of anger, disruptive behavior, and conduct problems. Anxiety levels correlated with lower levels of self-esteem.

One systematic review compared idiopathic and monogenic forms of dystonia.[55] This review encompassed 20 case control studies that included 1,275 individuals with idiopathic or monogenic (*ATP1A3*, *SGCE*, and *TOR1A*) dystonia. Compared with control individuals, there were higher rates of psychiatric comorbidities in both idiopathic and monogenic groups. There were also some gene-dependent differences. For example, most groups had higher rates of mood and anxiety disorders, but not major depressive disorder or obsessive-compulsive disorder. In contrast, individuals with genetic variants in *SGCE* also had a higher risk of major depression, obsessive-compulsive disorder, and alcohol dependence. A high risk of psychiatric disorders has also been reported in studies focusing only on *SGCE*.[85,86]

Specific Psychiatric Problems

ANXIETY DISORDERS

In addition to studies focusing on specific dystonia populations, other studies have focused on specific psychiatric problems. A systematic review and meta-analysis of the prevalence of anxiety-related disorders in adult-onset isolated dystonia from 34 studies estimated the overall prevalence of clinically significant anxiety to be 33.3%, with social phobia being the most common. More specific estimates were for cervical dystonia 40%, cranial dystonia 25%, laryngeal dystonia 26%, and upper limb dystonia 32% (Figure 11.1).[70]

Social phobia is classified among anxiety disorders and refers to discomfort and avoidance of social situations, such as interacting with others or even going out in public. It is not surprising that social phobia is common in dystonia because dystonia is often overtly apparent to others. For example, cervical dystonia is associated with abnormal head movements, blepharospasm is associated with abnormal facial movements, and laryngeal dystonia is associated with impaired communication. Several studies have indicated that social phobia is the most common psychiatric problem for several types of dystonia.[38,58,70]

For example, a study of 116 individuals with cervical dystonia found that 41% met DSM-IV criteria for social phobia as the main psychiatric problem.[38] Compared to prevalence in non-dystonia controls, individuals with cervical dystonia had a 10-fold increased prevalence of clinically relevant social phobia, 2.4-fold increase

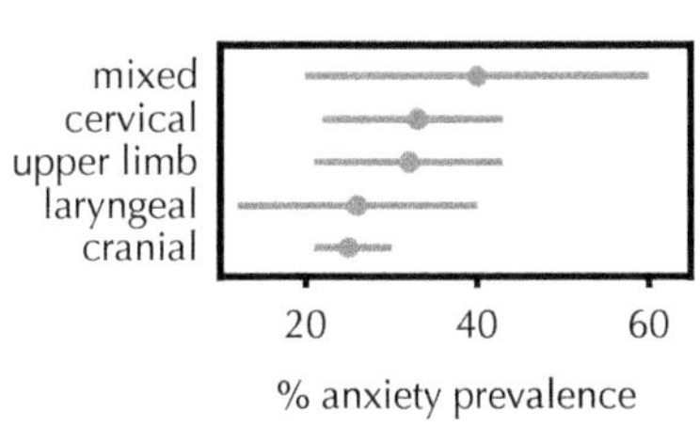

Figure 11.1. Meta-analysis of anxiety-related disorders in dystonia. This Forest plot shows the overall estimated prevalence as a point, with error bars depicting confidence intervals adapted from data spanning 14 prior articles.[70]

in mood disorders, and 2.6-fold increase in lifetime psychiatric comorbidity. Psychiatric comorbidity was associated with depressive coping behavior but not dystonia severity, pain or body image dissatisfaction.

MOOD DISORDERS

One systematic review addressed depression-related disorders in adult-onset focal dystonias across 54 studies.[71] The overall prevalence of clinically significant depression in the dystonia group was 33.6 %. More specific estimates were 31.5% for cervical dystonia and 29.2% for cranial dystonia with major depressive disorder more prevalent than dysthymia in cervical dystonia, and dysthymia more prevalent in cranial dystonia (Figure 11.2). In cervical dystonia, the prevalence of clinically significant depression was higher when screened by rating scales than with structured interviews.

Suicidal behavior was reported by 32.3% of 542 individuals with dystonia in an anonymous survey, significantly higher than rates of suicidal ideation (9.2%) and suicide attempt (2.7%) reported in the general population.[113] The prevalence of suicidality was higher in multifocal/segmental and generalized forms of dystonia (range 46–50%) compared to focal dystonias (range of 26–33%). Suicidality in focal dystonia is associated with a history of depression and anxiety.

Increased suicide risk was also found in a study of idiopathic dystonia and psychiatric outcomes extracted from the Swedish National Patient and Cause of Death Registers from 1997–2013, as well as the Multi-Generation Register.[69] Individuals with most forms of dystonia were approximately two times more likely than those without dystonia to have a diagnosis of depressive disorder, anxiety disorder, and suicide attempts/death by suicide combined. Full siblings of individuals with dystonia also had a higher likelihood of

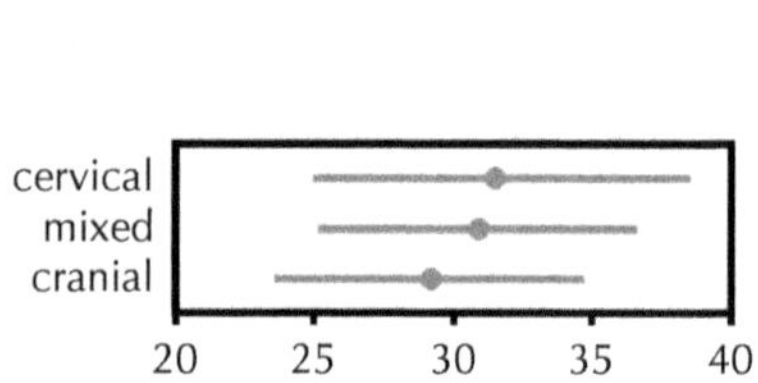

Figure 11.2. Meta-analysis of mood-related disorders in dystonia. This Forest plot shows the overall estimated prevalence as a point, with error bars depicting confidence intervals adapted from data provided in a prior article.[71]

these problems compared with siblings of individuals without dystonia.[69]

Overall, these many studies establish a high frequency of psychiatric illness among individuals with dystonia. The frequency and types of psychiatric illness may vary according to the methods of assessment, the type of dystonia, age at onset, duration of illness, and other factors such as sex or genetic etiology. Apparent differences among the studies are likely to reflect differences in populations studied or the way that psychiatric problems were evaluated. In many cases, the psychiatric problems emerged before overt dystonic movements.

Psychiatric Features of Dystonia: Cause, Consequence, or Endophenotype?

DO PSYCHIATRIC PROBLEMS CAUSE DYSTONIA?

Many individuals recall a particularly stressful event preceding the onset of their dystonia.[20,45,87,94] Examples include loss of a loved one or job, a severe medical illness, or an automobile accident. In fact, psychiatric diagnoses often predate dystonia diagnoses, particularly in the 12 months prior to diagnosis.[9] This sequence of events might imply that psychiatric problems may somehow trigger the movement disorder, and many individuals with dystonia ask whether their dystonia was caused by emotional stress. However, it is possible that the preceding diagnoses reflect a psychiatric disturbance arising from early symptoms of dystonia that eluded diagnosis, given that the diagnosis of dystonia is often delayed by many years.[12,23,48,54,67,102,111] In addition, epidemiological studies have suggested that the recollection of a stressful event can reflect recall bias, and they have failed to confirm a causal link between stress and most cases of dystonia.

While there is little epidemiological evidence that stress triggers the onset of dystonia in most cases, it is well known that stress may exaggerate dystonia,[45,93] just as it can exaggerate other movement disorders such as tremor or parkinsonism. Furthermore, many individuals with dystonia report benefit from stress-reduction methods such as meditation and stretching exercises.[13,35,50]

In addition to these more common examples, there are some rare examples where stress clearly triggers dystonia. For example, stress (either emotional or physical) can trigger the onset of dystonia in the rapid-onset dystonia-parkinsonism syndrome caused by pathogenic variants in the *ATP1A3* gene.[14,17,106] This association between stress and onset of dystonia is not spurious, as non-physical stress can also reliably trigger dystonia in mouse models with defects in the same gene.[17,25] Stress can also precipitate attacks of dystonia in the paroxysmal dyskinesias (see Chapter 17, "Dystonia and the Paroxysmal Dyskinesias") and in genetic mouse models of the paroxysmal dyskinesias.[36,89,97]

In short, there is little evidence that psychiatric problems trigger dystonia in most cases, but stress can certainly contribute to making it worse. In rare cases, however, stress may act as a biological trigger.

DOES DYSTONIA CAUSE PSYCHIATRIC PROBLEMS?

Dystonia is both physically disabling and overtly visible. As a result, it would not be surprising that dystonia might trigger depression, anxiety, or other psychiatric problems. In keeping with this possibility, there is an elevated rate of most psychiatric diagnoses after dystonia diagnosis, especially in the first year.[9] This sequence of events is compatible with the idea that dystonia causes psychiatric problems.

Another way of examining whether psychiatric problems are a cause or consequence of dystonia is to compare the incidence of these problems among individuals with other chronic diseases. One study compared 103 idiopathic isolated focal dystonia individuals with 78 consecutive hemifacial spasm individuals and 93 healthy control participants using the Yale-Brown Obsessive Compulsive Scale, the Beck Anxiety Inventory, and the Beck Depression Inventory.[57] All three psychiatric problems were more frequent in the dystonia group. A similar study also reported more psychiatric disorders in dystonia compared with hemifacial spasm.[34] These studies argue for a higher risk of psychiatric problems in dystonia compared with hemifacial spasm, although this difference could reflect how motor disorders of different severity might impact QoL.

In contrast, another study reported no differences in the prevalence of psychiatric disorders in a group of 85 individuals with cervical dystonia compared with 49 individuals with cervical spondylosis.[46] Depression in cervical dystonia was driven by self-referent negative thoughts such as self-blame, self-accusation, self-punitive thoughts, and negative body image.[46] The same investigators also found no difference in personality scales among individuals with cervical dystonia versus cervical spondylosis, but those with cervical dystonia were more likely to be single and unemployed due to permanent disability.[46] Another study addressed secondary social anxiety among 60 healthy controls and 20 individuals each with cervical dystonia, hemifacial spasm, and essential tremor. Social anxiety was similarly increased in all three disorders relative to controls, especially in younger individuals and those with depression.[82] Similar frequencies and severity, and a similar pattern of depression symptoms, were found in another study of 354 individuals with Parkinson disease, 83 with dystonia, and 53 with essential tremor using the Beck Depression Inventory.[72] The most common depressive symptoms were fatigability, difficulty with work, anhedonia, and sleep disturbance.

Another way to address whether psychiatric problems result from dystonia is to assess how psychiatric problems respond when the motor disorder is treated. Botulinum toxin therapy has been shown to effective therapy for most focal dystonias (see Chapter 30, "Botulinum Toxin Treatment for Dystonia"). Some of these studies have shown improvement in motor problems, psychiatric problems, and QoL.[52,80] However, many studies have shown improvement in motor problems with little or no improvement in psychiatric problems or QoL.[29,74,76] Similar results have been obtained for deep brain stimulation, which can be quite effective for the motor disorder for many types of dystonia (see Chapter 32, "Surgical Treatments for Dystonia"). Some studies of this surgery show improvement in motor features, psychiatric features, and QoL.[76] Other studies show improvements in motor features, but not psychiatric features or QoL.[47] A recent systematic review of 52 studies of deep brain stimulation for dystonia found significant improvement of pain, with no significant impact on anxiety, mood, or cognition.[31]

In summary, it seems likely that psychiatric features such as depression or anxiety may develop in response to the motor features of dystonia for some individuals with dystonia. However, the motor features do not appear to be responsible for the psychiatric features in all cases, and some other explanation is needed.

ARE PSYCHIATRIC PROBLEMS PART OF AN ENDOPHENOTYPE?

It is feasible that some innate biological factor (endophenotype) simultaneously predisposes to both dystonia and psychiatric problems. Some of the strongest evidence for this concept comes from genetic studies. One study addressed this possibility by taking advantage of the partial penetrance of *TOR1A*-associated dystonia among multiple families where there were a total of 96 symptomatic carriers, 60 non-symptomatic carriers, and 65 non-carriers. Using a standard psychiatric interview, the risk for recurrent major depressive disorder was increased approximately four-fold in both symptomatic and non-symptomatic carriers compared with non-carriers. Mutation carriers (both symptomatic and non-symptomatic) had an earlier age at onset of recurrent major depressive disorder than noncarriers, and the severity of motor signs was not associated with the likelihood of recurrent depression. Mutation carriers did not have an increased risk for other affective disorders, such as single major depression or bipolar disorder.[40] These results suggest a heritable tendency for depression that is not directly related to the motor phenotype, implying a genetically determined endophenotype for this disorder.

On the other hand, studies of dopa-responsive dystonia caused by genetic variants in the *GCH1* gene have revealed conflicting results regarding the prevalence of depression or anxiety.[3,15] Other studies have confirmed a high frequency of psychiatric problems in other monogenic dystonias caused by genetic variants in *ATP1A3* or *SGCE*.[55,85,86] However, the spectrum of psychiatric problems in these disorders varies from those associated with *TOR1A*. The specificity of the type of psychiatric problem according to dystonia gene again argues for a genetic predisposition.

An exploration of the role of serotonin in the pathogenesis of mood disorders in dystonia found differences in the methylation of the serotonin reuptake transporter (*SLC6A4*) between individuals with dopa-responsive dystonia and healthy controls but not idiopathic cervical dystonia or *SGCE*-associated myoclonus dystonia.[103] Methylation impacts the functional activity of the gene, by altering its level of transcription. Together, these findings imply that some but not all genes may have an influence on both dystonia and psychiatric problems. They also imply that psychiatric problems may be related not only genetic variants within specific genes but also the state of gene activation.

How these findings from genetic dystonias relate to the more common idiopathic dystonias is not clear. Other studies have sought evidence for an endophenotype influencing both dystonia and psychiatric problems by evaluating monoaminergic neurotransmitter systems (dopamine, serotonin, norepinephrine) implicated in both dystonia and psychiatric illnesses. One study compared monoamines in blood samples from individuals with cervical dystonia, myoclonus dystonia, or dopa-responsive dystonia.[104] Those with dystonia had higher 3-methoxytyramine (a dopamine metabolite) and reduced tryptophan (the precursor of serotonin). These results could not be attributed to treatment, implying a potential endogenous abnormality in monoamine metabolism.

Brain monoamine transmission has also been explored using neuroimaging tools, such as single photon emission CT (SPECT). One such study evaluated mood disorders and the dopamine transporter in isolated dystonia, Parkinson disease, and essential tremor.[28] For the dystonia cohort, there was an inverse correlation between the imaging marker for anxiety and depression scores in the left putamen. Another study revealed lower dopamine transporter binding in depressed individuals, compared with non-depressed individuals, who had cervical dystonia.[119] Similar studies targeting serotonin transporters have shown trends for reduced binding among individuals with cervical dystonia who also had difficulties with mood.[118] These results also imply differences in central monoamine transmission that may impact the expression of both dystonia and psychiatric features.

A study focusing on musician's dystonia reported higher anxiety and neuroticism scores than in healthy musicians and non-musician controls.[33] The psychiatric problems did not correlate with the duration of dystonia, suggesting a shared vulnerability to both, rather than the psychiatric problems being secondary to dystonia. Musicians with dystonia had higher levels of anxiety and perfectionism than healthy musician controls, and these issues predated dystonia.[44] A subgroup of both musicians with dystonia and golfers with "the yips" (thought to be a form of dystonia in at least some) were also reported to show increased perfectionistic, stress, and anxiety traits.[42,43] These studies imply an inherent predisposition to certain psychiatric or psychological factors and dystonia.

All together, these findings imply the existence of an endophenotype that predisposes to both dystonia and psychiatric illness. It seems likely that the relationship between dystonia and psychiatric problems varies among individuals. Some individuals who develop dystonia may later develop depression or anxiety purely as a consequence of the motor features. In other cases, psychiatric problems may trigger or contribute to dystonia. A third group may have an inherent predisposition to develop both problems, although both problems may not come at the same time. Further studies are needed to attempt to parse potential subgroups because the approach to therapy may vary.

Treatment of Psychiatric Problems in Dystonia

Psychiatric problems among individuals with dystonia do not always respond to treatment of the motor disorder. As a result, it is important to assess individuals with dystonia for coexisting psychiatric problems and provide more direct treatments for these problems. Such treatments may need to begin with counseling. The importance of illness perception and coping strategies has been suggested in a study where they explained 59% of variance in anxiety and 61% of variance in depression and QoL in cervical dystonia. This finding has therapeutic implications for counseling approaches for dystonia.[79]

The psychiatric problems among individuals with dystonia may also require medications. For depression, any of the commonly used antidepressants may be used. Selective serotonin reuptake inhibitors are commonly used, despite their rare association with acute dystonic reactions (see Chapter 19, "Dystonias Induced by Medications, Illicit Drugs, and Environmental Exposures").[59] One randomized and placebo-controlled trial compared escitalopram with placebo for the treatment of cervical dystonia regardless of coexisting psychiatric features.[117] Motor or psychiatric features were similar for both the treated and placebo groups, although an effect of treatment may have been masked by including individuals who did not have pre-existing depression.

Selective serotonin reuptake inhibitors may also be useful in certain types of anxiety disorders. For anxiety disorders, another option involves benzodiazepines, which can be simultaneously useful to suppress abnormal movements and for treatment of sleep-related problems (see Chapter 28, "Symptom-Targeted Oral Medications for Dystonia").

OTHER NON-MOTOR PROBLEMS

Clustering of Non-Motor Problems

Other non-motor problems are also frequent in dystonia. In a study of 102 individuals with idiopathic isolated dystonia from Brazil (61.8% adult onset, 82.8% focal or segmental), only 8 individuals reported no non-motor problems and 59.8% reported more than 5 problems.[24] The most prevalent problems were pain (72.5%) and anxiety (63.7%), followed by difficulty with recall (44.1%), sadness/anhedonia (41.2%), and sleep initiation insomnia (38.2%). A high prevalence of non-motor features (~95%) was also reported in a case-control study of 425 individuals with idiopathic blepharospasm from China.[115] Depression, cognitive dysfunction, and poor sleep quality were higher in females, while excessive daytime sleepiness was more common in males. A third study, from the United Kingdom, included 1,572 individuals with mixed types of dystonia and again reported increased anxiety, depression, pain, and sleep disturbances, with specific cognitive impairments of prospective memory and fluid intelligence.[109]

In the Brazilian study, the majority of non-motor problems correlated with each other but not with dystonia severity or botulinum toxin therapy.[24] This finding suggests the existence of subgroups of individuals who may have a high frequency of multiple non-motor problems. This possibility of subgroups was explored further in another study that involved two independent cohorts of adults with mixed types of dystonia; 114 individuals from the United Kingdom and 183 from the Dystonia Coalition.[108] This study again revealed a high frequency of multiple non-motor features in both cohorts. Cluster analyses implied the existence of two main subgroups driven by the existence of psychiatric symptoms. This result could imply that self-reports of multiple non-motor symptoms may be driven by underlying psychiatric problems. In fact, a recent study of cervical dystonia indicated that self-reports of motor symptoms were also influenced by coexisting psychiatric problems.[22]

Pain

Pain is not uncommon in some types of dystonia.[16,62] Pain is the most common non-motor symptom in some studies[24,53,112] and it often correlates with mood disturbance.[11,108,109] Pain is especially common in cervical dystonia, affecting 60–80% of all individuals. Pain involves mostly the neck and shoulders, although headache also is frequent, and arm pain may also occur.[61,92] Pain in cervical dystonia has been associated with greater opiate use[68] and it has a profound impact on QoL.[77,98]

Pain also occurs in the craniofacial dystonias.[95,96] The pain associated with blepharospasm is characterized by sensations of corneal irritation or eye pain with photophobia. Pain in oromandibular dystonia most prominently affects the jaw. Individuals with writer's cramp often describe sensations of soreness or aching in the hand or arm, sometimes even when motor abnormalities are not apparent.[116] Pain is also common in children with dystonia,[30] where it can be related to conduct problems.[9] However, pain is not universal among individuals with dystonia. Many individuals with severe and sometimes generalized dystonia leading to extremely abnormal movements and postures have surprisingly little pain.

Mechanisms responsible for pain vary. Pain from muscle pulling and spasms may respond to botulinum toxin treatments.[2,19] Pain may also result from secondary orthopedic problems such as degenerative joint disease of the spine in cervical dystonia. It can also result from tendonitis or fasciitis in limb dystonias. In these cases of orthopedic pain, the pain may persist even when abnormal movements are adequately treated. The perception of pain may also be related to other poorly understood psychological or psychiatric factors related to sensitization in the central nervous system.[92]

Treatment of the motor features of dystonia often alleviates pain, but not always.[92] As a result, therapies directed toward other causes of pain may be needed. The class of medications known as "muscle relaxants" may sometimes be useful, but these drugs will not alleviate pain from orthopedic processes. Orthopedic sources of pain may respond to nonsteroidal anti-inflammatory medications. A careful assessment of the source of the pain may help to guide therapeutic choices.

Sleep and Fatigue

In addition to studies that surveyed the types and frequencies of all non-motor features in dystonia, some studies have focused on more specific non-motor problems or more specific dystonia cohorts. Poor sleep and/or daytime fatigue have been shown to be increased in multiple types of dystonia[41] including cervical dystonia,[7,32,84,110,114] craniofacial dystonia,[7,84,90,110,114] writer's cramp,[116] and generalized dystonia.[60]

Sometimes problems going to sleep are related to abnormal movements that persist when lying down or to chronic pain from dystonia. However, sleep problems correlate poorly with the motor disorder of dystonia. Polysomnographic studies have shown that muscle activity of dystonia abates with sleep, but sleep disruption persists, indicating that sleep disruption is not always caused by the motor features of dystonia.[6] Problems relating to sleep sometimes persist even when the motor features are controlled with botulinum toxin treatments.[32] Sleep disruption and daytime fatigue may instead correlate with depression.[6,7,32,84,105,110]

Addressing sleep-related problems may require treatment of the movement disorder if this is the source of sleep disruption. Addressing sleep may also require treatment of co-existing pain and or psychiatric problems.

Cognition

There are numerous rare developmental disorders where dystonia is combined with cognitive impairments (see Chapter 18, "Dystonias Combined with Other Problems"). Cognitive impairments may take the form of non-progressive intellectual disability or progressive cognitive decline. Children with isolated dystonia are often treated with anticholinergics, sometimes very high doses.[37] Although such high doses are thought to be tolerated better by children than by adults, they often have an unrecognized impact on cognitive function in both age groups.[66,101] Therefore, anticholinergics can also be a source of cognitive impairment in children.

Cognitive impairments may also co-exist with dystonia for numerous degenerative or progressive disorders that emerge later in childhood or adults. Among the more common adult-onset idiopathic isolated focal dystonias, cognition is usually clinically normal. However, detailed neuropsychological testing often reveals potential subclinical cognitive impairments.[53,73,100] Numerous studies have reported apparent difficulties with specific neurocognitive tests,[63,114] or in specific cognitive domains such as executive functions (planning), detection or perception of sensory phenomena (proprioception, spatial and temporal discrimination),[21] mental representation of the body image or spatial orientation of body regions,[4,5,51] recognition of specific facial emotions such as disgust,[91] pseudobulbar affect,[81] apathy,[65] and others.

While comprehensive reviews of the many published articles regarding cognitive functions in dystonia acknowledge that some apparent deficits can be detected with specific cognitive tests,[1,78] deficits are often small, and they may be difficult to disentangle from co-existing psychiatric problems.

QUALITY OF LIFE

The non-motor features of dystonia have a great impact on QoL. In fact, numerous studies show QoL in dystonia is determined predominantly by the severity of non-motor symptoms, which correlate poorly with motor impairment. The Dystonia Coalition analyzed determinants of health-related QoL in an international cohort of 603 adults with various types of isolated dystonia and found that reduced QoL was strongly associated with the severity of symptoms of depression and anxiety. Increased severity of dystonia was also associated with worse physical and emotional functioning and social functioning.[49] In another study of 73 adults with isolated dystonia, QoL as assessed by the Medical Outcomes Study Short Form 36 questionnaire correlated most strongly with tiredness as well as depression and anxiety, but not with motor scores as measured by the Unified Dystonia Rating Scale.[99] The QoL of children with dystonia also is associated with psychiatric and behavioral symptoms but not motor scores.[30]

When comparing individuals with generalized dystonia to healthy controls, scores were lower for QoL, depression, anxiety, fatigue, and sleep quality.[60] Scores on psychiatric rating scales did not correlate with motor severity or disease duration. Another study showed that QoL scores were worse for generalized dystonia compared with focal dystonia. Functional disability, body concept, and depression were important predictors of QoL in dystonia.[83]

For different types of idiopathic focal dystonias, QoL has also been shown to vary. In a series of 157 consecutive individuals with adult-onset primary focal dystonia, QoL was best in writer's cramp, but pain was highest in cervical dystonia.[88] Overall, QoL was again correlated with depression and anxiety. Other studies have confirmed similar findings for more specific populations of blepharospasm[115] and cervical dystonia.[10,18,39,61,73,112] In a comparative study, QoL and mood were found to be similar in idiopathic focal dystonia and essential tremor, except that the prevalence of major depressive disorder was higher for dystonia.[56] QoL correlated with the severity of depression and anxiety in both groups.

SUMMARY AND FUTURE PROSPECTS

Non-motor problems are common among the dystonias. The most common are psychiatric problems relating to depression and/or anxiety, pain, sleep and fatigue, and sometimes specific cognitive processes. Several studies of large populations of different types of dystonia suggest that many of these non-motor problems may be linked, at least for a subgroup of individuals. In some cases, these problems may be a consequence of the motor features of dystonia. In other cases, these problems may cause or contribute to the motor features. In still others, there may be a biological endophenotype that predisposes to both motor and non-motor features. Further studies of the relationship between motor and non-motor problems in specific populations are needed to refine understanding of the directions of causation.

The motor features of dystonia are often easy to recognize, but the non-motor features may be less apparent unless a history is sought. The non-motor features are important to recognize because they have an impact on QoL that is greater than the impact of motor features. Treatment of the motor features of dystonia does not always alleviate the non-motor features, so therapies directed to both are often needed. Efforts are under way to develop screening tools for these non-motor features to make individuals who need directed therapy easier to identify.

REFERENCES

1. Aita SL, Del Bene VA, Marotta DA, Pizer JH, Hawley NA, Niccolai L, et al. Neuropsychological functioning in primary dystonia: Updated and expanded multidomain meta-analysis. Mov Disord 2022;37:1483–1494.
2. Albanese A, Wissel J, Jost WH, Castagna A, Althaus M, Comes G, et al. Pain reduction in cervical dystonia following treatment with incobotulinumtoxinA: A pooled analysis. Toxins (Basel) 2023;15:333.
3. Alves Junior AC, Daker MV, Machado AMC, Luna AS, Valladares Neto DC, Valadares ER. Neuropsychiatric and sleep study in autosomal dominant dopa-responsive dystonia. Mol Genet Metab Rep 2022;31:100870.
4. Anastasopoulos D, Bhatia K, Bisdorff A, Bronstein AM, Gresty MA, Marsden CD. Perception of spatial orientation in spasmodic torticollis. Part I: The postural vertical. Mov Disord 1997;12:561–569.
5. Anastasopoulos D, Nasios G, Psilas K, Mergner T, Maurer C, Lucking CH. What is straight ahead to a patient with torticollis? Brain 1998;121:91–101.
6. Antelmi E, Ferri R, Provini F, Scaglione CML, Mignani F, Rundo F, et al. Modulation of the muscle activity during sleep in cervical dystonia. Sleep 2017;40. doi:10.1093/sleep/zsx08.
7. Avanzino L, Martino D, Marchese R, Aniello MS, Minafra B, Superbo M, et al. Quality of sleep in primary focal dystonia: A case-control study. Eur J Neurol 2010;17:576–581.
8. Bailey GA, Rawlings A, Torabi F, Pickrell WO, Peall KJ. Longitudinal analysis of the relationship between motor and psychiatric symptoms in idiopathic dystonia. Eur J Neurol 2022;29:3513–3527.
9. Bates L, Taylor M, Lin JP, Gimeno H, Kingston J, Rudebeck SR. Mental health and behaviour in children with dystonia: Anxiety, challenging behaviour and the relationship to pain and self-esteem. Eur J Paediatr Neurol 2021;35:40–48.
10. Ben-Shlomo Y, Camfield L, Warner T. What are the determinants of quality of life in people with cervical dystonia? J Neurol Neurosurg Psychiatry 2002;72:608–614.
11. Berman BD, Junker J, Shelton E, Sillau SH, Jinnah HA, Perlmutter JS, et al. Psychiatric associations of adult-onset focal dystonia phentypes. J Neurol Neurosurg Psychiat 2017;88:505–602.
12. Bertram KL, Williams DR. Delays to the diagnosis of cervical dystonia. J Clin Neurosci 2015;25:62–64.
13. Boyce MJ, McCambridge AB, Bradnam LV, Canning CG, De Oliveira CQ, Verhagen AP. Botulinum toxin and conservative treatment strategies in people with cervical dystonia: An online survey. J Neural Transm 2023;131:43–51.
14. Brashear A, Dobyns WB, de Carvalho Aguiar P, Borg M, Frijns CJ, et al. The phenotypic spectrum of rapid-onset dystonia-parkinsonism (RDP) and mutations in the ATP1A3 gene. Brain 2007;130:828–835.
15. Bruggemann N, Stiller S, Tadic V, Kasten M, Munchau A, Graf J, et al. Non-motor phenotype of dopa-responsive dystonia and quality of life assessment. Parkinsonism Relat Disord 2014;20:428–431.
16. Bruno V, Achen B, Morgante F, Erro R, Fox SH, Edwards MJ, et al. The Pain in Dystonia Scale (PIDS): Development and validation in cervical dystonia. Mov Disord 2023;38:1175–1186.
17. Calderon DP, Fremont R, Kraenzlin F, Khodakhah K. The neural substrates of rapid-onset dystonia-parkinsonism. Nat Neurosci 2011;14:357–365.
18. Camfield L, Ben-Shlomo Y, Warner TT. Impact of cervical dystonia on quality of life. Mov Disord 2002;17:838–841.
19. Castelao M, Marques RE, Duarte GS, Rodrigues FB, Ferreira J, Sampaio C, Moore AP, Costa J. Botulinum toxin type A therapy for cervical dystonia. Cochrane Database Syst Rev 2017;12:CD003633.
20. Childs L, Rickert S, Murry T, Blitzer A, Sulica L. Patient perceptions of factors leading to spasmodic dysphonia: A combined clinical experience of 350 patients. Laryngoscope 2011;121:2195–2198.
21. Conte A, Defazio G, Hallett M, Fabbrini G, Berardelli A. The role of sensory information in the pathophysiology of focal dystonias. Nat Rev Neurol 2019;15:224–233.
22. Cotton AC, Scorr L, McDonald W, Comella C, Perlmutter JS, Goetz CG, et al. Assessing the severity of cervical dystonia: Ask the doctor or ask the patient. Mov Disord Clin Pract 2023;10:1399–1403.
23. Creighton FXJ, Hapner ER, Klein AM, Rosen A, Jinnah HA. Diagnostic delays in spasmodic dysphonia: A call for clinician education. J Voice 2015;29:592–594.
24. da Silva-Junior FP, Dos Santos Alves CO, Silva S, Borges V, Ferraz HB, Rocha MSG, et al. High prevalence of self-reported non-motor symptoms and lack of correlation with motor severity in adult patients with idiopathic isolated dystonia. Neurol Sci 2022;43:1061–1065.
25. DeAndrade MP, Yokoi F, van Groen T, Lingrel JB, Li Y. Characterization of Atp1a3 mutant mice as a model of rapid-onset dystonia with parkinsonism. Behav Brain Res 2011;216:659–665.
26. Defazio G, Gigante AF, Hallett M, Berardelli A, Perlmutter JS, Berman BD, et al. Motor and psychiatric features in idiopathic blepharospasm: A data-driven cluster analysis. Parkinsonism Relat Disord 2022;104:94–98.
27. Dias FM, Kummer A, Doyle FC, Harsányi E, Cardoso F, Fontenelle LF, Teixeira AL. Psychiatric disorders in primary focal dystonia and in Parkinson's disease. Neuropsychiatr Dis Treat 2011;7:111–116.
28. Di Giuda D, Camardese G, Bentivoglio AR, Cocciolillo F, Guidubaldi A, Pucci L, et al. Dopaminergic dysfunction and psychiatric symptoms in movement disorders: A 123I-FP-CIT SPECT study. Eur J Nucl Med Mol Imaging 2012;39:1937–1948.
29. Drexel SC, Klietz M, Kollewe K, Paracka L, Kutschenko A, Kopp B, et al. Caregiver burden and health-related quality of life in idiopathic dystonia patients under botulinum toxin treatment: A cross-sectional study. J Neural Transm (Vienna) 2020;127:61–70.
30. Eggink H, Coenen MA, de Jong R, Toonen RF, Eissens MH, Veenstra WS, et al. Motor and non-motor determinants of health-related quality of life in young dystonia patients. Parkinsonism Relat Disord 2019;58:50–55.
31. Eggink H, Szlufik S, Coenen MA, van Egmond ME, Moro E, Tijssen MAJ. Non-motor effects of deep

brain stimulation in dystonia: A systematic review. Parkinsonism Relat Disord 2018;55:26–44.
32. Eichenseer SR, Stebbins GT, Comella CL. Beyond a motor disorder: A prospective evaluation of sleep quality in cervical dystonia. Parkinsonism Relat Disord 2014;20:405–408.
33. Enders L, Spector JT, Altenmüller E, Schmidt A, Klein C, Jabusch HC. Musician's dystonia and comorbid anxiety: Two sides of one coin? Mov Disord 2011;26:539–542.
34. Fabbrini G, Berardelli I, Moretti G, Pasquini M, Bloise M, Colosimo C, et al. Psychiatric disorders in adult-onset focal dystonia: A case-control study. Mov Disord 2010;25:459–465.
35. Fleming BM, Schwab EL, Nouer SS, Wan JY, LeDoux MS. Prevalence, predictors, and perceived effectiveness of complementary, alternative and integrative medicine in adult-onset primary dystonia. Parkinsonism Relat Disord 2012;18:936–940.
36. Fureman BE, Jinnah HA, Hess EJ. Triggers of paroxysmal dyskinesias in the calcium channel mouse mutant tottering. Pharmacol Biochem Behav 2002;73:631–637.
37. Greene P, Shale H, Fahn S. Experience with high dosages of anticholinergic and other drugs in the treatment of torsion dystonia. Adv Neurol 1988;50:547–556.
38. Gundel H, Wolf A, Xidara V, Busch R, Ceballos-Baumann AO. Social phobia in spasmodic torticollis. J Neurol Neurosurg Psychiatry 2001;71:499–504.
39. Han V, Skorvanek M, Smit M, Turcanova Koprusakova M, Hoekstra T, van Dijk JP, et al. Prevalence of non-motor symptoms and their association with quality of life in cervical dystonia. Acta Neurol Scand 2020;142:613–622.
40. Heiman GA, Ottman R, Saunders-Pullman RJ, Ozelius LJ, Risch NJ, Bressman SB. Increased risk for recurrent major depression in DYT1 dystonia mutation carriers. Neurology 2004;63:631–637.
41. Hertenstein E, Tang NK, Bernstein CJ, Nissen C, Underwood MR, Sandhu HK. Sleep in patients with primary dystonia: A systematic review on the state of research and perspectives. Sleep Med Rev 2016;26:95–107.
42. Ioannou CI, Altenmüller E. Psychological characteristics in musician's dystonia: A new diagnostic classification. Neuropsychologia 2014;61:80–88.
43. Ioannou CI, Klämpfl MK, Lobinger BH, Raab M, Altenmüller E. Psychodiagnostics: Classification of the yips phenomenon based on musician's dystonia. Med Sci Sports Exerc 2018;50:2217–2225.
44. Jabusch HC, Muller SV, Altenmuller E. Anxiety in musicians with focal dystonia and those with chronic pain. Mov Disord 2004;19:1169–1175.
45. Jahanshahi M. Factors that ameliorate or aggravate spasmodic torticollis. J Neurol Neurosurg Psychiatry 2000;68:227–229.
46. Jahanshahi M, Marsden CD. Depression in torticollis: A controlled study. Psychol Med 1988;18:925–933.
47. Jahanshahi M, Torkamani M, Beigi M, Wilkinson L, Page D, Madeley L, et al. Pallidal stimulation for primary generalised dystonia: Effect on cognition, mood and quality of life. Psychol Med 2014;261:164–173.
48. Jog M, Chouinard S, Hobson D, Grimes D, Chen R, Bhogal M, Simonyi S. Causes for treatment delays in dystonia and hemifacial spasm: A Canadian survey. Can J Neurol Sci 2011;38:704–711.
49. Junker J, Berman BD, Hall J, Wahba D, Brandt V, et al. Quality of life in dystonia: Non-motor manifestations matter. J Neurol Neurosurg Psychiat 2021;92:622–628.
50. Junker J, Oberwittler C, Jackson D, Berger K. Utilization and perceived effectiveness of complementary and alternative medicine in patients with dystonia. Mov Disord 2004;19:158–161.
51. Konczak J, Aman JE, Chen YW, Li KY, Watson PJ. Impaired limb proprioception in adults with spasmodic dysphonia. J Voice 2015;29:777.e717–e723.
52. Kongsaengdao S, Maneeton N, Maneeton B. Long-term quality of life in cervical dystonia after treatment with abobotulinum toxin A: A 2-year prospective study. Neuropsychiatr Dis Treat 2018;14:1119–1124.
53. Kuyper DJ, Parra V, Aerts S, Okun MS, Kluger BM. Nonmotor manifestations of dystonia: A systematic review. Mov Disord 2011;26:1206–1217.
54. LaHue SC, Albers K, Goldman S, Lo RY, Gu Z, Leimpeter A, et al. Cervical dystonia incidence and diagnostic delay in a multiethnic population. Mov Disord 2019;35:450–456.
55. Lane V, Lane M, Sturrock A, Rickards H. Understanding psychiatric disorders in idiopathic and inherited (monogenic) forms of isolated and combined dystonia: A systematic review. J Neuropsychiatry Clin Neurosci 2021;33:295–306.
56. Lee S, Chung SJ, Shin HW. Neuropsychiatric symptoms and quality of life in patients with adult-onset idiopathic focal dystonia and essential tremor. Front Neurol 2020;11:1030.
57. Lehn A, Mellick G, Boyle R. Psychiatric disorders in idiopathic-isolated focal dystonia. J Neurol 2014;261:668–674.
58. Lencer R, Steinlechner S, Stahlberg J, Rehling H, Orth M, Baeumer T, et al. Primary focal dystonia: Evidence for distinct neuropsychiatric and personality profiles. J Neurol Neurosurg Psychiatry 2009;80:1176–1179.
59. Leo RJ. Movement disorders associated with the serotonin selective reuptake inhibitors. J Clin Psychiatry 1996;57:449–454.
60. Li S, Wang L, Yang Y, Qiao L, Zhang D, Wan X. Non-motor symptoms in Chinese patients with isolated generalized dystonia: A case-control study. Front Neurol 2020;11:209.
61. Liang Y, Lin J, Hou Y, Zhang L, Ou R, Li C, et al. Health-related quality of life in cervical dystonia using EQ-5D-5L: A large cross-sectional study in China. Front Neurol 2022;13:895272.
62. Listik C, Listik E, de Paiva Santos Rolim F, Meneses Cury Portela DM, Perez Lloret S, de Alves Araujo NR, et al. Development and validation of the Dystonia-Pain Classification System: A multicenter study. Mov Disord 2023;38:1163–1174.
63. Liu K, Hou Y, Ou R, Yang T, Yang J, Song W, et al. Cognitive impairment in Chinese patients with cervical dystonia. Front Neurol 2022;13:961563.
64. Lorentzos MS, Heyman I, Baig BJ, Coughtrey AE, McWilliams A, Dossetor DR, et al. Psychiatric comorbidity is common in dystonia and other movement disorders. Arch Dis Child 2021;106:62–67.
65. Louis ED, Huey ED, Gerbin M, Viner AS. Apathy in essential tremor, dystonia, and Parkinson's disease: A comparison with normal controls. Mov Disord 2012;27:432–434.
66. Lumsden DE, Kaminska M, Tomlin S, Lin JP. Medication use in childhood dystonia. Eur J Paediatr Neurol 2016;20:625–629.
67. Macerollo A, Superbo M, Gigante AF, Livrea P, Defazio G. Diagnostic delay in adult-onset dystonia: Data from

an Italian movement disorder center. J Clin Neurosci 2015;22:608–610.
68. Mahajan A, Jankovic J, Marsh L, Patel A, Jinnah HA, Comella C, et al. Cervical dystonia and substance abuse. J Neurol 2018;265:970–975.
69. Martino D, Brander G, Svenningsson P, Larsson H, de la Cruz LF. Association and familial coaggregation of idiopathic dystonia with psychiatric outcomes. Mov Disord 2020;35:2270–2278.
70. Medina Escobar A, Martino D, Goodarzi Z. The prevalence of anxiety in adult-onset isolated dystonia: A systematic review and meta-analysis. Eur J Neurol 2021;28:4238–4250.
71. Medina Escobar A, Pringsheim T, Goodarzi Z, Martino D. The prevalence of depression in adult onset idiopathic dystonia: Systematic review and metaanalysis. Neurosci Biobehav Rev 2021;125:221–230.
72. Miller KM, Okun MS, Fernandez HF, Jacobson CE, Rodriguez RL, Bowers D. Depression symptoms in movement disorders: Comparing Parkinson's disease, dystonia, and essential tremor. Mov Disord 2007;22:666–672.
73. Monaghan R, Cogley C, Burke T, McCormack D, O'Riordan S, Ndukwe I, et al. Non-motor features of cervical dystonia: Cognition, social cognition, psychological distress and quality of life. Clin Park Relat Disord 2021;4:100084.
74. Moriarty A, Rafee S, Ndukwe I, O'Riordan S, Hutchinson M. Longitudinal follow-up of mood in cervical dystonia and influence on age at onset. Mov Disord Clin Pract 2022;9:614–618.
75. Mula M, Strigaro G, Marotta AE, Ruggerone S, Tribolo A, Monaco R, Cantello F. Obsessive-compulsive-spectrum symptoms in patients with focal dystonia, hemifacial spasm, and healthy subjects. J Neuropsychiatry Clin Neurosci 2012;24:81–86.
76. Müller J, Kemmler G, Wissel J, Schneider A, Voller B, Grossmann J, et al. The impact of blepharospasm and cervical dystonia on health-related quality of life and depression. J Neurol 2002;249:842–846.
77. Ndukwe I, O'Riordan S, Walsh CB, Hutchinson M. Mood disorder affects age at onset of adult-onset cervical dystonia. Clin Park Relat Disord 2020;3:100049.
78. O'Connor S, Hevey D, Burke T, Rafee S, Pender N, O'Keeffe F. A systematic review of cognition in cervical dystonia. Neuropsychol Rev 2023;34:134–154.
79. O'Connor S, Hevey D, O'Keeffe F. Illness perceptions, coping, health-related quality of life and psychological outcomes in cervical dystonia. J Clin Psychol Med Settings 2022;30:129–142.
80. Ochudlo S, Bryniarski P, Opala G. Botulinum toxin improves the quality of life and reduces the intensification of depressive symptoms in patients with blepharospasm. Parkinsonism Relat Disord 2007;13:505–508.
81. Ospina-García N, Escobar-Barrios M, Rodríguez-Violante M, Benitez-Valenzuela J, Cervantes-Arriaga A. Neuropsychiatric profile of patients with craniocervical dystonia: A case-control study. Clin Neurol Neurosurg 2020;193:105794.
82. Ozel-Kizil ET, Akbostanci MC, Ozguven HD, Atbasoglu EC. Secondary social anxiety in hyperkinesias. Mov Disord 2008;23:641–645.
83. Page D, Butler A, Jahanshahi M. Quality of life in focal, segmental, and generalized dystonia. Mov Disord 2007;22:341–347.
84. Paus S, Gross J, Moll-Muller M, Hentschel F, Spottke A, Wabbels B, et al. Impaired sleep quality and restless legs syndrome in idiopathic focal dystonia: A controlled study. J Neurol 2011;258:1835–1840.
85. Peall KJ, Dijk JM, Saunders-Pullman R, Dreissen YE, van Loon I, Cath D, et al. Psychiatric disorders, myoclonus dystonia and SGCE: An international study. Ann Clin Transl Neurol 2016;3:4–11.
86. Peall KJ, Smith DJ, Kurian MA, Wardle M, Waite AJ, Hedderly T, et al. SGCE mutations cause psychiatric disorders: Clinical and genetic characterization. Brain 2013;136:294–303.
87. Peckham EL, Lopez G, Shamim EA, Richardson SP, Sanku S, Malkani R, et al. Clinical features of patients with blepharospasm: A report of 240 patients. Eur J Neurol 2011;18:382–386.
88. Pekmezovic T, Svetel M, Ivanovic N, Dragasevic N, Petrovic I, Tepavcevic DK, Kostic VS. Quality of life in patients with focal dystonia. Clin Neurol Neurosurg 2009;111:161–164.
89. Raike RS, Weisz C, Hoebeek FE, Terzi MC, De Zeeuw CI, van den Maagdenberg AM, et al. Stress, caffeine and ethanol trigger transient neurological dysfunction through shared mechanisms in a mouse calcium channelopathy. Neurobiol Dis 2013;50:151–159.
90. Ray S, Kutty B, Pal PK, Yadav R. Sleep and other non-motor symptoms in patients with idiopathic oromandibular dystonia and meige syndrome: A auestionnaire-based study. Ann Indian Acad Neurol 2021;24:351–355.
91. Rinnerthaler M, Benecke C, Bartha L, Entner T, Poewe W, Mueller J. Facial recognition in primary focal dystonia. Mov Disord 2006;21:78–82.
92. Rosales RL, Cuffe L, Regnault B, Trosch RM. Pain in cervical dystonia: Mechanisms, assessment and treatment. Expert Rev Neurother 2021;21:1125–1134.
93. Roze E, Soumare A, Pironneau I, Sangla S, de Cock VC, Teixeira A, et al. Case-control study of writer's cramp. Brain 2009;132:756–764.
94. Schweinfurth JM, Billante M, Courey MS. Risk factors and demographics in patients with spasmodic dysphonia. Laryngoscope 2002;112:220–223.
95. Scorr L, Cho HJ, Kilic-Berkmen G, McKay JL, Hallett M, Klein C, et al. Clinical features and evolution of blepharospasm: A multicenter international cohort and systematic literature review. Dystonia 2022;1:10359.
96. Scorr LM, Factor SA, Perez-Parra S, Kaye R, Paniello RC, Norris SA, et al. Oromandibular dystonia: A clinical examination of 2,020 cases. Front Neurol 2021;12:700714.
97. Shirley TL, Rao LM, Hess EJ, Jinnah HA. Paroxysmal dyskinesias in mice. Mov Disord 2008;23:259–264.
98. Smit M, Kamphuis ASJ, Bartels AL, Han V, Stewart RE, Zijdewind I, Tijssen MA. Fatigue, sleep disturbances, and their influence on quality of life in cervical dystonia patients. Mov Disord Clin Pract 2017;4:517–523.
99. Soeder A, Kluger BM, Okun MS, Garvan CW, Soeder T, Jacobson CE, et al. Mood and energy determinants of quality of life in dystonia. J Neurol 2009;256:996–1001.
100. Stamelou M, Edwards MJ, Hallett M, Bhatia KP. The non-motor syndrome of primary dystonia: Clinical and pathophysiological implications. Brain 2012;135:1668–1681.
101. Taylor AE, Lang AE, Saint-Cyr JA, Riley DE, Ranawaya R. Cognitive processes in idiopathic dystonia treated with high-dose anticholinergic therapy: Implications

for treatment strategies. Clin Neuropharmacol 1991;14:62–77.
102. Tiderington E, Goodman EM, Rosen AR, Hapner ER, Johns MM, 3rd, Evatt ML, et al. How long does it take to diagnose cervical dystonia? J Neurol Sci 2013;335:72–74.
103. Timmers ER, Plösch T, Smit M, Hof IH, Verkaik-Schakel RN, Tijssen MAJ, et al. Methylation of the serotonin reuptake transporter gene and non-motor symptoms in dystonia patients. Clin Epigenetics 2022;14:170.
104. Timmers ER, van Faassen M, Smit M, Kuiper A, Hof IH, Kema IP, et al. Dopaminergic and serotonergic alterations in plasma in three groups of dystonia patients. Parkinsonism Relat Disord 2021;91:48–54.
105. Tomic S, Kuric TG, Popovic Z, Zubonja TM. Fatigue is related to depression in idiopathic dystonia. Neurol Sci 2022;43:373–378.
106. Vezyroglou A, Akilapa R, Barwick K, Koene S, Brownstein CA, Holder-Espinasse M, et al. The phenotypic continuum of ATP1A3-related disorders. Neurology 2022;99:e1511–e1526.
107. Voon V, Butler TR, Ekanayake V, Gallea C, Ameli R, Murphy DL, Hallett M. Psychiatric symptoms associated with focal hand dystonia. Mov Disord 2010;25:2249–2252.
108. Wadon ME, Bailey GA, Yilmaz Z, Hubbard E, AlSaeed M, Robinson A, et al. Non-motor phenotypic subgroups in adult-onset idiopathic, isolated, focal cervical dystonia. Brain Behav 2021;11:e2292.
109. Wadon ME, Fenner E, Kendall KM, Bailey GA, Sandor C, Rees E, Peall KJ. Clinical and genotypic analysis in determining dystonia non-motor phenotypic heterogeneity: A UK Biobank study. J Neurol 2022;269:6436–6451.
110. Wagle Shukla A, Brown R, Heese K, Jones J, Rodriguez RL, Malaty IM, et al. High rates of fatigue and sleep disturbances in dystonia. Int J Neurosci 2016;126:928–935.
111. Weissbach A, Pauly MG, Herzog R, Hahn L, Halmans S, Hamami F, et al. Relationship of genotype, phenotype, and treatment in dopa-responsive dystonia: MDSGene review. Mov Disord 2021;2022:237–252.
112. Werle RW, Takeda SY, Zonta MB, Guimarães AT, Teive HA. The physical, social and emotional aspects are the most affected in the quality of life of the patients with cervical dystonia. Arq Neuropsiquiatr 2014;72:405–410.
113. Worthley A, Simonyan K. Suicidal ideations and attempts in patients with isolated dystonia. Neurology 2021;96:e1551–e1560.
114. Yang J, Shao N, Song W, Wei Q, Ou R, Wu Y, Shang HF. Nonmotor symptoms in primary adult-onset cervical dystonia and blepharospasm. Brain Behav 2017;7:e00592.
115. Yang J, Zhang L, Hou Y, Wei Q, Ou R, Lin J, et al. Sex related differences in nonmotor symptoms of patients with idiopathic blepharospasm. Sci Rep 2021;11:17856.
116. Zhang L, Hou Y, Lin J, Yang J, Cao B, Wei Q, et al. Comprehensive analysis of non-motor symptoms and their association with quality of life in writer's cramp. Parkinsonism Relat Disord 2022;100:37–40.
117. Zoons E, Booij J, Delnooz CCS, Dijk JM, Dreissen YEM, Koelman J, et al. Randomised controlled trial of escitalopram for cervical dystonia with dystonic jerks/tremor. J Neurol Neurosurg Psychiatry 2018;89:579–585.
118. Zoons E, Booij J, Speelman JD, Dreissen YEM, Smit M, Tijssen MAJ. Lower serotonin transporter binding in patients with cervical dystonia is associated with psychiatric symptoms. EJNMMI Res 2017;7:87.
119. Zoons E, Tijssen MAJ, Dreissen YEM, Speelman JD, Smit M, Booij J. The relationship between the dopaminergic system and depressive symptoms in cervical dystonia. Eur J Nucl Med Mol Imaging 2017;44:1375–1382.
120. Zurowski M, Marsh L, McDonald W. Psychiatric comorbidities in dystonia: Emerging concepts. Mov Disord 2013;28:914–920.

SECTION III

The Combined (Mixed) Dystonia Syndromes

Chapter 12

Dystonia and Tremor

INTRODUCTION

Tremor is characterized by rhythmical oscillation of a body region.[37,82] There are many types of tremors. The most common include the postural and kinetic tremors sometimes called *essential tremor* or the resting tremor of Parkinson disease. These common tremors typically have an oscillation that has a relatively steady tempo and a similar speed in both directions of oscillation, producing a rhythmical and sinusoidal movement.

Dystonia is characterized by involuntary muscle contractions leading to slow and prolonged twisting movements or sustained postures.[3] The clinical manifestations of tremor are therefore usually easy to distinguish from tremor. However, the contractions of dystonia are not always slow and prolonged. Sometimes, muscle contractions are very brief, appearing as a quick jerk. When these jerks occur in isolation, they may resemble myoclonus or tics. Dystonic jerks may recur and produce semi-rhythmical movements that may resemble a tremor.

In addition to repetitive dystonic jerks that mimic tremor, dystonia may coexist with more typical tremors. Therefore, it is possible to have a mixed disorder that includes both dystonia and tremor. There also are some movement abnormalities that fall in a gray area, such as isolated head or voice tremors or task-specific tremors. Expert opinions vary regarding whether these problems should be classified as subtypes of dystonia or as subtypes of tremor. These many areas of overlap between tremor and dystonia have been the subject of debate among experts for decades.[102]

EVOLVING TERMINOLOGY

The term *dystonic tremor* has been used in different ways over the years. The term was first used by Fahn to describe recurrent dystonic jerky movements resembling other tremors.[42] When a repetitive oscillatory movement was the dominant or sole manifestation of dystonia, the term *tremor-dominant dystonia* was applied.[42]

Early reports highlighted two major features that distinguished dystonic tremors from more common tremors. One feature was a jerky quality. This jerky quality was thought to differ from more common tremors, which are not usually jerky. The other feature of dystonic tremors was an irregular tempo. This irregularity also contrasted with the more rhythmical oscillations of more common tremors. Two other features also distinguished dystonic tremors from more common tremors. For example, dystonic tremors could be attenuated with a specific gesture, known as the *geste antagoniste*. Additionally, dystonic tremors often varied in amplitude, depending on position. They attenuated or disappeared in a specific position, referred to as the *null point*.

Fahn's original descriptions of dystonic tremors were later viewed as too subjective for reliable application. Oscillations that are very jerky or irregular are easy to identify by clinical exam, but more subtle jerkiness or irregularity can be more challenging to detect. Similarly, the *geste antagoniste* and null point sometimes produce incomplete responses that are difficult to interpret. As a result of the subjective quality of Fahn's criteria, expert committees of the Movement Disorders Society (MDS) recommended alternative criteria to define *dystonic tremor* in 1998 and again in 2018.[17,30] The MDS committees defined dystonic tremor as any tremor that occurred in a body region simultaneously affected with more obvious dystonic postures. They also defined a new entity, *tremor associated with dystonia*, to describe cases with dystonia in one body region and tremor in a different body region.

These two descriptions of dystonic tremor are very different. Fahn's criteria emphasized the phenomenology of repetitive movements of jerkiness and regularity, along with a *geste antagoniste* and a null point (Figure 12.1A). The coexistence of more obvious twisting or postural movements of dystonia was not required. In contrast, the MDS criteria required the coexistence of overt dystonia with the oscillatory movements, regardless of jerkiness or regularity (Figure 12.1B). One large study that compared these criteria in the same cohort of participants demonstrated that they produce very different results.[125]

The new MDS criteria have been criticized extensively and have not been universally adopted.[1,5,34,35,44,50,56,79,81,99,108,112,114] A concern about the MDS criteria was that assessing coexisting dystonic movements can be just as subjective as assessing jerkiness or irregularity.[97,125] Coexisting dystonia may be obvious, but mild dystonia is not always easy to identify or discriminate from potential compensatory motor behaviors, leading to frequent differences of interpretation.[11] The MDS criteria define any tremor in a dystonic body part as a dystonic tremor, implying that dystonic tremor can never coexist by chance with another type of tremor, such as a Parkinson tremor. Finally, the concept of tremor-dominant dystonia becomes challenging with the MDS criteria, especially if there is no coexisting dystonia.

Disagreement regarding criteria for dystonic tremor and tremor-dominant dystonia persists. Some experts use the MDS consensus criteria,[27]

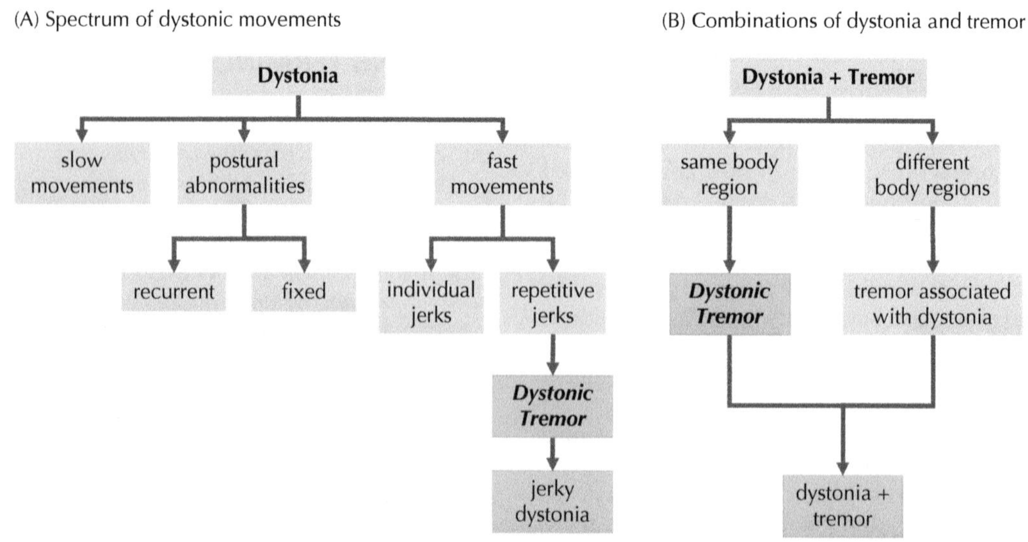

Figure 12.1. Dual use of the term *dystonic tremor*. Panel A shows the spectrum of abnormal movements in dystonia, and Panel B shows combinations of dystonia with tremor. The term *dystonic tremor* has been used to describe repetitive dystonic jerking that mimics tremor (Panel A) as well as coexistence of dystonia with a tremor that resembles essential tremor (Panel B). Clearer terminology may be preferable to avoid confusion regarding the meaning of dystonic tremor.

Table 12.1 **Different terms to describe combinations of tremor and dystonia**

Term	Explanation
Dystonia-tremor syndrome	A syndrome with two distinct movement abnormalities (dystonia and tremor) occurring in the same individual, synonymous with dystonia and tremor, or dystonia with tremor[52,68,76]
Dystonic tremor	Recurrent dystonic jerks with irregular timing that may be sufficiently regular to resemble a tremor, with or without other co-existing dystonic movements[41,42] Any tremor that occurs in the same body region that also has more obvious dystonic postures or movements[17,30]
Jerky dystonia	Rapid and repetitive dystonic movements that usually have an irregular tempo, but may be sufficiently regular to mimic a tremor[7,23,46]
Tremor associated with dystonia	A movement disorder where dystonia occurs in one body region, and tremor occurs in a different body region[17,30]
Tremulous dystonia	Dystonia with prominent co-existing tremor or other tremor-like movements[20,90]

Some terminology used to describe relationships between tremor and dystonia, along with representative citations.

while others use the Fahn criteria.[37,43,73,111] Other experts, dissatisfied with both criteria, have used alternative terminology, such as *tremulous dystonia, dystonia-tremor syndrome*, or others (Table 12.1).[20,90] Because the term *dystonic tremor* has been used to describe two very different types of movement, it probably should be avoided and replaced with less equivocal terminology.

COEXISTENCE OF DYSTONIA AND TREMOR

There is strong evidence that dystonia and tremor may coexist. Many large studies have described cohorts of individuals with dystonia, where 10–90% had a coexisting tremor (Table 12.2). The variations among these reports arise

Table 12.2 **Descriptive studies of dystonia cohorts**

Predominant type of dystonia	Study	Total cases	Percent with tremor
Blepharospasm	Jankovic et al., 1983[59]	100	31.0
Cervical dystonia	Chan et al., 1991[19]	266	27.9
	Jankovic et al., 1991[61]	300	71.3
	Deuschl et al., 1997[31]	55	60.0
	Pal et al., 2000[95]	114	68.4
	Godeiro-Junior, 2008[49]	118	42.4
	LeDoux et al., 2016[135]	1000	62.0
	Hvizdosova et al., 2020[57]	120	58.3
	Pandey et al., 2020[98]	293	57.6
Hand dystonia	Jhunjhunwala et al., 2015[63]	125	28.8
Laryngeal dystonia	Schweinfurth et al., 2002[124]	168	26.2
	Tisch et al., 2003[135]	169	13.1
	White et al., 2011[139]	146	32.0
Mixed dystonias	Dubinsky et al., 1993[33]	296	10.8
	Defazio et al., 2013[28]	429	16.7
	Rudzinska et al., 2013[120]	123	48.8
	Erro et al., 2013[39]	473	55.4
	Gigante et al., 2016[47]	173	34.0
	Williams et al., 2016[141]	375	16.8–23.8
	Pandey et al., 2017[100]	90	45.6
	Shaikh et al., 2020[125]	2362	53.3

This table summarizes the prevalence of tremor among dystonia cohorts with at least 50 participants published after 1980. The vast majority of cohorts included idiopathic adult-onset dystonias, although some also included cases secondary to known causes. Studies are grouped by predominant type of dystonia included, although many included segmental and multifocal patterns as well.

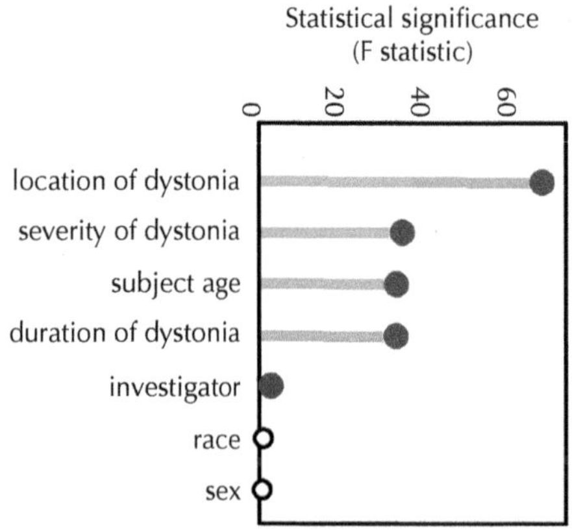

Figure 12.2. Factors influencing the coexistence of tremor and dystonia. This figure was adapted from an article that included a cohort of 2,362 participants with different forms of isolated dystonia, more than half of whom also had tremor.[125] Logistic regression revealed several variables associated with the risk of tremor, including (in order of impact) body location affected by dystonia, severity of dystonia, age at patient evaluation, duration of dystonia, and recruiting investigator. Sex and race did not have a significant impact on the frequency of tremor in dystonia subjects. The strength of each variable is estimated by the length of the line. Variables with a statistically significant impact are shown as solid circles, while those with no significant impact are shown as open circles.

from many factors, most notably the types of dystonias included in the study. For example, studies with large numbers of participants with cervical dystonia report higher frequencies of tremor than do cohorts focusing on laryngeal dystonia or blepharospasm. Variations in tremor frequency are also influenced by other factors, such as how dystonia and tremor were determined.

In one study, 2,362 participants with different types of dystonia were recruited across 37 centers.[125] Overall, the frequency of coexisting tremor was 53%, but this frequency depended on which body regions were affected with dystonia, dystonia severity and duration, and participant age (Figure 12.2). Coexisting tremor did not depend on sex or race. The frequency of coexisting tremor was also influenced by recruiting investigator, pointing to the subjectiveness of the clinical exam for diagnosis.

There are also many large studies that aimed to delineate the clinical features of individuals with a primary tremor disorder, often called "essential tremor" (Table 12.3). In these studies, the frequency of coexisting dystonia has varied from 0% to 47%. Differences among these studies are due to many of the same factors described for dystonia cohorts. However, for essential tremor cohorts, inclusion criteria also influence the results. Some investigators excluded any cases with dystonia because essential tremor traditionally was defined as a pure tremor disorder. Other investigators included participants who had a tremor resembling essential tremor, even if they had mild dystonia, a syndrome sometimes called *essential tremor-plus*.[17] Thus the overall prevalence of dystonia in studies of cohorts of "essential tremor" is lower than that reported for dystonia cohorts.

As noted above, the terminology used to describe tremor and tremor-like movements in dystonia is not consistently used (Table 12.1). Even the term *essential tremor* has been called into question.[13,32,44,48,81,82,97,114] Despite the limitations of the terminology and uncertainty of studies that depend on it, it is clear from many descriptive cohort studies that dystonia occurs along with a tremor that can resemble essential tremor far more frequently than predicted by

Table 12.3 **Descriptive studies of essential tremor cohorts**

Type of tremor	Study	Total cases	Percent with dystonia
Essential tremor	Lou & Jankovic, 1991[77]	350	47.1
Essential tremor	Koller et al.[67]	678	6.9
Essential tremor	Jankovic et al., 1997[60]	251	15.0
Essential tremor	Shatunov et al., 2006[129]	325	4.6
Essential tremor	Hedera et al., 2010[54]	463	21.1
Essential tremor	Rana et al., 2012[115]	274	0.0
Essential tremor	Louis et al., 2013[85]	100	15.0
Essential tremor	Lenka et al., 2015[73]	234	13.7

This table summarizes the prevalence of dystonia among essential tremor cohorts with at least 50 participants published after 1980. The numbers are likely to reflect an underestimate because some studies excluded dystonia participants, some reported only on specific types of dystonia, and some did not specify the types of dystonia evaluated.

chance alone. About half of all individuals presenting with dystonia or tremor will have both movement disorders. It remains unclear if these cases should be viewed as having a single disorder that combines dystonia and tremor or two coincidental movement disorders.

SOME GRAY AREAS: DYSTONIA OR TREMOR?

Task-Specific Tremors

The tremor of Parkinson disease occurs mostly at rest. Conversely, the tremor of essential tremor typically emerges with action, such as holding a specific posture or doing hand tasks. Some tremors occur only during performance of a specific task, such as writing. It is not entirely clear if these task-specific tremors should be considered as a task-specific jerky dystonia, an unusual subtype of essential tremor, or a distinct etiological group.[51,116]

The literature on task-specific writing tremors goes by several names, such as *essential writing tremor*, *dystonic writing tremor*, *writer's tremor*, *writing tremor*, or *primary writing tremor* (PWT). The largest studies are summarized in Table 12.4. Some of these studies imply that PWT is a subtype of essential tremor because individuals with these disorders share many features such as a

Table 12.4 **Reports of task-specific primary writing tremor**

Study	Participants studied	Findings
Kachi et al., 1985[65]	9	Clinical assessments revealed features of ET such as rhythmic and sinusoidal oscillations, and treatment with ET medications
Cohen et al., 1987[25]	1	Family study revealed 1 with PWT, 2 with ET, 2 with dystonic writer's cramp, and 1 with ET combined with dystonic writer's cramp
Rosenbaum et al., 1988[119]	10	Clinical assessments revealed some cases resembled dystonia, while others resembled ET, suggesting a heterogeneous group
Elble et al., 1990[36]	5	EMG and accelerometry revealed some cases resembled dystonia, some resembled ET, and some had two distinct but overlapping tremor-like oscillations
Jedynak et al., 1991[62]	5	Irregular EMG discharges were more consistent with dystonia than ET
Bain et al., 1995[8]	21	EMG and accelerometry revealed features distinct from dystonia or ET, implying a distinct nosological entity.
Soland et al., 1996[131]	9	Clinical assessments revealed subtle dystonia in 3 cases
Berg et al., 2000[15]	3	fMRI study revealed brain changes that were not typical for dystonic writer's cramp or ET
Modugno et al., 2002[92]	7	Physiological study showed normal cortical excitability and normal reciprocal inhibition, unlike dystonia writer's cramp
Ljubisavljevic et al., 2006[75]	6	EMG and TMS revealed features distinct from dystonic writer's cramp or ET
Papapetropoulos and Singer 2006[104]	5	Clinical study revealed 3 cases had mirror dystonia
Meunier et al., 2011[91]	9	Transcutaneous nerve stimulation worsened PWT, unlike improvement seen in dystonia writer's cramp
Ondo and Satija, 2012[94]	56	Longitudinal study showed that 43 developed tremors with other tasks, but none developed dystonia
Erro et al., 2015[38]	1	Family study revealed 1 with PWT, 1 with dystonic writer's cramp, and 1 with dystonic tremor that was not task-specific
Latorre et al., 2021[70]	7	PWT cases resembled dystonic tremor more than ET on several physiological measures (eyeblink conditioning, blink reflex recovery, transcranial magnetic stimulation)

This table is not a complete review of all reports of PWT. It includes only the most instructive reports that included more than one case of PWT and instructive families with PWT.

Abbreviations: EMG, electromyography; ET, essential tremor; PWT, primary writing tremor; TMS, transcranial magnetic stimulation.

rhythmical and sinusoidal movement pattern, a frequency of 4–7 cycles/second, responses to medications such as primidone or propranolol, responses to alcohol, or family history that includes different individuals with PWT or essential tremor.[8,36,65,119] Although some exceptions exist, these features are not typical of most types of dystonia. One longitudinal study of 53 cases of PWT revealed that 43 progressed to have tremors with other tasks as well, but none was reported to develop dystonia.[94] These observations argue that PWT may be an early manifestation of essential tremor.

On the other hand, other studies imply that PWT is a subtype of dystonia because PWT and dystonia share a jerky and irregular pattern of movement; coexisting soft signs of dystonia, such as mirroring or hyperextension of the wrist and fingers; response to anticholinergics or botulinum toxins; co-activation of antagonistic muscles on electromyography (EMG); or other physiological phenomena more consistent with dystonia than tremor.[36,62,70,104,119,131] Other studies have implied that PWT is an etiological entity distinct from either essential tremor or dystonia because physiological or imaging findings are atypical for either.[8,15,75,91,92,137]

It is important to emphasize that PWT is rare, and most of the literature consists of case reports or small series, usually reported from a single center. The largest studies suggest that PWT may not be a homogenous group.[8,36,119] In these larger studies, some individuals had features consistent with essential tremor while others had features consistent with dystonia. These studies imply that patients with PWT may sometimes reflect a tremor and other times may reflect jerky dystonia. Other studies imply that a single biological predisposition may produce varied clinical phenomenologies that appear as PWT, essential tremor, or dystonia. For example, one family had one individual with PWT; two with essential tremor, two with dystonic writer's cramp, and one with both essential tremor and writer's cramp.[25] In another report, a woman with PWT developed dystonic writer's cramp when she began writing with the other hand.[107]

Altogether, the literature on PWT suggests that the clinical phenomenology in individual cases varies and may resemble essential tremor or dystonia. However, some studies suggest that the varied clinical phenomenology comes from the same underlying biological predisposition.

Isolated Head Tremor

The diagnosis of essential tremor requires involvement of the upper limbs.[21] However, some individuals may have isolated tremors of the head, without upper limb involvement. It is not clear if individuals with isolated head tremors (IHT) should be considered as a rare type of essential tremor, a type of dystonia resembling tremor, or a distinct category.[3,5,112] Many individuals with IHT often have coexisting abnormal postures of the head, making a diagnosis of dystonia more likely. However, sometimes this head posturing is so subtle that it is not readily identifiable, and the diagnosis is less obvious.

The literature on IHT uses different terminology including *isolated head tremor*, *essential tremor of the head*, *essential head tremor*, or *head tremor* (Table 12.5). Some studies point to IHT as a tremor-dominant dystonia because patients with IHT may have an effective sensory trick[90] and abnormal temporal discrimination[26] consistent with dystonia. More importantly, numerous studies have described patients with IHT who later evolved to have more obvious cervical dystonia.[19,28,61,73,95,118] The simplest explanation in these cases is that IHT was an early manifestation of cervical dystonia, although it is feasible that dystonia may evolve after essential tremor, too. One longitudinal study of 20 cases of IHT revealed that 15 progressed to have cervical dystonia within 5 years.[45] In contrast, other studies imply that IHT could be a rare manifestation of essential tremor. Some individuals with IHT have features suggestive of essential tremor including regular and sinusoidal oscillations, responses to medications for essential tremor, and family studies that show members with both IHT and essential tremor. Furthermore, patients may present with complaints of a prominent head tremor that overshadow minor tremors of the hands.[83] Therefore, it is feasible that some patients with apparent IHT may actually be diagnosable with essential tremor when a thorough exam is conducted.

Similar to PWT, IHT probably reflects a heterogeneous group. Some cases of IHT may reflect essential tremor of the head with clinically minor hand tremors, or essential tremor of the head prior to emergence of hand tremors. Other cases may reflect tremor-dominant cervical dystonia, and more overt head turning or twisting may emerge later.

Table 12.5 **Reports of isolated head tremor**

Study	Participants studied	Findings
Rivest & Marsden 1990[117]	12	Clinical assessments of patients with severe head or trunk tremors revealed 5 with IHT, which the authors viewed as subtype of dystonia because many patients later developed more obvious dystonia
Jedynak et al., 1991[62]	45	EMG of patients with dystonia or tremor revealed 3 patients with IHT, which authors argued more closely resembled dystonia
Valls-Sole, 1997[136]	30	EMG of patients with prominent head tremor revealed 3 patients with IHT, which authors argued more closely resembled ET
Louis et al., 2000[84]	115	Clinical assessments of patients with ET revealed 2 patients with IHT
Masuhr et al., 2000[90]	60	EMG and accelerometry in patients with prominent head tremor revealed 3 with IHT
Pal et al., 2000[95]	114	Clinical assessments of patients with cervical dystonia revealed 8 with IHT, which authors viewed as a subtype of dystonia
Louis & Dogu, 2009[83]	583	Clinical assessments of patients with ET revealed no cases of IHT, but 2.7% had prominent head tremor with mild hand tremor
Conte et al., 2015[26]	61	Temporal discrimination revealed abnormalities in dystonia but not ET; 8 with IHT resembled dystonia
Prasad & Pal, 2019[108]	252	Clinical study of patients with ET revealed 5 with IHT
Ferrazzano et al., 2022[45]	20	Longitudinal study showing that 15 of 20 cases later developed cervical dystonia

Abbreviations: EMG, electromyography; ET, essential tremor; IHT, isolated head tremor; TMS, transcranial magnetic stimulation.

Isolated Voice Tremor

Like IHT, isolated voice tremor (IVT) may occur without tremor of the upper limbs. Also, like IHT, it is not clear if IVT is an unusual manifestation of essential tremor or dystonia. The literature on IVT employs several different terms including *essential voice tremor, essential vocal tremor, laryngeal essential tremor, isolated vocal tremor, primary vocal tremor*, and more.[9]

Many of the same phenomena described for IHT also apply to IVT. However, two additional issues must be considered. First, many studies have shown that vocal tremors and laryngeal dystonia often coexist, and experts cannot reliably tell them apart.[86,133] Second, different types of specialists who evaluate patients with voice disorders have fundamentally different viewpoints.[9] The concept of tremor-dominant dystonia is well accepted in the neurological literature, but otolaryngologists and speech-language pathologists do not recognize a tremor-dominant dystonia of the voice (see Chapter 7, "Laryngeal Dystonias," for more details). Thus, opinions regarding the place of IVT as a type of tremor or dystonia may vary among different types of specialists.

THE PROBLEM OF MISDIAGNOSIS

Misdiagnosis in the Clinic

Discriminating recurrent dystonic jerking movements from tremor is not purely an academic exercise. A precise diagnosis is important for counseling and treatment. Clinically, patients with dystonia and tremulous movements are frequently misdiagnosed with essential tremor or Parkinson tremor.[58,69,123] The consequence is that misdiagnosed individuals may be improperly treated with medications for essential tremor (e.g., primidone, propranolol) or medications for Parkinson disease (e.g., levodopa or dopamine agonists), sometimes for decades.[43]

Similarly, individuals may be offered inappropriate surgical procedures. The favored target for deep brain stimulation of most forms of dystonia is the internal segment of the globus pallidus. In contrast, the thalamus is the favored target for essential tremor.[103,106] Thus, the optimal surgical target depends on whether rapid and repetitive movement is a tremor or recurrent dystonic jerking that mimics tremor.

Misdiagnosis in Clinical Research

Misdiagnoses of tremor disorders in the clinic are common and have been ascribed to poor clinical recognition of the varied manifestations of different tremors. However, the clinical research literature implies misdiagnosis also is frequent among experts. There are numerous reviews and commentaries describing misdiagnosis, particularly for dystonic tremor.[2,5,18,27,34,58,66,69,88,99,121,122,134]

Misdiagnosis has obvious impacts on study results. One of the most thoroughly studied areas of misdiagnosis involves clinical trials of novel therapeutic agents in Parkinson disease, where positron emission tomography (PET) scans were used to document associated basal ganglia dopaminergic deficits. A clinical diagnosis of Parkinson disease was required for entry into each of these studies. However, many studies had a significant percentage of participants without evidence of any dopaminergic deficit on PET scan. These individuals were labeled as "SWEDD," for *scans without evidence of dopaminergic deficit.* Some examples of these Parkinson trials included the InSPECT trial, which aimed to compare levodopa and pramipexole therapy (13.3% SWEDDs)[138]; the European FP-CIT trial, which compared imaging to clinical features (19.6% SWEDDs)[14]; the Real-PET trial, which aimed to compare ropinirole with pramipexole (11.2% SWEDDs)[140]; the ELLDOPA trial, which compared early versus late levodopa therapy (14.7% SWEDDs)[101]; and PRECEPT trial, which evaluated a potential neuroprotective therapy (11.3% SWEDDs).[105] On repeat PET scans years later, a few of these cases had evidence for a dopaminergic deficit consistent with the diagnosis of Parkinson disease, but many did not. The majority of the remaining cases were later interpreted to be dystonic tremor or essential tremor clinically misdiagnosed at study entry.[10,40,89,122] Obviously, including misdiagnosed cases will have a significant impact on assessments of a clinical trial.

Another area where misdiagnosis has impacted results involves studies aiming to identify genes responsible for essential tremor. Because a single misdiagnosed family member can markedly alter outcomes, it has been suggested that misdiagnosis may explain the many failed attempts at identifying genes for essential tremor.[56,134] For example, many family studies of essential tremor have included members who also had dystonia.[54,60,85,129] One large study included 463 individuals across 97 families where a proband was diagnosed with essential tremor. Overall, 363 individuals were diagnosed with essential tremor, 88 had tremor combined with dystonia, and 10 had dystonia without tremor. Another study of essential tremor included 100 individuals across 28 families. Careful reexamination revealed that 10% of the probands with essential tremor also has dystonia, which was not recognized in most because it was so mild.[85]

In summary, misdiagnosis of tremor and dystonia is common, even among experts. One of the reasons for misdiagnosis is that the clinical manifestations of oscillatory movements in dystonia overlap with more common tremor disorders, such as essential tremor and Parkinson tremor. Another reason is that these problems may coexist.

LABORATORY-BASED ASSESSMENTS FOR TREMOR

One of the major limitations in understanding the relationship between tremor and dystonia relates to traditional strategies of relying on the clinical exam. Subtle or intermittent tremors are easy to miss. Other characteristics, such as regularity or jerkiness, are very subjective. Coexisting intermittent or very mild dystonia can also be subjective. The remarkable advances in digital technologies have the potential to provide more objective data. Many technologies are available including accelerometry, EMG, magnetic position detectors, gyroscopic devices, digital analysis of video recordings, and others.[53]

Although not yet widely used, these methods have provided some important insights regarding the relationships between tremor and dystonia. First, almost all sensor-based devices are more sensitive than the clinical exam. Second, many devices can provide quantitative measures that discriminate among different types of tremors, such as amplitude, regularity, or jerkiness. Third, some devices have implied that a single patient may have more than one type of oscillation. These characteristics have the potential to provide substantial insights into several confusing areas such as task-specific tremors or isolated head or voice tremors.

These issues have been studied in great detail for individuals with cervical dystonia using a magnetic head coil to track precise head positions.[16,126,127] The device was capable of detecting tremor-like oscillations of the head in all cases, including those who did not have obvious head tremor by clinical exam. The device was also capable of detecting two distinct types of tremor-like oscillations of the head, and sometimes these two types coexisted in the same individual. One type was typical of essential tremors of the hands because it was regular and sinusoidal, with a relatively low amplitude. The other type had features consistent with Fahn's original concept of dystonic tremor because it was irregular, jerky, and had a much greater amplitude. Although all of these studies focused on tremor-like oscillations of the head in cervical dystonia, other methods applied to other types of dystonia have also revealed two distinct tremor-like oscillations that can sometimes coexist in the same patient.[6,36,142]

BIOLOGICAL BASIS FOR TREMOR-DYSTONIA OVERLAP

The many overlapping clinical features for dystonia and tremor can probably be explained by overlapping biological mechanisms.[74] One frequent observation is that individuals with dystonia may later develop tremor.[28,61,95,121] Similarly, individuals with tremors frequently later develop dystonia.[19,28,61,62,73,95,118] This clinical evolution implies progression of a shared biological mechanism.

Additional evidence for a shared biology comes from family studies. Many families have individual members who have dystonia, tremor, or both.[54,60,67,76,85,129] These families imply a shared biological predisposition to either dystonia or tremor. In fact, individuals with genes typically associated with dystonia often have coexisting tremor (Figure 12.3).[96] In some cases of these cases, tremor is the main clinical finding, with little or no dystonia. Examples of this phenomenon include *ANO3*, *KMT2B*, *SCGE*, *THAP1*, and *TOR1A*.[18,22,24,40,66,72,130,132] These observations mean that the consequences of defects in "dystonia genes" may lead to dystonia or tremor, perhaps depending on some additional genetic or environmental factors.

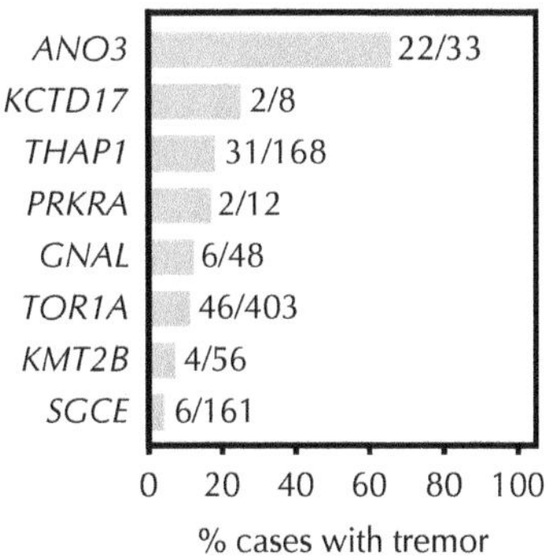

Figure 12.3. Percentage of individuals with tremor according to gene. This figure was adapted from data presented in a prior review and shows the risk of tremor according to specific genes associated with dystonia.[96]

Dystonia and tremor also appear to share certain neuroanatomical substrates in the brain. Dystonia is viewed as a disorder of a motor network that includes the basal ganglia, cerebellum, sensorimotor cortex, and potentially other regions.[64,93,109,128] The tremor of Parkinson disease is thought to arise from interactions between basal ganglia and cerebellum,[55] while essential tremor is viewed as a disorder of the cerebellum and its circuits.[80,113] When regional brain abnormalities are evaluated in dystonia or essential tremor with fluro-deoxyglucose PET[12] or functional MRI (fMRI),[29] there are many areas of overlap. Autopsy studies of dystonia[87,110] and essential tremor[78] demonstrate some similarities, too, such as loss of cerebellar Purkinje cells or abnormal inclusion bodies in the cerebellum. Thus, many studies addressing the neuroanatomical substrates for dystonia or tremor point to similar brain regions.

SYNOPSIS AND FUTURE PROSPECTS

Although dystonia is considered a disorder that is phenomenologically distinct from tremor, their clinical features and biological mechanisms overlap. By clinical exam, dystonia and tremor usually present with sufficiently distinct manifestations that make them easy to distinguish. However, their clinical phenomenology may sometimes overlap, and they are occasionally hard to discriminate with certainty. Expert opinion is divided in certain areas, such as best ways to describe the varied relationships between dystonia and tremor. Expert opinion also is divided regarding whether some disorders should be considered as subtypes of tremor or dystonia, including task-specific tremors or isolated tremors of the head or voice without simultaneous tremor of the upper limbs. Further work is needed to reach more consistent expert agreements in these areas.

Dystonia and tremor cannot be readily distinguished by any blood-based biomarkers or neuroimaging protocols. Some laboratory-based measures can discriminate dystonia and tremor, but they are not widely available for clinical diagnostic use. In the future, increasing use of these measures may provide some empirical evidence to address areas where expert opinion is currently divided.

Numerous observations suggest that the biological mechanisms responsible for dystonia and tremor overlap, at least in part. Further studies addressing these mechanisms may help to clarify similarities and differences and whether or not similar medical or surgical treatments may be applied under different circumstances.

REFERENCES

1. Albanese A. Classifying tremor: Language matters. Mov Disord 2018;33:3–4.
2. Albanese A, Lalli S. Is this dystonia? Mov Disord 2009;24:1725–1731.
3. Albanese A, Bhatia K, Bressman SB, DeLong MR, Fahn S, Fung VSC, et al. Phenomenology and classification of dystonia: A consensus update. Mov Disord 2013;28:863–873.
4. Albanese A, Bhatia KP, Cardoso F, Comella C, Defazio G, Fung VSC, et al. Isolated cervical dystonia: Diagnosis and classification. Mov Disord 2023;38:1367–1348.
5. Albanese A, Sorbo FD. Dystonia and tremor: The clinical syndromes with isolated tremor. Tremor Other Hyperkinet Mov (N Y) 2016;6:319.
6. Ansari KA, Webster DD. Quantitative measurements in spasmodic torticollis. Description of a method and results of measurement. Dis Nerv Syst 1974;35:44–47.
7. Asmus F, Langseth A, Doherty E, Nestor T, Munz M, Gasser T, et al. "Jerky" dystonia in children: Spectrum of phenotypes and genetic testing. Mov Disord 2009;24:702–709.
8. Bain PG, Findley LJ, Britton TC, Rothwell JC, Gresty MA, Thompson PD, Marsden CD. Primary writing tremor. Brain 1995;118:1461–1472.
9. Barkmeier-Kraemer JM. Isolated voice tremor: A clinical variant of essential tremor or a distinct clinical phenotype? Tremor Other Hyperkinet Mov (N Y) 2020;10. doi:10.7916/tohm.v0.738.
10. Batla A, Erro R, Stamelou M, Schneider SA, Schwingenschuh P, Ganos C, Bhatia KP. Patients with scans without evidence of dopaminergic deficit: A long-term follow-up study. Mov Disord 2014;29:1820–1825.
11. Becktepe J, Govert F, Balint B, Schlenstedt C, Bhatia K, Elble R, Deuschl G. Exploring interrater disagreement on essential tremor using a standardized tremor elements assessment. Mov Disord Clin Pract 2021;8:371–376.
12. Belenky V, Stanzhevsky A, Klicenko O, Skoromets A. Brain positron emission tomography with 2-18F-2-deoxi-D-glucose of patients with dystonia and essential tremor detects differences between these disorders. Neuroradiol J 2018;31:60–68.
13. Bellows ST, Jankovic J. Phenotypic features of isolated essential tremor, essential tremor plus, and essential tremor-Parkinson's disease in a movement disorders clinic. Tremor Other Hyperkinet Mov (N Y) 2021;11:12.
14. Benamer HT, Oertel WH, Patterson J, Hadley DM, Pogarell O, Hoffken H, et al. Prospective study of presynaptic dopaminergic imaging in patients with mild parkinsonism and tremor disorders: Part 1. Baseline and 3-month observations. Mov Disord 2003;18:977–984.
15. Berg D, Preibisch C, Hofmann E, Naumann M. Cerebral activation pattern in primary writing tremor. J Neurol Neurosurg Psychiatry 2000;69:780–786.
16. Beylergil SB, Singh AP, Zee DS, Jinnah HA, Shaikh AG. Relationship between jerky and sinusoidal oscillations in cervical dystonia. Parkinsonism Relat Disord 2019;66:130–137.
17. Bhatia KP, Bain P, Bajaj N, Elble RJ, Hallett M, Louis ED, et al. Consensus statement on the classification of tremors. from the task force on tremor of the International Parkinson and Movement Disorder Society. Mov Disord 2018;33:75–87.
18. Cardoso F. Difficult diagnoses in hyperkinetic disorders: A focused review. Front Neurol 2012;3:151.
19. Chan J, Brin MF, Fahn S. Idiopathic cervical dystonia: Clinical characteristics. Mov Disord 1991;6: 119–126.
20. Charlesworth G, Plagnol V, Holmstrom KM, Bras J, Sheerin UM, Preza E, et al. Mutations in ANO3 cause dominant craniocervical dystonia: Ion channel implicated in pathogenesis. Am J Hum Genet 2012;91:1041–1050.
21. Chen W, Hopfner F, Szymczak S, Granert O, Muller SH, Kuhlenbaumer G, Deuschl G. Topography of essential tremor. Parkinsonism Relat Disord 2017;40:58–63.
22. Cheng FB, Ozelius LJ, Wan XH, Feng JC, Ma LY, Yang YM, Wang L. THAP1/DYT6 sequence variants in non-DYT1 early-onset primary dystonia in China and their effects on RNA expression. J Neurol 2012;259:342–347.
23. Chinnery PF, Reading PJ, McCarthy EL, Curtis A, Burn DJ. Late-onset axial jerky dystonia due to the DYT1 deletion. Mov Disord 2002;17:196–198.
24. Cilia R, Reale C, Castagna A, Nasca A, Muzi-Falconi M, Barzaghi C, et al. Novel DYT11 gene mutation in patients without dopaminergic deficit (SWEDD) screened for dystonia. Neurology 2014;83:1155–1162.
25. Cohen LG, Hallett M, Sudarsky L. A single family with writer's cramp, essential tremor, and primary writing tremor. Mov Disord 1987;2:109–116.
26. Conte A, Ferrazzano G, Manzo N, Leodori G, Fabbrini G, Fasano A, et al. Somatosensory temporal discrimination in essential tremor and isolated head and voice tremors. Mov Disord 2015;30:822–827.
27. Defazio G, Conte A, Gigante AF, Fabbrini G, Berardelli A. Is tremor in dystonia a phenotypic feature of dystonia? Neurology 2015;84:1053–1059.

28. Defazio G, Gigante AF, Abbruzzese G, Bentivoglio AR, Colosimo C, Esposito M, et al. Tremor in primary adult-onset dystonia: Prevalence and associated clinical features. J Neurol Neurosurg Psychiatry 2013;84:404–408.
29. DeSimone JC, Archer DB, Vaillancourt DE, Wagle Shukla A. Network-level connectivity is a critical feature distinguishing dystonic tremor and essential tremor. Brain 2019;142:1644–1659.
30. Deuschl G, Bain P, Brin M. Consensus statement of the movement disorder society on tremor. Mov Disord 1998;13 Suppl. 3:2–23.
31. Deuschl G, Heinen F, Guschlbauer B, Schneider S, Glocker FX, Lucking CH. Hand tremor in patients with spasmodic torticollis. Mov Disord 1997;12:547–552.
32. Du W, Bain PG, Defazio G, Jankovic J, Kim CY, Tan EK, Vidailhet M, Louis ED. The conundrum of dystonia in essential tremor patients: How does one classify these cases? Tremor Other Hyperkinet Mov 2022;12:15.
33. Dubinsky RM, Gray CS, Koller WC. Essential tremor and dystonia. Neurology 1993;43:2382–2384.
34. Elble RJ. Defining dystonic tremor. Curr Neuropharmacol 2013;11:48–52.
35. Elble RJ. What is essential tremor? Curr Neurol Neurosci Rep 2013;13:353.
36. Elble RJ, Moody C, Higgins C. Primary writing tremor. A form of focal dystonia? Mov Disord 1990;5:118–126.
37. Elias WJ, Shah BB. Tremor. JAMA 2014;311:948–954.
38. Erro R, Ciocca M, Hirschbichler ST, Rothwell JC, Bhatia KP. Primary writing tremor is a dystonic trait: Evidence from an instructive family. J Neurol Sci 2015;356:210–211.
39. Erro R, Rubio-Agusti I, Saifee TA, Cordivari C, Ganos C, Batla A, Bhatia KP. Rest and other types of tremor in adult-onset primary dystonia. J Neurol Neurosurg Psychiatry 2013;85:965–968.
40. Erro R, Schneider SA, Stamelou M, Quinn NP, Bhatia KP. What do patients with scans without evidence of dopaminergic deficit (SWEDD) have? New evidence and continuing controversies. J Neurol Neurosurg Psychiatry 2016;87:319–323.
41. Fahn S. Atypical tremors, rare tremors and unclassified tremors. In: Findley LJ, Capildeo R, eds. *Movement Disorders: Tremor.* Palgrave Macmillan; 1984: 555–563.
42. Fahn S. The varied clinical expressions of dystonia. Neurol Clinics 1984;2:541–554.
43. Fasano A, Bove F, Lang AE. The treatment of dystonic tremor: A systematic review. J Neurol Neurosurg Psychiatry 2014;85:759–769.
44. Fasano A, Lang AE, Espay AJ. What is "essential" about essential tremor? A diagnostic placeholder. Mov Disord 2018;33:58–61.
45. Ferrazzano G, Belvisi D, De Bartolo MI, Baione V, Costanzo M, Fabbrini G, et al. Longitudinal evaluation of patients with isolated head tremor. Parkinsonism Relat Disord 2022;94:10–12.
46. Ghika J, Bogousslavsky J, Henderson J, Maeder P, Regli F. The "jerky dystonic unsteady hand": A delayed motor syndrome in posterior thalamic infarctions. J Neurol 1994;241:537–542.
47. Gigante AF, Berardelli A, Defazio G. Rest tremor in idiopathic adult-onset dystonia. Eur J Neurol 2016;23:935–939.
48. Gionco JT, Hartstone WG, Martuscello RT, Kuo SH, Faust PL, Louis ED. Essential tremor versus "ET-plus": A detailed postmortem study of cerebellar pathology. Cerebellum 2021;20:904–912.
49. Godeiro-Junior C, Felicio AC, Aguiar PC, Borges V, Silva SM, Ferraz HB. Head tremor in patients with cervical dystonia: Different outcome? Arq Neuropsiquiatr 2008;66:805–808.
50. Govert F, Deuschl G. Tremor entities and their classification: An update. Curr Opin Neurol 2015;28:393–399.
51. Hai C, Yu-ping W, Hua W, Ying S. Advances in primary writing tremor. Parkinsonism Relat Disord 2010;16:561–565.
52. Harrer P, Skorvanek M, Kittke V, Dzinovic I, Borngraber F, Thomsen M, et al. Dystonia linked to EIF4A2 haploinsufficiency: A disorder of protein translation dysfunction. Mov Disord 2023;38:1914–1924.
53. Haubenberger D, Abbruzzese G, Bain PG, Bajaj N, Benito-Leon J, Bhatia KP, et al. Transducer-based evaluation of tremor. Mov Disord 2016;31:1327–1336.
54. Hedera P, Phibbs FT, Fang JY, Cooper MK, Charles PD, Davis TL. Clustering of dystonia in some pedigrees with autosomal dominant essential tremor suggests the existence of a distinct subtype of essential tremor. BMC Neurol 2010;10:66.
55. Helmich RC, Janssen MJ, Oyen WJ, Bloem BR, Toni I. Pallidal dysfunction drives a cerebellothalamic circuit into Parkinson tremor. Ann Neurol 2011;69:269–281.
56. Hopfner F, Haubenberger D, Galpern WR, Gwinn K, Van't Veer A, White S, et al. Knowledge gaps and research recommendations for essential tremor. Parkinsonism Relat Disord 2016;33:27–35.
57. Hvizdosova L, Nevrly M, Otruba P, Hlustik P, Kanovsky P, Zapletalova J. The prevalence of dystonic tremor and tremor associated with dystonia in patients with cervical dystonia. Sci Rep 2020;10:1436.
58. Jain S, Lo SE, Louis ED. Common misdiagnosis of a common neurological disorder: How are we misdiagnosing essential tremor? Arch Neurol 2006;63:1100–1104.
59. Jankovic J, Ford J. Blepharospasm and orofacial-cervical dystonia: Clinical and pharmacological findings in 100 patients. Ann Neurol 1983;13:402–411.
60. Jankovic J, Beach J, Pandolfo M, Patel PI. Familial essential tremor in 4 kindreds. Prospects for genetic mapping. Arch Neurol 1997;54:289–294.
61. Jankovic J, Leder S, Warner D, Schwartz K. Cervical dystonia: Clinical findings and associated movement disorders. Neurology 1991;41:1088–1091.
62. Jedynak CP, Bonnet AM, Agid Y. Tremor and idiopathic dystonia. Mov Disord 1991;6:230–236.
63. Jhunjhunwala K, Lenka A, Pal PK. A clinical profile of 125 patients with writer's cramp. Eur Neurol 2015;73:316–320.
64. Jinnah HA, Neychev V, Hess EJ. The anatomical basis for dystonia: The motor network model. Tremor Other Hyperkinet Mov 2017;7:506.
65. Kachi T, Rothwell JC, Cowan JM, Marsden CD. Writing tremor: Its relationship to benign essential tremor. J Neurol Neurosurg Psychiatry 1985;48:545–550.
66. Klepitskaya O, Neuwelt AJ, Nguyen T, Leehey M. Primary dystonia misinterpreted as Parkinson disease: Video case presentation and practical clues. Neurol Clin Pract 2013:469–474.
67. Koller WC, Busenbark K, Miner K. The relationship of essential tremor to other movement disorders: Report on 678 patients. Essential Tremor Study Group. Ann Neurol 1994;35:717–723.
68. Kuukasjarvi A, Landoni JC, Kaukonen J, Juhakoski M, Auranen M, Torkkeli T, et al. IMPDH2: A new gene

associated with dominant juvenile-onset dystonia-tremor disorder. Eur J Hum Genet 2021;29:1833–1837.
69. Lalli S, Albanese A. The diagnostic challenge of primary dystonia: Evidence from misdiagnosis. Mov Disord 2010;25:1619–1626.
70. Latorre A, Rocchi L, Batla A, Berardelli A, Rothwell JC, Bhatia KP. The signature of primary writing tremor is dystonic. Mov Disord 2021;36:1715–1720.
71. LeDoux MS, Vemula SR, Xiao J, Thompson MM, Perlmutter JS, Wright LJ, et al. Clinical and genetic features of cervical dystonia in a large multicenter cohort. Neurol Genet 2016;2:e69.
72. LeDoux MS, Xiao J, Rudzinska M, Bastian RW, Wszolek ZK, Van Gerpen JA, et al. Genotype-phenotype correlations in THAP1 dystonia: Molecular foundations and description of new cases. Parkinsonism Relat Disord 2012;18:414–425.
73. Lenka A, Bhalsing KS, Jhunjhunwala KR, Chandran V, Pal PK. Are patients with limb and head tremor a clinically distinct subtype of essential tremor? Can J Neurol Sci 2015;42:181–186.
74. Lenka A, Pandey S. Dystonia and tremor: Do they have a shared biology? Int Rev Neurobiol 2023;169:413–439.
75. Ljubisavljevic M, Kacar A, Milanovic S, Svetel M, Kostic VS. Changes in cortical inhibition during task-specific contractions in primary writing tremor patients. Mov Disord 2006;21:855–859.
76. Loens S, Hamami F, Lohmann K, Odorfer T, Ip CW, Zittel S, et al. Tremor is associated with familial clustering of dystonia. Parkinsonism Relat Disord 2023;110:105400.
77. Lou JS, Jankovic J. Essential tremor: Clinical correlates in 350 patients. Neurology 1991;41:234–238.
78. Louis ED. Essential tremor: Evolving clinicopathological concepts in an era of intensive post-mortem enquiry. Lancet Neurol 2010;9:613–622.
79. Louis ED. The evolving definition of essential tremor: What are we dealing with? Parkinsonism Relat Disord 2018;46 Suppl:S87–S91.
80. Louis ED. Essential tremor and the cerebellum. Handb Clin Neurol 2018;155:245–258.
81. Louis ED. Essential tremor: "Plus" or "Minus". Perhaps now is the time to adopt the term "the essential tremors". Parkinsonism Relat Disord 2018;56:111–112.
82. Louis ED. Tremor. Continuum 2019;25:959–975.
83. Louis ED, Dogu O. Isolated head tremor: Part of the clinical spectrum of essential tremor? Data from population-based and clinic-based case samples. Mov Disord 2009;24:2281–2285.
84. Louis ED, Ford B, Barnes LF. Clinical subtypes of essential tremor. Arch Neurol 2000;57:1194–1198.
85. Louis ED, Hernandez N, Alcalay RN, Tirri DJ, Ottman R, Clark LN. Prevalence and features of unreported dystonia in a family study of "pure" essential tremor. Parkinsonism Relat Disord 2013;19:359–362.
86. Ludlow CL, Domangue R, Sharma D, Jinnah HA, Perlmutter JS, Berke G, et al. Consensus-based attributes for identifying patients with spasmodic dysphonia and other voice disorders. JAMA Otolaryngol Head Neck Surg 2018;144:657–665.
87. Ma K, Babij R, Cortes E, Vonsattel JP, Louis ED. Cerebellar pathology of a dual clinical diagnosis: Patients with essential tremor and dystonia. Tremor Other Hyperkinet Mov 2012;2:1–6.
88. Macerollo A, Superbo M, Gigante AF, Livrea P, Defazio G. Diagnostic delay in adult-onset dystonia: Data from an Italian movement disorder center. J Clin Neurosci 2015;22:608–610.
89. Marek K, Seibyl J, Eberly S, Oakes D, Shoulson I, Lang AE, et al. Longitudinal follow-up of SWEDD subjects in the PRECEPT Study. Neurology 2014;82:1791–1797.
90. Masuhr F, Wissel J, Muller J, Scholz U, Poewe W. Quantification of sensory trick impact on tremor amplitude and frequency in 60 patients with head tremor. Mov Disord 2000;15:960–964.
91. Meunier S, Bleton JP, Mazevet D, Sangla S, Grabli D, Roze E, Vidailhet M. TENS is harmful in primary writing tremor. Clin Neurophysiol 2011;122:171–175.
92. Modugno N, Nakamura Y, Bestmann S, Curra A, Berardelli A, Rothwell J. Neurophysiological investigations in patients with primary writing tremor. Mov Disord 2002;17:1336–1340.
93. Neychev VK, Gross R, Lehericy S, Hess EJ, Jinnah HA. The functional neuroanatomy of dystonia. Neurobiol Dis 2011;42:185–201.
94. Ondo WG, Satija P. Task-specific writing tremor: Clinical phenotypes, progression, treatment outcomes, and proposed nomenclature. Int J Neurosci 2012;122:88–91.
95. Pal PK, Samii A, Schulzer M, Mak E, Tsui JK. Head tremor in cervical dystonia. Can J Neurol Sci 2000;27:137–142.
96. Pandey S, Bhattad S, Dinesh S. Tremor in primary monogenic dystonia. Curr Neurol Neurosci Rep 2021;21:48.
97. Pandey S, Bhattad S, Hallett M. The problem of questionable dystonia in the diagnosis of "essential tremor-plus." Tremor Other Hyperkinet Mov (N Y) 2020;10:27.
98. Pandey S, Kreisler A, Druzdz A, Biering-Sorensen B, Slawek J, Tatu L, Jost WH. Tremor in idiopathic cervical dystonia - Possible implications for botulinum toxin treatment considering the col-cap classification. Tremor Other Hyperkinet Mov (N Y) 2020;10:13.
99. Pandey S, Sarma N. Tremor in dystonia. Parkinsonism Relat Disord 2016;29:3–9.
100. Pandey S, Sarma N. Tremor in dystonia: A cross-sectional study from India. Mov Disord Clin Pract 2017;4:858–863.
101. Panyakaew P, Cho HJ, Lee SW, Wu T, Hallett M. The pathophysiology of dystonic tremors and comparison with essential tremor. J Neurosci 2020;40:9317–9326.
102. Panyakaew P, Jinnah HA, Shaikh AG. Clinical features, pathophysiology, treatment, and controversies of tremor in dystonia. J Neurol Sci 2022;435:120199.
103. Paoli D, Mills R, Brechany U, Pavese N, Nicholson C. DBS in tremor with dystonia: VIM, GPi or both? A review of the literature and considerations from a single-center experience. J Neurol 2023;270:2217–2229.
104. Papapetropoulos S, Singer C. Treatment of primary writing tremor with botulinum toxin type a injections: Report of a case series. Clin Neuropharmacol 2006;29:364–367.
105. Parkinson Study Group. Mixed lineage kinase inhibitor CEP-1347 fails to delay disability in early Parkinson disease. Neurology 2007;69:1480–1490.
106. Paschen S, Becktepe JS, Hobert MA, Zeuner KE, Helmers AK, Berg D, Deuschl G. The challenge of choosing the right stimulation target for dystonic tremor: A series of instructive cases. Mov Disord Clin Pract 2023;10:1478–1484.
107. Pita Lobo P, Quattrocchi G, Jutras MF, Sangla S, Apartis E, Vidailhet M, Grabli D. Primary writing tremor and writer's cramp: Two faces of a same coin? Mov Disord 2013;28:1306–1307.
108. Prasad S, Pal PK. Reclassifying essential tremor: Implications for the future of past research. Mov Disord 2019;34:437.

109. Prudente CN, Hess EJ, Jinnah HA. Dystonia as a network disorder: What is the role of the cerebellum? Neuroscience 2014;260:23–35.
110. Prudente CN, Pardo CA, Xiao J, Hanfelt J, Hess EJ, LeDoux MS, Jinnah HA. Neuropathology of cervical dystonia. Exp Neurol 2012;241:95–104.
111. Puschmann A, Wszolek ZK. Diagnosis and treatment of common forms of tremor. Semin Neurol 2011;31:65–77.
112. Quinn NP, Schneider SA, Schwingenschuh P, Bhatia KP. Tremor - some controversial aspects. Mov Disord 2011;26:18–23.
113. Raethjen J, Deuschl G. The oscillating central network of essential tremor. Clin Neurophysiol 2012;123:61–64.
114. Rajalingam R, Breen DP, Lang AE, Fasano A. Essential tremor plus is more common than essential tremor: Insights from the reclassification of a cohort of patients with lower limb tremor. Parkinsonism Relat Disord 2018;56:109–110.
115. Rana AQ, Kabir A, Dogu O, Patel A, Khondker S. Prevalence of blepharospasm and apraxia of eyelid opening in patients with parkinsonism, cervical dystonia and essential tremor. Eur Neurol 2012;68:318–321.
116. Rana AQ, Vaid HM. A review of primary writing tremor. Int J Neurosci 2012;122:114–118.
117. Rivest J, Marsden CD. Trunk and head tremor as isolated manifestations of dystonia. Mov Disord 1990;5:60–65.
118. Rondot P, Marchand MP, Dellatorlas G. Spasmodic torticollis-review of 220 patients. Can J Neurol Sci 1991;18:143–151.
119. Rosenbaum F, Jankovic J. Focal task-specific tremor and dystonia: Categorization of occupational movement disorders. Neurology 1988;38:522–527.
120. Rudzinska M, Krawczyk M, Wojcik-Pedziwiatr M, Szczudlik A, Wasielewska A. Tremor associated with focal and segmental dystonia. Neurol Neurochir Pol 2013;47:223–231.
121. Schiebler S, Schmidt A, Zittel S, Baumer T, Gerloff C, Klein C, Munchau A. Arm tremor in cervical dystonia: Is it a manifestation of dystonia or essential tremor? Mov Disord 2011;26:1789–1792.
122. Schneider SA, Edwards MJ, Mir P, Cordivari C, Hooker J, Dickson J, et al. Patients with adult-onset dystonic tremor resembling parkinsonian tremor have scans without evidence of dopaminergic deficit (SWEDDs). Mov Disord 2007;22:2210–2215.
123. Schrag A, Munchau A, Bhatia KP, Quinn NP, Marsden CD. Essential tremor: An overdiagnosed condition? J Neurol 2000;247:955–959.
124. Schweinfurth JM, Billante M, Courey MS. Risk factors and demographics in patients with spasmodic dysphonia. Laryngoscope 2002;112:220–223.
125. Shaikh AG, Beylergil SB, Scorr L, Kilic-Berkmen G, Freeman A, Klein C, et al. Dystonia & tremor: A cross-sectional study of the Dystonia Coalition cohort. Neurology 2021;96:e563–e574.
126. Shaikh AG, Wong AL, Zee DS, Jinnah HA. Keeping your head on target. J Neurosci 2013;33:11281–11295.
127. Shaikh AG, Zee DS, Jinnah HA. Oscillatory head movements in cervical dystonia: Dystonia, tremor, or both? Mov Disord 2015;30:834–842.
128. Shakkottai VG, Batla A, Bhatia K, Dauer WT, Dresel C, Niethammer M, et al. Current opinions and areas of consensus on the role of the cerebellum in dystonia. Cerebellum 2017;16:577–594.
129. Shatunov A, Sambuughin N, Jankovic J, Elble R, Lee HS, Singleton AB, et al. Genomewide scans in North American families reveal genetic linkage of essential tremor to a region on chromosome 6p23. Brain 2006;129:2318–2331.
130. Shimazaki R, Ikezawa J, Okiyama R, Azuma K, Akagawa H, Takahashi K. Dystonic tremor in adult-onset DYT-KMT2B. Intern Med 2022;61:2357–2360.
131. Soland VL, Bhatia KP, Volonte MA, Marsden CD. Focal task-specific tremors. Mov Disord 1996;11:665–670.
132. Stamelou M, Charlesworth G, Cordivari C, Schneider SA, Kagi G, Sheerin UM, et al. The phenotypic spectrum of DYT24 due to ANO3 mutations. Mov Disord 2014;29:928–934.
133. Sulica L, Louis ED. Clinical characteristics of essential voice tremor: A study of 34 cases. Laryngoscope 2010;120:516–528.
134. Testa CM. Key issues in essential tremor genetics research: Where are we now and how can we move forward? Tremor Other Hyperkinet Mov (N Y) 2013;3:tre-03-105-1843-1.
135. Tisch SHD, Brake HM, Law M, Cole IE, Darveniza P. Spasmodic dysphonia: Clinical features and effects of botulinum toxin therapy in 169 patients - an Australian experience. J Clin Neurosci 2003;10:434–438.
136. Valls-Sole J, Tolosa ES, Nobbe F, Dieguez E, Munoz E, Sanz P, Valldeoriola F. Neurophysiological investigations in patients with head tremor. Mov Disord 1997;12:576–584.
137. Vives-Rodriguez A, Kim CY, Louis ED. Primary writing tremor. Tremor Other Hyperkinet Mov (N Y) 2018;8:586.
138. Vu JP, Lee HY, Chen Q, Cisneros E, Barbano RL, Goetz CG, et al. Head tremor and pain in cervical dystonia. J Neurol 2021;268:1945–1959.
139. White LJ, Klein AM, Hapner ER, Delgaudio JM, Hanfelt JJ, Jinnah HA, Johns MM, 3rd. Coprevalence of tremor with spasmodic dysphonia: A case-control study. Laryngoscope 2011;121:1752–1755.
140. Whone AL, Watts RL, Stoessl AJ, Davis M, Reske S, Nahmias C, et al. Slower progression of Parkinson's disease with ropinirole versus levodopa: The REAL-PET study. Ann Neurol 2003;54:93–101.
141. Williams L, McGovern E, Kimmich O, Molloy A, Beiser I, Butler JS, et al. Epidemiological, clinical and genetic aspects of adult onset isolated focal dystonia in Ireland. Eur J Neurol 2016;24:73–81.
142. Yanagisawa N, Goto A. Dystonia musculorum deformans: Analysis with electromyography. J Neurol Sci 1971;13:39–65.

Chapter 13

Dystonia and Parkinsonism

INTRODUCTION

Dystonia and parkinsonism are two distinct movement disorders. *Dystonia* is defined by excessive involuntary muscle contractions leading to involuntary abnormal movements and postures.[1] Parkinsonism is defined by several features, most commonly bradykinesia combined with rest tremor, rigidity, or both.[29] In clinical medicine, the term *bradykinesia* is used in two different ways. Strictly speaking, bradykinesia means slow movement. When referring to parkinsonism, some writers use the term to imply slowness that is also combined with akinesia (paucity of spontaneous movement) or hypometria (reduced amplitude of movements). Here we use the broader definition. In addition to these core features, numerous other features of parkinsonism are summarized in Table 13.1 including hypomimia, reduced blink rate, hypophonia, tachyphemia, reduced arm swing, gait festination or freezing, and postural instability.

The syndrome of dystonia-parkinsonism refers to the combination of dystonia with parkinsonism. This combined syndrome is common, with many different etiologies.[46,61] Dystonia and parkinsonism may occur simultaneously, or they may occur sequentially over time. Sometimes, dystonia affects one region of the body while parkinsonism occurs in another region. Either

Table 13.1 **Clinical characteristics of parkinsonism**

Characteristic	Description
Akinesia	Paucity of spontaneous movements
Bradykinesia	Slowness of movement
Festination	Gait abnormality described by tiny steps that progressively speed up
Freezing	Abnormality described by difficulty initiating the gait, or sudden stopping of the gait
Hypometria	Reduced amplitude of movements
Hypomimia	Reduced facial expression
Hypophonia	Reduced voice volume
Rigidity	Abnormally high muscle tone causing increased resistance to passive movement. Often, the term ***lead pipe*** resistance is used, to designate a velocity-independent resistance to passive movement, that distinguishes rigidity from spasticity (velocity-dependent, or ***clasp-knife*** phenomenon)
Rest tremor	Rest tremor is classically a 4-6 Hz tremor in the fully resting limb, which is suppressed during movement initiation
Tachyphemia	A stuttering type of speech, sometimes called *festination of speech*

dystonic or parkinsonian features may dominate. This chapter summarizes the most relevant causes, with a focus on frequent and/or treatable disorders. Additional syndromes of dystonia-parkinsonism are summarized in several Tables. The disorders are grouped by common pathogenic mechanisms, although these mechanisms sometimes overlap.

PATHOGENIC LINKS BETWEEN DYSTONIA AND PARKINSONISM

Several lines of evidence suggest that dystonia and parkinsonism share common biological links, mainly involving dopaminergic signaling or structural abnormalities in the basal ganglia. Case studies with lesions have shown that dystonia or parkinsonism emerges after lesions of the putamen, pallidum, and midbrain.[10,15,31] Pharmacological evidence comes from dopamine receptor-blocking drugs, which can cause dystonia, parkinsonism, or both combined (see Chapter 19, "Dystonia Induced by Medications, Illicit Drugs, and Environmental Exposures"). The main medications are antipsychotics such as haloperidol or risperidone, but they also include antiemetics such as metoclopramide. In addition, dystonia may occur in Parkinson disease (PD) when levodopa wears off, and it responds to a higher dose.

Genetic conditions demonstrate the importance of dopaminergic neurotransmission in both parkinsonism and dystonia.[30] These are mainly conditions that affect dopamine synthesis, transport, storage, or signal transduction. Most of these disorders are associated with dystonia and parkinsonism. For example, genetic variants in *GCH1* cause dystonia, parkinsonism, or both combined. Variants in *PRKN* cause early-onset PD that may manifest with a combination of parkinsonism and dystonia or only isolated dystonia.

Animal models similarly demonstrate a link between dystonia and parkinsonism. For example, in non-human primates treated with 1-methyl-4-phenyl-1,2,3,6-tetrahydropyridine (MPTP), dystonia develops several weeks before parkinsonism emerges.[51,67] In a mouse model of dopa-responsive dystonia associated with mutations in the *TH* gene encoding tyrosine hydroxylase, young animals exhibit dystonia, but parkinsonism develops as animals get older.[57]

Just as the pathogenesis of dystonia is not entirely understood, there remain also many open questions regarding the commonalities and differences in the pathophysiology of these two distinct movement disorders.[61] One interesting aspect, for example, involves the age-dependent effects of dopamine deficiency. Dystonia is more common when nigrostriatal dopamine deficiency emerges in early childhood, while parkinsonism is more likely when nigrostriatal dopamine deficiency begins in older adults. A clinical example is early-onset PD that may manifest purely with dystonia compared with classical, late-onset PD. An age-dependent effect can also be observed with dopamine receptor antagonists. These drugs tend to induce dystonia and particularly retrocollis in young adults, but they induce tardive dyskinesia in older adults.[59]

CLINICAL APPROACH

Introduction

The clinical and etiological spectrum of dystonia-parkinsonism syndromes is very broad, encompassing idiopathic neurodegenerative diseases, drug-related causes, genetic disorders, and autoimmune disease. The clinical approach is described here, and the most relevant conditions are summarized in more detail below. The differential diagnosis greatly depends on the age of onset (Figure 13.1). Early in life, from infancy to early adulthood, genetic causes are more frequent. Later in life, idiopathic neurodegenerative diseases are more common. Fortunately, most of these conditions can be diagnosed using imaging, metabolic studies, or genetic testing.

Age at Onset

In infants, disorders of dopamine synthesis are the first consideration. Common additional clinical signs include truncal hypotonia, oculogyric crises, a fast jittery tremor, and often autonomic dysfunction.[28,36,76] These disorders may also present later in childhood, when additional etiologies to consider include brain metal accumulation disorders, such as Wilson disease and neurodegeneration with brain iron accumulation (NBIA).[7,17,78] These other disorders are further suggested by the presence of prominent bulbar involvement,

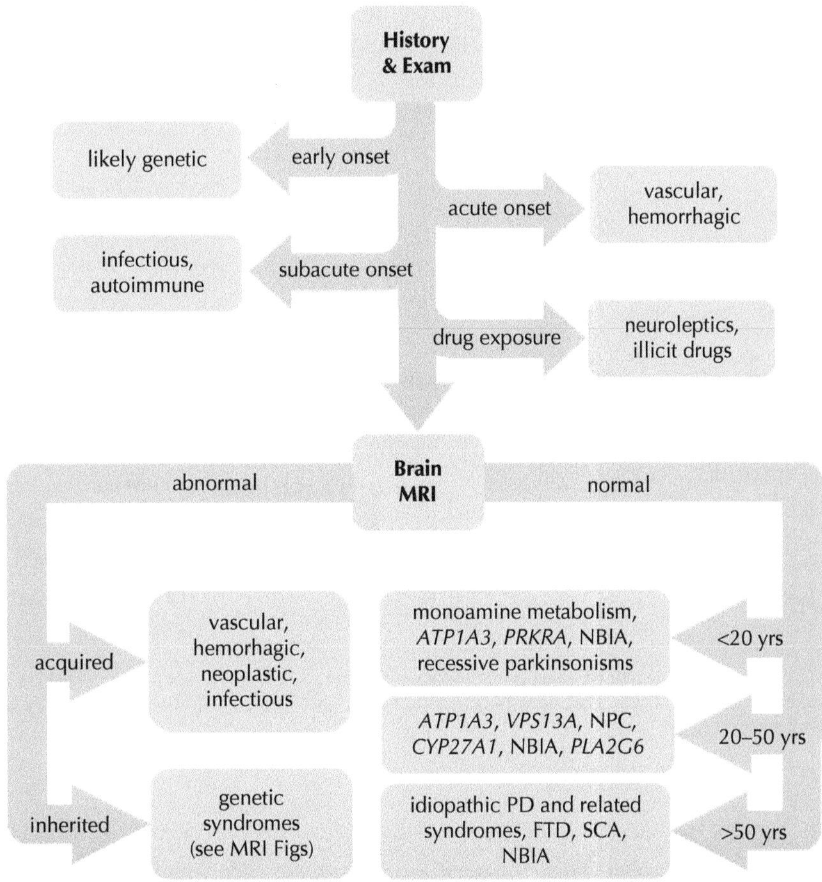

Figure 13.1. Algorithm for assessment of syndromes that combine dystonia and parkinsonism. This schematic provides only a general approach for diagnosis as exceptions may exist. Abbreviations: FTD, frontotemporal dementia; NBIA, neurodegeneration with brain iron accumulation; PD, Parkinson disease. Gene symbols: *ATP1A3*, rapid-onset dystonia-parkinsonism; *CYP27A1*, cerebrotendinous xanthomatosis; *PLA2G6*, *PLA2G6*-associated neurodegeneration, PLAN; *PRKRA*, previously DYT16; *VPS13A*, chorea-acanthocytosis.

cognitive or psychiatric impairment, ataxia, or oculomotor disturbance. Another important diagnosis to consider in adolescents and young adults is early-onset PD. Individuals with early-onset degenerative PD may be difficult to distinguish from non-degenerative metabolic disorders affecting the dopamine pathways because their clinical pictures can be indistinguishable.[52] While both conditions respond to levodopa, obtaining a definitive diagnosis is important for counseling regarding prognosis.

Later in life, when neurodegenerative causes become more prevalent, the pattern of dystonia as well as additional features can help to distinguish PD from multisystem atrophy, progressive supranuclear palsy, or corticobasal syndrome.[20,81] A careful drug history is always relevant because the syndrome of dystonia-parkinsonism can be caused by dopamine receptor antagonists as well as a range of other drugs (see Chapter 19).

Laboratory Evaluation

Brain imaging has a major role in dystonia-parkinsonism syndromes (Figure 13.2 and Figure 13.3). Brain MRI can show highly characteristic patterns, such as abnormal metal or mineral accumulation, or characteristic signal abnormalities confined to specific brain regions (see Chapter 27, "Workup of Dystonia").[47] Other recognizable patterns on

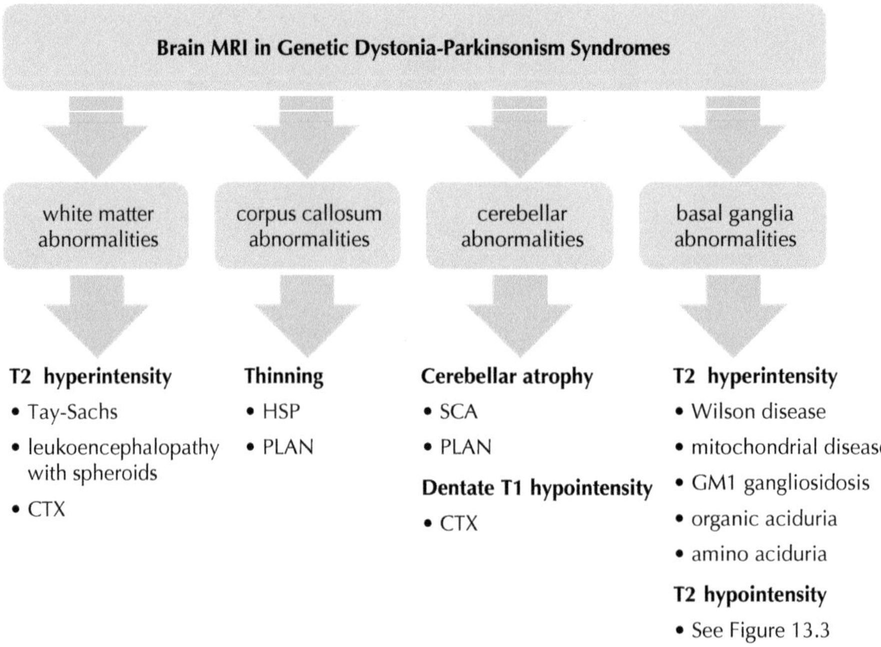

Figure 13.2. Brain MRI findings in genetic dystonia-parkinsonism syndromes. Some typical examples are provided. Abbreviations: CTX, cerebrotendinous xanthomatosis; HSP, hereditary spastic paraplegia; PLAN, PLAG2G6-associated neurodegeneration; SCA, spinocerebellar ataxia.

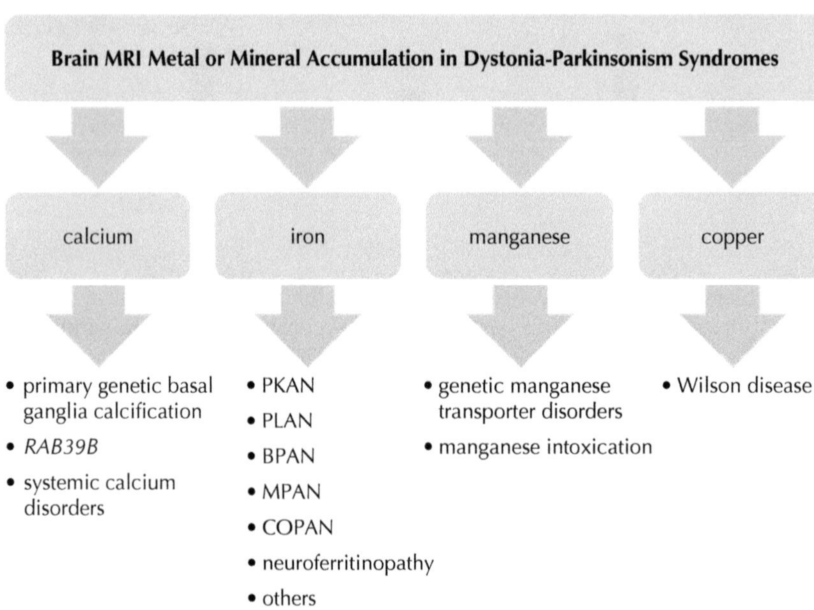

Figure 13.3. Brain MRI findings in genetic dystonia-parkinsonism syndromes associated with metal or mineral accumulation. Some typical examples are provided. Abbreviations: BPAN, beta-propeller protein–associated neurodegeneration (WDR45 gene); COPAN, coenzyme-A synthase protein–associated neurodegeneration (COASY gene); MPAN, mitochondrial membrane protein–associated neurodegeneration (C19orf12 gene); PKAN, pantothenate kinase–associated neurodeneration (PANK2 gene); PLAN, PLAG2G6–associated neurodegeneration (PLA2G6 gene).

brain MRI include certain infectious causes like West Nile virus, or autoimmune disorders such as anti-Ma2 encephalitis. Similarly, structural lesions causing dystonia-parkinsonism can be detected, which is particularly relevant for hemidystonia-hemiparkinsonism.[10,41]

Radionuclide scans that detect nigrostriatal axonal projections, such as dopamine transporter single photon emission CT (SPECT or DAT scan), can also be helpful. The DAT scan is usually normal in metabolic disorders of dopamine synthesis, while it is usually abnormal in neurodegenerative disorders such as PD and related parkinsonian syndromes. This scan can therefore be very helpful in discriminating early-onset PD from dopa-responsive dystonia. However, this test involves exposure to radiation, which should be avoided in young individuals. When using this scan, it also is important to recognize that false-positive and false-negative results may occur, and results may be confounded by recent use of medications that interact with dopaminergic transmission.

Historically, studies of cerebrospinal fluid (CSF) neurotransmitters were routinely recommended by experts for the workup of dystonia-parkinsonism in pediatric neurology (see Chapter 27). However, obtaining good results can be difficult. The sample needs to be collected in tubes with special preservatives, rapidly cooled, transported to the lab quickly, and protected from light. Such procedures are challenging in clinical practice. In addition, the results may be clouded by treatment with various drugs, including levodopa. An abnormal CSF result cannot reliably discriminate among subtypes of dopamine synthesis disorders, and results may be abnormal in disorders where there is nigrostriatal degeneration as well. Most disorders that may be revealed by abnormal CSF neurotransmitter studies can now be detected using genetic tests, which may also discriminate metabolic from degenerative disorders.

GENETIC DISORDERS CAUSING DYSTONIA AND PARKINSONISM

Monoamine Metabolism

Genetic disorders of monoamine metabolism (Figure 13.4) tend to manifest early in life.[28,76,79] The most common is dopa-responsive dystonia (Segawa syndrome), most often due to autosomal-dominant variants in *GCH1*. The disorder is characterized by childhood-onset diurnal fluctuation of dystonia that is worse in the evenings. It predominantly affects the lower limbs, and there is usually a good response to small doses of levodopa. Parkinsonism is typically minor but may dominate in some cases, particularly late-onset cases. Variants in *GCH1* are recognized as a risk factor for PD, too.[43]

There are also more complicated phenotypes due to variants in *TH, DDC, PTS*, and *SLC6A3* (Table 13.2 and Figure 13.4). While a minority of individuals with variants in these genes occasionally present with the dopa-responsive dystonia phenotype, they more often present in infancy with additional features such as encephalopathy, hypotonia, oculogyric crises, and autonomic dysfunction. Some cases respond to levodopa, but many do not.

Brain Metal or Mineral Accumulation

INTRODUCTION

The NBIA disorders that may present with dystonia-parkinsonism are defined by deposition of iron in the brain, and this deposition can be picked up on brain MRI (Table 13.3). The exact underlying pathomechanisms are not completely understood. In particular, it is not clear if the metal deposition is a cause or consequence of neurodegeneration. This group of disorders share some clinical characteristics and treatment principles that justify grouping them together.[17,78] Age at onset ranges from early childhood to early adulthood. Prominent bulbar involvement, leading to dysarthria or dysphagia, is common. Tongue protrusion dystonia, pushing the food out of the mouth, has been described as characteristic for NBIA, although it is not pathognomonic.[2,60] Similarly, a tendency to retrocollis or dystonic opisthotonos are other red flags for NBIAs.[64]

Pantothenate kinase-associated neurodegeneration (PKAN) is the most frequent NBIA. It is autosomal recessive. Genetic variants in *PANK2* cause a broad spectrum of disease.[26,27] The more severe typical cases have onset in early childhood with generalized dystonia, spasticity, parkinsonism, pigmentary retinopathy, and global developmental delay. Less severely affected atypical

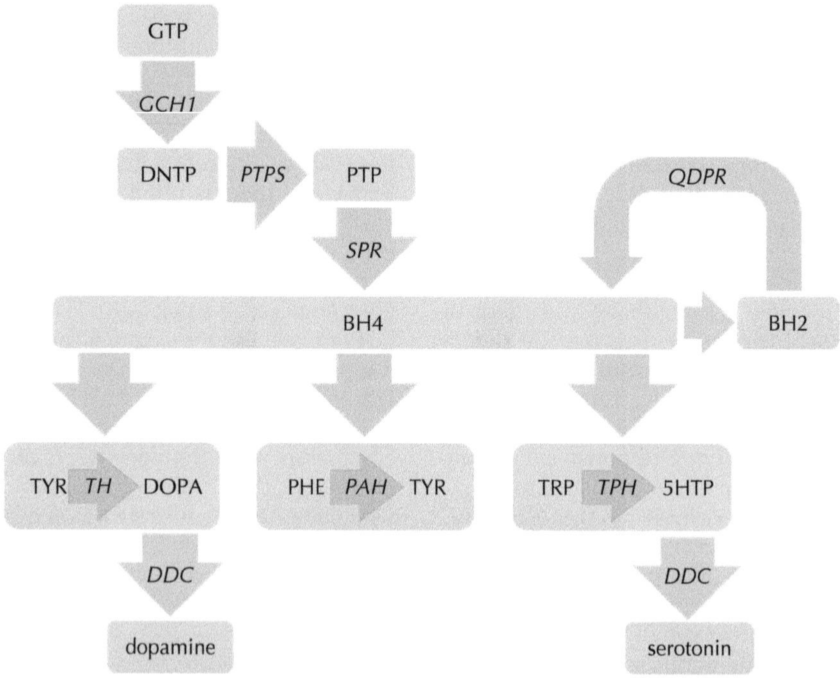

Figure 13.4. Inherited defects in biopterin metabolism associated with dystonia-parkinsonism syndromes. Metabolites are show in regular typeface and genes are shown in italics. Abbreviations: 5HTP, 5-hydroxytryptophan; BH2, biopterin; BH4, tetrahydrobiopterin; DDC, aromatic amino acid decarboxylase; DNTP, dihydroneopterin triphosphate; DOPA, levodopa; GCH1, GTP-cylohydrolase 1; GTP, guanosine triphosphate; PAH, phenylalanine hydroxylase; PHE, phenylalanine; PTP, pyrovoyl tetrahyropterin; PTPS, pyruvoyl tetrahydropterin synthase; QDPR, dihydopterin reductase; SPR, sepiapterin reductase; TH, tyrosine hydroxylase; TPH, tryptophan hydroxylase; TRP, tryptophan; TYR, tyrosine.

cases may present in adolescence or early adults as dystonia-parkinsonism, often with pronounced oromandibular involvement.

Genetic variants in *PLA2G6* cause PLAN (*PLA2G6*-associated neurodegeneration), which is also autosomal recessive with a broad spectrum of clinical phenotypes.[49] The most severe phenotype includes neuroaxonal dystrophy with infantile onset, while the least severe have adult-onset dystonia-parkinsonism. Individuals with dystonia-parkinsonism may have other features that include corticospinal or cerebellar signs or psychiatric or cognitive impairment, which, together with a retrocollic/opisthotonic component, are useful clinical clues. As in early-onset PD, individuals may experience a good response to levodopa, levodopa-induced dyskinesia, and rapid eye movement (REM) sleep behavior disorder. Iron deposition may not be detectable on brain MRI even when symptomatic.

Genetic variants in *ATP13A2*, which encode the ATPase cation transporting 13A2 protein, can also cause early-onset, dopa-responsive parkinsonism with dystonia. Some but not all patients feature iron deposition in the basal ganglia.[35] The presence of cognitive impairment, pyramidal signs, and a characteristic vertical supranuclear gaze palsy point to the diagnosis. Other NBIAs may manifest with dystonia and parkinsonism, but do so more rarely (Table 13.3).

MANGANESE

Variants in manganese transporters encoded by the genes *SLC30A10*[53,71] and *SLC39A14*[72] can cause a disorder with early-onset dystonia-parkinsonism, often with prominent dysarthria and dysphagia. Sometimes there is a gait disorder characteristic of manganism termed "cock-walk," where individuals walk with the front of the foot (metacarpophalangeal joint and toes) on the ground and the heel raised up off the ground.

Manganese deposition on brain MRI shows as T1-hyperintensity with T2-hypointensity in the pallidum, striatum, brainstem, and dentate nucleus. While chelation therapies in NBIA have

Table 13.2 **Genetic disorders affecting monoamine metabolism**

Disorder	Gene	Typical clinical features	Response to levodopa
6-pyruvoyl-tetrahydropterin synthase deficiency	*PTS* (AR)	Onset within the first months of life with hypokinetic-rigid syndrome, dystonia, encephalopathy, chorea, epilepsy.	Sometimes good
Aromatic l-amino acid decarboxylase deficiency	*DDC* (AR)	Onset within the first months of life with hypokinetic-rigid syndrome, dystonia, autonomic abnormalities, and oculogyric crises.	Rarely*
Dopa-responsive dystonia	*GCH1* (AD)	Onset before adolescence with dystonia and sometimes minor parkinsonism. Onset in adults with parkinsonism and sometimes minor dystonia.	Excellent
Dihydropteridine reductase deficiency	*QDPR* (AR)	Onset in the first months of life with motor delay, hypotonia, microcephaly, irritability and epilepsy. Some cases develop tremor or dystonia-parkinsonism.	Sometimes good
DNAJC12 deficiency	*DNAJC12* (AR)	Childhood onset intellectual disability, autism spectrum disorder, and sometimes dystonia-parkinsonism.	Excellent
Dopamine transporter deficiency	*SLC6A3* (AR)	Onset in infancy with dystonia-parkinsonism, anarthria/aphonia, dysphagia, dyskinesia, impaired saccades, and ocular flutter.	None
Sepiapterin reductase deficiency	*SPR* (AR)	Onset within the first year of life of motor delay, hypotonia, dystonia, paroxysmal stiffening, oculogyric crises, and sometimes parkinsonism.	Sometimes good
Tyrosine hydroxylase deficiency	*TH* (AR)	Type A has onset from infancy to early childhood with hypokinetic-rigid syndrome, hypotonia, and dystonia; Type B has onset in infancy with severe hypokinetic-rigid syndrome, dystonia, myoclonus, ptosis, oculogyric crises, and autonomic dysfunction.	Type A responds well, Type B does not
Vesicular monoamine transporter-2 deficiency	*SLC18A2* (AR)	Onset in infancy with hypotonia and oculogyric crises, facial dyskinesia with later anarthria and dystonia-parkinsonism.	Worse*

This table summarizes the typical clinical features of disorders of monoamine metabolism. The pattern of inheritance is shown below the gene as autosomal dominant (AD) or autosomal recessive (AR). Further details can be found in prior reviews and Figure 13.4.[46,76] Asterisks show conditions where there may be a response to dopamine agonists rather than levodopa.

Table 13.3 **Genetic disorders involving brain metal accumulation**

Disorder	Gene	Main metal	Typical clinical features
Beta-propeller protein-associated neurodegeneration (BPAN)	*WDR45* (XL)	Fe	Childhood-onset cognitive decline, seizures, autism, and dystonia-parkinsonism with aging
Coenzyme A synthase deficiency (COPAN)	*COASY* (AR)	Fe	Childhood-onset parkinsonism with oromandibular dystonia, corticospinal signs, neuropathy
Kufor-Rakeb disease	*ATP13A2*	Fe	Childhood-onset dystonia-parkinsonism with corticospinal signs, supranuclear gaze palsy, facial-faucial-finger myoclonus, psychiatric symptoms and cognitive decline
Mitochondrial membrane protein-associated neurodegeneration (MPAN)	*C19orf12* (AR)	Fe	Onset in childhood or young adults with corticospinal signs, dysarthria, intellectual disability, psychiatric features, and age-related dystonia-parkinsonism, optic atrophy, amyotrophy
Neuroferritinopathy	*FTL* (AR)	Fe	Adult-onset chorea and dystonia, with parkinsonism in some cases
Pantothenate kinase-associated neurodegeneration (PKAN)	*PANK2* (AR)	Fe	Childhood-onset corticospinal signs, cognitive decline, retinopathy, dystonia and parkinsonism; cases with later onset often have dystonia-parkinsonism
Phospholipase A2 Group VI (PLA2G6)-related neurodegeneration (PLAN)	*PLA2G6* (AR)	Fe	Dystonia-parkinsonism that may be levodopa responsive with levodopa-induced dyskinesia and REM-sleep behaviour disorder; dystonia often with retrocollic or opisthotonic component. Possible associated features: Cognitive/psychiatric, cerebellar, pyramidal signs.
Parkinsonism-dystonia with hypermanganesemia	*SLC30A10* (AR)	Mn	Childhood-onset dystonia-parkinsonism with dysarthria, dysphagia, liver disease, polycythemia, and sometimes a high-stepping gait
Childhood-onset parkinsonism-dystonia	*SLC39A14* (AR)	Mn	Childhood-onset dystonia-parkinsonism, with dysphagia and dysarthria
Wilson disease	*ATP7B (AR)*	Cu	Onset in childhood or young adults with liver disease, dystonia, parkinsonism, tremor, and cognitive or psychiatric features.

This table summarizes the typical clinical features of disorders associated with accumulation of metals in the brain. The pattern of inheritance is shown below the gene as autosomal dominant (AD) or autosomal recessive (AR). Further details can be found in Figure 13.3 and prior reviews[17,78]

no proven effect,[34,69] the response in manganese transportopathies is broad. Some cases with variants in *SLC30A1* respond well while others with *SLC39A14* variants do not.[19]

COPPER

The variable response of iron and manganese storage disorders to chelation therapies stands in stark contrast to Wilson disease, where chelation is usually effective. Wilson disease is an autosomal recessive disorder associated with genetic variants in the *ATP7B* gene that lead to copper deposition in liver, brain (mainly basal ganglia and cerebellum), cornea, and kidneys. It presents with a wide range of symptoms. Two main forms are recognized: a hepatic form with onset in early childhood, and a neurological form with onset in late childhood or early adolescence. However, mixed cases are common, and onset of symptoms may be as late as the age of 74 years.[16]

Neurological manifestations are quite varied, but dystonia and parkinsonism are the most common.[40,66] Dysarthria is common, too, along with tremor that characteristically has a "wing-beating" appearance in the upper limbs when the shoulders are abducted laterally and the elbows are flexed with the hands in front of the chin. Other features may include ataxia, chorea, myoclonus, or psychiatric disturbance. Risus sardonicus, a dystonic retraction of the upper lip and mouth, is also considered characteristic, but it is not pathognomonic. An important and characteristic finding is a corneal Kayser-Fleischer ring consisting of red-brown pigmentation around the edge of the iris due to deposition of copper in the Descemet's membrane, best seen on slit-lamp examination. Similarly, sunflower cataracts due to a radiating, red-brown pattern of copper deposition in the lens can point to the diagnosis.

Treatments include chelating agents and zinc. There can be a worsening of neurological problems after initiation of therapy, particularly with penicillamine. Lifelong treatment is essential and needs to be continued even when individuals become asymptomatic. Continuous monitoring and maintaining compliance are therefore important aspects of management. In rapidly progressive cases with hepatic failure, a liver transplant may be required.

CALCIUM

Fahr syndrome, also known as primary familial basal ganglia calcification, has been linked with a number of different genes (Table 13.4).[3] Calcium deposits occur in a number of different regions, particularly the basal ganglia, cerebellum, and deep white matter. Symptoms emerge in a very wide age range, and a substantial proportion remain symptom free for decades, even with an abnormal brain scan. Typical symptoms include cognitive impairment, dysarthria, and headaches. The most common movement disorder is parkinsonism. Dystonia occurs in a smaller proportion. Some individuals may respond to levodopa.[58]

Parkinson Disease and Related Conditions

A large number of genes can cause parkinsonism. These genes can be divided into distinct groups. One group includes genes that cause a clinical picture that resembles idiopathic PD. In a systematic review that aggregated published data from individually reported cases, the genes associated with autosomal dominant disease (*LRRK2*, *SNCA*, *VPS35*) tended to present at an age slightly earlier than idiopathic PD, and dystonia was uncommon (<10%).[70] In a similar systematic review of genes associated with autosomal recessive disease (*DJ1*, *PRKN*, *PINK1*), symptoms often emerged at an age much earlier than idiopathic PD, and dystonia was more common (18–48%).[32] The exact prevalence of dystonia associated with these genes cannot be determined from these studies because methodical assessments for dystonia were often lacking in the published reports surveyed, with a large amount of missing data. However, the results appear to echo large cohort studies focusing on individual genes, where dystonia appears to be more common in early-onset genetic PD.

Table 13.4 **Genetic disorders of primary familial basal ganglia calcification**

Gene	Total cases	Symptomatic (%)	Age at onset (range)	Dystonia (%)	Parkinsonism (%)	Other common features
JAM2 (AR)	11	91	37 (7–50)	50	80	Cognitive impairment, dysarthria, ataxia
MYORG (AR)	66	91	46 (8–87)	7	27	Dysarthria, ataxia, cognitive impairment
PDGFB (AD)	64	86	30 (1–70)	9	18	Headache, cognitive impairment, ataxia, chorea
PDGFRB (AD)	26	46	48 (6–78)	0	17	Headache, cognitive deficits, dysarthria, tremor
SLC20A2 (AD)	317	60	47 (1–84)	14	28	Cognitive impairment, headache, dysarthria, chorea, ataxia
XPR (AD)	32	94	44 (29–81)	5	29	Cognitive impairment, dysarthria, ataxia

This table summarizes clinical features from one large meta-analysis that involved aggregation of data from published reports.[3] The pattern of inheritance is shown below the gene as autosomal dominant (AD) or autosomal recessive (AR). Age at onset reflects median and range in parentheses. The results show that parkinsonism and dystonia are common, but actual figures must be interpreted with caution because of the small numbers of cases in some groups, and large numbers of reports where the movement disorder was not described.

Another group of genes associated with neurodegeneration has additional clinical features not typical of idiopathic PD. The most common atypical features include corticospinal signs, abnormalities of respiration, myoclonus, eye movement abnormalities, and seizures.[80] The genes include *ATP1A3, DCTN1, DNAJC6, FBXO7, PRKRA, SYNJ1, TAF1, VPS13*, and others. These disorders tend to present earlier than idiopathic PD and also include a high proportion of individuals with dystonia. A third group of genes is associated with early-onset metabolic disease where dystonia and parkinsonism are common.[46,47] A few of these are described here because dystonia is a prominent feature.

The *ATP1A3* gene is associated with the syndrome of *rapid-onset dystonia-parkinsonism*. The onset of symptoms is often abrupt, emerging over a period of hours or weeks.[12,74] Symptoms emerge in adolescents or young adults with specific triggers such as physical or psychological stress, alcohol binging, exercise, hyperthermia, uncomplicated surgery, or childbirth. Early studies emphasized a rostro-caudal (face > arm > leg) gradient of dystonia and parkinsonism with prominent bulbar involvement,[12] and more recent studies have called attention to arm dystonia, which may be paroxysmal.[5,25,83] *ATP1A3* encodes the alpha-3 subunit of the sodium-potassium ATPase pump, which is highly expressed in the basal ganglia, cerebellum, thalamus, hippocampus, and several areas of the brainstem. Neuropathology shows various degrees of neuronal loss, plaques, and neurofibrillary tangles.[48] Affected individuals do not respond to levodopa or deep brain stimulation.

The *TAF1* gene is associated with the syndrome of *X-linked dystonia-parkinsonism* (also called *Lubag*). The defect has been linked with an unusual genetic anomaly in which a retrotransposon is inserted into an intron. The typically affected individual is a Filipino man from the Panay region, but female carriers with skewed X-activation have been reported. Childhood onset has been reported, but usually it begins in adults. Craniocervical dystonia is the most common early feature. Over several years, dystonia generalizes and parkinsonism emerges.[50] Postmortem pathological studies have indicated the dystonia phase to be associated with relatively selective degeneration of the striosomal compartment of the striatum, while parkinsonism evolves when degeneration spreads to include the matrix compartment.[22] During life, the routine clinical brain MRI is normal. but voxel-based morphometry may reveal selective involvement of striosomes.[24] Most cases do not respond to levodopa, but the response to deep brain stimulation is often good.

Dystonia-parkinsonism due to variants in the *PRKRA* gene has been reported in a small number of families.[38] Onset occurs in childhood in about 70% of cases. Segmental dystonia commonly affects bulbar and axial musculature. Oromandibular dystonia and opisthotonus may be prominent early features, whereas parkinsonism develops later. Although brain MRI is frequently unremarkable, striatal hyperintensities have been reported in some cases. The gene encodes the protein kinase interferon-inducible double-stranded RNA-dependent activator. The disorder does not usually respond to levodopa but it may respond to deep brain stimulation.

DYSTONIA IN IDIOPATHIC PARKINSON DISEASE AND RELATED DISORDERS

Idiopathic Parkinson Disease

While dystonia is more prevalent in individuals with early-onset PD with a genetic cause, it is also a well-recognized feature of individuals with idiopathic PD.[61] Dystonia may be the first or most prominent manifestation of idiopathic PD, preceding other parkinsonian signs by a few years or even decades.[33,39] The most common presentation is dystonia of a lower limb,[14,42] and less commonly an upper limb or the neck.[4] Rarely, the face is involved. Although well-recognized, dystonia preceding PD is not common. One particularly methodical study described dystonia preceded other features of PD in only 5 of 207 cases.[39] However, methodical longitudinal studies are lacking.

Dystonia occurs more commonly in more advanced disease in relation to treatment with dopaminergic drugs. When a dose of levodopa is wearing off, dystonia is common, occurring in approximately one-third of PD individuals.[33] Blepharospasm can also be triggered in idiopathic PD following deep brain stimulation of the subthalamic nucleus.[75]

Parkinsonian Syndromes

Several retrospective studies of medical records have reported dystonia to be more common in the related neurodegenerative parkinsonian syndromes than idiopathic PD.[20,56] Estimates of dystonia in these studies are likely to be underestimates because methodical examination and recording was absent. In one prospective study of 1,278 individuals with parkinsonism, 176 also had dystonia.[81] The frequencies of dystonia were 11.0% in PD, 66.7% in corticobasal syndrome, 40.7% in progressive supranuclear palsy, and 20.9% in multiple system atrophy. Other studies focused on dystonia in specific subtypes of parkinsonian syndromes.

In a large series of 203 pathologically proven cases of multiple system atrophy, dystonia was noted in the medical records for 12%.[77] This figure may represent an underestimate because dystonia was not methodically evaluated or recorded for all cases. In fact, one systematic study of dystonia in 24 individuals with clinically probable multiple system atrophy described dystonia for 46%.[11] The most common features in this series included cervical dystonia (antecollis) and unilateral limb dystonia. This disorder is also associated with stridor and a characteristic strained voice. These phenomena have sometimes been attributed to laryngeal dystonia.[45] Individuals with this disorder also exhibit a high frequency of levodopa-induced facial dystonia.

In a similar series of 404 pathologically proven cases of corticobasal syndrome, dystonia was noted in the medical records for 38%, with the vast majority having dystonia of the upper limb.[63] However, a more methodical study focusing on 66 individuals with corticobasal syndrome found dystonia in 59%.[73] Commonly affected regions included the upper limb (92%) or lower limb (28%), although one-third also had dystonia in the craniofacial regions or trunk.

In a methodical study of dystonia in 83 cases of clinically probable progressive supranuclear palsy, 46% had dystonia.[8] The most common manifestations in this series included limb dystonia, blepharospasm, and axial dystonia. Limb dystonia was also reported as a characteristic finding in another series of 30 cases.[54] Blepharospasm and eyelid opening apraxia may be even more common.[18,21,37,55,82] Many cases of eyelid opening apraxia are thought to arise from dystonic contraction of muscles intrinsic to the eyelid (see Chapter 6, "Craniofacial Dystonias").[68]

Dystonic features are therefore not uncommon in idiopathic PD and related parkinsonian conditions. Similarly, parkinsonian features are not uncommon in idiopathic dystonia.[23] Although systematic studies are lacking, there are numerous studies describing slight slowness of movements in many idiopathic adult-onset non-degenerative focal dystonias, reduced arm swing in cervical dystonia, or gait abnormalities in blepharospasm. These abnormalities are often subtle, but they may be related to reduced dopamine transmission even when there is no evidence for neurodegeneration.[9,62]

AUTOIMMUNE CAUSES OF DYSTONIA AND PARKINSONISM

Autoimmune causes of dystonia-parkinsonism are rare, but they merit special attention because of their treatment potential (see Table 13.5 and Chapter 21, "Dystonia and Autoimmunity"). The classic scenario where dystonia and parkinsonism may be seen is anti-Ma2 encephalitis, a paraneoplastic syndrome with an association with testicular cancer. It is associated with a phenotype resembling progressive supranuclear palsy with supranuclear gaze palsy (vertical > horizontal), eye closure resembling apraxia of lid opening, hypothalamic-pituitary dysfunction, and prominent sleep disorders including excessive daytime sleepiness, REM behavior disorder, and narcolepsy-cataplexy.[6,65]

Brainstem encephalitis with anti-Ri antibodies is another paraneoplastic syndrome where jaw-closing dystonia with recurrent episodes of laryngospasm suggest the diagnosis. Respiratory difficulties are also a red flag for IgLON5 autoantibodies. A broad spectrum of other movement disorders has been described such as dystonia and parkinsonism, but these are typically associated with other signs like a characteristic non-REM parasomnia, prominent bulbar involvement, and gaze palsies.

Dystonia and parkinsonism may be seen in children with N-methyl-D-aspartate receptor (NMDAR) or dopamine D_2 receptor (D_2R) antibodies and may be part of other encephalitic syndromes where other signs (cognitive, psychiatric, seizures) are prominent.[6,65] Corticobasal-like phenotypes without an identifiable antibody have been also described as a paraneoplastic syndrome. Last, the combination of dystonia and

Table 13.5 **Autoimmune causes of dystonia-parkinsonism**

Antibody target	Typical clinical features
Ma2	Rapidly progressive; classic is a phenotype resembling progressive supranuclear palsy with supranuclear gaze palsy (vertical > horizontal) and apraxia of lid opening, hypothalamic-pituitary dysfunction, and prominent sleep disorders
Ri	Rapidly progressive parkinsonism and jaw-closing dystonia with recurrent episodes of laryngospasm.
IgLON5	Broad spectrum of movement disorders including dystonia and parkinsonism, typically associated with other signs such as non-REM parasomnia, dysarthria/ dysphagia, and oculomotor paresis.
NMDAR	Encephalopathy, sometimes with dystonia and parkinsonism, mainly in children and young adults
D2R	Encephalopathy, sometimes with dystonia and parkinsonism, mainly in children

More details can be found in prior reviews.[6,44,65]

parkinsonism is extremely rare in rheumatological disease with neurological manifestation, such as systemic lupus erythematosus or antiphospholipid syndrome.[44]

TOXIC AND METABOLIC CAUSES OF DYSTONIA AND PARKINSONISM

Apart from dopamine receptor antagonists, numerous other agents may cause dystonia-parkinsonism. One example is manganese intoxication, either due to environmental exposure (e.g., miners and welders) or illicit drug use (e.g., ephedrine contaminated with potassium permanganate). Another is carbon monoxide exposure from poorly ventilated gas cookers or clay ovens, gas or paraffin heaters, portable generators, running a car or other motor in an enclosed garage, or fires of wood or coal. Other toxins include methanol, cyanide, disulfiram, and mycotoxins. Most of these conditions are associated with lesions in the basal ganglia that can be visualized by MRI. All are described in more detail in Chapter 19.

SUMMARY AND FUTURE PROSPECTS

The links between dystonia and parkinsonism are manifold and stem from clinical observations, imaging studies, genetics, and animal models. The syndrome of dystonia-parkinsonism has various etiologies including medications or toxins, genetic disease, sporadic neurodegeneration, and autoimmune diseases. The most frequent causes encompass disorders of the dopamine synthesis pathway or dopamine homeostasis, genetic forms of PD or other early-onset parkinsonian conditions, and disorders of brain metal accumulation or mineralization, as well as rapid-onset dystonia-parkinsonism or X-linked dystonia-parkinsonism. Dystonia is also frequently seen in sporadic PD and the related sporadic neurodegenerative parkinsonian syndrome. Rarely, it may be the predominant phenotype in idiopathic or paraneoplastic autoimmune disease.

The frequent associations between dystonia and parkinsonism are likely to involve pathogenic mechanisms that are at least partly shared. The most obvious shared mechanisms relate to dopaminergic signaling, and they include both degenerative and non-degenerative metabolic causes. Understanding these relationships is important because medications effective for one condition may then be explored for the other. Numerous investigators have suggested that drugs interacting with dopaminergic pathways or drugs effective for levodopa-induced dyskinesias in PD may also be useful for dystonia.[13]

REFERENCES

1. Albanese A, Bhatia K, Bressman SB, DeLong MR, Fahn S, Fung VSC, et al. Phenomenology and classification of dystonia: A consensus update. Mov Disord 2013;28:863–873.
2. Bader B, Walker RH, Vogel M, Prosiegel M, McIntosh J, Danek A. Tongue protrusion and feeding dystonia:

A hallmark of chorea-acanthocytosis. Mov Disord 2010;25:127–129.
3. Balck A, Schaake S, Kuhnke NS, Domingo A, Madoev H, Margolesky J, et al. Genotype-phenotype relations in primary familial brain calcification: Systematic MDSGene review. Mov Disord 2021;36:2468–2480.
4. Balint B, Mulroy E, Govert F, Latorre A, Di Lazarro G, Erro R, et al. Development of parkinsonism after long-standing cervical dystonia: A cohort. J Neurol Sci 2021;427:117477.
5. Balint B, Stephen CD, Udani V, Sankhla CS, Barad NH, Lang AE, Bhatia KP. Paroxysmal asymmetric dystonic arm posturing: A less recognized but characteristic manifestation of ATP1A3-related disease. Mov Disord Clin Pract 2019;6:312–315.
6. Balint B, Vincent A, Meinck HM, Irani SR, Bhatia KP. Movement disorders with neuronal antibodies: Syndromic approach, genetic parallels and pathophysiology. Brain 2018;141:13–36.
7. Bandmann O, Weiss KH, Kaler SG. Wilson's disease and other neurological copper disorders. Lancet Neurol 2015;14:103–113.
8. Barclay CL, Lang AE. Dystonia in progressive supranuclear palsy. J Neurol Neurosurg Psychiatry 1997;62:352–356.
9. Berman BD, Hallett M, Herscovitch P, Simonyan K. Striatal dopaminergic dysfunction at rest and during task performance in writer's cramp. Brain 2013;136:3645–3658.
10. Bhatia KP, Marsden CD. The behavioral and motor consequences of focal lesions of the basal ganglia in man. Brain 1994;117:859–876.
11. Boesch SM, Wenning GK, Ransmayr G, Poewe W. Dystonia in multiple system atrophy. J Neurol Neurosurg Psychiatry 2002;72:300–303.
12. Brashear A, Dobyns WB, de Carvalho Aguiar P, Borg M, Frijns CJ, Gollamudi S, et al. The phenotypic spectrum of rapid-onset dystonia-parkinsonism (RDP) and mutations in the ATP1A3 gene. Brain 2007;130:828–835.
13. Calabresi P, Standaert DG. Dystonia and levodopa-induced dyskinesias in Parkinson's disease: Is there a connection? Neurobiol Dis 2019;132:104579.
14. Chang FC, Josephs KA. Levodopa responsiveness in adult-onset lower limb dystonia is associated with the development of Parkinson's disease. Tremor Other Hyperkinet Mov 2013:tre-03-150-3598-2. doi:10.7916/D8VD6X5M.
15. Corp DT, Greenwood C, Morrison-Ham J, Pullinen J, McDowall G, Younger E, et al. Clinical and structural findings in patients with lesion-induced dystonia: Descriptive and quantitative analysis of published cases. Neurology 2022;99:e1957–e1967.
16. Członkowska A, Rodo M, Gromadzka G. Late onset Wilson's disease: Therapeutic implications. Mov Disord 2008;23:896–898.
17. Di Meo I, Tiranti V. Classification and molecular pathogenesis of NBIA syndromes. Eur J Paediatr Neurol 2018;22:272–284.
18. Friedman DI, Jankovic J, McCrary JA, 3rd. Neuro-ophthalmic findings in progressive supranuclear palsy. J Clin Neuroophthalmol 1992;12:104–109.
19. Garg D, Yoganathan S, Shamim U, Mankad K, Gulati P, Bonifati V, et al. Clinical profile and treatment outcomes of hypermanganesemia with dystonia 1 and 2 among 27 Indian children. Mov Disord Clin Pract 2022;9:886–899.
20. Godeiro-Junior C, Felicio AC, Barsottini OG, Aguiar PM, Silva SM, Borges V, Ferraz HB. Clinical features of dystonia in atypical parkinsonism. Arq Neuropsiquiatr 2008;66:800–804.
21. Golbe LI, Davis PH, Lepore FE. Eyelid movement abnormalities in progressive supranuclear palsy. Mov Disord 1989;4:297–302.
22. Goto S, Lee LV, Munoz EL, Tooyama I, Tamiya G, Makino S, et al. Functional anatomy of the basal ganglia in X-linked recessive dystonia-parkinsonism. Ann Neurol 2005;58:7–17.
23. Haggstrom L, Darveniza P, Tisch S. Mild parkinsonian features in dystonia: Literature review, mechanisms and clinical perspectives. Parkinsonism Relat Disord 2017;35:1–7.
24. Hanssen H, Prasuhn J, Heldmann M, Diesta CC, Domingo A, Göttlich M, et al. Imaging gradual neurodegeneration in a basal ganglia model disease. Ann Neurol 2019;86:517–526.
25. Haq IU, Snively BM, Sweadner KJ, Suerken CK, Cook JF, Ozelius LJ, et al. Revising rapid-onset dystonia-parkinsonism: Broadening indications for ATP1A3 testing. Mov Disord 2019;34:1528–1536.
26. Hayflick SJ, Kurian MA, Hogarth P. Neurodegeneration with brain iron accumulation. Handb Clin Neurol 2018;147:293–305.
27. Hayflick SJ, Westaway SK, Levinson B, Zhou B, Johnson MA, Ching KH, Gitschier J. Genetic, clinical, and radiographic delineation of Hallervorden-Spatz syndrome. N Engl J Med 2003;348:33–40.
28. Himmelreich N, Blau N, Thony B. Molecular and metabolic bases of tetrahydrobiopterin (BH4) deficiencies. Mol Genet Metab 2021;133:123–136.
29. Jankovic J, Tan EK. Parkinson's disease: Etiopathogenesis and treatment. J Neurol Neurosurg Psychiatry 2020;91:795–808.
30. Jinnah HA, Sun YV. Dystonia genes and their biological pathways. Neurobiol Dis 2019;129:159–168.
31. Joutsa J, Horn A, Hsu J, Fox MD. Localizing parkinsonism based on focal brain lesions. Brain 2018;141:2445–2456.
32. Kasten M, Hartmann C, Hampf J, Schaake S, Westenberger A, Vollstedt EJ, et al. Genotype-phenotype relations for the Parkinson's disease genes Parkin, PINK1, DJ1: MDSGene systematic review. Mov Disord 2018;33:730–741.
33. Kidron D, Melamed E. Forms of dystonia in patients with Parkinson's disease. Neurology 1987;37:1009–1011.
34. Klopstock T, Tricta F, Neumayr L, Karin I, Zorzi G, Fradette C, et al. Safety and efficacy of deferiprone for pantothenate kinase-associated neurodegeneration: A randomised, double-blind, controlled trial and an open-label extension study. Lancet Neurol 2019;18:631–642.
35. Kruer MC, Paudel R, Wagoner W, Sanford L, Kara E, Gregory A, et al. Analysis of ATP13A2 in large neurodegeneration with brain iron accumulation (NBIA) and dystonia-parkinsonism cohorts. Neurosci Lett 2012;523:35–38.
36. Kurian MA, Gissen P, Smith M, Heales S, Jr., Clayton PT. The monoamine neurotransmitter disorders: An expanding range of neurological syndromes. Lancet Neurol 2011;10:721–733.
37. Lamberti P, De Mari M, Zenzola A, Aniello MS, Defazio G. Frequency of apraxia of eyelid opening in the general population and in patients with extrapyramidal disorders. Neurol Sci 2002;23 Suppl 2:S81–82.

38. Lange LM, Junker J, Loens S, Baumann H, Olschewski L, Schaake S, et al. Genotype-phenotype relations for isolated dystonia genes: MDSGene systematic review. Mov Disord 2021;36:1086–1103.
39. LeWitt PA, Burns RS, Newman RP. Dystonia in untreated Parkinsonism. Clinical Neuropharmacology 1986;9:293–297.
40. Machado A, Chien HF, Deguti MM, Cancado E, Azevedo RS, Scaff M, Barbosa ER. Neurological manifestations in Wilson's disease: Report of 119 cases. Mov Disord 2006;21:2192–2196.
41. Marsden CD, Obeso JA, Zarranz JJ. The anatomical basis of symptomatic hemidystonia. Brain 1985;108:463–483.
42. McKeon A, Matsumoto JY, Bower JH, Ahlskog JE. The spectrum of disorders presenting as adult-onset focal lower extremity dystonia. Parkinsonism Relat Disord 2008;14:613–619.
43. Mencacci NE, Isaias IU, Reich MM, Ganos C, Plagnol V, Polke JM, et al. Parkinson's disease in GTP cyclohydrolase 1 mutation carriers. Brain 2014;137:2480–2492.
44. Menozzi E, Mulroy E, Akbarian-Tefaghi L, Bhatia KP, Balint B. Movement disorders in systemic autoimmune diseases: Clinical spectrum, ancillary investigations, pathophysiological considerations. Parkinsonism Relat Disord 2021;88:116–128.
45. Merlo IM, Occhini A, Pacchetti C, Alfonsi E. Not paralysis, but dystonia causes stridor in multiple system atrophy. Neurology 2002;58:649–652.
46. Morales-Briceno H, Fung VSC, Bhatia KP, Balint B. Parkinsonism and dystonia: Clinical spectrum and diagnostic clues. J Neurol Sci 2022;433:120016.
47. Morales-Briceno H, Mohammad SS, Post B, Fois AF, Dale RC, Tchan M, Fung VSC. Clinical and neuroimaging phenotypes of genetic parkinsonism from infancy to adolescence. Brain 2020;143:751–770.
48. Oblak AL, Hagen MC, Sweadner KJ, Haq I, Whitlow CT, Maldjian JA, et al. Rapid-onset dystonia-parkinsonism associated with the I758S mutation of the ATP1A3 gene: A neuropathologic and neuroanatomical study of four siblings. Acta neuropathologica 2014;128:81–98.
49. Paisán-Ruiz C, Li A, Schneider SA, Holton JL, Johnson R, Kidd D, et al. Widespread Lewy body and tau accumulation in childhood and adult onset dystonia-parkinsonism cases with PLA2G6 mutations. Neurobiol Aging 2012;33:814–823.
50. Pauly MG, Ruiz López M, Westenberger A, Saranza G, Brüggemann N, Weissbach A, et al. Expanding data collection for the MDSGene database: X-linked dystonia-parkinsonism as use case example. Mov Disord 2020;35:1933–1938.
51. Perlmutter JS, Tempel LW, Black KJ, Parkinson D, Todd RD. MPTP induces dystonia and parkinsonism. Clues to the pathophysiology of dystonia. Neurology 1997;49:1432–1438.
52. Potulska-Chromik A, Hoffman-Zacharska D, Lukawska M, Kostera-Pruszczyk A. Dopa-responsive dystonia or early-onset Parkinson disease: Genotype-phenotype correlation. Neurol Neurochir Pol 2016;51:1–6.
53. Quadri M, Federico A, Zhao T, Breedveld GJ, Battisti C, Delnooz C, et al. Mutations in SLC30A10 cause parkinsonism and dystonia with hypermanganesemia, polycythemia, and chronic liver disease. Am J Hum Genet 2012;90:467–477.
54. Rafal RD, Friedman JH. Limb dystonia in progressive supranuclear palsy. Neurology 1987;37:1546–1549.
55. Rana AQ, Kabir A, Dogu O, Patel A, Khondker S. Prevalence of blepharospasm and apraxia of eyelid opening in patients with parkinsonism, cervical dystonia and essential tremor. Eur Neurol 2012;68:318–321.
56. Rivest J, Quinn N, Marsden CD. Dystonia in Parkinson's disease, multiple system atrophy, and progressive supranuclear palsy. Neurology 1990;40:1571–1578.
57. Rose SJ, Harrast P, Donsante C, Fan X, Joers V, Tansey MG, et al. Parkinsonism without dopamine neuron degeneration in aged l-dopa-responsive dystonia knockin mice. Mov Disord 2017;32:1694–1700.
58. Rücker M, Halder W, Kofler M, Ehling R, Brenneis C. Levodopa-responsive dystonia and parkinsonism in Fahr syndrome. Neurol Clin Pract 2019;9:527–529.
59. Savitt D, Jankovic J. Tardive syndromes. J Neurol Sci 2018;389:35–42.
60. Schneider SA, Aggarwal A, Bhatt MH, Dupont E, Tisch S, Limousin P, et al. Severe tongue protrusion dystonia: Clinical syndromes and possible treatment. Neurology 2006;67:940–943.
61. Shetty AS, Bhatia KP, Lang AE. Dystonia and Parkinson's disease: What is the relationship? Neurobiol Dis 2019;132:104462.
62. Simonyan K, Berman BD, Herscovitch P, Hallett M. Abnormal striatal dopaminergic neurotransmission during rest and task production in spasmodic dysphonia. J Neurosci 2013;33:14705–14714.
63. Stamelou M, Alonso-Canovas A, Bhatia KP. Dystonia in corticobasal degeneration: A review of the literature on 404 pathologically proven cases. Mov Disord 2012;27:696–702.
64. Stamelou M, Lai SC, Aggarwal A, Schneider SA, Houlden H, Yeh TH, et al. Dystonic opisthotonus: A "red flag" for neurodegeneration with brain iron accumulation syndromes? Mov Disord 2013;28:1325–1329.
65. Sturchio A, Dwivedi AK, Gastaldi M, Grimberg MB, Businaro P, Duque KR, et al. Movement disorders associated with neuronal antibodies: A data-driven approach. J Neurol 2022;269:3511–3521.
66. Svetel M, Kozic D, Stefanova E, Semnic R, Dragasevic N, Kostic VS. Dystonia in Wilson's disease. Mov Disord 2001;16:719–723.
67. Tabbal SD, Mink JW, Antenor JAV, Carl JL, Moerlein SM, Perlmutter JS. 1-methyl-4-phenyl-1,2,3,6-tetrahydropyridine-induced acute transient dystonia in monkeys with low striatal dopamine. Neurosci 2006;141:1281–1287.
68. Tawfik HA, Dutton JJ. Debunking the puzzle of eyelid apraxia: The muscle of Riolan hypothesis. Ophthalmic Plast Reconstr Surg 2023;39:211–220.
69. Thakur N, Klopstock T, Jackowski S, Kuscer E, Tricta F, Videnovic A, Jinnah HA. Rational design of novel therapies for pantothenate kinase-associated neurodegeneration. Mov Disord 2021;36:2005–2016.
70. Trinh J, Zeldenrust FMJ, Huang J, Kasten M, Schaake S, Petkovic S, et al. Genotype-phenotype relations for the Parkinson's disease genes SNCA, LRRK2, VPS35: MDSGene systematic review. Mov Disord 2018;33:1857–1870.
71. Tuschl K, Clayton PT, Gospe SM, Jr., Gulab S, Ibrahim S, Singhi P, et al. Syndrome of hepatic cirrhosis, dystonia, polycythemia, and hypermanganesemia caused by mutations in SLC30A10, a manganese transporter in man. Am J Hum Genet 2012;90:457–466.

72. Tuschl K, Meyer E, Valdivia LE, Zhao N, Dadswell C, Abdul-Sada A, et al. Mutations in SLC39A14 disrupt manganese homeostasis and cause childhood-onset parkinsonism-dystonia. Nat Commun 2016;7:11601.
73. Vanek Z, Jankovic J. Dystonia in corticobasal degeneration. Mov Disord 2001;16:252–257.
74. Vezyroglou A, Akilapa R, Barwick K, Koene S, Brownstein CA, Holder-Espinasse M, et al. The phenotypic continuum of ATP1A3-related disorders. Neurology 2022;99:e1511–e1526.
75. Weiss D, Wachter T, Breit S, Jacob SN, Pomper JK, Asmus F, et al. Involuntary eyelid closure after STN-DBS: Evidence for different pathophysiological entities. J Neurol Neurosurg Psychiatry 2010;81:1002–1007.
76. Weissbach A, Pauly MG, Herzog R, Hahn L, Halmans S, Hamami F, et al. Relationship of genotype, phenotype, and treatment in dopa-responsive dystonia: MDSGene review. Mov Disord 2021;2022:237–252.
77. Wenning GK, Tison F, Ben Shlomo Y, Daniel SE, Quinn NP. Multiple system atrophy: A review of 203 pathologically proven cases. Mov Disord 1997;12:133–147.
78. Wiethoff S, Houlden H. Neurodegeneration with brain iron accumulation. Handb Clin Neurol 2017;145:157–166.
79. Wijemanne S, Jankovic J. Dopa-responsive dystonia--clinical and genetic heterogeneity. Nat Rev Neurol 2015;11:414–424.
80. Wittke C, Petkovic S, Dobricic V, Schaake S, Respondek G, Weissbach A, et al. Genotype-phenotype relations for the atypical parkinsonism genes: MDSGene systematic review. Mov Disord 2021;36:1499–1510.
81. Yoon WT. Comparison of dystonia between Parkinson's disease and atypical parkinsonism: The clinical usefulness of dystonia distribution and characteristics in the differential diagnosis of parkinsonism. Neurol Neurochir Pol 2018;52:48–53.
82. Yoon WT, Chung EJ, Lee SH, Kim BJ, Lee WY. Clinical analysis of blepharospasm and aparxia of eyelid opening in patients with parkinsonism. J Clin Neurol 2005;1:159–165.
83. Zuniga-Ramirez C, Kramis-Hollands M, Mercado-Pimentel R, Gonzalez-Usigli HA, Saenz-Farret M, Soto-Escageda A, Fasano A. Generalized dystonia and paroxysmal dystonic attacks due to a novel ATP1A3 variant. Tremor Other Hyperkinet Mov (N Y) 2019;9. doi:10.7916/tohm.v0.

Chapter 14

Dystonia and Ataxia

INTRODUCTION

The term *ataxia* stems from the Greek ἀταξία, which means *lack of order*. Although many clinicians use this term to describe any disorganized movement, specialists in movement disorders reserve the term to describe a more specific syndrome resulting from dysfunction of the cerebellum or its connections. Individuals with cerebellar ataxia often have trouble regulating movement force, range, direction, velocity, and rhythm. These problems cause a range of clinical signs and symptoms that may affect the gait, more complex movements of the limbs, compensatory movements to stabilize posture, eye movements, and speech (Table 14.1).

There are many disorders where ataxia may be combined with dystonia. The most likely reason for the frequent association of these two problems is that dysfunction of the cerebellum contributes to ataxia, but it also is part of the broader motor network responsible for dystonia (see Chapter 23, "The Neuroanatomical Substrates of Dystonia").[13,39,50,54] Also, genes that cause ataxia or dystonia have overlapping biological functions involving neural development or neurotransmitter function.[52] For example, in a large exome sequencing study involving 1,100 individuals with different types of dystonia, 21% of cases had pathological genetic variants in genes found in ataxia panels rather than dystonia panels.[20]

There are many ways in which ataxia and dystonia may be combined. Ataxia and dystonia may manifest at the same time or sequentially over time. Ataxia and dystonia may affect the same body region, or each may occur in a different body region. Ataxia and dystonia may be equally severe, or one may be the dominant problem. Disorders that combine ataxia and dystonia can be grouped into several overlapping categories. The first category includes disorders where dystonia and ataxia often occur simultaneously as expected features, although one or the other problem may be more prominent. The second category includes disorders where ataxia is usually the defining problem but some individuals may also have minor coexisting dystonia. In this group, individuals may rarely have dystonia rather than ataxia as the main problem. The last category includes disorders with highly variable phenotypes in which ataxia or dystonia or both combined may occur in association with numerous other problems.

This chapter covers the most relevant syndromes with a focus on the most frequent (Table 14.2) and/or treatable disorders. The disorders are grouped by biological commonalities, although these mechanisms may overlap.

Table 14.1 **Signs of cerebellar dysfunction**

Sign	Description
Oculomotor abnormalities	The most specific features are saccadic hypermetria (overshooting the target when making a rapid eye movement) and nystagmus; other common features include hypometria and broken smooth pursuit
Dysarthria	Unclear speech, often with impaired prosody that is "scanning" (lack of prosody) or "explosive" (irregular prosody)
Dysmetria	Impaired distancing expressed as hypermetria (overshooting a target or past-pointing) or hypometria (undershooting a target)
Dysrhythmia	Impaired timing of a simple repetitive one-joint movement
Dysdiadochokinesis	Impaired timing of more complicated multi-joint movements
Tremor	The most characteristic tremor is the intention tremor, which worsens in amplitude as the limb comes closer to its target
Rebound	Difficulties in curbing a sudden movement
Titubation	A coarse tremor of the head and/or trunk
Gait ataxia	Difficulty walking characterized by a broad stance, irregular stepping in both orthogonal and lateral planes, difficulty with toe-heel-tandem walking, and often falling
Truncal ataxia	Unstable trunk, evident when walking or sitting
Hypotonia	Reduced muscle tone

GENETIC CAUSES OF DYSTONIA AND ATAXIA

Disorders of DNA Repair and Related Diseases

More than 100 genetic disorders are capable of causing dystonia and ataxia, and the number keeps expanding.[58] Each of these disorders is rare. Several disorders due to gene variants that affect DNA repair have a combination of ataxia and dystonia, often with additional neurological signs such as other movement disorders, neuropathy, or corticospinal signs. An interesting clinical sign particularly frequent in this group of disorders is *oculomotor apraxia*, difficulty with initiating voluntary saccades when reflexive saccades are relatively preserved. To overcome this problem, affected individuals tend to initiate eye movements first with a *head thrust*, which is a rapid movement of the head that facilitates redirection of the eyes. Long latency and hypometric saccades can also result in a dissociation of head and eye movements, evident as the eyes lagging behind head movements and catching up to their target late.

Ataxia telangiectasia, due to autosomal recessive pathogenic variants in the *ATM* gene, is a classical example and the most frequent cause of the syndrome of ataxia and oculomotor apraxia, accounting for approximately one-third of all cases. Ataxia telangiectasia provides an example in which ataxia is usually the defining characteristic, but many individuals may also have some dystonia.[43] In rare cases, dystonia may be the dominant feature, and sometimes dystonia occurs without the ataxia.[3,11,16,31,41,45,49,62,71] Other examples that combine ataxia with oculomotor apraxia include ataxia with oculomotor apraxia type 1 (autosomal recessive variants in *APTX*), type 2 (autosomal recessive variants in *SETX*), and type 4 (autosomal recessive variants in *PNKP)*.[1] Other rarer causes are ataxia-telangiectasia–like types 1 and 2, ataxia with oculomotor apraxia type 3 (autosomal recessive variants in *PIK3R5*) and type 5 (autosomal recessive variants in *XRCC1*), and xeroderma pigmentosum (autosomal recessive variants in *THIIF*).[2,17,56] Focal or generalized dystonia may occasionally occur in any of these disorders.

All these disorders manifest typically in childhood, but onset in adulthood is possible, too. Brain MRI usually shows cerebellar atrophy, and lab abnormalities are common including elevated alpha fetoprotein (*ATM* and *SETX*), low albumin (*APTX* and *PNKP*), low immunoglobulins (IgG or IgA), CD4/CD8 deficiency (*ATM*), high cholesterol (*APTX*), or elevated creatine kinase (*SETX* and *PNKP*).[56] All these conditions are progressive, but there are wide variations in rate of worsening and level of disability. While there are currently no specific treatments targeting disease

Table 14.2 **More common genetic dystonia–ataxia disorders**

Biological category	Gene	Typical onset			Associated features
		Infancy	Childhood/adolescence	Adulthood	
DNA repair and related diseases					
Ataxia-telangiectasia	*ATM*		■	■	Telangiectasias, oculomotor apraxia, chorea, peripheral neuropathy, cerebellar atrophy
Ataxia-oculomotor apraxia types 1-5	*APTX, SETX, PNKP*		■	■	Oculomotor apraxia, chorea, peripheral neuropathy, cerebellar atrophy
Ataxia-telangiectasia-like types 1-2	*MRE11A, PCNA*		■	■	Oculomotor apraxia, chorea, peripheral neuropathy, cerebellar atrophy
Xeroderma pigmentosum	*THIIF*		■	■	Oculomotor apraxia, chorea, peripheral neuropathy, skin lesions, cerebellar atrophy
Transportopathies and channelopathies					
Glucose transporter type 1 deficiency syndrome	*SLC2A1*	■	■		Global delay, migraine, alternating hemiplegia, spasticity, chorea, epilepsy; exercise-induced or persistent dystonia, fasting-induced symptoms
ATP1A3-related disorders	*ATP1A3*	■	■	■	Migraine, episodic ataxia or hemiplegia, paroxysmal dyskinesias epilepsy, cognitive impairment, rapid-onset or episodic worsening with physical or psychological stress
CACNA1A-related disorders	*CACNA1A*	■	■	■	Epilepsy, developmental delay, paroxysmal torticollis of infancy, paroxysmal tonic upward gaze; episodic ataxia
Neurometabolic disorders					
L-2-hydroxyglutaric aciduria	*L2HGDH*	■	■	■	Acute encephalopathic crises triggered by metabolic stress, macrocephaly
Abetalipoproteinemia	*MTTP*	■	■		Failure to thrive in infancy, diarrhoea, vomiting, acanthocytosis, anemia, hemolysis, retinitis pigmentosa, neuropathy, cognitive impairment
Niemann-Pick disease type C	*NPC1, NPC2*	■	■	■	Vertical gaze palsy, hepatomegaly or splenomegaly, cognitive decline, psychiatric problems, epilepsy
Gaucher disease, type III	*GBA*		■	■	Developmental delay, cognitive decline, horizontal gaze palsy, parkinsonism epilepsy, organomegaly, cytopenia

Continued

Table 14.2 **(cont.)**

Biological category	Gene	Typical onset			Associated features
		Infancy	Childhood/ adolescence	Adulthood	
Mitochondrial disorders					
Mitochondrial complex I and complex III deficiency (multiple genes), other mitochondrial disorders (due to genomic rearrangements, mitochondrial DNA depletion syndrome)	many	■	■	■	Stroke-like episodes, epilepsy, spasticity, dementia, optic atrophy, deafness, myopathy, polyneuropathy, short stature, diabetes, cardiomyopathy, other systemic manifestations.
POLG-related disorders	*POLG*		■	■	Prominent gaze palsies
Friedreich ataxia	*FXN*		■	■	Square wave jerks, head titubation, neuropathy, pes cavus, scoliosis
Disorders of brain metal accumulation					
Wilson disease	*ATP7B*		■	■	Parkinsonism, tremor, cognitive decline, psychiatric symptoms, Kayser-Fleischer ring, sunflower cataract, liver disease
PLA2G6-associated neurodegeneration	*PLA2G6*	■	■	■	Corticospinal signs, cognitive decline, optic atrophy, cerebellar atrophy and white matter disease
Other neurodegenerative disorders					
Spinocerebellar ataxias	Many		■	■	Spasticity, oculomotor disturbance, neuropathy, parkinsonism, myoclonus
SQSTIM1-related neurodegeneration	*SQSTIM1*		■		Vertical gaze palsy, cognitive decline
Hypomyelination with atrophy of the basal ganglia and the cerebellum	*TUBB4A*	■	■		Spasticity, dysarthria and dysphagia

mechanisms, the diagnosis has important implications for management. Because the underlying genetic defects impair DNA repair, affected individuals have a higher risk of malignancies. Hence, appropriate surveillance and avoidance of radiation (X-rays, CT) is warranted.

Transportopathies and Channelopathies

In some disorders where ataxia is combined with dystonia, the underlying mechanism is dysfunction of transporters or ion channels. One important transportopathy is glucose transporter 1 deficiency syndrome (also called GLUT1 deficiency syndrome) due to autosomal dominant variants in the *SLC2A1* gene. This disorder provides an example in which there is a broad spectrum of abnormalities. The manifestations may involve various combinations of epilepsy, developmental delay, cognitive impairment, microcephaly, migraine, alternating hemiplegia, spasticity, ataxia, dystonia, and chorea.[32,53] Ataxia may be constant, progressive, or episodic. Dystonia may be focal or generalized, constant or paroxysmal and sometimes triggered by exercise. Onset is typically in childhood, but atypical phenotypes with milder or later manifestations are well recognized. Low cerebrospinal fluid (CSF) glucose (<60 mg/dL) corroborates the diagnosis, which also can be verified by the identification of a heterozygous pathogenic variant in the *SLC2A1* gene. An early diagnosis facilitates early treatment, which consists of avoiding triggers associated with low glucose (fasting, exercise), use of a ketogenic diet, or triheptanoin (see Chapter 28, "Symptom-Targeted Oral Medications for Dystonia").[35,47] Early treatment is thought to provide better long-term outcomes. A similar clinical picture that includes low CSF glucose can rarely occur also with other variants in other genes.[60]

Dystonia and ataxia can also be seen with pathogenic variants in *ATP1A3*, the gene encoding the alpha-3 subunit of the sodium/potassium-ATPase transmembrane ion pump. This pump is exclusively expressed in neurons of various brain regions, including the basal ganglia, hippocampus, and cerebellum. This is another disorder with remarkably varied phenotypes. In one large review of 1,018 cases, approximately half had ataxia, dystonia, or both.[72] The classic *ATP1A3*-related syndromes include rapid-onset dystonia parkinsonism (see Chapter 13, "Dystonia and Parkinsonism"), which may sometimes emerge more slowly, or it may feature mostly dystonia or mostly parkinsonism. Other classical syndromes include alternating hemiplegia of childhood, CAPOS syndrome (cerebellar ataxia, areflexia, pes cavus, optic atrophy, and sensorineural hearing loss), RECA syndrome (relapsing encephalopathy with cerebellar ataxia), and developmental and epileptic encephalopathy.[72] Additional features that are frequently encountered are cognitive impairment and microcephaly. The phenotypic spectrum continues to expand, with many overlapping syndromes that do not fit originally defined clinical categories. Clues to the diagnosis include paroxysmal events or rapid-onset or episodic worsening (often with incomplete remission) with stress. The stress can be psychological (e.g., excessive noise or crowds), but it may also be physical and include environmental stressors (e.g., excessive heat or cold), strenuous exercise, illness and fever, lack of sleep, or alcohol binging. The management of *ATP1A3*-related disease includes avoidance of these triggers. Flunarizine can prevent episodes of worsening, along with topiramate, the ketogenic diet, and regular sleep. Symptomatic treatments for dystonia that were reported to be beneficial in some cases were benzodiazepines, levodopa, and dopamine agonists. The response to deep brain stimulation seems consistently poor (see Chapter 31, "Surgical Treatments for Dystonia").

Another example of a channelopathy with a very varied phenotype includes disorders related to the calcium channel subunit gene *CACNA1A*, which shows an autosomal-dominant pattern of inheritance.[37] The classic syndromes linked to *CACNA1A* include spinocerebellar ataxia type 6 (usually due to expansion of a triplet repeat), familial hemiplegic migraine (usually due to missense gain-of-function mutations), or episodic ataxia type 2 (usually due to variants causing a loss-of-function). However, these syndromes may overlap, and numerous additional phenotypes have been described, including migraine without hemiplegia, recurrent hemiplegia without migraine, various forms of epilepsy with or without encephalopathy, developmental delay, early-onset ataxia, paroxysmal tonic upgaze, and others. The recent literature suggests more of a continuum of mixed phenotypes rather than discrete syndromes.[37] Focal or generalized dystonia may occur along with these other features, and it may be relatively constant or paroxysmal.

Patients with episodic ataxia might also have dystonia during an ataxic episode. There are also reports of individuals presenting with episodic ataxia who developed persistent cervical dystonia or who first noted limb or cervical dystonia before ataxia became apparent.[25,65,66] Rarely, dystonia may be the main feature. For example, *CACNA1A* variants have been associated with adult-onset focal dystonia, early-onset paroxysmal dystonia, and paroxysmal torticollis of infancy.[33,36,37] Interestingly, *CACNA1A* is also associated with marked phenotypic heterogeneity in mice with dystonia or ataxia or both, which may be relatively constant or paroxysmal.[63] While treatment with acetazolamide or 4-aminopyridine may be effective in reducing the frequency and severity of episodic ataxia, the treatment of choice for *CACNA1A*-related dystonia is less clear. The response to acetazolamide varies, and some individuals responded to clonazepam or carbamazepine. Given that *CACNA1A*-related dystonia is often focal or segmental, treatment with botulinum toxin is also an option.

Neurometabolic Diseases

Inborn errors of metabolism encompass a group of disorders which, due to genetic defects, result in deficiency in a metabolic pathway that causes accumulation of a toxic substance or a reduced ability to produce an essential compound. There are more than 1,000 inborn errors, and most present in childhood.[22,23] However, later onset in adulthood and milder phenotypes that are missed until adulthood are increasingly recognized and relevant for adult neurologists as well. These heterogeneous and usually multisystem diseases manifest with systemic and neurological signs. Approximately 30% include some type of movement disorder.[21] Ataxia is the most common, followed by dystonia.[24,30] Additional clues for the diagnosis include a history of acute exacerbation in the setting of a catabolic state (precipitated by febrile illness, fasting, or physical exhaustion) or worsening after high-protein intake. Early diagnosis is important because some of these disorders can be treated (see Chapter 28).[38]

A classic example is glutaric aciduria type 1, an autosomal recessive disorder caused by deficiency of glutaryl-CoA dehydrogenase, an enzyme involved in the catabolism of lysine and tryptophan. Typically, a sudden encephalopathic crisis with acute striatal necrosis can be precipitated in childhood by febrile reactions to infection or vaccination, surgery, or some other metabolic stress.[15,67] The striatal damage results in dystonia, sometimes with ataxia, chorea, and cognitive-behavioral changes.[28] Milder phenotypes have been reported with adult onset, and some cases develop symptoms without any apparent metabolic crisis. Ideally, the disorder is diagnosed before symptoms develop, and neonatal screening is routinely conducted in a growing number of countries. However, neonatal screening is not conducted in all countries, and neurologists might have to make the diagnosis in those who have traveled from one of these countries. Prevention of crises is important and consists of a low-lysine diet, carnitine supplementation, and intensified supportive care during catabolic periods of metabolic stress. Treatment after symptom onset is less effective. After age 6 years, the dietary regimen is often relaxed, but individuals should be followed at centers specialized in metabolic disorders for late decompensations.

Both avoidance of triggers as well as dietary intervention also play a major role in GLUT1 deficiency syndrome, as outlined above. Dietary interventions are also key in abetalipoproteinemia, an autosomal recessive disorder due to variants in microsomal triglyceride transfer protein (*MTTP*). This disorder typically presents in infancy with failure to thrive, diarrhea, vomiting, and fat malabsorption. Malabsorption of fat-soluble vitamins (A, D, E, and K) can result in impaired blood clotting. Furthermore, the blood may show acanthocytosis, anemia, and hemolysis with hyperbilirubinemia. If not treated with dietary fat restriction and supplementation of vitamins A and E, the disorder will progress, and affected individuals are likely to develop retinitis pigmentosa and eventually blindness, neuropathy, sensory and cerebellar ataxia, dystonia, and cognitive impairment.[69]

Niemann Pick type C is an autosomal-recessively inherited lysosomal storage disorder associated with defects in intracellular cholesterol trafficking. Ataxia and dystonia are the most frequent movement disorders. A tell-tale sign is a vertical supranuclear gaze palsy, which can precede other neurological manifestations. Other frequent findings are neonatal icterus, deafness, hepatomegaly or splenomegaly, cognitive decline or psychiatric problems, epilepsy, and gelastic cataplexy. The clinical spectrum is very broad. Some individuals develop severe and life-threatening complications in early childhood, while others manifest a more slowly progressive disorder beginning later in childhood and even as late as 50 years of age.[75] N-butyl-deoxynojirimycin (Miglustat) is a synthetic glucose analog that inhibits glycosylceramide synthase, the enzyme responsible for the first step in the synthesis of glycosphingolipids that accumulate in lysosomes. Hence, the treatment reduces lysosomal storage products and results in a slower progression of the disease.[61]

The combination of dystonia and ataxia is less common in Gaucher disease type 3, where there is also cognitive decline, seizures, and a horizontal gaze palsy. Due to biallelic pathogenic variants in the gene encoding glucocerebrosidase (*GBA*), glucocerebrosides accumulate throughout the body, especially within the bone marrow, spleen, and liver. Individuals with Gaucher disease may also benefit from treatment with Miglustat.

Mitochondrial Disorders

The mitochondrial disorders encompass a large group of disorders with the pathophysiological commonality that mitochondrial function is impaired either through pathological gene variants in the nuclear or the mitochondrial genome (primary mitochondriopathies) or due to exogenous factors (secondary mitochondriopathies). More than 350 genes can affect mitochondria and cause disease. Because of the ubiquitous presence of mitochondria and their important role as powerhouses of all cells, multisystem disease is common.

The genetic mitochondrial disorders have a broad clinical spectrum ranging from severe, infantile-onset multisystem disease to relatively mild and oligosymptomatic presentations in adulthood only.[51] Central nervous system signs and symptoms encompass stroke-like episodes, epilepsy, corticospinal signs, and dementia. Movement disorders, including ataxia and dystonia, are common.[27,40,44] The eyes can be affected by cataracts, pigmentary retinopathy, and optic atrophy. Deafness is a red flag for mitochondrial disease. The peripheral nervous system can be compromised by myopathy or polyneuropathy. Signs of endocrinopathy are short stature, diabetes, hypogonadism, amenorrhea, and delayed puberty. Involvement of the heart (cardiomyopathy, heart failure, conduction abnormalities) can be life-threatening. Further manifestations may involve the gastrointestinal system (dysphagia, vomiting, diarrhea, hepatopathy, pseudo-obstruction) and kidneys (renal failure, cysts). Brain imaging may show leukoencephalopathy, basal ganglia hyperintensities, atrophy or calcifications.[48] Blood and CSF may show elevated lactate levels. The diagnosis is best secured with genetic testing. Depending on the phenotype and family history, some genes may be more likely to harbor the causative variant, but there is much phenotypic overlap and a huge number of potentially relevant genes.

One disorder that is not classically considered a mitochondrial disorder but that shares some biological features is Friedreich ataxia. It is an autosomal-recessive trinucleotide repeat disorder of the *FXN* gene, which results in a lack of frataxin, a small mitochondrial protein. It is the most common autosomal-recessive ataxia, with an estimated prevalence of 3 per 100,000. Onset is mostly in adolescence, but ranges from early childhood to manifestation in the sixth decade of life. Characteristic skeletal deformities are pes cavus and scoliosis. Affected individuals also suffer from cardiomyopathy and diabetes. The core neurological phenotype consists of cerebellar and sensory ataxia (often with ocular square wave jerks and head titubation) with neuropathy and an extensor plantar reflex. Dystonia may sometimes be also part of the picture, even though it is rarely the most prominent or troublesome symptom.[6,59]

Disorders of Brain Metal Accumulation

A number of disorders that share the hallmark feature of brain metal accumulation typically present with dystonia combined with parkinsonism but may sometimes instead manifest with dystonia and ataxia. Examples include Wilson disease[9] and *PLA2G6*-associated neurodegeneration.[19,74] The diagnosis may be suspected when brain MRI reveals evidence for metal accumulation, usually in the basal ganglia and cerebellum (see Chapter 13).

Other Genetic Neurodegenerative Disorders

Dystonia and ataxia, often associated with other features, are common in several of the spinocerebellar ataxias.[58] This is a large group of heterogeneous disorders, where neurodegeneration mainly affects the cerebellum. More than 40 subtypes have been identified, and many are due to repeat expansions in different genes (trinucleotide, pentanucleotide, or hexanucleotide). Although ataxia is the defining characteristic for this group of disorders, there is a very broad phenotypic spectrum, with either isolated ataxia or ataxia combined with corticospinal signs, dystonia, parkinsonism, myoclonus, oculomotor disturbances, neuropathy, and/or dementia. As expected for such a large group of diseases, onset and natural history are variable, but the most common presentations begin gradually in adulthood (20–80 years of age) with slow progression over many years.

Ataxia is combined with dystonia most commonly for genetic variants in *ATXN1* (also called SCA1), *ATXN2* (also called SCA2), *ATXN3* (also called SCA3), and *CACNA1A* (discussed above, with one allelic variant called SCA6). Sometimes dystonia may be the dominant feature, and occasionally ataxia is absent. Hypometric and slow saccades are suggestive of *ATXN2,* while ophthalmoparesis seems to be more common with *ATXN3*, and both may also feature neuropathy, as does *ATXN1.* The spectrum of dystonia in these conditions is very broad, including focal, segmental, hemi-, or generalized. Dystonia may be task-specific, episodic, or paroxysmal.[58]

In contrast to the above disorders, *SQSTIM1*-related neurodegeneration starts in childhood and has a characteristic phenotype of dystonia, ataxia, vertical gaze palsy, and cognitive decline. It is a relatively rare disorder. The protein encoded by *SQSTIM1* plays an important role in autophagy, an essential mechanism for removing abnormal proteins that may lead to neurodegeneration.

Hypomyelination with atrophy of the basal ganglia and cerebellum (HABC) is another childhood-onset disorder with progressive corticospinal signs, ataxia, dystonia, and marked dysarthria and dysphagia. The acronym HABC summarizes the distinct brain MRI features, and the diagnosis can be made by testing for pathogenic variants in the *TUBB4A* gene.[64] Interestingly, isolated dystonia (typically with prominent laryngeal involvement) may also occur. Genetic variants causing HABC destabilize microtubules, leading to impaired oligodendrocyte development, resulting in hypomyelination. On the other hand, variants responsible for the isolated dystonia phenotype appear to affect mainly postmitotic oligodendrocytes, where disturbed subsequent arborization and myelination might alter signal transduction.[42]

IDIOPATHIC NEURODEGENERATIVE CAUSES OF DYSTONIA AND ATAXIA

Multiple system atrophy (MSA) is an idiopathic, neurodegenerative disorder defined pathologically by accumulation of alpha synuclein aggregates in oligodendrocytes.[73] Onset is typically in the fifth decade, though rare cases have manifested as early as their thirties. The disease is progressive, with a survival time of approximately 6–9 years. Clinically it is characterized by parkinsonism, cerebellar signs, and/or signs of autonomic dysfunction such as orthostatic hypotension, erectile dysfunction, or urinary incontinence. MSA can be subdivided into MSA-P (parkinsonism-predominant) and MSA-C (cerebellar-predominant). Dystonia occurs in 20–30% of cases with MSA, most often the MSA-P subtype.[12,29,46,57,76] The dystonia of MSA has some characteristic features that may include prominent anterocollis or retrocollis, laryngeal dystonia, prominent orofacial involvement, or triggering of orofacial dystonia with levodopa (see Chapter 13).

The pattern of dystonia is somewhat different in progressive supranuclear palsy (PSP), a sporadic tauopathy that manifests typically in the seventh decade of life but may rarely occur much earlier.[14] A vertical supranuclear gaze palsy combined with parkinsonism and early postural instability are frequent defining features. Dystonia is common in PSP and encompasses frontalis overactivity leading to a fixed look of surprise; blepharospasm, often with apraxia of eyelid opening; anterocollis or retrocollis; or limb dystonia.[10,29,57,76] The clinical picture of dystonia and ataxia may be suggested by a gait with prominent instability and falling ("drunken sailor gait"). Moreover, there is a rare PSP subtype in which ataxia is more prominent than parkinsonism (PSP-C).

AUTOIMMUNE CAUSES OF DYSTONIA AND ATAXIA

Autoimmune causes of dystonia-ataxia are even rarer than genetic causes, but, as treatable disorders, they should not be missed (see Chapter 21, "Dystonia and Autoimmunity").[7] Encephalitis with antibodies directed to the N-methyl-D-aspartic acid (NMDA) glutamate receptor is a disease that affects mainly children and young adults (95% of cases are younger than 45 years). It is much more frequent in females (~80%) than males.[18,68] It may be paraneoplastic (associated with ovarian teratoma), idiopathic, or triggered by a preceding herpes simplex virus encephalitis. Dystonia with ataxia is not a classic presentation, but both can be seen, particularly in children.[70] Indeed, children present more often with movement disorders than do adults, and the picture is often a complex combination of various movement disorders (dystonia, chorea, stereotypies), behavioral disorders (catatonia, tonic or clonic perseveration), seizures, cognitive changes, and/or psychosis. The combination of symptoms should point to the diagnosis. Antibody testing (serum and CSF) can confirm clinical suspicion, but in clear cases immunotherapy should not be delayed by waiting for test results as early treatment has a better prognosis.

In adults, the antibody spectrum is very different.[68] Paraneoplastic cases are much more frequent. Ri-antibodies are associated with a characteristic brainstem syndrome that combines cerebellar ataxia and a jaw-opening dystonia, often with an underlying cancer (mostly lung or ovarian). Stiff person spectrum disorders can mimic axial or limb dystonia and also may have ataxia, particularly if associated with antibodies to glutamic acid decarboxylase.[4,5,6] Last, ataxia, sometimes combined with dystonia and other neurological features, can be seen with IgLON5-antibodies. These antibodies target a neuronal surface protein and seem to induce a tauopathy with a slowly progressive disease over years.[70] Cardinal features are sleep-related (movement disorders, sleep–wake cycle disturbance), respiratory (hypoventilation, stridor requiring tracheostomy), bulbar (dysphagia, dysarthria, vocal cord paresis) and oculomotor (gaze palsies, ptosis) problems. The spectrum of other neurological symptoms is very broad, including dementia, parkinsonism, chorea, motor neuron disease, and others (see Chapter 21).

DIAGNOSIS AND TREATMENT

Approach to Diagnosis

The main approach to the diagnosis of ataxia-dystonia syndromes is to carefully assess the history and exam for a syndromic pattern that might provide clues to the diagnosis.[58] One of the first steps is to consider the onset and progression of disease. Most of the inherited and idiopathic conditions begin insidiously and progress slowly. A subacute onset with rapid progression provides a clue for an autoimmune, metabolic, or acquired cause.

For the many genetic disorders that may combine dystonia and ataxia, the approach is different for children (Figure 14.1) versus adults (Figure 14.2) because the major conditions to consider are different. In either case, MRI is useful because it can disclose features that narrow the differential diagnosis. Many of these conditions may be uncovered by next-generation sequencing that involves broad ataxia panels or clinical exome sequencing. However, many of these disorders involve repeat expansions, which are not readily picked up using next-generation methods and may require additional testing.

Treatment

For dystonia-ataxia syndromes, the dystonia may respond to symptomatic oral medications (see Chapter 28) or the botulinum toxins (see Chapter 30, "Botulinum Toxin Treatment for Dystonia"). These interventions do not address the ataxia, which is treated with largely supportive strategies, including physiotherapy and occupational therapy. However, several dystonia-ataxia syndromes have specific interventions that may have a dramatic impact on the disorder (Table 14.3).

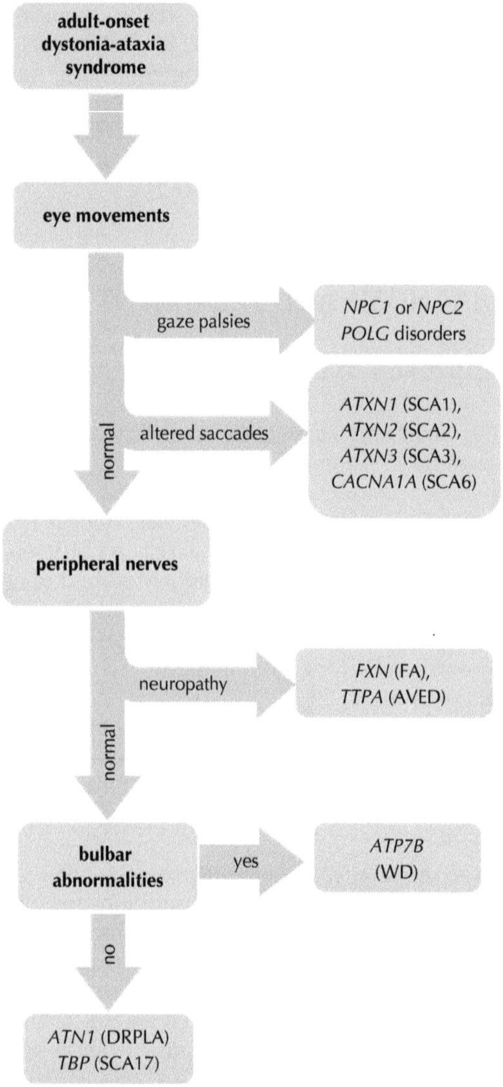

Figure 14.1. Algorithm for assessment of adult-onset syndromes that combine dystonia and ataxia. This schematic provides only a general approach for diagnosis, as exceptions may exist. Gene symbols (italics) and abbreviations: ATN1, dentatorubro-pallidalluysian atrophy (DRPLA); ATP7B, Wilson disease (WD): ATXN1, spinocerebellar ataxia type 1 (SCA1); ATXN2, spinocerebellar ataxia type 2 (SCA2); ATXN3, spinocerebellar ataxia type 3 (SCA3); FXN, Freidreich ataxia (FA); POLG, polymerase gamma; NPC1-2 (Niemann-Pick type C); TBP, TATA box binding protein, spinocerebellar ataxia type 17 (SCA17). TTPA, ataxia with vitamin E deficiency (AVED).

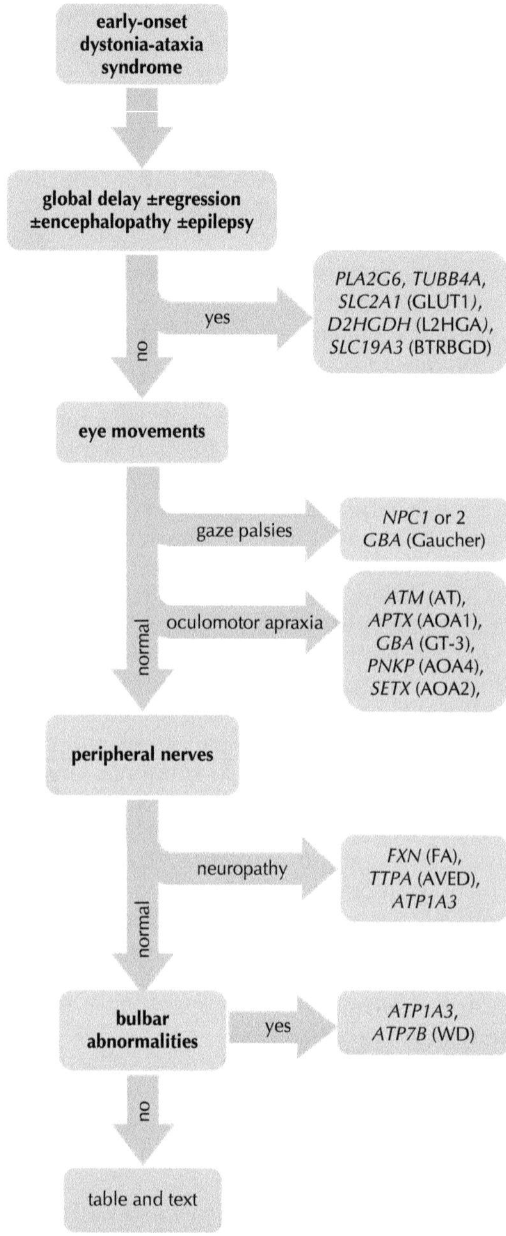

Figure 14.2. Algorithm for assessment of childhood-onset syndromes that combine dystonia and ataxia. This schematic provides only a general approach for diagnosis as exceptions may exist. Gene symbols (italics) and abbreviations: APTX, ataxia with ocular motor apraxia type 1 (AOA1); ATM, ataxia telangiectasia (AT); ATP7B, Wilson disease (WD); D2HGDH, L-2 hydroxy glutaric aciduria (L2HGA); FXN, Freidreich ataxia (FA); GBA, Gaucher disease type 3 (GT-3); NPC1-2, Niemann-Pick type C: PLA2G6, PLA2G6–associated neurodegeneration (PLAN); PNKP, ataxia with ocular motor apraxia type 4 (AOA4); SETX, ataxia with ocular motor apraxia type 2 (AOA2); SLC19A3, biotin-thiamin–responsive basal ganglia disease (BTRBGD); SLC2A1 (Glut1 deficiency syndromes); TTPA, ataxia with vitamin E deficiency (AVED).

Table 14.3 **Dystonia-ataxia syndromes with specific interventions**

Disease	Gene	Additional clinical features	Treatment
Ataxia with vitamin E deficiency	*TTPA*	Neuropathy, visual impairment	Vitamin E
Biotin-thiamine responsive basal ganglia disease	*SLC19A3*	Encephalopathy (often triggered by metabolic decompensation), psychomotor retardation, behavioural disorders, parkinsonism, spasticity, seizures	Biotin plus thiamine, avoid or treat triggers
Biotinidase deficiency	*BTD*	Developmental delay, corticospinal signs, seizures, visual and auditory impairment, skin changes	Biotin
Cerebral creatine deficiency	*GAMT, AGAT*	Developmental delay, chorea, epilepsy, behavioral deficits, myopathy	Creatine ± ornithine and dietary restriction of arginine
Cerebral folate deficiency	*FL1, SLC46A1*	Developmental delay, spasticity, seizures, psychiatric impairment	Folinic acid
Cerebrotendinous xanthomatosis	*CYP27A*	Spasticity, parkinsonism, myoclonus, tendon xanthomas, cataracts, neuropathy, seizures, cognitive impairment	Chenodeoxycholic acid
Cobalamin deficiency	multiple genes	Developmental delay, spasticity, encephalopathy, seizures (often triggered by metabolic decompensation)	Cobalamin derivates
Coenzyme Q10 deficiency	multiple genes	Parkinsonism, spasticity, seizures, intellectual disability, autonomic failure, deafness, optic atrophy, cardiac or renal involvement	Coenzyme Q10
Maple syrup urine disease	*BCKDHA, BCKDHB, DBT*	Developmental delay, episodic encephalopathy (often triggered by metabolic decompensation)	Avoid or treat triggers; dietary leucine restriction
Pyruvate dehydrogenase deficiency	*PDHA1, DLAT*	Developmental delay, encephalopathy, seizures	Thiamine, ketogenic diet, triheptanoin

SUMMARY AND FUTURE PROSPECTS

Even though they are rare, the large number of conditions that can cause the syndrome of dystonia with ataxia make it relevant in clinical practice. The frequent combination of dystonia and ataxia may be related to the role of the cerebellum in both of these movement disorders.

When evaluating patients with dystonia and ataxia, the differential diagnosis can be largely guided by the age of onset, additional neurological or systemic features, radiological findings, and other relevant studies. For some of these conditions, there are specific management implications in addition to the general symptomatic treatment for dystonia and physiotherapy for cerebellar ataxia. These treatments can have a large potential clinical impact if they are instituted early. As more is learned about the biological mechanisms responsible for ataxia and dystonia, it is likely that additional targeted therapeutics will be developed.

REFERENCES

1. Anheim M, Monga B, Fleury M, Charles P, Barbot C, Salih M, et al. Ataxia with oculomotor apraxia type 2: Clinical, biological and genotype/phenotype correlation study of a cohort of 90 patients. Brain 2009;132:2688–2698.
2. Anttinen A, Koulu L, Nikoskelainen E, Portin R, Kurki T, Erkinjuntti M, et al. Neurological symptoms and natural course of xeroderma pigmentosum. Brain 2008;131:1979–1989.

3. Arican P, Dundar NO, Kirbiyik O, Cavusoglu D, Yilmaz SB, Gencpinar P. Variant ataxia-telangiectasia in a child presenting with laryngeal dystonia. Turk J Pediatr 2020;62:491–494.
4. Balint B, Mahant N, Meinck HM, Fung V. Stiff limb syndrome mimicking corticobasal syndrome. Mov Disord Clin Pract 2014;1:354–356.
5. Balint B, Meinck HM. Pragmatic treatment of stiff person spectrum disorders. Mov Disord Clin Pract 2018;5:394–401.
6. Balint B, Meinck HM, Bhatia KP. Axial dystonia mimicking stiff person syndrome. Mov Disord Clin Pract 2016;3:176–179.
7. Balint B, Vincent A, Meinck HM, Irani SR, Bhatia KP. Movement disorders with neuronal antibodies: Syndromic approach, genetic parallels and pathophysiology. Brain 2018;141:13–36.
8. Bally JF, Camargos S, Oliveira Dos Santos C, Kern DS, Lee T, et al. DYT-TUBB4A (DYT4 Dystonia): New clinical and genetic observations. Neurology 2021;96:e1887–e1897.
9. Bandmann O, Weiss KH, Kaler SG. Wilson's disease and other neurological copper disorders. Lancet Neurol 2015;14:103–113.
10. Barclay CL, Lang AE. Dystonia in progressive supranuclear palsy. J Neurol Neurosurg Psychiatry 1997;62:352–356.
11. Bodensteiner JB, Goldblum RM, Goldman AS. Progressive dystonia masking ataxia in ataxia-telangiectasia. Arch Neurol 1980;37:464–465.
12. Boesch SM, Wenning GK, Ransmayr G, Poewe W. Dystonia in multiple system atrophy. J Neurol Neurosurg Psychiatry 2002;72:300–303.
13. Bologna M, Berardelli A. Cerebellum: An explanation for dystonia? Cerebellum Ataxias 2017;4:6.
14. Boxer AL, Yu JT, Golbe LI, Litvan I, Lang AE, Hoglinger GU. Advances in progressive supranuclear palsy: New diagnostic criteria, biomarkers, and therapeutic approaches. Lancet Neurol 2017;16:552–563.
15. Boy N, Mühlhausen C, Maier EM, Heringer J, Assmann B, Burgard P, et al. Proposed recommendations for diagnosing and managing individuals with glutaric aciduria type I: Second revision. J Inherit Metab Dis 2017;40:75–101.
16. Charlesworth G, Mohire MD, Schneider SA, Stamelou M, Wood NW, Bhatia KP. Ataxia telangiectasia presenting as dopa-responsive cervical dystonia. Neurology 2013;81:1148–1151.
17. da Costa SCG, de Rezende-Filho FC, de Freitas JL, de Assis Pereira Matos PCA, Della-Ripa B, Franca MC, Jr., et al. Clinical and genetic characterization of Brazilian patients with ataxia and oculomotor apraxia. Mov Disord 2022;37:1309–1316.
18. Dalmau J, Armangue T, Planaguma J, Radosevic M, Mannara F, Leypoldt F, et al. An update on anti-NMDA receptor encephalitis for neurologists and psychiatrists: Mechanisms and models. Lancet Neurol 2019;18:1045–1057.
19. Di Meo I, Tiranti V. Classification and molecular pathogenesis of NBIA syndromes. Eur J Paediatr Neurol 2018;22:272–284.
20. Dzinovic I, Boesch S, Skorvanek M, Necpal J, Svantnerova J, Pavelekova P, et al. Genetic overlap between dystonia and other neurologic disorders: A study of 1,100 exomes. Parkinsonism Relat Disord 2022;102:1–6.
21. Ferreira CR, Hoffmann GF, Blau N. Clinical and biochemical footprints of inherited metabolic diseases. I. Movement disorders. Mol Genet Metab 2019;127:28–30.
22. Ferreira CR, van Karnebeek CDM, Vockley J, Blau N. A proposed nosology of inborn errors of metabolism. Genet Med 2019;21:102–106.
23. Ferreira CR, Rahman S, Keller M, Zschocke J, Group IA. An international classification of inherited metabolic disorders (ICIMD). J Inherit Metab Dis 2021;44:164–177.
24. Garcia-Cazorla A, Wolf NI, Serrano M, Perez-Duenas B, Pineda M, Campistol J, et al. Inborn errors of metabolism and motor disturbances in children. J Inherit Metab Dis 2009;32:618–629.
25. Garcin B, Villain N, Mesrati F, Naccache L, Roze E, Degos B. A single-center series of 482 patients with functional motor disorders. J Psychosom Res 2021;148:110565.
26. Gelener P, Severino M, Diker S, Teralı K, Tuncel G, Tuzlalı H, et al. Adult-onset glutaric aciduria type I: Rare presentation of a treatable disorder. Neurogenetics 2020;21:179–186.
27. Ghaoui R, Sue CM. Movement disorders in mitochondrial disease. J Neurol 2018;265:1230–1240.
28. Gitiaux C, Roze E, Kinugawa K, Flamand-Rouviere C, Boddaert N, Apartis E, et al. Spectrum of movement disorders associated with glutaric aciduria type 1: A study of 16 patients. Mov Disord 2008;23:2392–2397.
29. Godeiro-Junior C, Felicio AC, Barsottini OG, Aguiar PM, Silva SM, Borges V, Ferraz HB. Clinical features of dystonia in atypical parkinsonism. Arq Neuropsiquiatr 2008;66:800–804.
30. Gouider-Khouja N, Kraoua I, Benrhouma H, Fraj N, Rouissi A. Movement disorders in neuro-metabolic diseases. Eur J Paediatr Neurol 2010;14:304–307.
31. Goyal V, Behari M. Dystonia as presenting manifestation of ataxia telangiectasia: A case report. Neurol India 2002;50:187–189.
32. Gras D, Roze E, Caillet S, Meneret A, Doummar D, Billette de Villemeur T, et al. GLUT1 deficiency syndrome: An update. Rev Neurol (Paris) 2014;170:91–99.
33. Gur-Hartman T, Berkowitz O, Yosovich K, Roubertie A, Zanni G, Macaya A, et al. Clinical phenotypes of infantile onset CACNA1A-related disorder. Eur J Paediatr Neurol 2021;30:144–154.
34. Haack TB, Ignatius E, Calvo-Garrido J, Iuso A, Isohanni P, Maffezzini C, et al. Absence of the autophagy adaptor SQSTM1/p62 causes childhood-onset neurodegeneration with ataxia, dystonia, and gaze palsy. Am J Hum Genet 2016;99:735–743.
35. Hainque E, Gras D, Meneret A, Atencio M, Luton MP, Barbier M, et al. Long-term follow-up in an open-label trial of triheptanoin in GLUT1 deficiency syndrome: A sustained dramatic effect. J Neurol Neurosurg Psychiatry 2019;90:1291–1293.
36. Hess EJ, Jen JC, Jinnah HA. Neuronal voltage-gated calcium channels: Brief overview of their function and clinical implications in neurology. Neurology 2010;75:937–938.
37. Indelicato E, Boesch S. From genotype to phenotype: Expanding the clinical spectrum of CACNA1A variants in the era of next generation sequencing. Front Neurol 2021;12:639994.
38. Jinnah HA, Albanese A, Bhatia KP, Cardoso F, Da Prat G, de Koning TJ, et al. Treatable inherited rare movement disorders. Mov Disord 2018;33:21–35.
39. Jinnah HA, Neychev V, Hess EJ. The anatomical basis for dystonia: The motor network model. Tremor Other Hyperkinet Mov 2017;7:506.
40. Jinnah HA, Sun YV. Dystonia genes and their biological pathways. Neurobiol Dis 2019;129:159–168.
41. Kim M, Kim AR, Park J, Kim JS, Ahn JH, Park WY, et al. Clinical characteristics of ataxia-telangiectasia

presenting dystonia as a main manifestation. Clin Neurol Neurosurg 2020;199:106267.
42. Krajka V, Vulinovic F, Genova M, Tanzer K, Jijumon AS, Bodakuntla S, et al. H-ABC- and dystonia-causing TUBB4A mutations show distinct pathogenic effects. Sci Adv 2022;8:eabj9229.
43. Levy A, Lang AE. Ataxia-telangiectasia: A review of movement disorders, clinical features and genotype correlations – Addendum. Mov Disord 2018;33:1238–1247.
44. Martikainen MH, Ng YS, Gorman GS, Alston CL, Blakely EL, Schaefer AM, et al. Clinical, genetic, and radiological features of extrapyramidal movement disorders in mitochondrial disease. JAMA Neurol 2016;73:668–674.
45. Meneret A, Ahmar-Beaugendre Y, Rieunier G, Mahlaoui N, Gaymard B, Apartis E, et al. The pleiotropic movement disorders phenotype of adult ataxia-telangiectasia. Neurology 2014;83:1087–1095.
46. Merlo IM, Occhini A, Pacchetti C, Alfonsi E. Not paralysis, but dystonia causes stridor in multiple system atrophy. Neurology 2002;58:649–652.
47. Mochel F, Hainque E, Gras D, Adanyeguh IM, Caillet S, Heron B, et al. Triheptanoin dramatically reduces paroxysmal motor disorder in patients with GLUT1 deficiency. J Neurol Neurosurg Psychiatry 2016;87:550–553.
48. Mohammad SS, Angiti RR, Biggin A, Morales-Briceno H, Goetti R, Perez-Duenas B, et al. Magnetic resonance imaging pattern recognition in childhood bilateral basal ganglia disorders. Brain Commun 2020;2:fcaa178.
49. Necpal J, Zech M, Skorvanek M, Havrankova P, Fecikova A, Winkelmann J, Jech R. Ataxia telangiectasia gene mutation in isolated segmental dystonia without ataxia and telangiectasia. Mov Disord Clin Pract 2018;5:89–91.
50. Neychev VK, Gross R, Lehericy S, Hess EJ, Jinnah HA. The functional neuroanatomy of dystonia. Neurobiol Dis 2011;42:185–201.
51. Ng YS, Bindoff LA, Gorman GS, Klopstock T, Kornblum C, Mancuso M, et al. Mitochondrial disease in adults: Recent advances and future promise. Lancet Neurol 2021;20:573–584.
52. Nibbeling EA, Delnooz CC, de Koning TJ, Sinke RJ, Jinnah HA, Tijssen MA, Verbeek DS. Using the shared genetics of dystonia and ataxia to unravel their pathogenesis. Neurosci Biobehav Rev 2017;75:22–39.
53. Pearson TS, Akman C, Hinton VJ, Engelstad K, De Vivo DC. Phenotypic spectrum of glucose transporter type 1 deficiency syndrome (Glut1 DS). Curr Neurol Neurosci Rep 2013;13:342.
54. Prudente CN, Hess EJ, Jinnah HA. Dystonia as a network disorder: What is the role of the cerebellum? Neuroscience 2014;260:23–35.
55. Rascol O, Fox S, Gasparini P, Kenney C, Di Paolo T, Gomez-Mancilla B. Use of metabotropic glutamate 5 receptor antagonists for treatment of levodopa-induced dyskinesias. Parkinsonism Rel Disord 2014;2014:947–956.
56. Renaud M, Tranchant C, Koenig M, Anheim M. Autosomal recessive cerebellar ataxias with elevated alpha-fetoprotein: Uncommon diseases, common biomarker. Mov Disord 2020;35:2139–2149.
57. Rivest J, Quinn N, Marsden CD. Dystonia in Parkinson's disease, multiple system atrophy, and progressive supranuclear palsy. Neurology 1990;40:1571–1578.
58. Rossi M, Balint B, Millar Vernetti P, Bhatia KP, Merello M. Genetic dystonia-ataxia syndromes: Clinical spectrum, diagnostic approach, and treatment options. Mov Disord Clin Pract 2018;5:373–382.
59. Rota S, Marchina E, Todeschini A, Nanetti L, Rinaldi F, Vanotti A, et al. Very late-onset friedreich ataxia with laryngeal dystonia. Case Rep Neurol 2014;6:287–290.
60. Sanchez-Lijarcio O, Yubero D, Leal F, Couce ML, Gonzalez Gutierrez-Solana L, Lopez-Laso E, et al. The clinical and biochemical hallmarks generally associated with GLUT1DS may be caused by defects in genes other than SLC2A1. Clin Genet 2022;102:40–55.
61. Santos-Lozano A, Villamandos Garcia D, Sanchis-Gomar F, Fiuza-Luces C, Pareja-Galeano H, Garatachea N, et al. Niemann-Pick disease treatment: A systematic review of clinical trials. Ann Transl Med 2015;3:360.
62. Saunders-Pullman R, Raymond D, Stoessl AJ, Hobson D, Nakamura T, Pullman S, et al. Variant ataxia-telangiectasia presenting as primary-appearing dystonia in Canadian Mennonites. Neurology 2012;78:649–657.
63. Shirley TL, Rao LM, Hess EJ, Jinnah HA. Paroxysmal dyskinesias in mice. Mov Disord 2008;23:259–264.
64. Simons C, Wolf NI, McNeil N, Caldovic L, Devaney JM, Takanohashi A, et al. A de novo mutation in the β-tubulin gene TUBB4A results in the leukoencephalopathy hypomyelination with atrophy of the basal ganglia and cerebellum. Am J Hum Genet 2013;92:767–773.
65. Spacey SD, Materek LA, Szczygielski BI, Bird TD. Two novel CACNA1A gene mutations associated with episodic ataxia type 2 and interictal dystonia. Arch Neurol 2005;62:314–316.
66. Stampfl B, Fee D. Novel mutation in CACNA1A associated with activity-induced dystonia, cervical dystonia, and mild ataxia. Case Rep Neurol Med 2021;2021.
67. Strauss KA, Williams KB, Carson VJ, Poskitt L, Bowser LE, Young M, et al. Glutaric acidemia type 1: Treatment and outcome of 168 patients over three decades. Mol Genet Metab 2020;131:325–340.
68. Sturchio A, Dwivedi AK, Gastaldi M, Grimberg MB, Businaro P, Duque KR, et al. Movement disorders associated with neuronal antibodies: A data-driven approach. J Neurol 2022;269:3511–3521.
69. Takahashi M, Okazaki H, Ohashi K, Ogura M, Ishibashi S, Okazaki S, et al. Current diagnosis and management of abetalipoproteinemia. J Atheroscler Thromb 2021;28:1009–1019.
70. Varley JA, Webb AJS, Balint B, Fung VSC, Sethi KD, Tijssen MAJ, et al. The movement disorder associated with NMDAR antibody-encephalitis is complex and characteristic: An expert video-rating study. J Neurol Neurosurg Psychiatry 2019;90:724–726.
71. Verhagen MM, Abdo WF, Willemsen MA, Hogervorst FB, Smeets DF, Hiel JA, et al. Clinical spectrum of ataxia-telangiectasia in adulthood. Neurology 2009;73:430–437.
72. Vezyroglou A, Akilapa R, Barwick K, Koene S, Brownstein CA, Holder-Espinasse M, et al. The phenotypic continuum of ATP1A3-related disorders. Neurology 2022;99:e1511–e1526.
73. Wenning GK, Tison F, Ben Shlomo Y, Daniel SE, Quinn NP. Multiple system atrophy: A review of 203 pathologically proven cases. Mov Disord 1997;12:133–147.
74. Wiethoff S, Houlden H. Neurodegeneration with brain iron accumulation. Handb Clin Neurol 2017;145:157–166.
75. Wu M, Ceponiene R, Bayram E, Litvan I. Two patients with Niemann Pick disease type C diagnosed in the seventh decade of life. Mov Disord Clin Pract 2020;7:961–964.
76. Yoon WT. Comparison of dystonia between Parkinson's disease and atypical parkinsonism: The clinical usefulness of dystonia distribution and characteristics in the differential diagnosis of parkinsonism. Neurol Neurochir Pol 2018;52:48–53.

Chapter 15

Dystonia and Myoclonus

INTRODUCTION

The term *myoclonus* describes sudden, brief, shock-like jerks.[13,66] Among normal individuals, examples of *physiological myoclonus* include hiccups or hypnic jerks. Myoclonus can also be pathological. Myoclonus may be the single or most prominent manifestation of certain disorders. Alternatively, myoclonus may be combined with other signs or symptoms, such as dystonia.

The combination of myoclonus with dystonia, or *myoclonus-dystonia syndrome*, is a relatively distinct, albeit rare, syndrome. The myoclonus-dystonia syndrome has a limited number of causes, many of which are genetic. For these conditions, the differential diagnosis is guided by the distribution of myoclonus and dystonia, accompanying clinical features, and age at onset. Apart from the syndromes dominated by myoclonus and dystonia, there is another group of syndromes which manifest myoclonus and dystonia along with other symptoms or signs. For these conditions, other features are often more prominent.

In addition to clinical syndromes in which myoclonus and dystonia may be combined, there is a related condition, *myoclonic dystonia*. Dystonia itself may sometimes be jerky, with jerks coming in isolation or in semi-rhythmical trains resembling a tremor (see Chapter 12, "Dystonia and Tremor"). These jerky movements may be the dominant manifestation of dystonia, and the term *myoclonic dystonia* is sometimes used to describe them.

This chapter begins with a description of myoclonus itself. The main focus is on syndromes where myoclonus is combined with dystonia. Also included is a brief summary of how dystonic jerks resembling myoclonus (myoclonic dystonia) can be discriminated from true myoclonus.

MYOCLONUS

Myoclonus is clinically defined by movements that are brief, sudden, and shock-like.[13,66] In more common language, myoclonus is a movement described as a *jerk*. The jerks of myoclonus may be caused by a sudden muscle contraction (*positive myoclonus*) or a sudden brief loss of muscle tone (*negative myoclonus*) as seen in asterixis.

There are many types of myoclonus, which can be classified in many ways (Table 15.1). Myoclonus is clinically classified according to the main body area affected (proximal, distal), distribution of body areas affected (focal, segmental, multifocal, generalized), or inducing factors (spontaneous, on action, stimulus-sensitive or reflex myoclonus, and orthostatic). Myoclonus

Table 15.1 **Categories of myoclonus**

Category	Subtypes
Body distribution	Focal Segmental Multifocal Generalized
Etiology	Physiological Epileptic Symptomatic Psychogenic Essential
Inducing factor	Spontaneous Action-induced Stimulus-sensitive Orthostatic
Neuroanatomical source	Cortical Subcortical Brainstem Spinal cord Peripheral nerve

can also be classified by etiology as physiological (occurring in normal individuals), essential (myoclonus is the only problem), epileptic (associated with epilepsy), symptomatic (from a known or presumed cause), or psychogenic (functional). Another classification approach considers the neuroanatomical origin of myoclonus as cortical, subcortical, brainstem, spinal, or peripheral.

Sudden jerks are not always myoclonus.[6,46] Sudden jerks are typical of startle syndromes and may be triggered by auditory, somatosensory, or visual sensory stimuli. Sudden jerks may also reflect tics, with some common examples being sudden jerks of the head, quick shoulder shrugs, or brief twitches of the face. Jerky movements are not uncommon among individuals with psychogenic (functional) disorders, as described in Chapter 25, "Psychogenic (Functional) Dystonia." Sudden jerks can also be a manifestation of dystonia. These movements are sometimes called *myoclonic dystonia*, as described further below.

Electrophysiological investigations can aid in the discrimination of myoclonus from other types of jerks, and they can point to potential etiologies or neuroanatomical origins.[36] Electromyography (EMG) is useful to establish whether myoclonic jerks are positive or negative, and whether they are stimulus sensitive. EMG is also useful to establish the duration of jerks. Bursts of 50–75 msec or shorter are generally seen in cortical myoclonus, while longer bursts of 250 msec are seen in subcortical myoclonus. Electroencephalography (EEG) can be useful to detect associated epileptic discharges from the cerebral cortex in myoclonic epilepsy. Sometimes there is a clear association between epileptiform discharges and jerks. At other times, the technique of back-averaging, where jerks are time-locked to cortical discharges is needed to obtain a clear signal. Other features typical of cortical myoclonus include giant somatosensory evoked potentials and an enhanced C-reflex, a long-loop reflex mediated by the sensorimotor cortex. A slow rising potential called the *Bereitschaftspotential* (pre-movement potential) is indicative of a psychogenic jerk.

GENETIC CAUSES OF MYOCLONUS-DYSTONIA

SGCE

The most frequent cause of the myoclonus-dystonia syndrome is related to pathogenic genetic variants in *SGCE*.[12,42] Heterozygous loss-of-function variants in *SGCE* are found in 20–50% of cases with the myoclonus-dystonia syndrome. More than 100 different pathogenic variants have been described, including missense mutations, nonsense mutations, small insertions or deletions, and larger deletions affecting one or more exons.

Inheritance is autosomal dominant, but penetrance is determined by the parent of origin.[52] Paternal inheritance is nearly always penetrant, while maternal inheritance is usually not penetrant. The complex pattern of inheritance results from imprinting of the maternal allele, resulting in it being silenced. This imprinting can make identification of patterns of inheritance challenging. Indeed, a family history may be lacking because of multiple skipped generations. For example, a mother may pass a pathological allele to a son, who will not manifest symptoms. Yet this son may then pass the allele to his son, who will be affected. The disorder has been reported from all regions of the globe, with an estimated prevalence of about 2 per million in Europe.[5]

Myoclonus-dystonia relating to *SGCE* typically manifests in childhood (mean age of onset 6 years, range 1 year through adulthood). Myoclonus is the most prominent feature of the condition. Myoclonic movements are distinct, very brief, or lightning-like in appearance. Myoclonus characteristically involves the upper part of the body (neck, trunk, limb), and proximal more than distal muscles. More rarely, myoclonus might affect face, larynx, or lower limbs. It is typically most prominent on action and posture, and movements can be aggravated by stress. On the other hand, myoclonus can be suppressed by alcohol. Clinical and electrophysiological features suggest that the myoclonus associated with *SGCE* is of subcortical origin.[36,39,57]

Myoclonus may be the only problem with *SGCE*, and then the condition is called *essential myoclonus*. Dystonia is a frequent but variable feature (Figure 15.1). Dystonia may be very subtle, but it can be severe and disabling. Rarely, dystonia occurs without myoclonus. Dystonia most frequently affects the neck or the hands (often as writer's cramp in children), but it can also involve the craniofacial regions. Affected children often have dystonia in the lower limbs. Interestingly, lower limb dystonia emerging in children commonly abates or disappears spontaneously over time.[51] Tremor of the upper limbs may be an additional feature in some individuals.[42]

Apart from the distinctive motor symptoms, the non-motor features of this condition merit special mention. Psychiatric disturbances occur in approximately 65% of cases and include anxiety-related disorders such as specific phobias (33%) or social phobia (31%) and obsessive-compulsive disorder (21%).[47,48] Carriers of a pathogenic *SGCE* variant are 10-12 times more likely than normal individuals to have obsessive-compulsive disorder or social phobia. In addition, alcohol abuse is common and estimated to affect

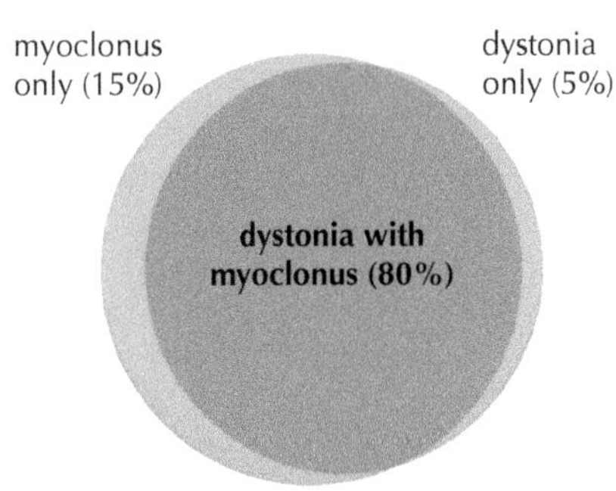

Figure 15.1. Overlap of myoclonus and dystonia associated with the *SGCE* gene. This schematic was prepared from data for 281 individuals in the MDSgene database. Most individuals have varying degrees of both myoclonus and dystonia, although a small proportion has only one of these problems.

31% of cases.[47,48] This problem may be related to observations that myoclonus tends to be alcohol-sensitive, leading to self-medication.[30,68]

The pathogenesis of abnormal movements and psychiatric features in *SGCE*-related myoclonus-dystonia syndrome is not well-understood. The gene encodes a member of the sarcoglycan family, epsilon. These sarcoglycans are components of the dystrophin-glycoprotein complex, which link the actin cytoskeleton to the extracellular matrix in muscle. Most sarcoglycans are expressed predominantly in muscle, but the epsilon member is broadly expressed, including the brain. Within the brain, there are particularly high levels in the cerebellum, especially in Purkinje neurons and neurons of the dentate nucleus.[54] Brain-exclusive isoforms are enriched in presynaptic and postsynaptic membranes, suggesting a role in synaptic function.[54,60]

The pathophysiological correlate for myoclonus and its alcohol responsiveness likely lies in alterations of cerebello-thalamic pathway activity, possibly related to a gamma aminobutyric acid (GABA)ergic deficit affecting Purkinje neuron dysfunction.[68] Accordingly, deep brain stimulation of the thalamic receiving zone of the thalamus (ventral intermediate nucleus) modulates myoclonus.[73] While *SGCE*-related myoclonus was classically considered subcortical, recent research described increased intrinsic excitability of cortical glutamatergic neurons, highlighting the fact that regions other than the cerebellum are likely to be involved.[60]

There are several treatments for *SGCE*-related myoclonus-dystonia that are at least partly effective. Apart from the usual symptomatic treatments for dystonia (see Chapter 28, "Symptom-Targeted Oral Medications for Dystonia"), abnormal movements may respond to clonazepam or zonisamide.[29] There are also case reports describing success with tetrabenazine,[37] carbamazepine, and perampanel.[9] Among severe and medically refractory cases, improvements in both dystonia and myoclonus have also been achieved with deep brain stimulation of the internal pallidum[3,33] or thalamus.[43,73]

KCTD17

The *SGCE* gene is the most common gene responsible for the myoclonus-dystonia syndrome, but other genes have also been described (Table 15.2). Pathogenic variants in *KCTD17*

Table 15.2 **Genes implicated in myoclonus–dystonia syndromes**

Gene	Typical age at onset	Features of dystonia	Features of myoclonus	Additional clinical clues
ADCY5	Childhood	Usually mixed with other movements; isolated dystonia is rare	Usually mixed with other movements; isolated myoclonus is rare	Chorea, hypotonia, ataxia, facial twitching, marked waxing-waning of symptoms, persist during sleep, developmental delay
ANO3	Young adult	Often cranio-cervical distribution, and very jerky	Jerky dystonia difficult to discriminate from myoclonus	Action-induced, tremor
ATM	Childhood	May occur in isolation but more commonly mixed with other movements	Not usually particularly prominent	Ataxia, chorea, ocular telangiectasias, association with malignancy
ATP1A3	Childhood	Rapid-onset following physical or psychological stress	Other problems usually more prominent	Rapid-onset, often with parkinsonism
CACNA1B	Childhood	Cervical and axial distribution	High frequency leg myoclonus on standing, alcohol responsive	Cardiac arrhythmia, painful cramps, anxiety
CAMTA1	Childhood	Cervical	Stimulus-sensitive	Intellectual disability
GCH1	Childhood or young adult	Dystonia > myoclonus, dopa-responsive	Dystonia > myoclonus	Parkinsonism
GNAL	Childhood	Neck, larynx, upper limbs	Alcohol-responsive	Tremor
GNB1	Childhood	Generalized	High amplitude myoclonus	Global delay, hypotonia, limited up-gaze, ocd
KCNN2	Childhood	Myoclonus > dystonia	Myoclonus > dystonia	Fast upper limb tremor, facial twitching, cerebellar signs, anxiety
KCTD17	Childhood	Often cranio-cervical with upper limb distribution, progressive	Myoclonus usually earlier and worse than dystonia	Anxiety, depression, ocd
PRKCG	Childhood	Cervical and truncal distribution	Generalized	Progressive cerebellar signs
RELN	Childhood	Distribution affects neck, trunk, upper limbs	Neck, trunk, upper limbs	Anxiety, depression, exaggerated startle
SGCE	Childhood or young adult	Cervical and upper limb distribution	Action-induced, alcohol-responsive	Anxiety, depression, ocd, tremor
TH	Infancy	Severe and generalized with severe spasms; sometimes levodopa-responsive	Generalized myoclonus	Infantile encephalopathy, hypotonia, oculogyric crises
TITF	Childhood	Myoclonus > dystonia	Myoclonus > dystonia	Chorea usually comes first
TTPA	Childhood	Cervical and axial distribution	Mostly limbs	Sensory deficits, cerebellar signs
TUBB2B	Adolescence	Cranio-cervical distribution	Upper body	Global delay, epilepsy, adhd
VPS16	Childhood	Generalized	Upper limbs	Worse with anxiety
YY1	Childhood	Other problems usually more prominent	Other problems usually more prominent	Global delay, dysmorphism

This table summarizes the clinical features of disorders that may be associated with myoclonus and dystonia, some reported as single unconfirmed cases.

Abbreviations: ADHD, attention-deficit hyperactivity disorder; OCD, obsessive-compulsive disorder.

also are rare causes of the myoclonus-dystonia syndrome.[38,40] The disorder may be sporadic or inherited in an autosomal dominant manner. In contrast to *SGCE*-related myoclonus-dystonia, the myoclonus is milder and less disabling. Also unlike *SGCE*, dystonia associated with *KCTD17* is progressive and often functionally very disabling. The psychiatric comorbidities that are characteristic of *SGCE*-related myoclonus dystonia are uncommon with *KCTD17*-related myoclonus-dystonia. However, the clinical spectrum may not yet be fully appreciated because only small numbers of cases have been reported.

KCNN2

Pathogenic variants in *KCCN2* have been reported in a family with autosomal-dominant, early-onset dystonia predominantly affecting the neck and hands, and a fast tremor with superimposed myoclonus and, in some individuals, subtle cerebellar signs.[8] Subsequent reports confirmed the gene as a relevant cause of myoclonus-dystonia syndrome and expanded the clinical spectrum to encompass more complex neurodevelopmental disorders.[19,34,44]

Other Genes Sometimes Causing Myoclonus-Dystonia Syndrome

Some disorders may occasionally manifest with myoclonus and dystonia, although other clinical features are usually more common. One of these is the Silver-Russell syndrome, which is characterized by growth retardation, body asymmetry, macrocephaly with prominent forehead, and feeding difficulties. Other common but less consistent features include micrognathia with crowded teeth, triangular face, clinodactyly of the fifth finger, hypoglycemia, and developmental delay. It is genetically heterogeneous, but a handful of cases have been reported with genomic abnormalities that span a large region of chromosome 7 that include *SGCE*. Most of these cases have resulted from maternal uniparental disomy affecting portions of chromosome 7, where both copies of the gene were inherited from the mother, and the copy from the father is missing. Some cases have had the myoclonus-dystonia syndrome, with reports of cases with only myoclonus or focal dystonia, too.

Another condition in this category involves pathogenic variants in *TITF1* (also known as *NKX2-1*), which is more commonly associated with benign hereditary chorea or the brain-thyroid-lung syndrome.[4,7,32] Another involves pathogenic variants in *ADCY5*, which is more typically associated with a complex phenotype with multiple abnormal movements, most notably chorea (see Chapter 17, "Dystonia and the Paroxysmal Dyskinesias"). However, some cases may present with a phenotype resembling myoclonus-dystonia syndrome.[1,11,16] Genetic variants in *TH* are most commonly associated with a developmental encephalopathy, but occasionally with dopa-responsive dystonia and rarely with a phenotype resembling the myoclonus-dystonia syndrome.[63] Ataxia-telangiectasia due to pathogenic variants in *ATM* are classically associated with a mixed movement disorder that usually includes ataxia. However, occasional patients present instead with a phenotype dominated by dystonia or chorea, and rarely the myoclonus-dystonia syndrome.[20] Isolated reports have described phenotypes resembling myoclonus-dystonia with pathogenic variants in a number of other genes such as *ATP1A3*,[70] *CACNA1B*,[26] *CAMTA1*,[17] *GCH1*,[35] *RELN*,[27] and *YY1*.[14]

Because these conditions are very rare, additional studies may be needed to confirm how often these genes are associated with the myoclonus-dystonia syndrome. For many of these disorders, it may be difficult to discriminate true myoclonus from the rapid jerks sometimes associated with chorea or dystonia. For example, the movements of benign hereditary chorea often include a mixture of very fast small movements and slower larger movements, and the phenotype can be difficult to discriminate from myoclonus-dystonia.[4] The same challenge holds for jerky dystonic movements sometimes called myoclonic dystonia (see below).

Other Genes Causing Complex Phenotypes That May Include Myoclonus and Dystonia

Myoclonus and dystonia may be combined with a plethora of other signs and symptoms in a large number of other syndromes. Included are metabolic disorders, mitochondrial disease, storage disorders, and others. In most of these conditions, features other than myoclonus and dystonia are more prominent and therefore play a more important role in diagnosis (see Chapter 18, "Dystonias Combined with Other Features"). Most can be diagnosed by identifying syndromic patterns with a careful history and exam, together with laboratory findings (bloodwork, urine, MRI).

NON-GENETIC CAUSES OF MYOCLONUS-DYSTONIA

Acquired Syndromes

Myoclonus and dystonia are not uncommon in certain encephalopathies caused by infection. One example is subacute sclerosing panencephalitis, a chronic measles infection causing a lethal encephalopathy with characteristic rhythmic, hung-up jerks.[21]

Myoclonus and dystonia may also be seen with several post-infectious syndromes presumably resulting from autoimmune processes, such as acute disseminated encephalomyelitis[58] and steroid-responsive autoimmune encephalopathy associated with autoimmune thyroiditis.[56] For most of these conditions, myoclonus and dystonia may be accompanying features, but a severe encephalopathy is usually the main problem.

Idiopathic Syndromes

Among adults, the most common examples in which myoclonus and dystonia may be combined with other features include degenerative parkinsonian conditions (see Chapter 13, "Dystonia and Parkinsonism"). Stimulus-sensitive myoclonus and dystonia of one limb are not uncommon in corticobasal syndrome.[25,55,61,67,72] Cervical dystonia (particularly anterocollis) and stimulus-sensitive myoclonus may occur in multiple system atrophy.[10,25,55,69,72] Myoclonus with dystonia of a limb or the neck may rarely occur in progressive supranuclear palsy.[25,55,72] For all of these conditions, dystonia and myoclonus are not usually the most prominent features.

MYOCLONIC DYSTONIA

There has been widespread agreement on the usage of certain terms such as *myoclonus* or *dystonia*, as well as *myoclonus-dystonia syndrome* when both coexist. The term *myoclonic dystonia* also appears in the literature to refer dystonic movements that have a very jerky quality.[18,45,50,51] These jerky movements may occur in adult-onset focal dystonia as well as early-onset genetic dystonias.

One series of 14 cases reported as myoclonic dystonia described jerks occurring in isolation or in trains resembling tremor.[45] However, the jerks tended to be less brisk than true myoclonus. Additionally, they occurred in the same body region as dystonia, often when the individual's dystonia worsened by moving the dystonic body part away from its most comfortable (null) position. In contrast, myoclonic jerks and dystonia in the myoclonus-dystonia syndromes often occur independently in separate body regions.

It is important to emphasize that the jerks of myoclonic dystonia are dystonic jerks that mimic myoclonus, rather than true myoclonic jerks. It can sometimes be difficult to distinguish dystonic jerks from myoclonic jerks clinically. However, dystonic jerks often appear less abrupt on exam, and EMG usually reveals a longer duration than typical myoclonic jerks. Physiological measures are sometimes required to discriminate these types of jerks, although in some cases dystonic jerks and myoclonic jerks may coexist, for example in association with genetic variants in *ANO3* or *GNAL*.[15,62,71]

The value of the term *myoclonic dystonia* has been questioned,[50,51] and its use probably should be avoided. The term is too easily confused with the closely related term *myoclonus-dystonia*, and both terms are sometimes used interchangeably,[22,49,71] even though they refer to different conditions. It also causes confusion among patients and non-specialist clinical providers, who are not sure if the problem is myoclonus, dystonia, or both combined as in myoclonus-dystonia. The term *jerky dystonia* may be preferable over myoclonic dystonia.

DIAGNOSIS AND TREATMENT

Approach to Diagnosis

The recognition and differential diagnosis of syndromes that combine dystonia and myoclonus relies on recognizing a syndromic pattern from a careful history and exam.[42] Key features include age at onset, manner of progression, and whether there are associated findings. Most inherited or degenerative disorders begin insidiously and progress slowly. A subacute onset or rapid progression raises suspicion for an autoimmune or acquired cause.

When a genetic disorder is suspected, it is useful to know that the *SGCE* gene is the most common, accounting for up to 50% of cases. It may therefore be reasonable to begin with single-gene testing. Deletions and insertions are not uncommon, so gene dosage analyses, such as multiple ligation-dependent probe amplification, are an important part of *SGCE* testing.[42] Beyond *SGCE*, there are many other potential genes, so broader panels or clinical exome sequencing may be required.

Treatment

For myoclonus-syndromes, the dystonia may respond to symptomatic oral medications (see Chapter 28) or the botulinum toxins (see Chapter 30, "Botulinum Toxin Treatment for Dystonia"). One double-blind placebo-controlled trial reported success with zonisamine[29] and some reports have described success with carbamazepine, perampanel, or tetrabenazine.[2,9,37] However, experience is limited. The inherited myoclonus-dystonia syndromes also respond well to deep brain stimulation surgery (see Chapter 31, "Surgical Treatments for Dystonia").

SYNOPSIS AND FUTURE PROSPECTS

Myoclonus and dystonia are distinct movement disorders, but they may coexist. Syndromes that are dominated by the combination of myoclonus and dystonia are most commonly genetic, the most frequent involving genetic variants in *SGCE*. An even broader list of genes may include a combination of myoclonus, dystonia, and other neurological and medical features. However, the other clinical features are usually more prominent for these conditions. Knowledge of the syndromic patterns associated with these conditions facilitates diagnosis and workup. Identifying the cause is important because some have specific interventions.

The number of genes associated with the combination of myoclonus and dystonia continues to grow. In addition, the phenotypic spectrum linked with genes already known to cause the combination of myoclonus and dystonia continues to grow. Additionally, a number of non-genetic causes are recognized. Our understanding of the pathogenesis of these disorders is still in its infancy, and additional treatments are likely to be forthcoming as more is learned.

REFERENCES

1. Agarwal PA, Ramprasad VL. Adult-onset myoclonus-dystonia syndrome preceding characteristic facial myoclonus in Indian ADCY5-related dyskinesia. Mov Disord Clin Pract 2019;6:267–268.
2. Aljabri MF, Kamal NM, Alghamdi A, Alghamdi H, Alomairi N. Favorable response to carbamazepine therapy in genetically proven myoclonus-dystonia child. Ital J Pediatr 2021;47:33.
3. Artusi CA, Dwivedi A, Romagnolo A, Bortolani S, Marsili L, Imbalzano G, et al. Differential response to pallidal deep brain stimulation among monogenic dystonias: Systematic review and meta-analysis. J Neurol Neurosurg Psychiatry 2020;91:426–433.
4. Asmus F, Devlin A, Munz M, Zimprich A, Gasser T, Chinnery PF. Clinical differentiation of genetically proven benign hereditary chorea and myoclonus-dystonia. Mov Disord 2007;22:2104–2109.
5. Asmus F, Gasser T. Dystonia-plus syndromes. Eur J Neurol 2010;17 Suppl 1:37–45.
6. Asmus F, Langseth A, Doherty E, Nestor T, Munz M, Gasser T, et al. "Jerky" dystonia in children: Spectrum of phenotypes and genetic testing. Mov Disord 2009;24:702–709.
7. Balicza P, Grosz Z, Molnar V, Illes A, Csaban D, Gezsi A, et al. NKX2-1 new mutation associated with myoclonus, dystonia, and pituitary involvement. Front Genet 2018;9:335.
8. Balint B, Guerreiro R, Carmona S, Dehghani N, Latorre A, Cordivari C, et al. KCNN2 mutation in autosomal-dominant tremulous myoclonus-dystonia. Eur J Neurol 2020;27:1471–1477.
9. Belli E, Del Prete E, Unti E, Mazzucchi S, Palermo G, Ceravolo R. Perampanel as a novel treatment for subcortical myoclonus in myoclonus-dystonia syndrome. Neurol Sci 2023;44:2943–2945.
10. Boesch SM, Wenning GK, Ransmayr G, Poewe W. Dystonia in multiple system atrophy. J Neurol Neurosurg Psychiatry 2002;72:300–303.
11. Bohlega SA, Abou-Al-Shaar H, AlDakheel A, Alajlan H, Bohlega BS, Meyer BF, et al. Autosomal recessive ADCY5-related dystonia and myoclonus: Expanding the genetic spectrum of ADCY5-related movement disorders. Parkinsonism Relat Disord 2019;64:145–149.
12. Carecchio M, Magliozzi M, Copetti M, Ferraris A, Bernardini L, Bonetti M, et al. Defining the epsilon-sarcoglycan (SGCE) gene phenotypic signature in myoclonus-dystonia: A reappraisal of genetic testing criteria. Mov Disord 2013;28:787–794.
13. Caviness JN. Myoclonus. Continuum 2019;25:1055–1080.

14. Chawla T, Kumar NK, Goyal V. Heterozygous YY1 mutation: A mimicker of SGCE-myoclonus-dystonia. Parkinsonism Relat Disord 2023:117:105846.
15. Di Luca DG, Grippe TC, Adams J, Chen R, Fasano A, Lozano A, Lang AE. Generalized dystonia with tremor and myoclonus associated with ANO3 variant. Can J Neurol Sci 2023:1–3. doi:10.1017/cjn.2023.282.
16. Douglas AG, Andreoletti G, Talbot K, Hammans SR, Singh J, Whitney A, et al. ADCY5-related dyskinesia presenting as familial myoclonus-dystonia. Neurogenetics 2017;18:111–117.
17. Dzinovic I, Serranova T, Prouteau C, Colin E, Ziegler A, Winkelmann J, et al. Myoclonic dystonia phenotype related to a novel calmodulin-binding transcription activator 1 sequence variant. Neurogenetics 2021;22:137–141.
18. Fahn S. The varied clinical expressions of dystonia. Neurol Clinics 1984;2:541–554.
19. Fearon C, Grippe TC, Chen R, Lang AE. Early-onset neurodevelopmental movement disorder secondary to novel mutation in KCNN2. Mov Disord Clin Pract 2022;9:S9–S12.
20. Ganguly J, Bernaola MT, Goobie S, Prasad A, Jog M. Myoclonus-dystonia presentation of ATM gene mutation in a Canadian mennonite. Mov Disord Clin Pract 2022;9:264–267.
21. Garg D, Kakkar V, Kumar A, Kapoor D, Abbey P, Pemde H, et al. Spectrum of movement disorders among children with subacute sclerosing panencephalitis: A cross-sectional study. J Child Neurol 2022;37:491–496.
22. Gazzina S, Alberici A, Padovani A, Borroni B. Myoclonic dystonia (DYT11) responsive to insulin therapy: A case report. Neurology 2017;89:517–518.
23. Geiger JT, Schindler AB, Blauwendraat C, Singer HS, Scholz SW. TUBB2B mutation in an adult patient with myoclonus-dystonia. Case Rep Neurol 2017;9:216–221.
24. Geoghegan AR, Al Hussona M, Beauchamp NJ, Hutchinson M, Sean O'Riordan MB, Lynch T, Webb D. A novel GNAL mutation in familial dystonia presenting with childhood tremor and myoclonus. Mov Disord 2019;34:923–924.
25. Godeiro-Junior C, Felicio AC, Barsottini OG, Aguiar PM, Silva SM, Borges V, Ferraz HB. Clinical features of dystonia in atypical parkinsonism. Arq Neuropsiquiatr 2008;66:800–804.
26. Groen JL, Andrade A, Ritz K, Jalalzadeh H, Haagmans M, Bradley TE, et al. CACNA1B mutation is linked to unique myoclonus-dystonia syndrome. Hum Mol Genet 2015;24:987–993.
27. Groen JL, Ritz K, Jalalzadeh H, van der Salm SM, Jongejan A, Mook OR, et al. RELN rare variants in myoclonus-dystonia. Mov Disord 2015;30:415–419.
28. Gu X, Lin J, Hou Y, Zhang L, Shang H. De novo missense mutation of VPS16 in a Chinese patient with generalized dystonia with myoclonus. Mov Disord Clin Pract 2022;9:551–552.
29. Hainque E, Vidailhet M, Cozic N, Charbonnier-Beaupel F, Thobois S, Tranchant C, et al. A randomized, controlled, double-blind, crossover trial of zonisamide in myoclonus-dystonia. Neurology 2016;86:1729–1735.
30. Hess CW, Raymond D, Aguiar Pde C, Frucht S, Shriberg J, Heiman GA, et al. Myoclonus-dystonia, obsessive-compulsive disorder, and alcohol dependence in SGCE mutation carriers. Neurology 2007;68:522–524.
31. Jones HF, Morales-Briceno H, Barwick K, Lewis J, Sanchis-Juan A, Raymond FL, et al. Myoclonus-dystonia caused by GNB1 mutation responsive to deep brain stimulation. Mov Disord 2019;34:1079–1080.
32. Koht J, Lostegaard SO, Wedding I, Vidailhet M, Louha M, Tallaksen CM. Benign hereditary chorea, not only chorea: A family case presentation. Cerebellum Ataxias 2016;3:3.
33. Kosutzka Z, Tisch S, Bonnet C, Ruiz M, Hainque E, Welter ML, et al. Long-term GPi-DBS improves motor features in myoclonus-dystonia and enhances social adjustment. Mov Disord 2019;34:87–94.
34. Lavenstein B, McGurrin P, Attaripour S, Vial F, Hallett M. KCNN2 mutation in pediatric temor myoclonus dystonia syndrome with electrophysiological evaluation. Tremor Other Hyperkinet Mov (N Y) 2022;12:2.
35. Leuzzi V, Carducci C, Carducci C, Cardona F, Artiola C, Antonozzi I. Autosomal dominant GTP-CH deficiency presenting as a dopa-responsive myoclonus-dystonia syndrome. Neurology 2002;59:1241–1243.
36. Li JY, Cunic DI, Paradiso G, Gunraj C, Pal PK, Lang AE, Chen R. Electrophysiological features of myoclonus-dystonia. Mov Disord 2008;23:2055–2061.
37. Luciano AY, Jinnah HA, Pfeiffer RF, Truong DD, Nance MA, LeDoux MS. Treatment of myoclonus-dystonia syndrome with tetrabenazine. Parkinsonism Relat Disord 2014;20:1423–1426.
38. Marce-Grau A, Correa M, Vanegas MI, Munoz-Ruiz T, Ferrer-Aparicio S, Baide H, et al. Childhood onset progressive myoclonic dystonia due to a de novo KCTD17 splicing mutation. Parkinsonism Relat Disord 2019;61:7–9.
39. Marelli C, Canafoglia L, Zibordi F, Ciano C, Visani E, Zorzi G, et al. A neurophysiological study of myoclonus in patients with DYT11 myoclonus-dystonia syndrome. Mov Disord 2008;23:2041–2048.
40. Mencacci NE, Rubio-Agusti I, Zdebik A, Asmus F, Ludtmann MH, Ryten M, et al. A missense mutation in KCTD17 causes autosomal dominant myoclonus-dystonia. Am J Hum Genet 2015;96:938–947.
41. Menon PJ, Nilles C, Silveira-Moriyama L, Yuan R, de Gusmao CM, Munchau A, et al. Scoping review on ADCY5-related movement disorders. Mov Disord Clin Pract 2023;10:1048–1059.
42. Menozzi E, Balint B, Latorre A, Valente EM, Rothwell JC, Bhatia KP. Twenty years on: Myoclonus-dystonia and epsilon-sarcoglycan: Neurodevelopment, channel, and signaling dysfunction. Mov Disord 2019;34:1588–1601.
43. Mercado-Pimentel R, Piedimonte F, Micheli F, Montilla-Uzcategui V, Barbosa N, Ramirez-Gomez C, Zuniga-Ramirez C. Successful unilateral surgical approach to internal globus pallidus and ventral intermediate nucleus of the thalamus in 3 cases of myoclonus-dystonia syndrome. Stereotact Funct Neurosurg 2021;99:250–255.
44. Mochel F, Rastetter A, Ceulemans B, Platzer K, Yang S, Shinde DN, et al. Variants in the SK2 channel gene (KCNN2) lead to dominant neurodevelopmental movement disorders. Brain 2020;143:3564–3573.
45. Obeso JA, Rothwell JC, Lang AE, Marsden CD. Myoclonic dystonia. Neurology 1983;33:825–830.
46. Park J, Reilaender A, Petry-Schmelzer JN, Stobe P, Cordts I, Harmuth F, et al. Transcript-specific loss-of-function

variants in VPS16 are enriched in patients with dystonia. Neurol Genet 2022;8:e644.
47. Peall KJ, Dijk JM, Saunders-Pullman R, Dreissen YE, van Loon I, Cath D, et al. Psychiatric disorders, myoclonus dystonia and SGCE: An international study. Ann Clin Transl Neurol 2016;3:4–11.
48. Peall KJ, Smith DJ, Kurian MA, Wardle M, Waite AJ, Hedderly T, et al. SGCE mutations cause psychiatric disorders: Clinical and genetic characterization. Brain 2013;136:294–303.
49. Pueschel SM, Friedman JH, Shetty T. Myoclonic dystonia. Childs Nerv Syst 1992;8:61–66.
50. Quinn NP. Essential myoclonus and myoclonic dystonia. Mov Disord 1996;11:119–124.
51. Quinn NP, Rothwell JC, Thompson PD, Marsden CD. Hereditary myoclonic dystonia, hereditary torsion dystonia and hereditary essential myoclonus: An area of confusion. Adv Neurol 1988;50:391–401.
52. Raymond D, Saunders-Pullman R, de Carvalho Aguiar P, Schule B, Kock N, Friedman J, et al. Phenotypic spectrum and sex effects in eleven myoclonus-dystonia families with epsilon-sarcoglycan mutations. Mov Disord 2008;23:588–592.
53. Reyes NGD, Di Luca DG, McNiven V, Lang AE. Dystonia with myoclonus and vertical supranuclear gaze palsy associated with a rare GNB1 variant. Parkinsonism Relat Disord 2023;106:105239.
54. Ritz K, van Schaik BD, Jakobs ME, van Kampen AH, Aronica E, Tijssen MA, Baas F. SGCE isoform characterization and expression in human brain: Implications for myoclonus-dystonia pathogenesis? Eur J Hum Genet 2011;19:438–444.
55. Rivest J, Quinn N, Marsden CD. Dystonia in Parkinson's disease, multiple system atrophy, and progressive supranuclear palsy. Neurology 1990;40:1571–1578.
56. Rozankovic PB, Rozankovic M, Susak I, Vlahovic I, Sporis D. Steroid-responsive autoimmune encephalopathy associated with autoimmune thyroiditis (SREAT) presenting with myoclonus-dystonia syndrome. J Neurol Sci 2015;354:110–111.
57. Roze E, Apartis E, Clot F, Dorison N, Thobois S, Guyant-Marechal L, et al. Myoclonus-dystonia: Clinical and electrophysiologic pattern related to SGCE mutations. Neurology 2008;70:1010–1016.
58. Sa M, Thornton R, Chong WK, Kaliakatsos M, Hacohen Y. Paediatric MOG antibody-associated ADEM with complex movement disorder: A case report. Mult Scler 2019;25:125–128.
59. Schmitz-Hubsch T, Lux S, Bauer P, Brandt AU, Schlapakow E, Greschus S, et al. Spinocerebellar ataxia type 14: Refining clinicogenetic diagnosis in a rare adult-onset disorder. Ann Clin Transl Neurol 2021;8:774–789.
60. Sperandeo A, Tamburini C, Noakes Z, de la Fuente DC, Keefe F, Petter O, et al. Cortical neuronal hyperexcitability and synaptic changes in SGCE mutation-positive myoclonus dystonia. Brain 2023;146:1523–1541.
61. Stamelou M, Alonso-Canovas A, Bhatia KP. Dystonia in corticobasal degeneration: A review of the literature on 404 pathologically proven cases. Mov Disord 2012;27:696–702.
62. Stamelou M, Charlesworth G, Cordivari C, Schneider SA, Kagi G, Sheerin UM, et al. The phenotypic spectrum of DYT24 due to ANO3 mutations. Mov Disord 2014;29:928–934.
63. Stamelou M, Mencacci NE, Cordivari C, Batla A, Wood NW, Houlden H, et al. Myoclonus-dystonia syndrome due to tyrosine hydroxylase deficiency. Neurology 2012;79:435–441.
64. Timsina J, Dinasarapu AR, Kilic-Berkmen G, Wang L, Budde J, Sung YJ, et al. Blood-based proteomics for adult-onset focal dystonias. Ann Neurol 2024;96:110–120.
65. Todisco M, Gana S, Cosentino G, Errichiello E, Arceri S, Avenali M, Valente EM, Alfonsi E. KCTD17-related myoclonus-dystonia syndrome: Clinical and electrophysiological findings of a patient with atypical late onset. Parkinsonism Relat Disord 2020;78:129–133.
66. van der Veen S, Caviness JN, Dreissen YEM, Ganos C, Ibrahim A, Koelman J, et al. Myoclonus and other jerky movement disorders. Clin Neurophysiol Pract 2022;7:285–316.
67. Vanek Z, Jankovic J. Dystonia in corticobasal degeneration. Mov Disord 2001;16:252–257.
68. Weissbach A, Werner E, Bally JF, Tunc S, Lons S, Timmann D, et al. Alcohol improves cerebellar learning deficit in myoclonus-dystonia: A clinical and electrophysiological investigation. Ann Neurol 2017;82:543–553.
69. Wenning GK, Tison F, Ben Shlomo Y, Daniel SE, Quinn NP. Multiple system atrophy: A review of 203 pathologically proven cases. Mov Disord 1997;12:133–147.
70. Williams L, Waller SE, Bradley M, Lockhart A, Narayanan RK, Kumar KR, et al. ATP1A3 related disease manifesting as rapid onset dystonia-parkinsonism with prominent myoclonus and exaggerated startle. Parkinsonism Relat Disord 2023;117:105864. doi:10.1016/j.parkreldis.2023.105864.
71. Wu MC, Chang YY, Lan MY, Chen YF, Tai CH, Lin YF, et al. A clinical and integrated genetic study of isolated and combined dystonia in Taiwan. J Mol Diagn 2022;24:262–273.
72. Yoon WT. Comparison of dystonia between Parkinson's disease and atypical parkinsonism: The clinical usefulness of dystonia distribution and characteristics in the differential diagnosis of parkinsonism. Neurol Neurochir Pol 2018;52:48–53.
73. Zhang YQ, Wang JW, Wang YP, Zhang XH, Li JP. Thalamus stimulation for myoclonus dystonia syndrome: Five cases and long-term follow-up. World Neurosurg 2019;122:e933–e939.

Chapter 16

Dystonia and Cerebral Palsy

INTRODUCTION

The term *cerebral palsy* (CP) has carried different meanings over the years. Early studies focused on a characteristic motor disorder resulting from early brain injury arising from a non-progressive brain injury such as stroke, hypoxia-ischemia, structural damage, or infection. More recent studies have recognized that a significant proportion of cases have a genetic cause. As a result, the concept of CP has evolved. Currently, the term is applied as a purely descriptive diagnosis that refers to a non-progressive motor disorder that begins at an early age, regardless of cause.[37] Indeed, for many cases with the motor disorder characteristics of CP, a cause may not be known.

There is a broad range of severity, from mild clumsiness of a single limb to incapacitating dysfunction affecting the entire body. The motor disorder is usually divided into three subgroups according to the predominant motor signs: spastic CP, dyskinetic CP, or ataxic CP. Although three main subtypes are recognized, the motor disorder is often mixed. Dystonia may be the sole feature in dyskinetic CP, but most cases have some spasticity too. Spasticity dominates the clinical picture in spastic CP, but most cases also have some dystonia. Dystonia may also occur in ataxic CP.

CP is common, occurring in approximately 0.1–0.5% of live births. Despite its high prevalence, treatments that are broadly effective are lacking. Most affected individuals are treated symptomatically, with a combination of oral medications, physical and occupational therapy, and sometimes surgery. However, rare cases may have an etiology with a highly effective treatment, so careful evaluation of all cases is essential.

This chapter addresses the evolution of the concept of CP, the epidemiology of CP, differences in how dystonia is described in the CP literature, how to identify dystonia among individuals with CP, etiologies, and treatment.

DEFINITION OF CEREBRAL PALSY

Cerebral palsy traditionally has been defined according to the *Rosenbaum criteria* as "a group of permanent disorders of the development of movement and posture, causing activity limitation, that are attributed to non-progressive disturbances that occurred in the developing fetal or infant brain."[52] The definition emphasizes abnormalities in movement and posture which may disrupt fine and/or gross motor function. There may be difficulties with walking, use of the hands, speaking, eating, and swallowing.

Although defined by its motor features, CP is frequently accompanied by disturbances of sensation, perception, cognition, behavior, vision and eye movements, or epilepsy. With age, there may be secondary musculoskeletal problems, such as contractures or joint dislocations, particularly in more severely affected cases.

The motor disorder is divided into subgroups according to the predominant motor signs. The three main groups include spastic CP (corticospinal signs, often more prominent in the lower limbs and sometimes unilateral), dyskinetic CP (dystonia, chorea, and/or athetosis), or ataxic CP (cerebellar signs). Although three main subtypes are recognized, the motor disorder is often mixed.[32,37] Dystonia may be the sole feature in dyskinetic CP, but the majority of individuals with dyskinetic CP also have some corticospinal signs, hypotonia, or ataxia. Similarly, dystonia is common in spastic CP, but it is not the most prominent feature (Table 16.1). Although mixed phenotypes are common, it has been a tradition to classify cases according to the dominant motor disorder, and any additional motor abnormalities are listed as secondary.[52]

The syndrome of CP has different etiologies, but the etiology must be *non-progressive*. Classic examples include stroke, transient hypoxia-ischemia, structural damage, or infection. This requirement usually means that the motor syndrome also is non-progressive. However, the motor syndrome may evolve over the first few years of life as the nervous system develops and matures. For example, the earliest signs of CP are often reflected by hypotonia with motor delay in the first months of life. Spasticity and dystonia emerge within the first year, but they may continue to evolve over the next few years of life. The strength of abnormal movements may also appear to worsen as muscle mass increases around puberty. Secondary contractures and other orthopedic problems develop even later, particularly in more severely affected cases.

In addition to the Rosenbaum criteria described above, an earlier definition of CP recommended in 2000 by the Surveillance of Cerebral Palsy in Europe (SCPE) also remains in widespread use, especially in some longitudinal registries.[16] This definition includes the following key elements: (1) it is an umbrella term for a group of disorders; (2) the condition is permanent but not unchanging; (3) it involves a disorder of movement and/or posture and of motor function; (4) it is due to a non-progressive interference, lesion, or abnormality; and (5) it arises in the developing brain.

Decision trees have been provided to guide operationalization of SCPE criteria for classifying CP into subgroups. Affected individuals are first classified into groups according to the dominant abnormality in *muscle tone*. The first group has persistent hypertonia and consists of bilateral or unilateral *spastic* CP. The second group has persistent hypotonia with ataxia and constitutes the *ataxic* CP group. The third group, *dyskinetic* CP, is defined by variable muscle tone. Dyskinetic CP may be subdivided into a group with variable hypertonia with reduced activity (*dystonic* CP) and another group with variable hypertonia and increased activity (*choreoathetotic* CP). The applicability of these criteria with regard to more recent genetic advances was reviewed in 2014, with the recommendation that individuals with genetic etiologies (including inborn errors of metabolism, chromosomal abnormalities, or genes causing static developmental defects) be included under the rubric of CP provided their clinical presentations otherwise met the diagnostic criteria.[57] However, these recommendations are not universally followed.[5]

Table 16.1 **Dystonia in spastic cerebral palsy**

Study	Cases (N)	Inclusion criteria	Dystonia (%)
Odding 2006	40	Spastic CP with isolated PVL	94
Rice 2017	128	Spastic CP defined by SCPE criteria	80
Papadimitriou 2021	31	Very severe spastic CP with PVL	100
Tedroff 2022	97	Unilateral upper limb spastic CP only	70
Ueda 2023	85	Spastic CP with isolated PVL	59

This table describes the percentage of individuals diagnosed with spastic cerebral palsy (CP) who also had dystonia, from some of the largest and most detailed studies published.

Abbreviations: PVL, periventricular leukomalacia; SCPE, Surveillance of Cerebral Palsy in Europe.

It is worth emphasizing that the traditional SCPE approach for classifying motor disorders differs substantially from the classification and definition of motor disorders in the movement disorders literature, for both children and adults.[2,55] For example, dystonia is not defined in the movement disorders literature chiefly by variable hypertonia with reduced activity. Perhaps not surprisingly, a recent systematic review found poor adherence with SCPE operational diagnostic criteria in genetic studies of CP.[47] In addition, the natural history of many recently discovered genetic etiologies is not well enough delineated to be certain that they are not progressive. Furthermore, there is sometimes phenotypic heterogeneity with the same genetic etiology, with individual cases being non-progressive while other cases are progressive. Thus, the traditional SCPE approach has seen increasing conflicts with recent scientific advances.

EPIDEMIOLOGY

The global prevalence of all types of CP has been estimated from a systematic analysis of data from 41 regions in 27 countries across 5 continents. The prevalence is higher in low- and middle-income countries, estimated at 3.4 per 1,000 live births; in high-income countries, the estimate was 1.6 per 1,000 live births.[33] The prevalence of prenatal and perinatal CP has declined significantly compared with a previous systematic review published in 2013, mainly derived using data from high-income countries, where the estimate was 2.1 per 1,000 live births.[41]

Within the broader CP population, there are significant differences in the prevalence of the three main subgroups. Spastic CP is the most common subtype, accounting for 80–90% of all cases. Dyskinetic CP is the second most common, accounting for 5–15% of cases. Ataxic CP is the least common, usually fewer than 1–2% of all cases. These estimates come from early studies using the SCPE classification system with data collected from a network of 14 centers across 8 countries in Europe,[16] and from systematic reviews of the literature.[40]

More recent studies have confirmed these early findings. A retrospective single-center study of 243 children with CP from Australia revealed spastic CP was the most common subgroup (75%) with smaller numbers of dyskinetic CP (23%).[50] Dyskinetic CP made up only 7.9% of another cohort of 1,165 CP cases from a Danish nationwide register.[48] In another retrospective single-center study of 384 individuals from Germany, spastic CP was again the most common (62% bilateral, 34% unilateral), with smaller numbers of dyskinetic (3.4%) and ataxic (0.6%) subgroups.[34] Although three main CP subtypes are recognized based on the dominant motor problem, the majority of cases have a mixed motor disorder. Many patients with dyskinetic CP have some corticospinal signs, and many with spastic CP also have some dystonia. Indeed, the majority of individuals with CP have a mixed motor disorder that includes dystonia, although dystonia may not be the most prominent feature (Table 16.1).

Risk factors for spastic and dyskinetic CP overlap, but they are not identical. In a study from the Danish nationwide CP register, when compared with spastic CP, children with dyskinetic CP had experienced more peri- or neonatal adverse events, as evidenced by very low Apgar scores and neonatal seizures. Individuals with dyskinetic CP also had more motor impairment, neurodevelopmental impairment, visual impairment (39%), and epilepsy (51%).[48] Basal ganglia lesions were more prevalent in dyskinetic compared to bilateral spastic CP (28% vs. 13%).

Another study from the SCPE group evaluated 578 children with dyskinetic CP born between 1976 and 1996.[23] Severe learning disability was present in 52%, epilepsy in 51%, severe visual impairment in 19%, and hearing impairment in 6%. There was a correlation between comorbidity and greater motor impairment. Compared with those with bilateral spastic CP, individuals with dyskinetic CP were more likely to have evidence of perinatal adverse events, as indicated by a low Apgar score or convulsions in the first 72 hours. Children with dyskinetic cerebral palsy also had more severe cognitive and motor impairments compared with those with bilateral spastic CP.[3]

TERMINOLOGY DIFFERENCES

There has been a long-standing mismatch regarding how dystonia and related terms have been used in the literature. Definitions used in movement disorders literature are different from those used in CP literature. In many articles, dystonia is frequently incorrectly labeled as spasticity, or the two are combined under the rubric of *hypertonia.*

The current conceptualization of *dystonia* recognizes that it can be associated with either sustained *or* intermittent muscle contractions, it can produce abnormal movements or postures, and movements are often slow but sometimes quite rapid.[2] Abnormalities of muscle tone are not required, although they may sometimes occur. Dystonia is more often categorized as a *hyper*kinetic disorder, not a *hypo*kinetic disorder. This modern conceptualization of dystonia contrasts with traditional definitions of dystonic CP, which is described as variable muscle tone with *reduced activity.*[52,57]

In the neurological and movement disorders literature, *spasticity* is conceptualized as a syndrome that arises from pathology of the corticospinal system and leads to velocity-dependent hypertonia as one of its components. Spasticity may be variable rather than constant, and it may be non-detectable when the limb is at rest or only slowly moved. This view contrasts with the CP definition of spastic CP, where hypertonia is said to be persistent. Other components of corticospinal dysfunction can be helpful in these cases, including hyperreflexia, clonus, and a positive extensor plantar reflex.

Similarly, the hybrid term *choreoathetosis* is no longer recommended in the field of movement disorders because of ambiguities in the meaning of the term *athetosis.*[39] Historically, *athetosis* has been used to describe different movement disorders including dystonia, chorea, and fine writhing movements.[54] It is now used in the movement disorders literature to refer to a specific type of movement affecting the distal extremities or face.[38] Chorea is considered a distinct movement disorder, although it can coexist with athetosis or dystonia. The modern conceptualization of chorea and athetosis does not require abnormalities of muscle tone, although they may coexist. These modern conceptualizations of athetosis and chorea conflict with long-standing use of similar terms in the CP literature, where dyskinetic choreoathetoid CP is defined as a motor disorder of "variable muscle tone with increased activity."[52,57]

These very different uses of similar terminology across the movement disorders literature and the CP literature can be confusing. Achieving consistency in concepts and terminology is progressing but remains a process in evolution.[2,55] The differences are important to acknowledge until there is more universal harmonization of the language. Recognizing that some ambiguities exist, the ensuing sections use the terms as they appeared in the original published literature.

IDENTIFYING DYSTONIA IN CEREBRAL PALSY

Assessing Motor Function

Dystonia can be assessed using a number of rating scales.[3] The most common scale used in pediatrics and CP is the Barry-Albright Dystonia Rating Scale.[58] This rating scale has a number of clinimetric flaws, and it is not commonly used in the movement disorders literature, where the Burke-Fahn-Marsden Dystonia Rating Scale is more popular.[3] However, neither scale was designed to discriminate dystonia from other motor problems.

The syndrome of CP often reflects a mix of distinct motor problems[32,36,37,50,61] and discriminating dystonia from other movement disorders requires a high level of expertise, especially when the motor syndrome is mixed.[6,14,25,51,59] These observations have led to increasing popularity of scales that assess overall motor function, such as the Gross Motor Function Classification System (GMFCS), rather than scales that address the nature of the underlying motor disorder. However, discrimination of the component motor features is important because their pathogenesis and treatment vary.[56] For example, deep brain stimulation surgery may be useful for dystonia, but it is not useful for spasticity.

Discriminating Subtypes of Increased Muscle Tone

For both dyskinetic and spastic CP, dystonia often is combined with spasticity. The Hypertonia Assessment Tool was developed to discriminate different types of increased muscle tone including spasticity, dystonia, and rigidity.[25] In one detailed cross-sectional study, 151 individuals with CP were evaluated by several experts using this tool.[51] Among all cases, 85% were classified using SCPE criteria as spastic CP, with 14% dyskinetic CP, and 1% ataxic CP. As expected, 100% of individuals classified with dyskinetic CP had dystonia. However, about 80% of individuals classified with spastic CP as the major

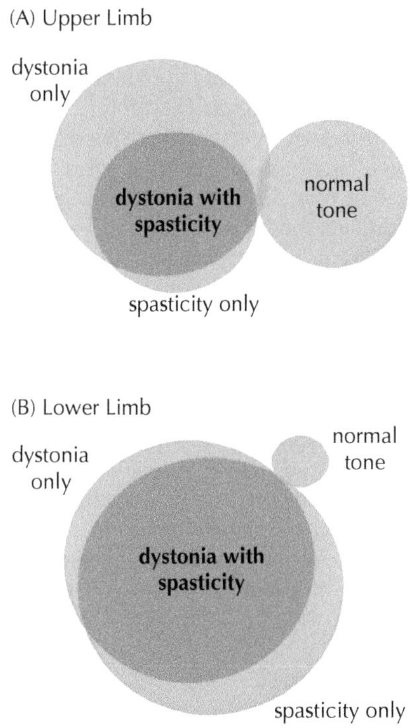

Figure 16.1. Overlap of spasticity and dystonia in cerebral palsy. This figure was adapted from results obtained using the Hypertonia Assessment Tool to discriminate spasticity from dystonia among 151 individuals with cerebral palsy.[51] The top panel shows the overlap of spasticity and dystonia for upper limb, and the bottom panel shows the lower limb.

motor problem also had dystonia in the legs, and approximately 60% had dystonia in the arms (Figure 16.1). Interestingly, rigidity was not found in this cohort.

Another retrospective videotape analysis assessed 85 predominantly pediatric individuals classified as having unilateral or bilateral spastic CP associated with the classic radiological findings of periventricular leukomalacia and lacking radiological evidence of basal ganglia and thalamic injury.[61] Dystonia was defined operationally as an intermittent abnormal movement or posture of varying amplitude that was triggered by purposeful movement of the same or another body part. It was further distinguished from spasticity by its variable amplitude and variable presence with purposeful movements, whereas abnormal posturing that was more constant in severity and amplitude was assumed to be spasticity. In this population with presumably predominant spasticity, dystonia was observed in 59%, present only in the upper limbs in 11%, lower limbs in 44%, and in both upper and lower limbs in 5%.[61]

In a similarly designed study of 31 more severely affected individuals with CP, including approximately 25% unable to walk without assistance, all patients were assessed as having coexistent dystonia, with 30 in the upper limbs, 30 in the lower limbs, 22 axial (cervical and/or trunk), 15 oromandibular, and 5 periocular.[42] The severity of dystonia and spasticity were closely correlated, but only dystonia correlated with motor disability. Another study of 97 children with unilateral spastic CP affecting the upper limb revealed 70% had coexisting dystonia, and dystonia correlated with higher levels of disability.[60]

Criteria typically used by experts to distinguish dystonia from spasticity were explicitly probed in another study by three pediatric movement disorder experts asked to identify dystonia in gait videos of 40 individuals with spastic CP and periventricular leukomalacia. A unanimous consensus about the presence of dystonia was achieved for 34 out of 40 videos, with unilateral leg or foot adduction that was variable over time being the main distinguishing feature.[6] However, the difficulty of this task was highlighted by the second main finding, which was difficulty in identifying dystonia in this population. These types of studies indicate that discriminating spasticity from dystonia requires a high level of expertise, and sometimes experts do not agree. This challenge is reflected in many studies, which have shown that many community practitioners do not use these terms consistently.[5] Overall, it seems spasticity may be more readily detected by clinicians using current operational criteria, but dystonia appears to be more functionally disabling.[59]

Discriminating Dystonia and Choreoathetosis

Dystonia is assessed in a number of clinical scales, but only the Dyskinesia Impairment Scale attempts to discriminate dystonia and choreoathetosis.[58] A cross-sectional study of 55 children and young adults diagnosed with dyskinetic CP were assessed using this scale.[36] Dystonia and choreoathetosis were frequently combined, with dystonia (70%) being more common than choreoathetosis (27%).[36] Motor impairment assessed with the GMFS correlated with the severity of dystonia, but not choreoathetosis.[36]

However, the definitions of dystonia and choreoathetosis used in the Dyskinesia Impairment Scale overlap, potentially mixing the two problems. Dystonia in CP was described as "dominated by abnormal postures (may give the impression of hypokinesia) and muscle tone that is fluctuating (but with easily elicitable tone increase)." Characteristics are "involuntary movements, distorted voluntary movements, and abnormal postures due to sustained muscle contractions." Choreoathetosis, by comparison, is defined as being "dominated by hyperkinesia and tone fluctuating (but mainly decreased)." Chorea means "rapid involuntary jerky, often fragmented movements." Athetosis means "slower, constantly changing writhing or contorting movements." These definitions and descriptions overlap, producing some uncertainty when discriminating dystonia from choreoathetosis, especially considering both are often combined.

ETIOLOGY

Acquired Brain Injury

Traditionally, CP was thought to reflect an acquired but static insult to the developing nervous system. Etiological factors for dyskinetic and spastic CP overlap but are not identical. For spastic CP, the most common etiologies were thought to include early stroke, hypoxia-ischemia, or brain infection. Spastic CP is most often associated with white matter injury in the periventricular regions on brain MRI.[61] Periventricular leukomalacia has been associated with a number of maternal or fetal risk factors in preterm infants. A systematic review and meta-analysis addressed the certainty of evidence across 186 studies covering a total of 16,569 individuals with periventricular leukomalacia and found significant but moderate evidence for intraventricular hemorrhage as a contributor.[1] This study also found significant but limited evidence for several other causes including perinatal asphyxia, shock/hypotension, circulatory collapse, patent ductus arteriosus, neonatal surgery, sepsis, necrotizing enterocolitis, hypocarbia, chorioamnionitis, multifetal pregnancy reduction, and antenatal medications.

In contrast, dyskinetic CP is more likely to be associated with basal ganglia and thalamic injury on MRI. Lesions in these regions are present in up to 70% of individuals.[36,37] Common causes include perinatal hypoxia-ischemia, neonatal hyperbilirubinemia (kernicterus), intracranial hemorrhage, perinatal stroke, or cerebral infection.[37] In developed countries, kernicterus is now uncommon, but it is still relatively common in underdeveloped countries. If a clear history of neonatal jaundice is not available, there may be other features suggestive of kernicterus such as upward gaze palsy, deafness, and globus pallidus and subthalamic nucleus hyperintensities.[53] In contrast, perinatal asphyxia is more commonly associated with putaminal, thalamic, and periventricular lesions.[53] In a study of 4- to 5-day-old neonates treated with therapeutic hypothermia for hypoxic-ischemic encephalopathy, MRI findings suggestive of abnormal diffusion in the thalamus and basal ganglia were highly predictive for the subsequent development of dystonia.[11]

Genetic Causes

In addition to the well-recognized acquired causes for CP, numerous recent studies have suggested that genetic factors play a role. Some experts believe that genetic disorders such as inborn errors of metabolism or chromosomal abnormalities should be included under the rubric of CP provided that their clinical features meet diagnostic criteria for CP.[31,57] However, other experts prefer to exclude genetic etiologies and instead label these individuals as "mimics" of CP.[4,44,65] In the genetics community, terminology other than CP is often preferred once a responsible gene is found. Individuals may be given a diagnosis based on the name of the gene or a more specific category of disease such as neurodevelopmental disorder, developmental encephalopathy, epilepsy-dyskinesia, or developmental and epileptic encephalopathy.[12,13,43,45]

With these caveats in mind, one meta-analysis summarized results from 13 independent exome sequencing studies that included 2,612 individuals who had a diagnosis of CP.[20] A pathogenic gene defect was disclosed for 31.1% of all cases. The likelihood of finding a gene defect depended on criteria used to define CP, age of the population, and several associated features. The most notable feature increasing the chance of an inherited disorder appears to be the absence of a definitive history of perinatal injury.[4,44,65] Other red flags include a family history of cerebral palsy, developmental regression, presence of other neurological abnormalities, paroxysmal fluctuations of symptoms, marked exacerbations of motor impairment with intercurrent illness, isolated generalized hypotonia, or prominent ataxia. Of course, there may be other systemic signs of an inherited disorder, such as dysmorphism.

The typical findings of periventricular leukomalacia or lesions of the thalamus and basal ganglia are supportive of an acquired etiology for CP, although these lesions may be mimicked by some genetic diseases.[35] Prominent basal ganglia hyperintensities, cystic or mixed lesions, and diffuse leukoencephalopathy should prompt a search for underlying metabolic or genetic disease.

TREATMENT

Overview

Individuals with CP suffer chronic motor impairments, and effective therapy can be a challenge. A variety of treatments have been evaluated, often with variable results, in part because of the clinical and etiological heterogeneity of CP. There are only limited data from large randomized controlled trials, and most of these trials have focused on spastic CP because it is more common than dyskinetic CP. In the absence of evidence-based medicine, treatments are often guided by physician experience, tailored to the specific handicaps of each individual. A multidisciplinary approach is often recommended, including a neurologist, physiatrist, and sometimes pain medicine or surgical specialists.

Oral Medications

Several systematic reviews of oral therapies for CP have been published.[8,17,22] However, there are few randomized controlled trials, most based on relatively small numbers of individuals. As a result, these systematic reviews often fail to reach criteria to make definitive recommendations. Among the many oral agents used, the anticholinergic trihexyphenidyl has received most attention, and it is often recommended for other types of dystonia (see Chapter 28, "Symptom-Targeted Oral Medications for Dystonia").

A 2018 systematic review of the treatment of dystonia in CP addressed oral baclofen, benzodiazepines, clonidine, gabapentin, levodopa, and trihexyphenidyl.[17] Outcomes assessed included motor function, pain, or facilitation of care. For dystonia in CP, trihexyphenidyl was determined to be *possibly ineffective*, with insufficient evidence to make recommendations for any of the other oral agents. Another systematic review focusing specifically on trihexyphenidyl also found insufficient evidence to recommend trihexyphenidyl for treating dystonia or overall motor function.[22] A more recent systematic review and meta-analysis of treatment of dystonia in CP again did not find sufficient evidence to recommend trihexyphenidyl and instead concluded it may increase adverse events.[8] However, a more recent open-label prospective 12-week study of 41 individuals (of whom only 34 completed) suggested that trihexyphenidyl could be useful for improving dystonia, motor function, and overall development.[49] The discrepancies for trihexyphenidyl likely reflect the clinical and etiological heterogeneity of CP, combined with how dystonia and its severity were assessed.

Another oral agent that has received considerable attention has been levodopa. The motor disorder of dopa-responsive dystonia may resemble spasticity, and many individuals with this inherited disorder are first diagnosed with CP.[18,24,30] The classic phenotype is most often caused by genetic variants in *GCH1*, and less commonly in the genes *TH*, *PTS*, *QPR*, and *SPR*.[62] These other genes more often cause dystonia combined with additional neurological features, such as encephalopathy or abnormal eye movements. Levodopa can be nearly curative for the classic phenotype, and it may be at least partially helpful in the more complex phenotypes.[26] Benefits may emerge with a very low dose, although some patients require higher doses up to 20 mg/kg/d (see Chapter 29, "Special Interventions for Certain Types of Dystonia"). Dyskinesias are uncommonly observed in the classical phenotype, even after years of therapy, but they may occur rapidly with the more complex phenotypes. Although these disorders are all rare, a trial of levodopa should be considered mandatory in all children with a diagnosis of dyskinetic or spastic CP, especially when there is not definitive evidence of perinatal birth injury on imaging.

An Australian survey of 25 clinicians who together cared for a cohort of 77 children with CP found that only 16 prescribed new medications for dystonia over the study period.[21] Baclofen and gabapentin were prescribed most, followed by levodopa, trihexyphenidyl, and diazepam.[21] However, the apparent benefits of these drugs may reflect an effect on coexisting spasticity rather than dystonia. It is no surprise that the discovery and evaluation of new therapies were among the major priorities identified in a recent study of the most important research themes in a community-driven research agenda for dystonic CP.[19] In the absence of stronger evidence, treatment often involves a trial-and-error process.

Botulinum Toxins

Despite the widespread use and demonstration of effectiveness of botulinum toxins for many forms of dystonia and spasticity in adults, the evidence to support their use for dyskinetic CP is mixed. Several systematic reviews have suggested efficacy for spastic CP,[29,63] but similar reviews for dyskinetic CP have concluded there is insufficient evidence for recommending its use.[8,17] This somewhat surprising finding may again reflect the clinical and etiological heterogeneity of dyskinetic CP, the types of CP included in the trials, and how spasticity and dystonia (and any improvements) were ascertained.

For CP, relaxing muscles with botulinum toxin may also unmask underlying weakness, with the overall result of worsening functional outcomes despite the alleviation of dystonia or spasticity. Thus, treatment may address problems such as painful muscle spasms and stiffness without improving motor function.

Given its safety and proven efficacy for dystonia or spasticity in other clinical settings, it is reasonable to provide a trial of botulinum toxin in individuals with dyskinetic CP, especially selectively targeting the more severely affected areas. For example, a small randomized controlled study showed efficacy for treating cervical dystonia in adults with dyskinetic CP, with an outcome similar to that for adult-onset idiopathic cervical dystonia.[64]

Intrathecal Baclofen

Baclofen can be useful for both spasticity and dystonia, so it is often used in CP[21,32] and it has been explored extensively in numerous studies. In systematic reviews of oral pharmacotherapy for dyskinetic CP, none of the many articles on oral baclofen met quality criteria for inclusion.[17] One of the limitations may be that the oral doses required to produce benefit also cause many side effects, such as sedation or dizziness.

Despite the mixed results for oral baclofen, intrathecal baclofen was concluded to be potentially useful in dyskinetic CP for improving dystonia, goal attainment, pain and comfort, ease of caregiving, and quality of life.[8] This recommendation was based on low or very low-level evidence. One multicenter, randomized, double-blind, placebo-controlled trial of 36 adults and children with severe dyskinetic CP reported significant improvement in goal achievement, but dropout rate was very high.[9]

Physical and Occupational Therapy

A recent review highlighted the value of early intervention and rehabilitation strategies as well as judicious use of assisted technologies in the management of CP.[7] A focus on functional outcomes is often recommended. Stretching and other exercises are likely to be valuable as well.

Additional strategies thought to be useful include gait training, strength and power training, constraint-induced movement therapy, bimanual therapy, action observation therapy, and goal-directed training. However, most of these interventions have been evaluated for spastic CP, and their value for dyskinetic CP is less clear. In addition, most of these interventions have been studied in less severely affected children, with little data on more severely affected children or adults. Further information regarding physiotherapy in CP can be found in Chapter 32, "Physiotherapy and Complementary Medicine for Dystonia."

Surgical Interventions

Individuals with CP often undergo palliative surgical procedures to reduce contractures or prevent joint dislocations. There also are numerous studies describing the treatment of dyskinetic CP with functional neurosurgery targeting the globus pallidus, thalamus, or cerebellum.[10,15,28,46] An early meta-analysis encompassing 20 different articles that included a total of 68 individuals with dyskinetic CP treated with deep brain stimulation reported overall mean improvements of 24% for

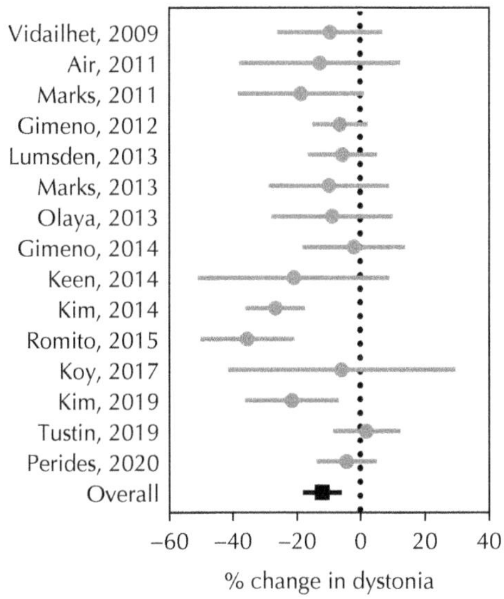

Figure 16.2. Meta-analysis of deep brain stimulation efficacy for cerebral palsy. This figure was adapted from a prior review that summarized the percentage of change in the Burke-Fahn Marsden Dystonia Rating Scale scores for 15 separate studies and a total of 168 cerebral palsy patients.[8] The overall percentage of improvement averaged 17%.

dystonia and 9% for disability using the Burke-Fahn-Marsden Dystonia Rating Scale.[27] A more recent 2021 meta-analysis using slightly different inclusion criteria encompassed 168 cases across 15 studies and reported 17% improvement on the Burke-Fahn-Marsden dystonia rating scale.[8] Other studies have described improvements of quality of life,[28] pain,[46] and facilitation of care.

It is worth noting that the degree of benefit with deep brain stimulation varies widely among cases and centers (Figure 16.2). This heterogeneity in responses is probably related to selection of surgical candidates. Meta-analyses spanning all types of treatments for dyskinetic CP found only low levels of evidence to support deep brain stimulation,[8,17] in part because of enormous variations in reported outcomes and the relatively higher risk of surgical complications in CP compared to other types of dystonia.

SYNOPSIS AND FUTURE PROSPECTS

For both children and adults, CP is one of the most common conditions where dystonia may occur. Traditionally, CP has been classified according to the dominant motor problem into three subgroups that include spastic CP, dyskinetic CP, and ataxic CP. Dyskinetic CP is further subdivided into dystonic and choreoathetoid forms. However, mixed motor disorders are common, and most individuals with spastic CP or choreoathetoid CP also have coexisting dystonia. Studies of functional disability have indicated that impairment correlates more with dystonia, rather than spasticity or choreoathetosis. Overall, it is likely that dystonia has a greater overall functional impact in CP than traditionally appreciated.

One of the challenges in appreciating the research relevant to dystonia in CP relates to the obscuration of distinct motor abnormalities with an overly simplified classification for all types of CP. Another challenge relates to the inconsistent use of terminology to define similar problems. The most common definitions of dystonia used for CP are quite different from the definitions of dystonia used in movement disorders. Together, the oversimplified classification system and conflicting uses of terminology make it challenging to know the precise characteristics of the individuals studied. Some long-held traditional approaches for classification and terminology may need to be revised.

Traditional beliefs regarding the etiologies for CP have also been undergoing change. The major change has been relatively recent recognition of genetic causes in addition to the historically recognized acquired causes. While many of these cases may continue to carry a descriptive diagnosis of CP, there has been increasing tendency to move toward more specific diagnoses rather than using only the broad umbrella term of CP. These other diagnoses may be based on more specific descriptive phenotypic subgroups, or on a more specific gene-based syndrome. Treatment, and particularly counseling, is often different for acquired versus genetic etiologies for CP.

Treatment of CP remains a challenge. Oral medications and neurosurgical procedures often useful for other types of dystonia do not always have the same effects for dystonia in CP. The evidence-based literature often produces inconclusive results, most likely relating to the underlying clinical and etiological heterogeneity of CP. Nevertheless, several treatments appear to produce benefit when cases are properly selected. They include oral agents, physiotherapy, intrathecal baclofen, and neurosurgical procedures. The identification of better treatments is a high priority, and it may need to focus on more specific populations, or more specific motor abnormalities in CP.

REFERENCES

1. Abiramalatha T, Bandyopadhyay T, Ramaswamy VV, Shaik NB, Thanigainathan S, Pullattayil AK, Amboiram P. Risk factors for periventricular leukomalacia in preterm infants: A systematic review, meta-analysis, and GRADE-based assessment of certainty of evidence. Pediatr Neurol 2021;124:51–71.
2. Albanese A, Bhatia K, Bressman SB, DeLong MR, Fahn S, Fung VSC, et al. Phenomenology and classification of dystonia: A consensus update. Mov Disord 2013;28:863–873.
3. Albanese A, Sorbo FD, Comella C, Jinnah HA, Mink JW, Post B, et al. Dystonia rating scales: Critique and recommendations. Mov Disord 2013;28:874–883.
4. Appleton RE, Gupta R. Cerebral palsy: Not always what it seems. Arch Dis Child 2019;104:809–814.
5. Aravamuthan BR, Fehlings D, Shetty S, Fahey M, Gilbert L, Tilton A, Kruer MC. Variability in cerebral palsy diagnosis. Pediatrics 2021;147:e2020010066.
6. Aravamuthan BR, Ueda K, Miao H, Gilbert L, Smith SE, Pearson TS. Gait features of dystonia in cerebral palsy. Dev Med Child Neurol 2021;63:748–754.
7. Bekteshi S, Monbaliu E, McIntyre S, Saloojee G, Hilberink SR, Tatishvili N, Dan B. Towards functional improvement of motor disorders associated with cerebral palsy. Lancet Neurol 2023;22:229–243.
8. Bohn E, Goren K, Switzer L, Falck-Ytter Y, Fehlings D. Pharmacological and neurosurgical interventions for individuals with cerebral palsy and dystonia: A systematic review update and meta-analysis. Dev Med Child Neurol 2021;63:1038–1050.
9. Bonouvrie LA, Becher JG, Vles JSH, Vermeulen RJ, Buizer AI, Group IS. The effect of intrathecal baclofen in dyskinetic cerebral palsy: The IDYS trial. Ann Neurol 2019;86:79–90.
10. Cajigas I, Morrison MA, Luciano MS, Starr PA. Cerebellar deep brain stimulation for the treatment of movement disorders in cerebral palsy. J Neurosurg 2023;139:605–614.
11. Chintalapati K, Miao H, Mathur A, Neil J, Aravamuthan BR. Objective and clinically feasible analysis of diffusion MRI data can help predict dystonia after neonatal brain injury. Pediatr Neurol 2021;118:6–11.
12. Dzinovic I, Boesch S, Skorvanek M, Necpal J, Svantnerova J, Pavelekova P, et al. Genetic overlap between dystonia and other neurologic disorders: A study of 1,100 exomes. Parkinsonism Relat Disord 2022;102:1–6.
13. Dzinovic I, Skorvanek M, Necpal J, Boesch S, Svantnerova J, Wagner M, et al. Dystonia as a prominent presenting feature in developmental and epileptic encephalopathies: A case series. Parkinsonism Relat Disord 2021;90:73–78.
14. Eggink H, Kremer D, Brouwer OF, Contarino MF, van Egmond ME, Elema A, et al. Spasticity, dyskinesia and ataxia in cerebral palsy: Are we sure we can differentiate them? Eur J Paediatr Neurol 2017;21:703–706.
15. Elia AE, Bagella CF, Ferre F, Zorzi G, Calandrella D, Romito LM. Deep brain stimulation for dystonia due to cerebral palsy: A review. Eur J Paediatr Neurol 2018;22:308–315.
16. European Cerebal Palsy Surveillance. Surveillance of cerebral palsy in Europe: A collaboration of cerebral palsy surveys and registers. Surveillance of Cerebral Palsy in Europe (SCPE). Dev Med Child Neurol 2000;42:816–824.
17. Fehlings D, Brown L, Harvey A, Himmelmann K, Lin JP, Macintosh A, et al. Pharmacological and neurosurgical interventions for managing dystonia in cerebral palsy: A systematic review. Dev Med Child Neurol 2018;60:356–366.
18. Furukawa Y, Graf WD, Wong H, Shimadzu M, Kish SJ. Dopa-responsive dystonia simulating spastic paraplegia due to tyrosine hydroxylase (TH) gene mutations. Neurology 2001;56:260–253.
19. Gilbert LA, Fehlings DL, Gross P, Kruer MC, Kwan W, Mink JW, et al. Top 10 research themes for dystonia in cerebral palsy: A community-driven research agenda. Neurology 2022;99:237–245.
20. Gonzalez-Mantilla PJ, Hu Y, Myers SM, Finucane BM, Ledbetter DH, Martin CL, Moreno-De-Luca A. Diagnostic yield of exome sequencing in cerebral palsy and implications for genetic testing guidelines: A systematic review and meta-analysis. JAMA Pediatr 2023;177:472–478.
21. Harvey A, Bear N, Rice J, Antolovich G, Waugh MC. National surveillance of oral medication prescription for children with dystonic cerebral palsy. J Paediatr Child Health 2021;57:1222–1227.
22. Harvey AR, Baker LB, Reddihough DS, Scheinberg A, Williams K. Trihexyphenidyl for dystonia in cerebral palsy. Cochrane Database Syst Rev 2018;5:CD012430.
23. Himmelmann K, McManus V, Hagberg G, Uvebrant P, Krageloh-Mann I, Cans C, et al. Dyskinetic cerebral palsy in Europe: Trends in prevalence and severity. Arch Dis Child 2009;94:921–926.
24. Jan MMS. Misdiagnoses in children with dopa-responsive dystonia. Pediatr Neurol 2004;31:298–303.
25. Jethwa A, Mink J, Macarthur C, Knights S, Fehlings T, Fehlings D. Development of the Hypertonia Assessment Tool (HAT): A discriminative tool for hypertonia in children. Dev Med Child Neurol 2010;52:e83–87.
26. Kim R, Jeon B, Lee WW. A systematic review of treatment outcome in patients with dopa-responsive dystonia (DRD) and DRD-plus. Mov Disord Clin Pract 2016;3:435–442.
27. Koy A, Hellmich M, Pauls KA, Marks W, Lin JP, Fricke O, Timmermann L. Effects of deep brain stimulation in dyskinetic cerebral palsy: A meta-analysis. Mov Disord 2013;28:647–654.
28. Koy A, Kuhn AA, Huebl J, Schneider GH, van Riesen AK, Eckenweiler M, et al. Quality of life after deep brain stimulation of pediatric patients with dyskinetic cerebral palsy: A prospective, single-arm, multicenter study with a subsequent randomized double-blind crossover (STIM-CP). Mov Disord 2022;37:799–811.
29. Kumar D, Kumar R, Mudgal SK, Ranjan P, Kumar S. The effects of botulinum toxin and casting in spastic children with cerebral palsy: A systematic review and meta-analysis. Cureus 2023;15:e36851.
30. Lee WW, Jeon BS. Clinical spectrum of dopa-responsive dystonia and related disorders. Curr Neurol Neurosci Rep 2014;14:461.
31. Lewis SA, Shetty S, Wilson BA, Huang AJ, Jin SC, Smithers-Sheedy H, et al. Insights from genetic studies of cerebral palsy. Front Neurol 2020;11:625428.
32. Lumsden DE, Crowe B, Basu A, Amin S, Devlin A, DeAlwis Y, et al. Pharmacological management of

abnormal tone and movement in cerebral palsy. Arch Dis Child 2019;104:775–780.
33. McIntyre S, Goldsmith S, Webb A, Ehlinger V, Hollung SJ, McConnell K, et al. Global prevalence of cerebral palsy: A systematic analysis. Dev Med Child Neurol 2022;64:1494–1506.
34. Metz C, Jaster M, Walch E, Sarpong-Bengelsdorf A, Kaindl AM, Schneider J. Clinical phenotype of cerebral palsy depends on the cause: Is it really cerebral palsy? A retrospective study. J Child Neurol 2022;37:112–118.
35. Mohammad SS, Angiti RR, Biggin A, Morales-Briceno H, Goetti R, Perez-Duenas B, et al. Magnetic resonance imaging pattern recognition in childhood bilateral basal ganglia disorders. Brain Commun 2020;2:fcaa178.
36. Monbaliu E, de Cock P, Ortibus E, Heyrman L, Klingels K, Feys H. Clinical patterns of dystonia and choreoathetosis in participants with dyskinetic cerebral palsy. Dev Med Child Neurol 2016;58:138–144.
37. Monbaliu E, Himmelmann K, Lin JP, Ortibus E, Bonouvrie L, Feys H, et al. Clinical presentation and management of dyskinetic cerebral palsy. Lancet Neurol 2017;16:741–749.
38. Morris JG, Grattan-Smith P, Jankelowitz SK, Fung VS, Clouston PD, Hayes MW. Athetosis II: The syndrome of mild athetoid cerebral palsy. Mov Disord 2002;17:1281–1287.
39. Morris JG, Jankelowitz SK, Fung VS, Clouston PD, Hayes MW, Grattan-Smith P. Athetosis I: Historical considerations. Mov Disord 2002;17:1278–1280.
40. Odding E, Roebroeck ME, Stam HJ. The epidemiology of cerebral palsy: Incidence, impairments and risk factors. Disabil Rehabil 2006;28:183–191.
41. Oskoui M, Coutinho F, Dykeman J, Jette N, Pringsheim T. An update on the prevalence of cerebral palsy: A systematic review and meta-analysis. Dev Med Child Neurol 2013;55:509–519.
42. Papadimitriou I, Dalivigka Z, Outsika C, Scarmeas N, Pons R. Dystonia assessment in children with cerebral palsy and periventricular leukomalacia. Eur J Paediatr Neurol 2021;32:8–15.
43. Papandreou A, Danti FR, Spaull R, Leuzzi V, McTague A, Kurian MA. The expanding spectrum of movement disorders in genetic epilepsies. Dev Med Child Neurol 2020;62:178–191.
44. Pearson TS, Pons R, Ghaoui R, Sue CM. Genetic mimics of cerebral palsy. Mov Disord 2019;34:625–636.
45. Perez-Duenas B, Gorman K, Marce-Grau A, Ortigoza-Escobar JD, Macaya A, Danti FR, et al. The genetic landscape of complex childhood-onset hyperkinetic movement disorders. Mov Disord 2022;37:2197–2209.
46. Perides S, Lin JP, Lee G, Gimeno H, Lumsden DE, Ashkan K, et al. Deep brain stimulation reduces pain in children with dystonia, including in dyskinetic cerebral palsy. Dev Med Child Neurol 2020;62:917–925.
47. Pham R, Mol BW, Gecz J, MacLennan AH, MacLennan SC, Corbett MA, et al. Definition and diagnosis of cerebral palsy in genetic studies: A systematic review. Dev Med Child Neurol 2020;62:1024–1030.
48. Preel M, Rackauskaite G, Larsen ML, Laursen B, Lorentzen J, Born AP, et al. Children with dyskinetic cerebral palsy are severely affected as compared to bilateral spastic cerebral palsy. Acta Paediatr 2019;108:1850–1856.
49. Rajkumar L, Ventatakrishnan A, Sairam S, Khosla M, Khanna R, Das B, et al. Trihexyphenidyl in young children with dystonic cerebral palsy: A single arm study. J Pediatr Rehabil Med 2023;16:115–124.
50. Reid SM, Meehan EM, Reddihough DS, Harvey AR. Dyskinetic vs spastic cerebral palsy: A cross-sectional study comparing functional profiles, comorbidities, and brain imaging patterns. J Child Neurol 2018;33:593–600.
51. Rice J, Skuza P, Baker F, Russo R, Fehlings D. Identification and measurement of dystonia in cerebral palsy. Dev Med Child Neurol 2017;59:1249–1255.
52. Rosenbaum P, Paneth N, Leviton A, Goldstein M, Bax M, Damiano D, et al. A report: The definition and classification of cerebral palsy April 2006. Dev Med Child Neurol Suppl 2007;109:8–14.
53. Saini AG, Sankhyan N, Malhi P, Ahuja C, Khandelwal N, Singhi P. Hyperbilirubinemia and asphyxia in children with dyskinetic cerebral palsy. Pediatr Neurol 2021;120:80–85.
54. Salam-Adams M, Adams RD. Athetotic syndromes. In: Vinken PJ, Bruyn GW, Klawans HL, eds. *Handbook of Clinical Neurology 49: Extrapyramidal Disorders.* Elsevier Science Publishers; 1997: 381–389.
55. Sanger TD, Chen D, Fehlings DL, Hallett M, Lang AE, Mink JW, et al. Definition and classification of hyperkinetic movements in childhood. Mov Disord 2010;25:1538–1549.
56. Sanger TD, Delgado MR, Gaebler-Spira D, Hallett M, Mink JW, Task F. Classification and definition of disorders causing hypertonia in childhood. Pediatrics 2003;111:89–97.
57. Smithers-Sheedy H, Badawi N, Blair E, Cans C, Himmelmann K, Krageloh-Mann I, et al. What constitutes cerebral palsy in the twenty-first century? Dev Med Child Neurol 2014;56:323–328.
58. Stewart K, Harvey A, Johnston LM. A systematic review of scales to measure dystonia and choreoathetosis in children with dyskinetic cerebral palsy. Dev Med Child Neurol 2017;59:786–795.
59. Stewart K, Tavender E, Rice J, Harvey A. Identification, classification and assessment of dyskinesia in children with cerebral palsy: A survey of clinicians. J Paediatr Child Health 2018;54:432–438.
60. Tedroff K, Lidbeck C, Lowing K. Dystonia during hand activity in children with spastic unilateral cerebral palsy, an observational study. Eur J Paediatr Neurol 2022;41:36–40.
61. Ueda K, Aravamuthan BR, Pearson TS. Dystonia in individuals with spastic cerebral palsy and isolated periventricular leukomalacia. Dev Med Child Neurol 2023;65:94–99.
62. Weissbach A, Pauly MG, Herzog R, Hahn L, Halmans S, Hamami F, et al. Relationship of genotype, phenotype, and treatment in dopa-responsive dystonia: MDSGene review. Mov Disord 2021;2022:237–252.
63. Yang H, Chen S, Shen J, Chen Y, Lai M, Chen L, Fang S. Safety and efficacy of botulinum toxin type A in children with spastic cerebral palsy aged <2 Years: A systematic review. J Child Neurol 2023;38:454–465.
64. Yi YG, Kim K, Yi Y, Choi YA, Leigh JH, Bang MS. Botulinum toxin type A injection for cervical dystonia in adults with dyskinetic cerebral palsy. Toxins (Basel) 2018;10:203.
65. Zouvelou V, Yubero D, Apostolakopoulou L, Kokkinou E, Bilanakis M, Dalivigka Z, et al. The genetic etiology in cerebral palsy mimics: The results from a Greek tertiary care center. Eur J Paediatr Neurol 2019;23:427–437.

Chapter 17

Dystonia and the Paroxysmal Dyskinesias

INTRODUCTION

The paroxysmal dyskinesias (PxD) are a heterogenous group of disorders characterized by recurrent but transient periods of involuntary abnormal movements. They are both clinically and etiologically distinct from epilepsy. The episodes are intermittent, lasting from a few seconds or hours and, rarely, up to several days. They are frequently described by patients or caregivers as "attacks," often with identifiable triggers. These episodes may occur in an individual who is neurologically normal at baseline, or they may occur in an individual who has some neurological abnormalities at baseline. The limbs are the most frequently affected region of the body, sometimes a single limb or the ipsilateral upper and lower limb. Involvement may instead affect only the neck, trunk, face, tongue, or chin. They may also be more generalized in many body regions.

The PxD are considered here because dystonia is a frequent feature. Dystonia may be combined with other abnormal movements, most notably chorea, but occasionally also ballismus, tremor, myoclonus, or ataxia. Sometimes one of these other movement disorders may dominate. However, dystonia is often the most consistent movement abnormality, the dominant abnormality, or the only abnormality. For example, a review of 500 cases reported in the literature described a combination of dystonia and chorea in 66% and dystonia alone in 20%.[36] In another summary of 600 cases from a multicenter consortium devoted to PxD in China, 34% had a mixed movement disorder and 61% had only dystonia.[53] In series of cases reported from centers specializing in movement disorders, the proportion of cases with dystonia alone is even higher.[29,66]

The PxD are probably best viewed as clinical syndromes rather than specific disease entities. Numerous genes are now known to cause PxD, or PxD may be acquired from insults to the nervous system such as autoimmune or cerebrovascular disease. Although the PxD are rare, they are important to recognize because specific treatments are highly effective for certain subtypes.

BRIEF HISTORY

Scattered cases of potential PxD have been described repeatedly since the 1800s, but they were usually considered forms of epilepsy, with terms such as *striatal epilepsy*, *extrapyramidal epilepsy*, *subcortical epilepsy*, or *reflex epilepsy*.[38] In 1940, Mount and Reback introduced the term *paroxysmal choreoathetosis* to describe a non-epileptic movement disorder in a 23-year-old man with sudden episodes of "choreodystonia" that began in childhood.[87] There were 27 similarly affected family members spanning 5 generations, suggesting an inherited disorder. Attacks lasted 5 minutes to 2 hours, and they could be triggered by stress, alcohol, or coffee. Descriptions of similar cases followed, and the term *paroxysmal dystonic choreoathetosis* was later suggested.[97]

A subgroup of the initially described cases had a distinct phenotype. In these cases, attacks were shorter, ranging from a few seconds to 2 minutes. In addition, these attacks were triggered by sudden movement or startle. In 1968, Kertesz described seven additional cases and coined the term *paroxysmal kinesigenic choreoathetosis* to distinguish these cases from the other cases.[63] Although the term *choreoathetosis* was used, early reports often used the term *athetosis* as a synonym for dystonia, and many of his cases were described using terminology that would be considered dystonia today.[86,99]

In 1977, Lance reviewed 100 previously reported PxD cases and described a new family with a third type of PxD that was triggered not by sudden movement, but by lengthier periods of exercise.[69] Episodes had a duration that was intermediate between paroxysmal dystonic choreoathetosis or paroxysmal kinesigenic dyskinesia, usually 10 minutes to an hour. All the cases had dystonic postures as the major or the only feature. Lance used the term *dystonic seizures* because of the episodic nature of predominantly dystonic movements. Numerous subsequent cases were reported and the condition was later called *paroxysmal exertional dyskinesia*.[10,29,38]

For all the preceding syndromes, attacks of abnormal movements usually occurred during wakefulness and abated with rest or sleep. However, some cases had attacks when sleeping. These cases became known as *paroxysmal nocturnal dyskinesia* or *paroxysmal hypnogogic dyskinesia*. The abnormal movements in many of these cases were subsequently linked with epilepsy, so this subgroup was initially considered a subtype of epilepsy, not PxD.[29] However, more recent studies have indicated some of these cases may actually have non-epileptic PxD. They may have both epileptic seizures or PxD attacks at different times, or they share abnormalities in genes linked with other known PxD.

Numerous reviews of PxD have appeared over the years, and the descriptions of their phenotypes and etiologies have evolved as more has been learned. Exactly how to define PxD has evolved, too. Currently, the most commonly used nomenclature and classification plan comes from a large series describing 46 new cases along with a literature review.[29] They include *paroxysmal kinesigenic dyskinesia* (PKD, corresponding to paroxysmal kinesigenic choreoathetosis), *paroxysmal non-kinesigenic dyskinesia* (PNKD, corresponding to paroxysmal dystonic choreoathetosis), *paroxysmal exertional dyskinesia* (PED), and *paroxysmal nocturnal dyskinesia* (PND). However, there have been repeated calls for revision of definitions and classification,[8,9,29,34,38,81,127,129] so it is likely that terminology will continue to evolve as more is learned.

CLINICAL MANIFESTATIONS

Classic Phenotypes

The classic syndromes are clinically distinguished by a combination of factors including age at onset, attack triggers, frequency and duration of attacks, and whether attacks occur during sleep (Table 17.1). PKD typically arises in infants or early childhood, but it may rarely begin in teenagers or adults. There may be many attacks per day, sometimes more than 100. Attacks are short, often 10–60 seconds, although they may last for several minutes. Attacks are triggered by sudden movement and sometimes by startle.

In comparison, PNKD typically starts in the same age range as PKD, although attacks are longer and less frequent. Attacks usually last 20–120 minutes, although attacks lasting for days have been reported. The frequency ranges from several per day to less than one per month. Triggers include fatigue, stress, alcohol, coffee, and tea.

PED usually first begins in children who are older than those with PKD or PNKD and, not infrequently, in young adults. Since attacks are triggered by exercise, their frequency depends on the level of exertion. Typical durations are 15–60 minutes. PND refers to attacks that occur during sleep.

It is important to recognize that individual cases may not precisely match any of these

Table 17.1 **Classical phenotypes of paroxysmal dyskinesias**

Aspect	Paroxysmal kinesigenic dyskinesia	Paroxysmal non-kinesigenic dyskinesia	Paroxysmal exertional dyskinesia	Paroxysmal nocturnal dyskinesia
Abbreviation	PKD	PNKD	PED	PND
Age at onset	Infancy to 20 years	Infancy to early childhood	Early childhood to late adulthood	Infancy to childhood
Triggers	Sudden movement, startle	Fatigue, alcohol, coffee, tea	10+ minutes of continued activity	While sleeping or falling asleep
Attack frequency	Up to dozens per day	A few per day to a few per month	Depends on level of exertion	A few per day to a few per month
Attack duration (minutes)	<2	10–240	5–60	5–120
Treatments	Carbamazepine, phenobarbital, diphenylhydantoin	Benzodiazepines, occasionally psychostimulants or caffeine	Depends on cause	Benzodiazepines

This table shows the typical features, although many exceptions and overlap cases exist. Paroxysmal nocturnal dyskinesia is sometimes also called paroxysmal hypnogogic dyskinesia (PHD).

classic phenotypes. Some cases have clinical features that fall between two classic phenotypes. Others may have variable attacks, with some attacks fitting criteria for one type of PxD and other attacks fitting a different PxD. PND may occur among individuals with other PxD that occur while awake.

Overlap with Action Dystonia

The phenotypes of PxD have been reported for numerous conditions typically associated with more typical non-PxD phenotypes. Clinical distinctions between PxD and action dystonia can sometimes be hard to make. For example, dystonic hand movements in writer's cramp may appear only after writing for several minutes, suggestive of PED. Alternatively, abnormal hand movements may emerge suddenly when attempting to write or even immediately after assuming a writing posture. These phenomena may resemble PKD. However, these examples are probably best viewed as manifestations of action dystonia. For typical action dystonias, the same trigger reliably produces a similar dystonic movement, and dystonia usually abates within seconds when the triggering activity is stopped. In PxD, the same trigger on different occasions might or might not induce an attack, and the attack often continues when the triggering activity stops.

Among individuals with generalized dystonia at baseline, there may be sudden and extreme exacerbations. Transient exacerbations may be triggered by a specific posture or voluntary action; stress, such as pain or unrecognized urinary tract infection. Sometimes they emerge with no obvious trigger. For example, sudden and extreme transient periods of backward head jerking that may occur on a baseline of dyskinetic cerebral palsy may suggest a PxD.[98] Similarly, the transient but severely abnormal leg postures that may occur among individuals with inherited disorders with dystonia who try to walk may also suggest a PxD.[17] Among individuals with dopa-responsive dystonia, the diurnal variations in severity may cause a severely disabling gait disorder each evening, whereas walking during the daytime is normal. Perhaps the most extreme example is the "dystonic storm," a life-threatening exacerbation of the condition in an individual with pre-existing dystonia. Although these phenomena are sometimes described as PxD,[68] most of these examples are probably best viewed as fluctuations in the severity of pre-existing dystonia, not PxD.

There also are numerous examples of PxD phenotypes in inherited disorders where there is a predisposition to dystonia but little or no dystonia at baseline. Examples include dopa-responsive dystonia,[27,37,68] Parkinson disease,[64] and GLUT1 deficiency.[71,94] Problems may begin immediately upon standing (resembling PKD), or they may emerge slowly only after walking for an extended period (resembling PED). The emergence of dystonia when the baseline neurological condition is apparently normal may suggest PxD. Whether these examples should be labeled PxD or a transient emergence of dystonia among predisposed individuals without baseline dystonia is not always clear. These examples suggest phenomenological and etiological overlaps between action dystonia and PxD and that strict distinctions between them are not always clinically obvious.

Overlap with Other Episodic Disorders

Numerous other episodic neurological disorders sometimes have a phenotype that overlaps with PxD. For example, epilepsy is often characterized by transient motor abnormalities. Epilepsy can be readily recognized when there are recurrent clonic movements, but predominantly tonic movements with a torsional character may resemble PxD. A good example is the *faciobrachial dystonic seizure* associated with antineuronal antibodies (see Chapter 21, "Dystonia and Autoimmunity").[2,6] Electroencephalography (EEG) does not reveal epileptiform activity in PxD. In contrast, epileptic seizures are defined by abnormal EEG activity, although this activity may not always be detectable with surface electrodes. In addition, it is important to recognize that PxD and epilepsy are distinct disorders, but occasional cases may have both PxD and epileptic seizures occurring at different times.[35]

Transient periods of ataxia occur in the *episodic ataxias*. The episodic ataxias are similar to PxD, but the main motor abnormality is ataxia rather than dystonia. The episodic ataxias are sometimes difficult to discriminate from PxD, especially when attacks are not apparent during a clinic visit and described only in the history. Individuals may describe attacks in ways that make it hard to determine if the movement disorder is ataxia, dystonia, or chorea. Some individuals with episodic ataxia may have a mixed motor disorder in which ataxia and dystonia are combined. Historically, the nature of an attack relied on the history if it could not be observed directly. Nowadays, individuals can be asked to record their attacks on video and present them in the clinic. Occasionally, individuals who carry a gene linked with episodic ataxia have attacks that are dystonic rather than ataxic (see Chapter 14, "Dystonia and Ataxia").[127,129] In short, there are both phenomenological and etiological overlaps between the episodic ataxias and PxD.

Migraine is another episodic neurological disorder characterized predominantly by transient headache rather than abnormal movement. Some individuals with migraine also have the transient appearance of motor manifestations such as hemiplegia or monoplegia, ataxia, or dystonia.[127,129] Some genes typically linked with migraine may produce only the motor manifestations. The lack of a strict correlation between genes and phenotypes sometimes produces a confusing situation when an individual is diagnosed genetically with *familial hemiplegic migraine* yet the observed phenotype resembles episodic ataxia or PxD. A related disorder is *alternating hemiplegia of childhood*, where the genes often produce minor weakness combined with ataxia or dystonia, not paralysis. To avoid confusion in such cases, it may be preferable to label the disorder according to the responsible gene rather than the historically defined phenotype.

There are numerous other episodic disorders in which the motor abnormalities resemble PxD. These other disorders historically were given distinct labels which are still in use today. Examples include benign paroxysmal torticollis of infancy, paroxysmal head shaking, paroxysmal lingual dystonia, paroxysmal orthostatic dystonia, shivering or shuddering attacks, limb-shaking attacks, hereditary geniospasm, hyperekplexia, and others. Occasionally, a single gene can be linked with PxD and one of these other disorders. Because of both phenotypic and etiologic overlap, it seems feasible that some of these conditions are related.

ETIOLOGIES

Genetic Causes

Pathogenic variants in many unrelated genes can cause PxD, and more genes continue to be found. The PxD phenotype is typical of certain genes described below and depicted in Figure 17.1. For many other genes, the more common phenotype is not PxD, but PxD may occasionally occur.

PRRT2 encodes the proline-rich transmembrane protein 2. It was the first gene to be linked with PxD.[23,122] *PRRT2* is responsible for several

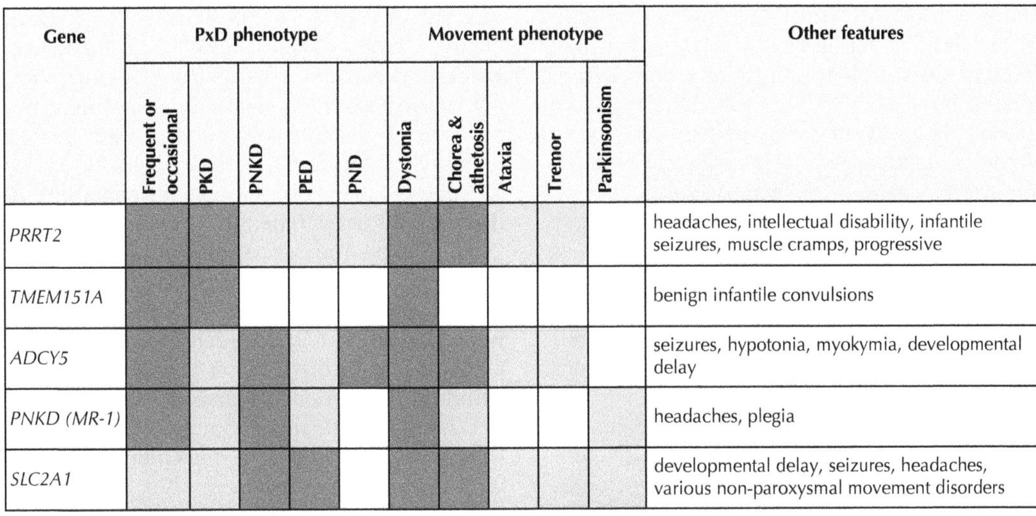

Figure 17.1. Frequency of the paroxysmal dyskinesia phenotypes associated with specific genes. Dark blue indicates the item is common, light blue indicates the feature is occasional, and empty indicates absent or rare. Note that dystonia is the most common movement abnormality for all these genes.

distinct phenotypes. In one large series of 1,444 cases, 39% had PKD, 42% had benign familial infantile epilepsy, and 14% had the syndrome of infantile convulsions combined with choreoathetosis.[32] Rarely, *PRRT2* may be associated with other PxD phenotypes, episodic ataxia, migraine with or without hemiplegia, or benign torticollis of infancy. Currently, *PRRT2* remains the most common gene found for PKD, accounting for a substantial proportion of cases in both Asians and Caucasians.[36,44,53,66,79] Inheritance is autosomal dominant, but sporadic mutations are common, and about half of affected individuals do not have a family history. Individuals usually have a normal baseline, although there may be a history of benign infantile epilepsy. Attacks are triggered by movement or startle, although some may also be triggered by stress or exertion. Attacks occur only rarely with sleep. The predominant movement abnormality during an attack is dystonia, sometimes combined with chorea. Involvement may affect all limbs bilaterally, it may be asymmetric or affect only the ipsilateral arm and leg, or it may affect a single limb. Affected individuals often have many attacks per day, most lasting less than a minute. Approximately half of the cases describe a sensory aura before an attack, and some individuals can predict when they are particularly susceptible to attacks. Onset is usually in early childhood and only rarely in adults. The frequency of attacks decreases with age, and attacks often remit entirely by the third or fourth decade. Anticonvulsants that block sodium channels (especially carbamazepine and oxcarbazepine) are highly effective for controlling attacks, often at very low doses.

A related condition is microdeletion of 16p11.2, a syndrome that results from this region of the genome being particularly vulnerable. This region encompasses *PRRT2*, but the clinical consequences are often broader because of deletion of nearby genes. The syndrome is typically associated with baseline abnormalities such as mild developmental delay, autistic features, and occasionally mild underlying dystonia. Some cases also have PKD, or they may rarely have PKD without other features.[25,120]

Variants in *TMEM151A*, which encodes a transmembrane protein of unknown function, are also linked with PKD.[112] These cases have a slightly different phenotype compared with *PRRT2*. Problems associated with *TMEM151A* tend to emerge in older children, attacks are shorter, and a history of benign infantile epilepsy is less likely.[24] This gene was found when studying a cohort of individuals with PxD who did not harbor *PRRT2* variants. It has not been extensively studied in cohorts with other phenotypes, so the full spectrum of phenotypes may expand as more cases are identified.

PNKD (formerly *MR-1* for myofibrillogenesis regulator protein 1) has been linked predominantly with PNKD, and only rarely with PKD or PED.[70,96] This gene is a very rare cause of PxD, and most available information comes from isolated families.[13,21,39,45,52,73,95,107,124] Inheritance is autosomal dominant. Most individuals have a normal baseline with attacks triggered by alcohol, coffee, stress, or fatigue. Attacks reflect a combination of dystonia and chorea, and they may last 30 minutes to several hours. Onset is in childhood, and the duration and frequency of attacks decrease with age. Onset in adolescence or adulthood is very rare. Carbamazepine is not usually effective, but clonazepam and other benzodiazepines may be useful.

ADCY5 has been linked with varied abnormal movements that include various combinations of chorea, dystonia, myoclonus, hypotonia, ataxia, weakness, and a gait disorder.[15,20,22,83] Motor delay is common, and onset of abnormal movements occurs usually in infancy or childhood. Approximately 90% of individuals have a baseline movement disorder. The severity of the baseline problems varies considerably, and more than 90% also have significant fluctuations in severity. Very prominent fluctuations result in a phenotype suggestive of PxD, but attacks do not always fit the classic PxD phenotypes. Most attacks resemble PNKD, but PKD and PED may also occur. Sometimes different PxD phenotypes may occur in the same individual during different attacks. Attacks may last only a few seconds, or they may last for several hours. Stress and anxiety may trigger attacks, although spontaneous attacks also occur. A helpful clue to the diagnosis is worsening with drowsiness or attempts to sleep, or occurrence during sleep, phenomena that are uncommon with other PxD genes.[4,82] Another helpful feature is facial dyskinesias, which are common with *ADCY5* but uncommon with other PxD genes.

There are numerous other genes that typically cause non-PxD phenotypes, but they may occasionally produce a PxD phenotype. Table 17.2 provides a list of these genes, along with their common phenotypes and occasional association with a PxD phenotype. For example, *PRKN* is typically associated with early-onset Parkinson disease often with dystonia, and *GCH1* is typically associated with dopa-responsive dystonia. Both genes have occasionally been reported to cause the PED phenotype. Other genes are associated with more severe phenotypes such as early-onset encephalopathy, movement disorders, and seizures. Examples include *ECHS1* and the genes associated with pyruvate dehydrogenase deficiency, which typically cause Leigh syndrome. Milder phenotypes resembling PxD occasionally occur with these genes. Finally, some genes have been linked with quite varied clinical phenotypes including *ATP1A3*, *CACNA1A*, and *SLC2A1*. Occasionally, these genes can also produce a PxD phenotype, for example the paroxysmal dystonic arm posturing associated with *ATP1A3*.[5] Among these genes, *SLC2A1* deserves special mention. Although PxD is not a "classic" phenotype for GLUT1-deficiency syndromes associated with this gene, it is one of the more common genes found in large genetic studies of PxD cohorts.[36] The more common phenotypes of GLUT-deficiency include developmental delay with intellectual or motor disability, seizures of various types, non-PxD movement disorders (typically spasticity and ataxia), or various combinations of these problems.[47,94]

Acquired Causes

Although the subgrouping of PxD into its classic phenotypes has been driven largely by cases with a known or presumed genetic cause, there are numerous reports of PxD phenotypes associated with acquired insults to the nervous system (Table 17.3). Acquired causes may be associated with attacks that resemble one of the classic PxD phenotypes, but episodes are more often mixed. Acquired cases of PxD also tend to occur more often in older adults.

Two overlapping reports described the largest series of acquired PxD, with 20 original cases and a review 130 previously cases.[11,12] The most common causes were demyelinating diseases such as multiple sclerosis, transient cerebral ischemia or stroke, trauma, and endocrine disorders. Since this summary, there has been increasing recognition of rare autoimmune causes[34] including acute disseminated encephalomyelitis, neuromyelitis optica spectrum disorders, systemic lupus erythematosus, specific neuronal autoantibodies, Hashimoto encephalopathy, antiphospholipid syndrome, and cryopyrin-associated periodic syndrome. Less common acquired causes may include anoxic brain injury, kernicterus, encephalitis, and neoplasm (Table 17.3).

The PxD phenotype is especially well-recognized in multiple sclerosis and neuromyelitis optica spectrum disorders. It has been described using a variety of terms including *tonic*

Table 17.2 **Genes occasionally associated with paroxysmal dyskinesias**

Gene	Disorder(s)	Typical phenotype(s)	Paroxysmal dyskinesia(s)
ALDH5A1[92,93]	Succinic semialdehyde dehydrogenase deficiency	Developmental delay, intellectual disability, behavioral problems, hypotonia, ataxia, seizures	PED[72]
ATP1A2[30,117]	AHC, FHM, developmental epileptic encephalopathy	Hemiplegia with or without migraine, developmental delay, epilepsy	BPTI[26]
ATP1A3[51,118]	RDP, AHC, CAPOS	Although three classic phenotypes are recognized, many cases have phenotypes that are overlapping, partial or otherwise atypical	PNKD[130]
ATP7B[74,109]	Wilson disease	Childhood onset liver disease and movement disorder, usually with dystonia	PKD[65]
BCKD complex[16]	Maple syrup urine disease	Spectrum of severity ranging from early encephalopathy to mild developmental delay, sometimes with seizures and various movement disorders	PNKD[110]
CACNA1A[55]	EA2, SCA6, FHM	Although three classic phenotypes are recognized, many cases have partial or overlapping phenotypes or variant phenotypes	PNKD, BPTI[26,105,106,119]
ECHS1[76,90]	Leigh syndrome; mitochondrial short-chain enoyl-CoA hydratase deficiency	Infantile encephalopathy with global delay and regression, dystonia, hypotonia, opisthotonos, chorea, ataxia, tremor, and abnormal MRI.	PED[75,76,89]
FGF14[116]	SCA12	Progressive and/or episodic ataxia, tremor	PNKD, BPTI[54,104]
GCH1[123]	Dopa-responsive dystonia	Childhood-onset dystonia, sometimes with parkinsonism	PED[27,68]
GNAO1[100]	Infantile epileptic encephalopathy type 17	Infantile epileptic encephalopathy, developmental delay and/or hyperkinetic movement disorder	PNKD[67,100]
HPRT1[56]	Lesch-Nyhan disease	Severe generalized dystonia, intellectual disability, self-injurious behaviors	PKD[17]
KCNA1[91]	Episodic ataxia type 1	Ataxia, myokymia, and/or epilepsy	PKD, BPTI[54,60,125]
KCNMA1[84]	*KCNMA1*-associated channelopathies, Liang-Wang syndrome	Epilepsy and/or developmental delay sometimes with cerebellar atrophy and often with various movement disorders	PNKD[14,31,126]
PDGFB[3]	Familial brain calcification	Adult-onset parkinsonism, chorea, ataxia, dystonia	PNKD[121]
PDHA1, PDHX, DLAT[28]	Pyruvate dehydrogenase complex deficiency	Leigh syndrome, early-onset encephalopathy with lactic acidosis, episodic ataxia or weakness	PNKD, PED[18,50,78]
PRKN[59]	Parkinson disease	Early-onset parkinsonism, often with dystonia	PED[64]
SCN8A[57]	Spectrum of epilepsy and early developmental phenotypes	Early onset epilepsy sometimes with developmental delay or encephalopathy, or infantile seizures with choreoathetosis	PNKD, PKD[43]
SLC16A[48,77]	MCT8 deficiency	Global developmental delay with hypokinesia, hypotonia, dystonia or spasticity	PKD[77]
SLC2A1[94]	GLUT1-related syndromes	Glut1 deficiency syndromes	PED, PNKD[108]
SLC20A2[3]	Familial brain calcification	Adult-onset parkinsonism, dystonia, ataxia	PNKD[128]
SLC3A1 or SLC7A9[33,61]	Cystinuria	Nephrolithiasis, sometimes intellectual disability or movement disorders	PNKD[19]
WASH5C (also *KIAA0196*)[46,102]	SPG8	Progressive spastic paraplegia	PED[88]

Further details and citations can be found in prior reviews.[34]

Abbreviations: AHC, alternating hemiplegia of childhood; BCKD, branched chain alpha-keto dehydrogenase; CAPOS, syndrome of cerebellar ataxia, areflexia, pes cavus, optic atrophy, and sensorineural hearing loss; BPTI, benign paroxysmal torticollis of infancy; EA2, episodic ataxia type 2; FHM, familial hemiplegic migraine; MCT8, monocarboxylate transporter type 8; RDP, rapid onset dystonia parkinsonism; SCA, spinocerebellar ataxia; SPG, spastic paraplegia.

Table 17.3 **Causes for acquired paroxysmal dyskinesias**

Category	Reported examples
Autoimmune	Acute disseminated encephalomyelitis
	Anti-caspr2 syndrome
	Anti-phospholipid syndrome
	Cryopyrin-associated periodic syndrome
	Hashimoto encephalitis
	Multiple sclerosis
	Neuromyelitis optica
	Parry-Rhomberg syndrome
	Voltage-gated calcium channel syndrome
Cerebrovascular	Carotid atherosclerosis
	Moyamoya disease
	Stroke
	Transient ischemic attack
Endocrine	Hyperglycemia
	Hyperthyroidism
	Hypocalcemia
	Hypoglycemia
	Hypothyroidism
Others	Basal ganglia calcification
	Brain tumor
	Cerebral palsy
	Viral encephalitis
	Kernicterus
	Neurodegenerative disease
	Trauma (central or peripheral)

Further details and citations can be found in prior reviews.[11,34]

spasms, *extensor spasms*, or *tonic seizures*. One systematic survey of 83 individuals with multiple sclerosis found PxD to be the most common of all types of movement disorders.[114] Another survey found PxD in 11 of 64 individuals (17%) with multiple sclerosis.[103] The PxD in multiple sclerosis most closely resemble PKD because episodes are usually short and frequent, and they can be triggered by voluntary movement. However, unlike typical PKD, episodes in multiple sclerosis can also be triggered by sensory stimulation or hyperventilation, and they are often painful. Episodes may respond to medications that suppress ephaptic transmission from demyelination, such as carbamazepine or oxcarbazepine.

Cerebrovascular disease is another well-recognized cause for PxD, including transient limb-shaking attacks. It may reflect a delayed consequence of stroke in a variety of regions including the thalamus, putamen, and brainstem. Ischemia or hypoperfusion may also cause PxD, including orthostatic PxD. The underlying cause may be Moyamoya disease or critical carotid atherosclerosis, where carotid endarterectomy may eliminate the problem.

Trauma to the central or peripheral nervous system has also been reported to cause PxD. A causal association can be difficult to establish because attacks may emerge weeks or months following the trauma. The movement disorder may be associated with prominent autonomic signs, or it may spread from the initially affected areas to adjacent ones (see Chapter 20, "Dystonia and Trauma").

The PxD phenotype can also rarely be seen with a variety of acquired endocrine abnormalities including hyperglycemia or hypoglycemia, and hyperthyroidism or hypothyroidism. In transient hypoglycemia due to insulinoma, episodes are often associated with autonomic features such as sweating, and they may be triggered by fasting. These conditions are important to recognize because correction of the underlying metabolic abnormality can prevent further attacks.

DIAGNOSIS

Workup

For early-onset PxD, the history can be useful to differentiate among the common phenotypes by delineating attack frequency, duration, triggers, and whether abnormal movements occur with sleep. The exam is useful to identify any potential baseline abnormalities. If attacks are not observed directly in the clinic, the family can be asked to bring a video recording.

Brain MRI can be helpful to identify some of the more common acquired causes of PxD, such as multiple sclerosis. Bloodwork focusing on endocrinopathies or autoimmune disorders can be useful, too, if the history and exam are suggestive. A family history of PxD or a related condition (episodic ataxia, migraine, recurrent unexplained hemiplegia) may point to an inherited cause, but many genetic cases are sporadic. Some experts advocate starting the genetic evaluation only with the more common genes, but the wide variety of potential genes and continued reports of new genes may require broader clinical exome sequencing.

For adult-onset PxD, the workup must focus more on potential acquired causes, including demyelination, endocrinopathy, and cerebral ischemia. A large proportion of cases of adult-onset PxD are psychogenic, as described further in Chapter 25, "Psychogenic (Functional) Dystonia."[41] Most genetically determined PxD begin in childhood, but adult-onset cases may occur. Genetic testing may therefore still be warranted especially if there is a family history of PxD or a related condition.

Differential Diagnosis

When confronted with an individual with episodic abnormal movements, epileptic seizures are often the first concern. Some useful clinical clues for PxD rather than epileptic seizure include the more varied types of abnormal movements in PxD, lack of recurrent clonic movements, often lengthy attacks with preserved sensorium, and lack of post-attack confusion. The EEG can be very useful to discriminate epileptic events from PxD. However, the EEG can produce false-negative and false-positive results. The EEG may fail to detect epileptiform discharges, especially when the abnormal movements are focal, and particularly when the epileptic focus is deep in the temporal or frontal lobe. Conversely, the EEG may detect epileptiform activity that does not correlate with the abnormal movements because some individuals may have both epilepsy and PxD. Because of false negatives and false positives, the EEG must be interpreted with caution.

Another frequent concern when confronted with an individual with episodic abnormal movements is a psychogenic process. Many individuals with PxD are first misdiagnosed with *non-epileptic seizures* or *pseudoseizures*, terms that often imply a psychogenic disorder. Conversely, psychogenic movement disorders are often paroxysmal.[41] Several clues may help to identify a psychogenic paroxysmal movement disorder.[40] Most of the inherited PxD begin in early childhood or the teenage years, while individuals with psychogenic paroxysmal movement disorders tend to be older. Individuals with psychogenic paroxysmal movement disorders also have more varied attacks in terms of their frequency, duration, and movement phenomenology. A temporal course of sudden onset of multiple daily attacks lasting days or weeks at a time, sometimes interspersed with days or weeks of complete remission, should raise suspicion for a psychogenic etiology. Individuals with psychogenic paroxysmal movement disorders also may have atypical triggers, unusual tricks for stopping attacks, or suggestibility. A search for additional unexplained somatic symptoms or psychogenic signs can be helpful.

Acute dystonic reactions to drugs are often paroxysmal, and they may be recurrent (see Chapter 19, "Dystonias Induced by Medications, Illicit Drugs and Environmental Exposures").[111] The diagnosis can usually be made by obtaining a history of exposure to a responsible medication or illicit drug. Acute dystonic reactions usually respond to diphenhydramine or benzodiazepines, while PxD rarely respond to these interventions.

PND may be mistaken for parasomnias such as rapid eye movement (REM) behavior disorder. However, the genetic disorders causing PxD with sleep typically begin in young children while REM behavior disorders usually begins in older adults. In addition, abnormal movements in PND often occur when first trying to sleep or during non-REM sleep, so a polysomnogram may be useful to discriminate them.[4,82]

Tics can come in "attacks" or a single complex tic may last a long time. These phenomena may resemble PKD. Tics can usually be discriminated from PKD by the lack of typical triggers and voluntary suppressibility.[7,42] Premonitory sensations may cause confusion because they are common in tics and may also occur in PxD. However, premonitory sensations in PxD are not typically described as an urge. In rare cases, PxD may be combined with tics.

TREATMENT

Counseling

Counseling and education play an important role in treatment. The PxD are rare and not well recognized. The diagnosis is often delayed for many years, individuals may be first misdiagnosed with epilepsy or a psychogenic disorder, and they may have tried many therapies without benefit. As a result, many individuals become skeptical that the medical system can understand their problem or help them. Anxiety and social phobia are common in PxD because attacks are often embarrassing. It can be very helpful to acknowledge the diagnostic odyssey and offer counseling as needed.

Education regarding the etiologies and the natural history of PxD can also be useful. Some of them, particularly the genetically determined PKD, resolve spontaneously as children get older. Others may be more persistent or even progressive. Counseling is valuable to set expectations. Education regarding known triggers can also be helpful. While many triggers are impossible to avoid, some can be managed. For example, avoidance of long periods of fasting can reduce periods of hypoglycemia that may trigger attacks associated with *GLUT1*. Avoidance of stress and anxiety can also be a goal for many.

Medications

Certain medications can be highly effective for specific subtypes of PxD. Although PKD is not considered a type of epilepsy, it can be very responsive to certain anticonvulsants that block sodium channels, such as carbamazepine, oxcarbazepine, phenytoin, or phenobarbital. Attacks may be controlled with very low doses, for example 50 mg/d carbamazepine. Sometimes higher doses are required. Other anticonvulsants have limited benefit.

Individuals with PED related to Parkinson disease or dopa-responsive dystonia often respond to levodopa. The PED associated with GLUT1-related disorders may respond to a ketogenic diet[58,71] or triheptanoin.[49,85] Although caffeine and tea may trigger PNKD, caffeine can suppress the attacks observed in *ADCY5*-related dyskinesias.[80,101] Individuals with PNKD are the most difficult to treat. Some of them respond to benzodiazepines, anticholinergics, baclofen, levodopa, vigabatrin, or other drugs often used to treat dystonia. PNKD associated with variants in *KCNMA1* may respond to amphetamine-related stimulants.[62,126]

Surgery

Severe and medically refractory PxD may respond to deep brain stimulation surgery (see Chapter 31, "Surgical Treatments for Dystonia").[1,113] There are isolated reports of success for *ADCY5*,[20] *GNAO1*,[67] and *ATP1A3*,[130] and PNKD without an identified molecular cause. However· experience with surgering in PxD remains limited.[115]

SUMMARY AND FUTURE PROSPECTS

The PxD are a growing group of heterogenous disorders characterized by transient and recurrent episodes of abnormal movements. Attacks of abnormal movements historically were called *dyskinesias* because of their mixed phenomenology, but dystonia is a frequent and often dominant feature.

The phenotype of PxD sometimes overlaps with action dystonia, and it is frequently mistaken for epilepsy. The phenotype also shares some similarities with other intermittent conditions, such as the episodic ataxias and complicated migraine syndromes. Dystonia may occur in these other episodic disorders, too, but it is not usually a defining feature.

There are numerous causes for PxD, both inherited and acquired. A thorough workup can often disclose a cause. Knowing the etiology is valuable because effective treatments are available for specific subtypes. Genes responsible for

PxD have only recently been identified, and more continue to be identified. As is often the case for genetic disorders, the discovery of new genes broadens understanding of the spectrum of phenotypes. The same phenotype may result from different genes, and specific genes may cause different phenotypes, both PxD and non-PxD. It seems likely that the definitions and classification of this group of disorders will be revised as more as learned.

REFERENCES

1. Artusi CA, Dwivedi A, Romagnolo A, Bortolani S, Marsili L, Imbalzano G, et al. Differential response to pallidal deep brain stimulation among monogenic dystonias: Systematic review and meta-analysis. J Neurol Neurosurg Psychiatry 2020;91:426–433.
2. Baizabal-Carvallo JF, Jankovic J. Autoimmune and paraneoplastic movement disorders: An update. J Neurol Sci 2018;385:175–184.
3. Balck A, Schaake S, Kuhnke NS, Domingo A, Madoev H, Margolesky J, et al. Genotype-phenotype relations in primary familial brain calcification: Systematic MDSGene review. Mov Disord 2021;36:2468–2480.
4. Balint B, Antelmi E, Mencacci NE, Batla A, Eriksson SH, Walker MC, et al. Oculomotor apraxia and disrupted sleep with nocturnal ballistic bouts in ADCY5-related disease. Parkinsonism Relat Disord 2018;54:103–106.
5. Balint B, Stephen CD, Udani V, Sankhla CS, Barad NH, Lang AE, Bhatia KP. Paroxysmal asymmetric dystonic arm posturing: A less recognized but characteristic manifestation of ATP1A3-related disease. Mov Disord Clin Pract 2019;6:312–315.
6. Balint B, Vincent A, Meinck HM, Irani SR, Bhatia KP. Movement disorders with neuronal antibodies: Syndromic approach, genetic parallels and pathophysiology. Brain 2018;141:13–36.
7. Balint B, Wiethoff S, Martino D, Del Gamba C, Latorre A, Ganos C, et al. Quick flicks: Association of paroxysmal kinesigenic dyskinesia and tics. Mov Disord Clin Pract 2018;5:317–320.
8. Bhatia KP. The paroxysmal dyskinesias. J Neurol 1999;246:149–155.
9. Bhatia KP. Paroxysmal dyskinesias. Mov Disord 2011;26:1157–1165.
10. Bhatia KP, Soland VL, Bhatt MH, Quinn NP, Marsden CD. Paroxysmal exercise induced dystonia: Eight new sporadic cases and a review of the literature. Mov Disord 1997;12:1007–1012.
11. Blakeley J, Jankovic J. Secondary causes of paroxysmal dyskinesia. Adv Neurol 2002;89:401–420.
12. Blakeley J, Jankovic J. Secondary paroxysmal dyskinesias. Mov Disord 2002;17:726–734.
13. Bruno MK, Hallett M, Gwinn-Hardy K, Sorensen B, Considine E, Tucker S, et al. Clinical evaluation of idiopathic paroxysmal kinesigenic dyskinesia: New diagnostic criteria. Neurology 2004;63:2280–2287.
14. Buckley C, Williams J, Munteanu T, King M, Park SM, Meredith AL, Lynch T. Status dystonicus, oculogyric crisis and paroxysmal dyskinesia in a 25 year-old woman with a novel KCNMA1 variant, K457E. Tremor Other Hyperkinet Mov (N Y) 2020;10:49.
15. Carecchio M, Mencacci NE, Iodice A, Pons R, Panteghini C, Zorzi G, et al. ADCY5-related movement disorders: Frequency, disease course and phenotypic variability in a cohort of paediatric patients. Parkinsonism Relat Disord 2017;41:37–43.
16. Carecchio M, Schneider SA, Chan H, Lachmann R, Lee PJ, Murphy E, Bhatia KP. Movement disorders in adult surviving patients with maple syrup urine disease. Mov Disord 2011;26:1324–1328.
17. Casa-Fages B, Perez-Sanchez JR, Grandas F. Paroxysmal kinesigenic dystonia in a Lesch-Nyhan disease variant. Mov Disord Clin Pract 2014;1:123–124.
18. Castiglioni C, Verrigni D, Okuma C, Diaz A, Alvarez K, Rizza T, et al. Pyruvate dehydrogenase deficiency presenting as isolated paroxysmal exercise induced dystonia successfully reversed with thiamine supplementation. Case report and mini-review. Eur J Paediatr Neurol 2015;19:497–503.
19. Cavanaugh NPC, Bicknell J, Howard F. Cystinuria with mental retardation and paroxysmal dyskinesia in 2 brothers. Arch Dis Child 1974;49:662–664.
20. Chang FC, Westenberger A, Dale RC, Smith M, Pall HS, Perez-Duenas B, et al. Phenotypic insights into ADCY5-associated disease. Mov Disord 2016;31:1033–1040.
21. Chen DH, Matsushita M, Rainier S, Meaney B, Tisch L, Feleke A, et al. Presence of alanine-to-valine substitutions in myofibrillogenesis regulator 1 in paroxysmal nonkinesigenic dyskinesia: Confirmation in 2 kindreds. Arch Neurol 2005;62:597–600.
22. Chen DH, Meneret A, Friedman JR, Korvatska O, Gad A, Bonkowski ES, et al. ADCY5-related dyskinesia: Broader spectrum and genotype-phenotype correlations. Neurology 2015;85:2026–2035.
23. Chen WJ, Lin Y, Xiong ZQ, Wei W, Ni W, Tan GH, et al. Exome sequencing identifies truncating mutations in PRRT2 that cause paroxysmal kinesigenic dyskinesia. Nat Genet 2011;43:1252–1255.
24. Chen YL, Chen DF, Li HF, Wu ZY. Features differ between paroxysmal kinesigenic dyskinesia patients with PRRT2 and TMEM151A variants. Mov Disord 2022;37:608–613.
25. Chen YL, Chen DF, Ke HZ, Zhao SY, Li HF, Wu ZY. Paroxysmal kinesigenic dyskinesia caused by 16p11.2 microdeletion and related clinical features. Neurol Genet 2022;8:e659.
26. Cuenca-Leon E, Corominas R, Fernandez-Castillo N, Volpini V, Del Toro M, Roig M, et al. Genetic analysis of 27 Spanish patients with hemiplegic migraine, basilar-type migraine and childhood periodic syndromes. Cephalalgia 2008;28:1039–1047.
27. Dale RC, Melchers A, Fung VS, Grattan-Smith P, Houlden H, Earl J. Familial paroxysmal exercise-induced dystonia: Atypical presentation of autosomal dominant GTP-cyclohydrolase 1 deficiency. Dev Med Child Neurol 2010;52:583–586.
28. De Meirleir L. Disorders of pyruvate metabolism. Handb Clin Neurol 2013;113:1667–1673.
29. Demirkiran M, Jankovic J. Paroxysmal dyskinesias: Clinical features and classification. Ann Neurol 1995;38:571–579.
30. Di Stefano V, Rispoli MG, Pellegrino N, Graziosi A, Rotondo E, Napoli C, et al. Diagnostic and therapeutic

aspects of hemiplegic migraine. J Neurol Neurosurg Psychiatry 2020;91:764–771.
31. Du W, Bautista JF, Yang H, Diez-Sampedro A, You SH, Wang L, et al. Calcium-sensitive potassium channelopathy in human epilepsy and paroxysmal movement disorder. Nature Genet 2005;37:733–738.
32. Ebrahimi-Fakhari D, Saffari A, Westenberger A, Klein C. The evolving spectrum of PRRT2-associated paroxysmal diseases. Brain 2015;138:3476–3495.
33. Ekinci B, Apaydin H, Vural M, Ozekmekci S. Two siblings with homocystinuria presenting with dystonia and parkinsonism. Mov Disord 2004;19:962–964.
34. Erro R, Bhatia KP. Unravelling of the paroxysmal dyskinesias. J Neurol Neurosurg Psychiatry 2019;90:227–234.
35. Erro R, Bhatia KP, Espay AJ, Striano P. The epileptic and nonepileptic spectrum of paroxysmal dyskinesias: Channelopathies, synaptopathies, and transportopathies. Mov Disord 2017;32:310–318.
36. Erro R, Sheerin UM, Bhatia KP. Paroxysmal dyskinesias revisited: A review of 500 genetically proven cases and a new classification. Mov Disord 2014;29:1108–1116.
37. Fahn S. Clinical variants of idiopathic torsion dystonia. J Neurol Neurosurg Psychiatry 1989;Suppl:96–100.
38. Fahn S, Marsden CD. The paroxysmal dyskinesias. In: Marsden CD, Fahn S, eds. *Movement Disorders 3*. Butterworth-Heinemann, 1994: 310–347.
39. Friedman A, Zakrzewska-Pniewska B, Domitrz I, Lee HY, Ptacek L, Kwiecinski H. Paroxysmal non-kinesigenic dyskinesia caused by the mutation of MR-1 in a large Polish kindred. Eur Neurol 2009;61:39–41.
40. Ganos C, Aguirregomozcorta M, Batla A, Stamelou M, Schwingenschuh P, Munchau A, et al. Psychogenic paroxysmal movement disorders: Clinical features and diagnostic clues. Parkinsonism Relat Disord 2014;20:41–46.
41. Ganos C, Edwards MJ, Bhatia KP. The phenomenology of functional (psychogenic) dystonia. Mov Disord Clin Pract 2014;1:36–44.
42. Ganos C, Mencacci N, Gardiner A, Erro R, Batla A, Houlden H, Bhatia KP. Paroxysmal kinesigenic dyskinesia may be misdiagnosed in co-occurring Gilles de la Tourette syndrome. Mov Disord Clin Pract 2014;1:84–86.
43. Gardella E, Becker F, Moller RS, Schubert J, Lemke JR, Larsen LH, et al. Benign infantile seizures and paroxysmal dyskinesia caused by an SCN8A mutation. Ann Neurol 2016;79:428–436.
44. Gardiner AR, Jaffer F, Dale RC, Labrum R, Erro R, Meyer E, et al. The clinical and genetic heterogeneity of paroxysmal dyskinesias. Brain 2015;138:3567–3580.
45. Ghezzi D, Viscomi C, Ferlini A, Gualandi F, Mereghetti P, DeGrandis D, Zeviani M. Paroxysmal non-kinesigenic dyskinesia is caused by mutations of the MR-1 mitochondrial targeting sequence. Hum Mol Genet 2009;18:1058–1064.
46. Ginanneschi F, D'Amore A, Barghigiani M, Tessa A, Rossi A, Santorelli FM. SPG8 mutations in Italian families: Clinical data and literature review. Neurol Sci 2020;41:699–703.
47. Gras D, Roze E, Caillet S, Meneret A, Doummar D, Billette de Villemeur T, et al. GLUT1 deficiency syndrome: An update. Rev Neurol 2014;170:91–99.
48. Groeneweg S, van Geest FS, Abaci A, Alcantud A, Ambegaonkar GP, Armour CM, et al. Disease characteristics of MCT8 deficiency: An international, retrospective, multicentre cohort study. Lancet Diabetes Endocrinol 2020;8:594–605.
49. Hainque E, Gras D, Meneret A, Atencio M, Luton MP, Barbier M, et al. Long-term follow-up in an open-label trial of triheptanoin in GLUT1 deficiency syndrome: A sustained dramatic effect. J Neurol Neurosurg Psychiatry 2019;90:1291–1293.
50. Head RA, Brown RM, Zolkipli Z, Shahdadpuri R, King MD, Clayton PT, Brown GK. Clinical and genetic spectrum of pyruvate dehydrogenase deficiency: Dihydrolipoamide acetyltransferase (E2) deficiency. Ann Neurol 2005;58:234–241.
51. Heinzen EL, Arzimanoglou A, Brashear A, Clapcote SJ, Gurrieri F, Goldstein DB, et al. Distinct neurological disorders with ATP1A3 mutations. Lancet Neurol 2014;13:503–514.
52. Hempelmann A, Kumar S, Muralitharan S, Sander T. Myofibrillogenesis regulator 1 gene (MR-1) mutation in an Omani family with paroxysmal nonkinesigenic dyskinesia. Neurosci Lett 2006;402:118–120.
53. Huang XJ, Wang SG, Guo XN, Tian WT, Zhan FX, Zhu ZY, et al. The phenotypic and genetic spectrum of paroxysmal kinesigenic dyskinesia in China. Mov Disord 2020;35:1428–1437.
54. Humbertclaude V, Krams B, Nogue E, Nagot N, Annequin D, Tourniaire B, et al. Benign paroxysmal torticollis, benign paroxysmal vertigo, and benign tonic upward gaze are not benign disorders. Dev Med Child Neurol 2018;60:1256–1263.
55. Indelicato E, Boesch S. From genotype to phenotype: Expanding the clinical spectrum of CACNA1A variants in the era of next generation sequencing. Front Neurol 2021;12:639994.
56. Jinnah HA, Visser JE, Harris JC, Verdu A, Larovere L, Ceballos-Picot I, et al. Delineation of the motor disorder of Lesch-Nyhan disease. Brain 2006;129:1201–1217.
57. Johannesen KM, Liu Y, Koko M, Gjerulfsen CE, Sonnenberg L, Schubert J, et al. Genotype-phenotype correlations in SCN8A-related disorders reveal prognostic and therapeutic implications. Brain 2022;145:2991–3009.
58. Kass HR, Winesett SP, Bessone SK, Turner Z, Kossoff EH. Use of dietary therapies amongst patients with GLUT1 deficiency syndrome. Seizure 2016;35:83–87.
59. Kasten M, Hartmann C, Hampf J, Schaake S, Westenberger A, Vollstedt EJ, et al. Genotype-phenotype relations for the Parkinson's disease genes Parkin, PINK1, DJ1: MDSGene systematic review. Mov Disord 2018;33:730–741.
60. Kegele J, Kruger J, Koko M, Lange L, Marco Hernandez AV, Martinez F, et al. Genetics of paroxysmal dyskinesia: Novel variants corroborate the role of KCNA1 in paroxysmal dyskinesia and highlight the diverse phenotypic spectrum of KCNA1- and SLC2A1-related disorders. Front Neurol 2021;12:701351.
61. Kempster PA, Brenton DP, Gale AN, Stern GM. Dystonia in homocystinuria. J Neurol Neurosurg Psychiatry 1988;51:859–862.
62. Keros S, Heim J, Hakami W, Zohar-Dayan E, Ben-Zeev B, Grinspan Z, et al. Lisdexamfetamine therapy in paroxysmal non-kinesigenic dyskinesia associated with the KCNMA1-N999S variant. Mov Disord Clin Pract 2022;9:229–235.
63. Kertesz A. Paroxysmal kinesigenic choreoathetosis. An entity within the paroxysmal choreoathetosis syndrome. Description of 10 cases, including 1 autopsied. Neurology 1967;17:680–690.

64. Khan NL, Graham E, Critchley P, Schrag AE, Wood NW, Lees AJ, et al. Parkin disease: A phenotypic study of a large case series. Brain 2003;126:1279–1292.
65. Kim HJ, Yoon JH. A case of Wilson's disease presenting with paroxysmal dystonia. Neurol Sci 2017;38:1881–1882.
66. Kim SY, Lee JS, Kim WJ, Kim H, Choi SA, Lim BC, et al. Paroxysmal dyskinesia in children: From genes to the clinic. J Clin Neurol 2018;14:492–497.
67. Koy A, Cirak S, Gonzalez V, Becker K, Roujeau T, Milesi C, et al. Deep brain stimulation is effective in pediatric patients with GNAO1 associated severe hyperkinesia. J Neurol Sci 2018;391:31–39.
68. Kurian MA, Gissen P, Smith M, Heales S, Jr., Clayton PT. The monoamine neurotransmitter disorders: An expanding range of neurological syndromes. Lancet Neurol 2011;10:721–733.
69. Lance JW. Familial paroxysmal dystonic choreoathetosis and its differentiation from related syndromes. Ann Neurol 1977;2:285–293.
70. Lee HY, Xu Y, Hunag Y, Ahn AH, Auburger GWJ, Pandolfo M, et al. The gene for paroxysmal non-kinesigenic dyskinesia encodes an enzyme in a stress response pathway. Hum Mol Genet 2004;13:3161–3170.
71. Leen WG, Mewasingh L, Verbeek MM, Kamsteeg EJ, van de Warrenburg BP, Willemsen MA. Movement disorders in GLUT1 deficiency syndrome respond to the modified Atkins diet. Mov Disord 2013;28:1439–1442.
72. Leuzzi V, Di Sabato ML, Deodato F, Rizzo C, Boenzi S, Carducci C, et al. Vigabatrin improves paroxysmal dystonia in succinic semialdehyde dehydrogenase deficiency. Neurology 2007;68:1320–1321.
73. Liang S, Yu X, Zhang S, Tai J. A case of familial paroxysmal nonkinesigenic dyskinesia due to mutation of the PNKD gene in Chinese Mainland. Brain Res 2015;1595:120–126.
74. Machado A, Chien HF, Deguti MM, Cancado E, Azevedo RS, Scaff M, Barbosa ER. Neurological manifestations in Wilson's disease: Report of 119 cases. Mov Disord 2006;21:2192–2196.
75. Mahajan A, Constantinou J, Sidiropoulos C. ECHS1 deficiency-associated paroxysmal exercise-induced dyskinesias: Case presentation and initial benefit of intervention. J Neurol 2017;264:185–187.
76. Marti-Sanchez L, Baide-Mairena H, Marce-Grau A, Pons R, Skouma A, Lopez-Laso E, et al. Delineating the neurological phenotype in children with defects in the ECHS1 or HIBCH gene. J Inherit Metab Dis 2021;44:401–414.
77. Masnada S, Sarret C, Antonello CE, Fadilah A, Krude H, Mura E, et al. Movement disorders in MCT8 deficiency/Allan-Herndon-Dudley syndrome. Mol Genet Metab 2022;135:109–113.
78. McWilliam CA, Ridout CK, Brown RM, McWilliam RC, Tolmie J, Brown GK. Pyruvate dehydrogenase E2 deficiency: A potentially treatable cause of episodic dystonia. Eur J Paediatr Neurol 2010;14:349–353.
79. Meneret A, Grabli D, Depienne C, Gaudebout C, Picard F, Durr A, et al. PRRT2 mutations: A major cause of paroxysmal kinesigenic dyskinesia in the European population. Neurology 2012;79:170–174.
80. Meneret A, Mohammad SS, Cif L, Doummar D, DeGusmao C, Anheim M, et al. Efficacy of caffeine in ADCY5-related dyskinesia: A retrospective study. Mov Disord 2022;37:1294–1298.
81. Meneret A, Roze E. Paroxysmal movement disorders: An update. Rev Neurol (Paris) 2016;172:433–445.
82. Meneret A, Roze E, Maranci JB, Dodet P, Doummar D, Riant F, et al. Sleep in ADCY5-related dyskinesia: Prolonged awakenings caused by abnormal movements. J Clin Sleep Med 2019;15:1021–1029.
83. Menon PJ, Nilles C, Silveira-Moriyama L, Yuan R, de Gusmao CM, et al. Scoping review on ADCY5-related movement disorders. Mov Disord Clin Pract 2023;10:1048–1059.
84. Miller JP, Moldenhauer HJ, Keros S, Meredith AL. An emerging spectrum of variants and clinical features in KCNMA1-linked channelopathy. Channels (Austin) 2021;15:447–464.
85. Mochel F, Hainque E, Gras D, Adanyeguh IM, Caillet S, Heron B, et al. Triheptanoin dramatically reduces paroxysmal motor disorder in patients with GLUT1 deficiency. J Neurol Neurosurg Psychiatry 2016;87:550–553.
86. Morris JG, Jankelowitz SK, Fung VS, Clouston PD, Hayes MW, Grattan-Smith P. Athetosis I: Historical considerations. Mov Disord 2002;17:1278–1280.
87. Mount LA, Reback S. Familial paroxysmal chreoathetosis. Arch Neurol 1940;44:841–847.
88. Mulroy E, Magrinelli F, Mohd Fauzi NA, Kutty SK, Latorre A, Bhatia KP. Paroxysmal, exercise-induced, diurnally fluctuating dystonia: Expanding the phenotype of SPG8. Parkinsonism Relat Disord 2021;85:26–28.
89. Olgiati S, Skorvanek M, Quadri M, Minneboo M, Graafland J, Breedveld GJ, et al. Paroxysmal exercise-induced dystonia within the phenotypic spectrum of ECHS1 deficiency. Mov Disord 2016;31:1041–1048.
90. Ozlu C, Chelliah P, Dahshi H, Horton D, Edgar VB, Messahel S, Kayani S. ECHS1 deficiency and its biochemical and clinical phenotype. Am J Med Genet A 2022;188:2908–2919.
91. Paulhus K, Ammerman L, Glasscock E. Clinical spectrum of KCNA1 mutations: New insights into episodic ataxia and epilepsy comorbidity. Int J Mol Sci 2020;21:2802.
92. Pearl PL, Gibson KM, Acosta MT, Vezina LG, Theodore WH, Rogawski MA, et al. Clinical spectrum of succinic semialdehyde dehydrogenase deficiency. Neurology 2003;60:1413–1417.
93. Pearl PL, Novotny EJ, Acosta MT, Jakobs C, Gibson KM. Succinic semialdehyde dehydrogenase deficiency in children and adults. Ann Neurol 2003;54 Suppl 6:S73–80.
94. Pearson TS, Akman C, Hinton VJ, Engelstad K, De Vivo DC. Phenotypic spectrum of glucose transporter type 1 deficiency syndrome (Glut1 DS). Curr Neurol Neurosci Rep 2013;13:342.
95. Pons R, Cuenca-Leon E, Miravet E, Pons M, Xaidara A, Youroukos S, Macaya A. Paroxysmal non-kinesigenic dyskinesia due to a PNKD recurrent mutation: Report of two Southern European families. Eur J Paediatr Neurol 2012;16:86–89.
96. Rainier S, Thomas D, Tokarz D, Ming L, Bui M, Plein E, et al. Myofibrillogenesis regulator 1 gene mutations cause paroxysmal dystonic choreoathetosis. Arch Neurol 2004;61:1025–1029.
97. Richards RN, Barnett HJ. Paroxysmal dystonic choreoathetosis. A family study and review of the literature. Neurology 1968;18:461–469.
98. Rosenfeld M, Friedman JH. Cervical stenosis and dystonic cerebral palsy. Mov Disord 1999;14:194–195.

99. Sanger TD, Chen D, Fehlings DL, Hallett M, Lang AE, Mink JW, et al. Definition and classification of hyperkinetic movements in childhood. Mov Disord 2010;25:1538–1549.
100. Schirinzi T, Garone G, Travaglini L, Vasco G, Galosi S, Rios L, et al. Phenomenology and clinical course of movement disorder in GNAO1 variants: Results from an analytical review. Parkinsonism Relat Disord 2019;61:19–25.
101. Shetty K, Sarma AS, Devan M, Dalal A, Dash GK, Jannabhatla A, Patil SJ. Recurrent ADCY5 mutation in mosaic form with nocturnal paroxysmal dyskinesias and video Eeectroencephalography documentation of dramatic response to caffeine treatment. J Mov Disord 2020;13:238–240.
102. Shi Y, Wang A, Chen B, Wang X, Niu S, Li W, et al. Clinical features and genetic spectrum of patients with clinically suspected hereditary progressive spastic paraplegia. Front Neurol 2022;13:872927.
103. Shibasaki H, Kuroiwa Y. Painful tonic seizure in multiple sclerosis. Arch Neurol 1974;30:47–51.
104. Shimojima K, Okumura A, Natsume J, Aiba K, Kurahashi H, Kubota T, et al. Spinocerebellar ataxias type 27 derived from a disruption of the fibroblast growth factor 14 gene with mimicking phenotype of paroxysmal non-kinesigenic dyskinesia. Brain Dev 2012;34:230–233.
105. Shin M, Douglass LM, Milunsky JM, Rosman NP. The genetics of benign paroxysmal torticollis of infancy: Is there an association with mutations in the CACNA1A gene? J Child Neurol 2016;31:1057–1061.
106. Stampfl B, Fee D. Novel mutation in CACNA1A associated with activity-induced dystonia, cervical dystonia, and mild ataxia. Case Rep Neurol Med 2021;7797770.
107. Stefanova E, Djarmati A, Momcilovic D, Dragasevic N, Svetel M, Klein C, Kostic VS. Clinical characteristics of paroxysmal nonkinesigenic dyskinesia in Serbian family with Myofibrillogenesis regulator 1 gene mutation. Mov Disord 2006;21:2010–2015.
108. Suls A, Dedeken P, Goffin K, Van Esch H, Dupont P, Cassiman D, et al. Paroxysmal exercise-induced dyskinesia and epilepsy is due to mutations in SLC2A1, encoding the glucose transporter GLUT1. Brain 2008;131:1831–1844.
109. Svetel M, Kozic D, Stefanova E, Semnic R, Dragasevic N, Kostic VS. Dystonia in Wilson's disease. Mov Disord 2001;16:719–723.
110. Temudo T, Martins E, Pocas F, Cruz R, Vilarinho L. Maple syrup disease presenting as paroxysmal dystonia. Ann Neurol 2004;56:749–750.
111. Testini P, Factor SA. Treatment of tardive dystonia: A review. Dystonia 2023;2:10957.
112. Tian WT, Zhan FX, Liu ZH, Liu Z, Liu Q, Guo XN, et al. TMEM151A variants cause paroxysmal kinesigenic dyskinesia: A large-sample study. Mov Disord 2022;37:545–552.
113. Tisch S, Kumar KR. Pallidal deep brain stimulation for monogenic dystonia: The effect of gene on outcome. Front Neurol 2021;11:630391.
114. Tranchant C, Bhatia KP, Marsden CD. Movement disorders in multiple sclerosis. Mov Disord 1995;10:418–423.
115. van Coller R, Slabbert P, Vaidyanathan J, Schutte C. Successful treatment of disabling paroxysmal nonkinesigenic dyskinesia with deep brain stimulation of the globus pallidus internus. Stereotact Funct Neurosurg 2014;92:388–392.
116. van Swieten JC, Brusse E, de Graaf BM, Krieger E, van de Graaf R, de Koning I, et al. A mutation in the fibroblast growth factor 14 gene is associated with autosomal dominant cerebellar ataxia. Am J Hum Genet 2003;72:191–199.
117. Vetro A, Nielsen HN, Holm R, Hevner RF, Parrini E, Powis Z, et al. ATP1A2- and ATP1A3-associated early profound epileptic encephalopathy and polymicrogyria. Brain 2021;144:1435–1450.
118. Vezyroglou A, Akilapa R, Barwick K, Koene S, Brownstein CA, Holder-Espinasse M, et al. The phenotypic continuum of ATP1A3-related disorders. Neurology 2022;99:e1511–e1526.
119. Vila-Pueyo M, Gene GG, Flotats-Bastardes M, Elorza X, Sintas C, Valverde MA, et al. A loss-of-function CACNA1A mutation causing benign paroxysmal torticollis of infancy. Eur J Paediatr Neurol 2014;18:430–433.
120. Vlaskamp DRM, Callenbach PMC, Rump P, Giannini LAA, Brilstra EH, Dijkhuizen T, et al. PRRT2-related phenotypes in patients with a 16p11.2 deletion. Eur J Med Genet 2019;62:265–269.
121. Wang C, Ma X, Xu X, Huang B, Sun H, Li L, et al. A PDGFB mutation causes paroxysmal nonkinesigenic dyskinesia with brain calcification. Mov Disord 2017;32:1104–1106.
122. Wang JL, Cao L, Li XH, Hu ZM, Li JD, Zhang JG, et al. Identification of PRRT2 as the causative gene of paroxysmal kinesigenic dyskinesias. Brain 2011;134:3493–3501.
123. Weissbach A, Pauly MG, Herzog R, Hahn L, Halmans S, Hamami F, et al. Relationship of genotype, phenotype, and treatment in dopa-responsive dystonia: MDSGene review. Mov Disord 2021;2022:237–252.
124. Yeh TH, Lin JJ, Lai SC, Wu-Chou YH, Chen AC, Yueh KC, et al. Familial paroxysmal nonkinesigenic dyskinesia: Clinical and genetic analysis of a Taiwanese family. J Neurol Sci 2012;323:80–84.
125. Yin XM, Lin JH, Cao L, Zhang TM, Zeng S, Zhang KL, et al. Familial paroxysmal kinesigenic dyskinesia is associated with mutations in the KCNA1 gene. Hum Mol Genet 2018;27:625–637.
126. Zhang G, Gibson RA, McDonald M, Liang P, Kang PW, Shi J, et al. A gain-of-function mutation in KCNMA1 causes dystonia spells controlled with stimulant therapy. Mov Disord 2020;35:1868–1873.
127. Zhang XJ, Xu ZY, Wu YC, Tan EK. Paroxysmal movement disorders: Recent advances and proposal of a classification system. Parkinsonism Relat Disord 2019;59:131–139.
128. Zhu M, Zhu X, Wan H, Hong D. Familial IBGC caused by SLC20A2 mutation presenting as paroxysmal kinesigenic dyskinesia. Parkinsonism Relat Disord 2014;20:353–354.
129. Zima L, Ceulemans S, Reiner G, Galosi S, Chen D, Sahagian M, et al. Paroxysmal motor disorders: Expanding phenotypes lead to coalescing genotypes. Ann Clin Transl Neurol 2018;5:996–1010.
130. Zuniga-Ramirez C, Kramis-Hollands M, Mercado-Pimentel R, Gonzalez-Usigli HA, Saenz-Farret M, Soto-Escageda A, Fasano A. Generalized dystonia and paroxysmal dystonic attacks due to a novel ATP1A3 variant. Tremor Other Hyperkinet Mov (N Y) 2019;9. doi:10.7916/tohm.v0.723.

Chapter 18

Dystonias Combined with Other Features

INTRODUCTION

The dystonias comprise a very heterogenous group of disorders with numerous recognized distinct syndromes.[3] The term *syndrome* refers to a characteristic combination of symptoms and signs that tend to cluster together.[18] For the *isolated dystonia syndromes*, dystonia is the only problem. The most common of the isolated dystonia syndromes are covered in separate chapters. In the *combined dystonia syndromes*, dystonia coexists with other relevant clinical problems. These other problems may include another movement disorder, another neurological problem, systemic disease, or characteristic neuroimaging findings (Figure 18.1).

The term *combined dystonia* refers to dystonia combined with another *relevant* problem that constitutes a syndromic combination, not a spurious association of dystonia with a coincidental problem. For example, an individual with a typical adult-onset focal dystonia and coincidental neuropathy would not be considered a combined dystonia syndrome. Neuropathy is common in adults, so the association of dystonia with neuropathy may be coincidental. On the other hand, a child with dystonia who also has a neuropathy might point to a syndromic pattern because neuropathy is uncommon in children. When confronted with an individual who has dystonia along with other clinical problems, it can sometimes be challenging to know if the additional problems are coincidental or elements of a defined syndrome.

Dystonia can be combined with many different problems. The majority of combined dystonia syndromes are relatively uncommon, but identifying a specific etiology can be valuable. Many combined dystonias do not yet have a specific treatment available, and management is symptomatic and supportive. However, some causes do have disease-modifying or disease-specific treatment implications and therefore the diagnosis should not be missed (see Chapter 29, "Special Interventions for Certain Types of Dystonia").

This chapter focuses on dystonia combined with other problems, where the lists of additional clinical problems and potential etiologies is very long. The most common movement disorder syndromes include dystonia combined with tremor, parkinsonism, ataxia, myoclonus, or spasticity for cerebral palsy. Each of these associations of dystonia with other movement

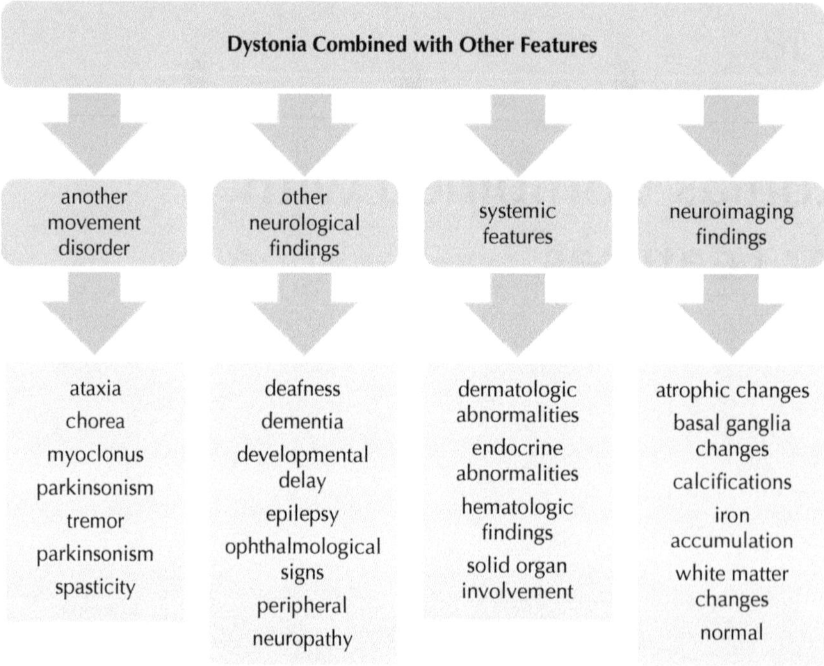

Figure 18.1. Combined dystonia syndromes. Dystonia may be combined with another movement disorder, other neurological problems, systemic disease, or neuroimaging findings.

disorders is covered in separate chapters. This chapter focuses on syndromes where dystonia is combined with other neurological or systemic abnormalities. Rather than attempt to provide exhaustive lists, this chapter summarizes some of the more common combinations as examples, especially those with specific treatments, along with a broader strategy useful for addressing all potential combinations.

SYNDROMIC APPROACH TO DIAGNOSIS

Overall Strategy

With only a few exceptions, the phenomenological manifestations of dystonia overlap among different syndromes regardless of underlying etiology. Because dystonia has so many different etiologies, it is not feasible to conduct a full investigation of all potential causes for every affected individual. A stepwise approach for characterizing the dystonia syndrome helps to narrow the list of possible causes to investigate. The stepwise process involves classification of the phenomenology of the movement disorder, formulation of the syndrome, and then generation of an etiological differential diagnosis. This process is described in more detail in Chapter 2 ("Defining the Clinical Features of Dystonia") and Chapter 3 ("Classification and Diagnostic Strategy for Dystonia").

In brief, the first step is to determine if the movement disorder falls into the category of dystonia by identifying its characteristic clinical features and excluding potential mimics. Important features to consider are age at onset, body regions affected, certain characteristics of the dystonia, and manner of onset and progression over time. The next step is to determine if the dystonia is combined with another relevant clinical problem, to distinguish the isolated dystonia syndromes from the combined dystonia syndromes. If dystonia is combined with another movement disorder, it can be useful to determine which movement disorder is dominant.[1,18] Many acquired and genetic movement disorders are associated with characteristic motor phenotypes, and identification of the dominant motor problem may guide the differential diagnosis. For example, for an individual with prominent ataxia and minor dystonia, a workup for ataxia should be considered first. In contrast, for an individual who has prominent dystonia and mild ataxia, a workup for dystonia should be prioritized.

If there are other neurological or systemic features, it becomes important to consider whether they are coincidental or if they reflect different elements of a known dystonia syndrome. A number of resources have been published over the past decade summarizing the clinical approach to the many combined dystonia syndromes.[6,11,18,25,57,58,62] For example, one prior review summarized more than 200 combined dystonia syndromes in 18 tables organized according to the main associated feature.[18] However, relentless advances in genetics and immunology have led to a constant expansion of potential etiologies, making it challenging to keep pace with these types of lists. Ultimately, a clinical strategy that does not depend on lists from review articles is needed. One very simple approach is to characterize the syndromic features and use these terms in varying combinations in internet search engines such as PubMed or Google Scholar. Undoubtedly the growth of artificial intelligence-based medical diagnostic tools will make this process more efficient and effective with the development of phenotyping tools.[2]

Isolated Versus Combined Dystonia

The sporadic, adult-onset, focal or segmental isolated dystonias are the most common dystonia syndromes. Almost all cases are idiopathic (of unknown etiology), and their natural history is well-understood. These conditions are each discussed in separate chapters. Neuroimaging is typically normal, or it shows findings unrelated to the dystonia syndrome. Bloodwork also is normal, or it shows coincidental findings. Rarely, affected individuals may have an underlying monogenic cause in the absence of a family history, but even in those with other family members affected, a causative gene is found in 2% to 5%. Therefore, the yield from most investigations is low, and the focus is usually on symptomatic management (see Chapter 27, "Workup of Dystonia").

In contrast, an identifiable cause is more likely in combined dystonia syndromes. The additional syndromic features are used to refine the differential diagnosis and guide investigations and treatment. More extensive investigation is generally warranted to determine whether a specific etiological diagnosis can be identified and whether a disease-modifying treatment is available (see Chapter 29).

The best recognized combined syndromes are those where dystonia coexists with another movement disorder such as tremor, parkinsonism, myoclonus, or ataxia. These more common combined syndromes are addressed in separate chapters. This chapter focuses on dystonia syndromes combined with other features not covered in these other chapters, especially syndromes where dystonia is combined with other neurological or systemic features.

DYSTONIA COMBINED WITH OTHER MOVEMENT DISORDERS

Dystonia and Chorea

Dystonia is commonly combined with chorea. In some cases, it may be difficult to discriminate dystonia from chorea. For example, very mobile forms of dystonia may resemble chorea, and chorea can sometimes be sufficiently repetitive and patterned to resemble dystonia. The term *choreoathetosis* is commonly used in the literature to reflect the combination of chorea and dystonia. Dystonia and chorea may occur simultaneously in the same or different body regions, or one movement disorder may precede another over time.

The large number of conditions that combine dystonia and chorea may relate to observations that both may arise from dysfunction of subregions of the basal ganglia (putamen, caudate, and pallidum). Many developmental or degenerative disorders affect all three subregions but to different degrees, leading to various combinations of dystonia and chorea. Studies based on focal lesions have suggested that selective involvement of the putamen and globus pallidus commonly cause dystonia rather than chorea, whereas lesions of the caudate cause both chorea and dystonia.[9] Another example is Huntington disease, where chorea is usually the dominant movement disorder in early stages when the caudate is primarily affected, but dystonia may dominate in later stages when the putamen also is affected.[34] There also may be age-related differences in neuroplasticity that affect whether dystonia or chorea is more prominent.[45]

The frequent coexistence of dystonia and chorea means that it is not practical to generate a comprehensive list of all potential etiologies. In recent years, the largest numbers of newly recognized etiologies has come from genetic studies of individuals with developmental and epileptic encephalopathies, many of whom also have dystonia and chorea and sometimes additional problems such as myoclonus and stereotypies.[40,42,56] Dystonia and chorea also frequently occur together among individuals with dyskinetic cerebral palsy (see Chapter 16, "Dystonia and Cerebral Palsy"), neurodegeneration with brain iron accumulation, and autoimmune movement disorders (see Chapter 21, "Dystonia and Autoimmunity").[7,21,60]

One useful way to approach the many different syndromes that combine dystonia and chorea is to consider their temporal course and potential mechanisms of disease (Table 18.1). Another useful strategy involves seeking additional relevant features that can narrow the list. For example, the majority of disorders listed in Table 18.1 have dystonia and chorea along with other neurological or systemic features. Although most of these conditions are rare, specific treatments are available for some, such as Wilson disease, GLUT1 deficiency, autoimmune conditions, and some developmental epileptic encephalopathies.[25]

Dystonia and Spasticity

Among individuals who have dystonia combined with spasticity, the most important clinical clue is the age of onset. By far the most common cause of infantile (0–2 years) onset dystonia combined with spasticity is cerebral palsy (see Chapter 16). Cerebral palsy itself is a syndrome rather than an etiological diagnosis, defined as a predominantly motor disorder that begins at an early age and is relatively non-progressive. The importance of this syndromic diagnosis is that cerebral palsy is usually caused by acquired perinatal or early infantile monophasic cerebral insults with a static encephalopathy. A diagnosis of cerebral palsy is supported by a history of perinatal stroke or infection, infantile prematurity or hypoxia, and delayed motor or speech milestones. There are also classic findings in neuroimaging, such as perinatal cerebral hemorrhage or MRI evidence of early basal ganglia lesions or periventricular leukomalacia. A history of perinatal insult and/or typical neuroimaging abnormalities is absent in some cases diagnosed with dystonic cerebral palsy. It is increasingly recognized that a substantial portion of these cases have an underlying genetic cause, leading some to propose the

Table 18.1 **Dystonia with chorea**

Onset of condition	Etiology	Examples
Acute (minutes-hours)	Vascular	Basal ganglia stroke, critical stenosis of internal cerebral or middle cerebral arteries, Moyamoya syndrome
	Drug-induced	Acute dystonic reactions from neuroleptics, anti-emetics, propofol
	Metabolic	Hypoglycemia, hyperglycemia
	Genetic	Paroxysmal dyskinesias, *ATP1A3*-associated disorders (rapid-onset dystonia parkinsonism), *SLC2A1* (GLUT1-deficiency), inborn errors of metabolism (many genes)
Subacute (days-weeks)	Autoimmune	Anti-neuronal antibodies (NMDA receptor, CV2/CRMP5, $GABA_A$ receptor, Lgi/CASPR2, Sydenham's chorea, systemic lupus erythematosus
	Demyelinating	Acute disseminated encephalomyelitis
Gradual (months-years)	Drug-induced	Tardive dystonia from neuroleptics or anti-emetics
	Metabolic	Hypocalcemia, hypoparathyroidism
	Genetic	Wilson disease (*ATP7B*), NBIA (several genes), atypical dopa-responsive dystonia (several genes), developmental and epileptic encephalopathies (many genes)
Congenital	Acquired	Perinatal brain injury (e.g., vascular, infectious, trauma)
	Genetic	Numerous genes

Abbreviations: NBIA, neurodegeneration with brain iron accumulation; NMDA, N-methyl-D-aspartic acid.

term *genetic cerebral palsy*,[33,50] or *cerebral palsy mimic*.[42,67]

The typical course is early motor delay, followed by the development of corticospinal signs and a movement disorder within the first year of life. While dystonia is usually present from early childhood, dystonia may emerge following a delay of months or even years.[46,48]

When dystonia combined with spasticity develops later in childhood or in adulthood, it can be useful to determine whether spasticity is the dominant feature and if there are additional family members affected (Table 18.2). Dystonia is not uncommon among several disorders classically classified as *hereditary spastic paraparesis*. There are now more than 80 subtypes of hereditary spastic paraparesis recognized, historically designated numerically starting with *SPG*. Many of these disorders combine corticospinal signs with other movement disorders. In one systematic review of 192 articles encompassing 1,413 individuals with a gene linked to hereditary spastic paraparesis, 9% had dystonia.[17] The percentage of cases with dystonia varied according to the subtype. In this series, dystonia was observed in more than 20% of cases with SPG11 and SPG35, and in 5–10% of patients with SPG7 and SPG26. Dystonia was less common for the other genotypes.

Sometimes genes associated with hereditary spastic paraplegia are associated with a phenotype where dystonia is more prominent than spasticity. In a whole-exome sequencing study of a large cohort of individuals diagnosed with isolated or combined dystonia that included 76 individuals diagnosed with dystonic cerebral palsy, pathogenic variants in *SPAST* (SPG4) was the single most common monogenic cause, accounting for 5 of 37 in whom a genetic diagnosis was made.[14] In a detailed cross-sectional study of 40 children or young adults with *SPAST* gene variants, focal or segmental dystonia was present in 28%.[37]

Another useful feature to look for is parkinsonism because a relatively large subgroup of conditions includes dystonia, spasticity, and parkinsonism (Table 18.2). Several terms have been used to describe this combination including *pallidopyramidal disease*, *pallidopyramidal syndrome*, or *parkinsonian-pyramidal syndrome*.[38,53,54] Although rare, they should not be missed because several of them respond to levodopa. One treatable cause of dystonia with spasticity that should not be missed involves *GCH1*, the most common cause of autosomal dominant dopa-responsive dystonia (Segawa disease). The classic presentation includes dystonia with prominent gait impairment and diurnal variation in childhood. Sometimes initial manifestations first appear in late childhood or in early adulthood, with a combination of dystonia and parkinsonism, and sometimes parkinsonism is the dominant problem. However, spasticity can be the most prominent or the sole motor impairment.[59,61] Spasticity can sometimes be a prominent feature associated with other genes

Table 18.2 **Dystonia with spasticity**

Subgroup	Etiology	Examples
Spasticity with parkinsonism	Autosomal dominant	Dopa-responsive dystonia (*GCH1*)
	Autosomal recessive	Cerebrotendinous xanthomatosis, Parkinson disease (***PRKN, PRKRA, DJ-1***), Kufor-Rakeb disease, ***FBXOX***, PKAN, MPAN, PLAN, SPG11, dopa-responsive dystonia (***TH***)
	X-linked	BPAN
Spasticity without parkinsonism	Autosomal recessive	Hereditary spastic paraparesis (***SPG7, 11, 13, 15, 35, 64; PEX16);*** cerebrotendinous xanthomatosis, GM1 and GM2 gangliosidosis, manganese transporter deficiency, MPAN, PKAN, PLAN, xeroderma pigmentosum
	Autosomal dominant	***SPG4, ATP5MC3***
	X-linked	Partington X-linked mental retardation syndrome (***ARX***); Allan-Herndon-Dudley syndrome (***MCT8***)
	Acquired	Cerebral palsy

Abbreviations: BPAN, beta-propellor associated neurodegeneration; MPAN, mitochondrial protein associated neurodegeneration; PKAN, pantothenate kinase associated neurodegeneration; PLAN, *PLA2G6*-associated neurodegeneration; SPG, spastic paraplegia.

associated with dopa-responsive dystonia.[65] A trial of levodopa is therefore warranted in all individuals with dystonia and spasticity, even when the cause is not known.

Dystonia and Tics

Tics are a distinct movement disorder characterized by recurrent and usually sudden movements or vocalizations.[49] Some common examples of simple tics include eye blinking, eye or neck rolling, shoulder shrugging, facial contractions, sniffing, or sudden short vocalizations or sounds. Complex tics are defined by combinations of simple tics, and tics may sometimes be sustained for several seconds. Tourette syndrome is defined by a combination of multiple motor and audible tics that often change character over time.

Tics can usually be discriminated from dystonia by several features. Tics are often preceded by some type of premonition, whereas dystonia is not. Tics may be voluntarily suppressed by will, while dystonia cannot be suppressed without physical restraint. Tics are often brief and sudden, while movements of dystonia are often more persistent. Voluntary movements often attenuate tics yet they worsen dystonia.

Tics are relatively common in normal children, but they often abate with age. Occasionally, tics may begin in older adults. The most common tic disorders are *primary tic disorders*, where an etiology often is not known. Occasionally, a cause can be identified, including certain developmental and degenerative disorders.

While tics and dystonia are distinct disorders, they may sometimes be combined in the same individual. In an early study of 224 individuals with primary tic disorders, 20 also had dystonia, most often cervical dystonia.[13] Either problem may occur years before the second one develops, although most cases with both problems had onset in adulthood. Tics and dystonia may also be combined in some adult-onset neurodegenerative conditions, such as neuroacanthocytosis and Huntington disease.

Another situation where tics and dystonia are considered together involves a type of tic called the *dystonic tic*.[4,16,24] These tics are often slower and more sustained than typical tics, and they therefore have a dystonic appearance. Because they are recurrent, they may be easily confused with dystonia. In one study of 156 individuals with Tourette syndrome, 57% had at least one dystonic tic.[24] Another cohort of 201 individuals with Tourette syndrome described dystonic tics in 36%.[4] The most common examples included facial twitches resembling craniofacial dystonias, neck muscle contractions resembling cervical dystonia, or eye rolling resembling oculogyric deviations of acute dystonic reactions.

Although the term *dystonic tic* is common in the literature, its use in the clinic should probably be discouraged. Individuals given this diagnosis often search the internet, and they may become confused regarding whether they have a tic disorder or dystonia. The term *tonic tic* may therefore be preferable, to more clearly refer to a tic disorder.[26]

DYSTONIA COMBINED WITH OTHER NEUROLOGICAL FEATURES

Overview

There are numerous syndromes where dystonia is combined with other features.[18] At times, additional neurological features are clinically obvious, but sometimes they require examination by a specialist, such as an ophthalmologist to define specific retinal abnormalities. Therefore consultation with other specialists can be useful when additional clinical features are found and their significance is uncertain. Often specialized testing may be needed to document or define these clinical features, such as nerve conduction studies to detect neuropathy or audiometry to assess hearing loss and differentiate cochlear from neural deafness.[18]

Ophthalmological Signs

Ophthalmological signs can provide a useful clue in individuals who also have dystonia.[64] Ophthalmological problems may be divided into those that affect the cornea, lens (including specific cataract types), retina (including specific patterns of retinopathy such as cherry red spots or retinitis pigmentosa), or optic nerve (especially atrophy). Each of these problems may delineate specific syndromes associated with dystonia (Table 18.3).

The presence of an abnormality of eye movement is one of the most important clues that argues against a diagnosis of idiopathic dystonia, whether in a child or adult.[27] It also may be one

Table 18.3 **Dystonia with eye signs**

Type	Subgroup	Examples
Retinal	Cherry red spot	GM1 or GM2 gangliosidosis; MLD; neuronal ceroid lipofuscinosis; PKAN
	Pigmentary retinopathy	Aceruloplasminemia, ALD, Boucher-Neuhauser syndrome, MLD, mitochondrial disease, PKAN, SCA (e.g., SCA7)
	Optic atrophy	ALD, CASK mutation, CTX, FAHN, MLD, methylmalonic aciduria (multiple genes), mitochondrial disease, MPAN, Mohr-Tranebjaerg syndrome, PLAN, SPG7, SCA (e.g., SCA2 and 3)
	Vascular malformations	cerebral microangiopathy with calcifications and cysts
Anterior compartment	Lens cataracts	4H leukodystrophy, ALD, CTX, ***FBX07*** mutation, GM1 gangliosidosis, homocystinuria, Marinesco-Sjogren syndrome, mitochondrial disease, Wilson disease
	Corneal defects	GM1 gangliosidosis (corneal clouding), Wilson disease (Kayser-Fleischer rings); xeroderma pigmentosa (corneal clouding)
Supranuclear gaze palsy	Mostly vertical	Glutaric aciduria, kernicterus, Kufor-Rakeb disease, Niemann-Pick type C, PKAN, phosphoglycerate kinase deficiency, PLAN, prion disease, progressive supranuclear palsy, SPG7 or 11, tau-gene associated frontotemporal degeneration, gene mutations (*ADCY5, EIF2AK2, FBXO7*)
	Multi-directional	*AFG3L2* mutation, Huntington disease; neuroacanthocytosis, SCA (SCA2 and 3)
	Oculomotor apraxia	Ataxia-telangiectasia, ataxia-telangiectasia-like; ataxia with oculomotor apraxia (several genes), corticobasal degeneration; Gaucher disease; GM2 gangliosidosis
External ophthalmoplegia	Mitochondrial disease	Many genes

Abbreviations: 4H leukodystrophy (hypomyelination, hypodontia and hypogonadotropic hypogonadism); ALD, adrenoleukodystrophy; CTX, cerebrotendinous xanthomatosis; MLD, metachromatic leukodystrophy; FAHN, fatty acid hydroxylase associated neurodegeneration; MPAN, mitochondrial protein associated neurodegeneration; PKAN, pantothenate kinase associated neurodegeneration; SCA, spinocerebellar ataxia.

of the earliest and subtle signs in the evolution of a neurodegenerative disease that presents with dystonia, whether apparently isolated or combined with other movement disorders or neurological features. Some signs may be nonspecific, such as the nystagmus associated with cerebellar involvement, but some may be highly suggestive of a particular condition associated with dystonia. Examples include impaired initiation of saccades in early Huntington disease, impaired downward saccades in Niemann Pick type C, or oculomotor apraxia associated with several conditions of ataxia with oculomotor apraxia that often also include dystonia.

Hearing Loss

Hearing loss provides another important diagnostic clue in an individual who has dystonia, and may have multiple potential causes (Table 18.4).[18,31] Hearing impairment may only be detectable on audiometric testing. The differentiation between cochlear and neural deafness can have important diagnostic but also therapeutic implications, such as suitability for cochlear implantation. One of the earliest deafness-dystonia syndromes to be recognized was the Mohr-Tranebjaerg syndrome caused by pathogenic variants in *TIMM8A*. For this gene, some cases may have dystonia without deafness.[22,29,52] Numerous other genes and nongenetic causes for the dystonia-deafness syndrome, often with additional clinical features, are also recognized.[12,15,63]

Peripheral Neuropathy

Peripheral neuropathy can also provide a useful indicator among individuals with dystonia (Table 18.5).[19] Nerve conduction and

Table 18.4 **Dystonia with deafness**

Etiology	Subgroup	Examples
Inherited	Dominant	*ACTB* (β actin)
	Recessive	*ATP1A3*, C2orf37 (Woodhouse-Sakati syndrome), Cockayne syndrome (several genes), *NPHS1* (congenital nephrotic syndrome, Finnish); *SERAC1* (MEGDEL syndrome), *SUCLA2*, methylmalonic aciduria (multiple genes), xeroderma pigmentosa (several genes)
	X-linked	*CASK, TIMM8A* (Mohr-Tranebjaerg syndrome)
	Mitochondrial	Many genes
	Chromosomal	Deletion of 10p, 18q, or xq28
Acquired	Perinatal brain injury	Kernicterus
	Later brain injury	Trauma, meningoencephalitis

Abbreviations: MEGDEL (3-methylglutaconic aciduria with sensorineural deafness, encephalopathy, and Leigh-like syndrome).

electromyography can be useful to detect subclinical neuropathy and to define axonal versus demyelinating subtypes. The age at evaluation plays an important role because peripheral neuropathy is common in older adults with dystonia, and it may therefore be coincidental. However, peripheral neuropathy in a child with dystonia is uncommon and warrants consideration that it may reflect a syndrome where these two problems coexist. It also is important to keep in mind that some focal neuropathies may mimic dystonia because they result in abnormal posturing. Additionally, several peripheral nerve hyperexcitability syndromes may mimic dystonia. These mimics are covered in more detail in Chapter 26, "Pseudodystonia and Differential Diagnosis."

DYSTONIA COMBINED WITH SYSTEMIC DISEASE

Solid Organ Involvement

There are numerous syndromes in which dystonia is associated with systemic disease. Perhaps the most widely recognized is Wilson disease. It was among the earliest inherited syndromes to be recognized, there are telltale clinical features,

Table 18.5 **Dystonia with neuropathy**

Etiology	Subgroup	Examples
Inherited	Dominant	*NOTCH2NLC* (neuronal intranuclear inclusion disease), spinocerebellar ataxias (e.g., SCA1, SCA3, SCA11), *VPS16*
	Recessive	*ARG1* (argininemia); *ARSA* (metachromatic leukodystrophy); *ATM* (ataxia-telangiectasia); *DDP1* (Mohr-Tranebjaerg syndrome); *ATP13A2* (Kufor-Rakeb syndrome); ataxia-oculomotor apraxia (several genes), *CTX* (cerebrotendinous xanthomatosis, *ERCC6* or *8* (Cockayne syndrome); *FXN* (Friedreich ataxia); *GALC* (Krabbe disease); *HEXA* (Tay-Sachs disease); *LYST* (Chediak-Higashi disease); *SCP2* (sterol carrier protein X); *NPC1* or *2* (Niemann-Pick type C); *VPS13A* (choreoacanthocytosis); Xeroderma pigmentosum (several genes); additional genes (*AFG3L2, COA7, NDUFA9, NGLY1, OPA1, PLA2G6, POLG, TXN20, VPS16*)
	Mitochondrial	Many genes
	Chromosomal	Deletion of 18q
Acquired	Infection	Human immunodeficiency virus
	Autoimmune	Multifocal motor neuropathy

Abbreviations: MEGDEL (3-methylglutaconic aciduria with sensorineural deafness, encephalopathy, and Leigh-like syndrome).

and it can be treated effectively with agents that reduce copper stores. Liver disease is common in Wilson disease, and dystonia is the most common movement disorder.[8,35,51] Often liver disease is recognized first, but some individuals first come to medical attention because of dystonia, and liver involvement is recognized only later. Individuals with this condition may also have additional problems including renal impairment and hematologic changes. Perhaps the best recognized additional clinical finding involves Kayser-Fleischer rings in the cornea, which are present in the vast majority (but not all) of individuals with neurological Wilson disease,[66] These rings are not pathognomonic of Wilson disease, as they are present also in other diseases, such as primary biliary cholangitis.

In addition to Wilson disease, there are a number of other conditions that combine liver disease and dystonia, often with other clinical problems, too.[39] They include defects in manganese transport,[43,44,55] multiple genes associated with Aicardi-Goutiere syndrome, and others (Table 18.6).

There also are conditions where dystonia is combined with disease affecting other organs, including the kidneys and lung.[10] Some examples of these other disorders are provided in Table 18.6. This table does not provide an exhaustive list. Instead, it serves as a reminder that further consideration of a syndromic pattern should be considered whenever dystonia is combined with routine laboratory studies that suggest the possible existence of underlying disease affecting the liver, kidney, or lung. These routine laboratory studies are readily overlooked but sometimes provide an early clue to the diagnosis.

Dermatological Abnormalities

The skin is another place where certain features can be very helpful in reaching a diagnosis in an individual with dystonia (Table 18.7).[32] For example, signs of early skin aging and cutaneous malignancy are frequent in disorders affecting DNA repair, such as xeroderma pigmentosum or ataxia telangiectasia. For both conditions, dystonia is usually combined with other problems that help to point to the diagnosis. Multiple scars may result from self-picking or self-biting, and they provide a clue for several conditions such as Lesch-Nyhan disease, complex dopa-responsive dystonia, glutaric aciduria, and antibodies to N-methyl-D-aspartic acid (NMDA) receptors.

Other abnormalities can point to more specific conditions such as telangiectasias in ataxia-telangiectasia, tendon xanthomas in cerebrotendinous xanthomatosis, angiokeratomas in fucosidosis, or autonomic signs with atrophic changes of the skin or nails in complex regional pain syndrome.

The skin is an easy place to search for abnormalities. It also is easy to overlook abnormalities unless they are sought. For example, tendon xanthomas are easily missed because they may be small or limited to tendons of the feet. Telangiectasias are often limited to the sclera, but they may also occur in the earlobes or pharynx. In other cases, skin abnormalities may be

Table 18.6 **Dystonia with solid organ involvement**

Organ	Disease	Examples
Liver	Cirrhosis, liver failure	Heptato-cerebral degeneration, manganese transporter deficiency (*SLC30A10* or *SLC39A14*), Wilson disease (*ATP7B*)
	Hepatosplenomegaly	Aicardi-Goutiere syndrome (multiple genes), fucosidosis (*FUCA1*), Gaucher disease, Niemann-Pick type C (*NPC1, NPC2*), methylmalonic aciduria (multiple genes), propionic aciduria (*PCCA* and *PCCB*)
Kidney	Renal failure	Glutaric aciduria (*GCDH*), Lesch-Nyhan disease (*HPRT1*), methylmalonic aciduria (multiple genes), nephrin mutation, Wilson disease (*ATP7B)*
	Nephrolithiasis	Lesch-Nyhan disease (*HPRT1*)
Lung	Interstitial lung disease	Ataxia-telangiectasia (*ATM*), benign hereditary chorea (*NKX2-1*), Niemann-Pick type C (*NPC1, NPC2*)
	Lung cancer	Paraneoplastic syndromes

more obvious, but they may be mistaken for a common rash. Consultation with the appropriate specialists can be useful when there is some unusual or unexplained dermatological finding.

Endocrine Abnormalities

Dystonia may sometimes be associated with abnormalities found in blood tests, such as routine hematology (e.g., anemia, leukopenia, polycythemia, thrombocytopenia) or chemistry profiles (e.g., calcium, glucose, liver enzymes, renal function).[41] Many of the conditions associated with these abnormalities are reviewed in Chapter 9, "Workup of Dystonia." There are also several conditions where dystonia is associated with specific endocrine disorders (Table 18.8).

There are several well-recognized syndromes that combine dystonia with thyroid disease.[47] *NKX2-1* has been associated with a spectrum of syndromes from very severe (brain-lung-thyroid syndrome) to much milder (benign hereditary chorea). More severely affected cases have hypothyroidism, pulmonary dysfunction, and developmental delay with a variety of movement disorders. Chorea may be most common, but dystonia and myoclonus also occur. Some cases may have only mild and non-progressive chorea, without signs of systemic disease, but other movement disorders also occur.[5,30]

Another well-recognized condition is the Allan-Herndon-Dudley syndrome, also called MCT8 deficiency. It is linked to genetic defects in a transporter that allows thyroid hormone to penetrate into the brain, resulting in peripheral hyperthyroidism with cerebral hypothyroidism and leukoencephalopathy. Affected individuals have global developmental delay, often with parkinsonism and dystonia.[36]

In addition to these inherited disorders, thyroid disease is associated with adult-onset focal dystonias.[23,28] It has also been associated with adult-onset acquired paroxysmal dyskinesias.[47] The reasons for these links are currently unknown, although autoimmune mechanisms have been suspected.

There also are specific syndromes in which dystonia may be combined with hypogonadism[20] or abnormalities of calcium or glucose metabolism (Table 18.8). Several of these syndromes are caused by defects in specific genes. Most are quite rare and typically present in childhood. Other syndromes are acquired and may present instead in adults. For example, both hypoglycemia (caused by insulinoma or overdose) and hyperglycemia (as in diabetes mellitus) have been associated with movement disorders in adults, including dystonia.

Table 18.7 **Dystonia with dermatologic abnormalities**

Condition	Cause	Skin finding	Therapeutic implications
6-Pyruvoyl-tetrahydropertin synthase deficiency	*PTPS*	Self-injury scarring	Levodopa
Ataxia-telangiectasia	*ATM*	Telangiectasia, progeric changes, malignancy, cutaneous granulomatosis, hypertrichosis	Avoidance of radiation and cancer surveillance
Biotinidase deficiency	*BTD*	Erythematous or seborrheic dermatitis, alopecia	Biotin
Cerebrotendinous xanthomatosis	*CYP27A1*	Tendon xanthomas	Chenodeoxycholic acid
Fucosidosis	*FUCA1*	Angiokeratomas	Bone marrow transplantation
Ehlers-Danlos syndrome	Multiple	Skin fragility	Aneurysm screening
Hartnup disease	*SLC6A19*	Photosensitive rash	High protein diet
Lesch-Nyhan disease	HPRT1	Self-injury scarring	
NMDA-receptor encephalitis	Autoimmune	Self-injury scarring	Immunosuppression
Xeroderma pigmentosum	multiple genes	Progeric changes, malignancy	Avoidance of radiation and cancer surveillance

Table 18.8 **Dystonia with endocrine abnormalities**

Abnormality	Subgroup	Examples
Calcium	Hypocalcemia	Hypocalcemia, hypoparathyroidism, chr10p deletion
	Hypercalcemia	Russell-Silver syndrome (multiple genes)
Glucose	Hypoglycemia	β-ketothiolase deficiency (*ACAT*), glutaric aciduria (*GCDH*), insulinoma or overdose, short chain acyl coa dehydrogenase deficiency,
	Hyperglycemia	Aceruloplasminemia (*CP*), chr18q deletion, diabetic uremia, mitochondrial disease, non-ketotic hyperglycemia, Woodhouse-Sakati syndrome (*DCAF17*)
Hypogonadism	Hypogonadotropic	Benign hereditary chorea (*NKX2-1*), Woodhouse-Sakati syndrome (*DCAF17*)
	Hypergonadotropic	Ataxia telangiectasia (*ATM*), galactosemia (multiple genes)
Thyroid hormone	Hypothyroidism	Allan-Herndon-Dudley syndrome (*SLC16A2*), benign hereditary chorea (*NKX2-1*), manganese transporter deficiency (*SLC30A10*), Woodhouse-Sakati syndrome (*DCAF17*)
	Hyperthyroidism	Adult-onset isolated focal dystonias, paroxysmal kinesigenic dyskinesia

SYNOPSIS AND FUTURE PROSPECTS

There is a vast array of potential causes of syndromes of dystonia combined with other movement disorders, other neurological features, and systemic disease. It is impossible to remember all potential syndromes, and new ones are discovered very often. The syndromic approach allows a narrowing of the differential diagnosis. At times, this will allow generation of a limited etiological differential diagnosis via use of search tools such as Google Scholar or PubMed. The arrival of artificial intelligence-based information systems will vastly improve this process, but clinical acumen and skills will still be required to extract the right information from the clinical scenario to enter into the search tool, no matter how advanced.

For the many genetic causes of combined dystonia syndromes, phenotypic variability and atypical phenotypes are increasingly recognized. As a result, whole-exome and whole-genome sequencing are preferred over single-gene testing or focused gene panels. Both forward and reverse phenotyping will remain essential clinical skills because of limited access to next-generation sequencing techniques in many parts of the world and results from these techniques that require clinical interpretation and additional phenotype information. Both now and in the future, good clinical recognition of these combined dystonia syndromes is essential because some of them are treatable.

REFERENCES

1. Abdo WF, van de Warrenburg BP, Burn DJ, Quinn NP, Bloem BR. The clinical approach to movement disorders. Nat Rev Neurol 2010;6:29–37.
2. Al-Antari MA. Artificial intelligence for medical diagnostics: Existing and future AI technology! Diagnostics 2023;13:688.
3. Albanese A, Bhatia K, Bressman SB, DeLong MR, Fahn S, Fung VSC, et al. Phenomenology and classification of dystonia: A consensus update. Mov Disord 2013;28:863–873.
4. Baizabal-Carvallo JF, Alonso-Juarez M, Jankovic J. Dystonic motor and phonic tics in Tourette syndrome. J Neurol 2022;269:5312–5318.
5. Balicza P, Grosz Z, Molnar V, Illes A, Csaban D, Gezsi A, et al. NKX2-1 new mutation associated with myoclonus, dystonia, and pituitary involvement. Front Genet 2018;9:335.
6. Balint B, Mencacci NE, Valente EM, Pisani A, Rothwell J, Jankovic J, et al. Dystonia. Nat Rev Dis Primers 2018;4:25.
7. Balint B, Vincent A, Meinck HM, Irani SR, Bhatia KP. Movement disorders with neuronal antibodies: Syndromic approach, genetic parallels and pathophysiology. Brain 2018;141:13–36.
8. Bandmann O, Weiss KH, Kaler SG. Wilson's disease and other neurological copper disorders. Lancet Neurol 2015;14:103–113.
9. Bhatia KP, Marsden CD. The behavioral and motor consequences of focal lesions of the basal ganglia in man. Brain 1994;117:859–876.
10. Bhowmick SS, Lang AE. Movement disorders and renal diseases. Mov Disord Clin Pract 2020;7:763–779.
11. Bukhari-Parlakturk N, Frucht SJ. Isolated and combined dystonias: Update. Handb Clin Neurol 2023;196:425–442.
12. Chouksey A, Pandey S. ATP1A3 mutation presenting as CAPOS syndrome + dystonia phenotype. Parkinsonism Relat Disord 2020;78:192–194.

13. Damasio J, Edwards MJ, Alonso-Canovas A, Schwingenschuh P, Kagi G, Bhatia KP. The clinical syndrome of primary tic disorder associated with dystonia: A large clinical series and a review of the literature. Mov Disord 2011;26:679–684.
14. Dzinovic I, Boesch S, Skorvanek M, Necpal J, Svantnerova J, Pavelekova P, et al. Genetic overlap between dystonia and other neurologic disorders: A study of 1,100 exomes. Parkinsonism Relat Disord 2022;102:1–6.
15. Eggink H, van Egmond ME, Verschuuren-Bemelmans CC, Schonherr MC, de Koning TJ, Oterdoom DL, et al. Dystonia-deafness syndrome caused by a beta-actin gene mutation and response to deep brain stimulation. Mov Disord 2017;32:162–165.
16. Erro R, Martino D, Ganos C, Damasio J, Batla A, Bhatia KP. Adult-onset primary dystonic tics: A different entity? Mov Disord Clin Pract 2014;1:62–66.
17. Fereshtehnejad SM, Saleh PA, Oliveira LM, Patel N, Bhowmick S, Saranza G, Kalia LV. Movement disorders in hereditary spastic paraplegia (HSP): A systematic review and individual participant data meta-analysis. Neurol Sci 2023;44:947–959.
18. Fung VS, Jinnah HA, Bhatia K, Vidailhet M. Assessment of the patient with dystonia: An update on dystonia syndromes. Mov Disord 2013;28:889–898.
19. Gentile F, Bertini A, Priori A, Bocci T. Movement disorders and neuropathies: Overlaps and mimics in clinical practice. J Neurol 2022;269:4646–4662.
20. Gonzalez-Latapi P, Sousa M, Lang AE. Movement disorders associated with hypogonadism. Mov Disord Clin Pract 2021;8:997–1011.
21. Govert F, Leypoldt F, Junker R, Wandinger KP, Deuschl G, Bhatia KP, Balint B. Antibody-related movement disorders - a comprehensive review of phenotype-autoantibody correlations and a guide to testing. Neurol Res Pract 2020;2:6.
22. Ha AD, Parratt KL, Rendtorff ND, Lodahl M, Ng K, Rowe DB, et al. The phenotypic spectrum of dystonia in Mohr-Tranebjaerg syndrome. Mov Disord 2012;27:1034–1040.
23. Idrissi S, Velucci V, Esposito M, Trinchillo A, Habestwallner F, Belvisi D, et al. Does thyroid disease contribute to the natural history of idiopathic adult-onset dystonia? Data from the Italian Dystonia Registry. J Neural Transm 2024;131:369–375.
24. Jankovic J, Stone L. Dystonic tics in patients with Tourette's syndrome. Mov Disord 1991;6:248–252.
25. Jinnah HA, Albanese A, Bhatia KP, Cardoso F, Da Prat G, de Koning TJ, et al. Treatable inherited rare movement disorders. Mov Disord 2018;33:21–35.
26. Kaczynska J, Janik P. Tonic tics in Gilles de la Tourette syndrome. Neuropediatrics 2021;52:370–376.
27. Kassavetis P, Kaski D, Anderson T, Hallett M. Eye movement disorders in movement disorders. Mov Disord Clin Pract 2022;9:284–295.
28. Kilic-Berkmen G, Scorr LM, Rosen A, Wu E, Freeman A, Silver M, et al. Thyroid disease in cervical dystonia. Parkinsonism Relat Disord 2023;107:10524.
29. Kim HT, Edwards MJ, Tyson J, Quinn NP, Bintner-Glindzicz M, Bhatia KP. Blepharospasm and limb dystonia caused by Mohr-Tranebjaerg syndrome with a novel splice site mutation in the deafness/dystonia peptide gene. Mov Disord 2007;22:1328–1331.
30. Koht J, Lostegaard SO, Wedding I, Vidailhet M, Louha M, Tallaksen CM. Benign hereditary chorea, not only chorea: A family case presentation. Cerebellum Ataxias 2016;3:3.
31. Kojovic M, Parees I, Lampreia T, Pienczk-Reclawowicz K, Xiromerisiou G, Rubio-Agusti I, et al. The syndrome of deafness-dystonia: Clinical and genetic heterogeneity. Mov Disord 2013;28:795–803.
32. Kulcsarova K, Baloghova J, Necpal J, Skorvanek M. Skin conditions and movement disorders: Hiding in plain sight. Mov Disord Clin Pract 2022;9:566–583.
33. Lewis SA, Shetty S, Wilson BA, Huang AJ, Jin SC, Smithers-Sheedy H, et al. Insights from genetic studies of cerebral palsy. Front Neurol 2020;11:625428.
34. Louis ED, Lee P, Quinn L, Marder K. Dystonia in Huntington's disease: Prevalence and clinical characteristics. Mov Disord 1999;14:95–101.
35. Machado A, Chien HF, Deguti MM, Cancado E, Azevedo RS, Scaff M, Barbosa ER. Neurological manifestations in Wilson's disease: Report of 119 cases. Mov Disord 2006;21:2192–2196.
36. Masnada S, Sarret C, Antonello CE, Fadilah A, Krude H, Mura E, et al. Movement disorders in MCT8 deficiency/Allan-Herndon-Dudley syndrome. Mol Genet Metab 2022;135:109–113.
37. Mo A, Saffari A, Kellner M, Dobler-Neumann M, Jordan C, Srivastava S, et al. Early-onset and severe complex hereditary spastic paraplegia caused by de novo variants in SPAST. Mov Disord 2022;37:2440–2446.
38. Morales-Briceno H, Fung VSC. Is pallido-pyramidal syndrome still a useful concept? No. Mov Disord Clin Pract 2020;7:27–29.
39. Mulroy E, Baschieri F, Magrinelli F, Latorre A, Cortelli P, Bhatia KP. Movement disorders and liver disease. Mov Disord Clin Pract 2021;8:828–842.
40. Papandreou A, Danti FR, Spaull R, Leuzzi V, McTague A, Kurian MA. The expanding spectrum of movement disorders in genetic epilepsies. Dev Med Child Neurol 2020;62:178–191.
41. Patel RA, Hall DA, Eichenseer S, Bailey M. Movement disorders and hematologic diseases. Mov Disord Clin Pract 2021;8:193–207.
42. Pearson TS, Pons R, Ghaoui R, Sue CM. Genetic mimics of cerebral palsy. Mov Disord 2019;34:625–636.
43. Quadri M, Federico A, Zhao T, Breedveld GJ, Battisti C, Delnooz C, et al. Mutations in SLC30A10 cause parkinsonism and dystonia with hypermanganesemia, polycythemia, and chronic liver disease. Am J Hum Genet 2012;90:467–477.
44. Riley LG, Cowley MJ, Gayevskiy V, Roscioli T, Thorburn DR, Prelog K, et al. A SLC39A8 variant causes manganese deficiency, and glycosylation and mitochondrial disorders. J Inherit Metab Dis 2017;40:261–269.
45. Romito LM, Leta V, Garavaglia B, Panteghini C, Zorzi G, Elia AE, et al. ANO3 as a cause of early-onset chorea combined with dystonia: Illustration of phenotypic evolution. Mov Disord 2024;39:220–221.
46. Saint Hilaire MH, Burke RE, Bressman SB, Brin MF, Fahn S. Delayed-onset dystonia due to perinatal or early childhood asphyxia. Neurology 1991;41:216–222.
47. Schneider SA, Tschaidse L, Reisch N. Thyroid disorders and movement disorders: A systematic review. Mov Disord Clin Pract 2023;10:360–368.
48. Scott BL, Jankovic J. Delayed-onset progressive movement disorders after static brain lesions. Neurology 1996;46:68–74.
49. Singer HS. Tics and Tourette syndrome. Continuum 2019;25:936–958.

50. Smithers-Sheedy H, Badawi N, Blair E, Cans C, Himmelmann K, Krageloh-Mann I, et al. What constitutes cerebral palsy in the twenty-first century? Dev Med Child Neurol 2014;56:323–328.
51. Svetel M, Kozic D, Stefanova E, Semnic R, Dragasevic N, Kostic VS. Dystonia in Wilson's disease. Mov Disord 2001;16:719–723.
52. Swerdlow RH, Wooten GF. A novel deafness/dystonia peptide gene mutation that causes dystonia in female carriers of Mohr-Tranebjaerg syndrome. Ann Neurol 2001;50:537–540.
53. Tranchant C. Is pallido-pyramidal syndrome still a useful concept? Yes. Mov Disord Clin Pract 2020;7:25–26.
54. Tranchant C, Koob M, Anheim M. Parkinsonian-pyramidal syndromes: A systematic review. Parkinsonism Relat Disord 2017;39:4–16.
55. Tuschl K, Clayton PT, Gospe SM, Jr., Gulab S, Ibrahim S, Singhi P, et al. Syndrome of hepatic cirrhosis, dystonia, polycythemia, and hypermanganesemia caused by mutations in SLC30A10, a manganese transporter in man. Am J Hum Genet 2012;90:457–466.
56. van der Veen S, Tse GTW, Ferretti A, Garone G, Post B, Specchio N, et al. Movement disorders in patients with genetic developmental and epileptic encephalopathies. Neurology 2023;101:e1884–e1892.
57. van Egmond ME, Kuiper A, Eggink H, Sinke RJ, Brouwer OF, Verschuuren-Bemelmans CC, et al. Dystonia in children and adolescents: A systematic review and a new diagnostic algorithm. J Neurol Neurosurg Psychiatry 2014;86:774–781.
58. van Egmond ME, Lagrand TJ, Lizaitiene G, Smit M, Tijssen MAJ. A novel diagnostic approach for patients with adult-onset dystonia. J Neurol Neurosurg Psychiatry 2022;93:1039–1048.
59. Varghaei P, Yoon G, Estiar MA, Veyron S, Leveille E, Dupre N, et al. GCH1 mutations in hereditary spastic paraplegia. Clin Genet 2021;100:51–58.
60. Varley JA, Webb AJS, Balint B, Fung VSC, Sethi KD, Tijssen MAJ, et al. The movement disorder associated with NMDAR antibody-encephalitis is complex and characteristic: An expert video-rating study. J Neurol Neurosurg Psychiatry 2019;90:724–726.
61. Wassenberg T, Schouten MI, Helmich RC, Willemsen M, Kamsteeg EJ, van de Warrenburg BPC. Autosomal dominant GCH1 mutations causing spastic paraplegia at disease onset. Parkinsonism Relat Disord 2020;74:12–15.
62. Weissbach A, Saranza G, Domingo A. Combined dystonias: Clinical and genetic updates. J Neural Transm 2021;128:417–429.
63. Whalen S, Shaw M, Mignot C, Heron D, Bastaraud SC, Walti CC, et al. Further delineation of BCAP31-linked intellectual disability: Description of 17 new families with LoF and missense variants. Eur J Hum Genet 2021;29:1405–1417.
64. Wilson D, Hallett M, Anderson T. An eye on movement disorders. Mov Disord Clin Pract 2021;8:1168–1180.
65. Wittke C, Petkovic S, Dobricic V, Schaake S, Respondek G, Weissbach A, et al. Genotype-phenotype relations for the atypical parkinsonism genes: MDSGene systematic review. Mov Disord 2021;36:1499–1510.
66. Youn J, Kim JS, Kim HT, Lee JY, Lee PH, Ki CS, Cho JW. Characteristics of neurological Wilson's disease without Kayser-Fleischer ring. J Neurol Sci 2012;323:183–186.
67. Zouvelou V, Yubero D, Apostolakopoulou L, Kokkinou E, Bilanakis M, Dalivigka Z, et al. The genetic etiology in cerebral palsy mimics: The results from a Greek tertiary care center. Eur J Paediatr Neurol 2019;23:427–437.

SECTION IV

Etiology and Pathogenesis

Chapter 19

Dystonia Induced by Medications, Illicit Drugs, and Environmental Toxins

INTRODUCTION

There are many known causes for the dystonias, both inherited and acquired. This chapter reviews dystonia that is acquired from chemicals an individual may be exposed to, intentionally or inadvertently. It covers common prescription medications, illicit drugs, and exposure to environmental toxins.

By far the most commonly implicated prescription medications are the dopamine receptor inhibitors, with the best recognized being the neuroleptics or antipsychotics. These medications are widely used for conditions other than psychosis, so neuroleptic-induced dystonia is still commonly encountered. There are many other less well-recognized drugs that also inhibit dopamine receptors, most notably metoclopramide and related drugs commonly used for nausea or migraine. Dystonia resulting from these drugs is also frequent.

Dystonic reactions to illicit drugs and environmental toxins may also occur. Although such reactions are rare, they are valuable to recognize because a key aspect of treatment involves limiting further exposure.

ACUTE DYSTONIC REACTIONS

Epidemiology

Acute dystonic reactions may emerge suddenly following treatment with a variety of medications. The onset of an acute dystonic reaction after taking an antipsychotic is usually quick, within 10 minutes to a few hours of dosing, rapidly reaching peak severity within a few minutes.

The most commonly implicated medications are those that inhibit central dopamine transmission, most notably the antipsychotics. A number of additional commonly used medications that inhibit dopamine transmission are frequently overlooked but equally important causes. They include metoclopramide or prochlorperazine, which may be used for gastrointestinal motility, nausea, and migraine. Dopamine receptor blockers are sometimes also (perhaps inappropriately) prescribed for insomnia, vertigo, and other nonspecific complaints. Dopamine receptor blockers are occasionally combined with antidepressants, where they are believed to augment effectiveness. Domperidone is a dopamine receptor blocker that does not usually cause acute dystonic reactions because it does not cross the blood–brain barrier, except in very young children where the barrier may be more leaky.[30]

There are a number of additional less common causes for acute dystonic reactions. Included in this list are almost all antidepressants, especially the selective serotonin uptake inhibitors, where several hundred cases have been reported.[67,68] An increased risk of dystonia was reported in one study of a large post-marketing database containing 29,253 reports of various movement disorders following antidepressant exposure.[95] There was a small increase in risk of dystonia associated with serotonin reuptake inhibitors as a group, and especially amoxepine, fluoxetine, fluvoxamine, and paroxetine. However, the type of dystonia was not reported. Many additional drugs have been reported to cause acute dystonic reactions. However, most are quite rare and described only in case reports where a causal association may be difficult to establish (Table 19.1).

The reported risk of medication-induced acute dystonic reactions varies widely, depending on multiple factors. The most important factor is the type of medication (Figure 19.1).[73] The risk appears to be highest with first-generation antipsychotics (dopamine receptor antagonists), also known as *typical* antipsychotics (e.g., haloperidol, fluphenazine). Early studies reported the risk of acute dystonic reactions with these drugs to be 10–60% of initial exposures.[2,22,57,74,94,114] The risk is lower with certain second-generation antipsychotics, also known as *atypical* antipsychotics, such as olanzepine, quetiapine, and clozapine (Figure 19.1).[73] In fact the risk with clozapine is almost negligible, although some case reports have been published.[56,81] Also implicated are third-generation antipsychotics such as aripiprazole, which have complex mechanisms of action that involve partial agonism of dopamine receptors.

The risk of an acute dystonic reaction also depends on prior exposures. Acute dystonic reactions are far more common among individuals with their first exposure to an antipsychotic compared to individuals who have had prior exposures. In one large study of 1,152 individuals receiving initial treatment with a first-generation antipsychotic, 116 (10.1%) experienced an acute dystonic reaction.[114] A total of 85% of acute dystonic reactions occurred within 4 days of starting an antipsychotic, and 96% occurred within 15 days after starting. Acute dystonic reactions are less common when individuals are premedicated with anticholinergics as a preventive strategy. Conversely, acute dystonic reactions with dopamine receptor inhibitors appear to be more common among individuals who have previously used cocaine.[50,127]

Age also has a strong impact on the risk of an acute dystonic reaction. One study of 49 individuals who had an acute dystonic reaction within 4 days of initial dosing with a first-generation antipsychotic reported a risk of approximately 60% among individuals younger than 20 years, dropping to less than 5% among those older than 50 years.[57] Risk

Table 19.1 **Non-antipsychotic drugs reported to cause acute dystonic reactions**

Albendazole	Cimetidine	General anesthesia	Prochlorperazine
Amphetamine	Clomipramine	Ketamine	Promethazine
Amitriptyline	Cloperastine	Lamivudine	Propofol
Amiodiaquine	Cocaine	Lamotrigine	Ranitidine
Amoxapine	Cyclizine	MDMA Metoclopramide	Rivastigmine
AMPT	Diazepam	Methotrimeprazine	Sertraline
Benzquinamide	Diphenhydramine	Methylphenidate	Sumatriptan
Benztropine	Doxepin	Mirtazapine	Tetrabenazine
Bethanechol	Escitalopram	Nitroxazepine	Tiagabine
Buproprion	Felbamate	Ondansetron	Tranylcypramine
Butamirate Citrate	Flunarizine	Oxatomide	Trazodone
Cefalexin	Fluvoxamine	Paroxetine	Varenicline
Cefixime	Fluoxetine	Phencyclidine	Venlafaxine
Ceftirazine	Foscarnet	Phenylzine	
Chloroquine	Gabapentin		

This table does not include the antipsychotics, all of which can cause acute dystonic reactions. Because information for some of these drugs is obtained from a handful of case reports, a true causal relationship may be difficult to establish.

Abbreviations: AMPT, alpha-methyl paratyrosine; MDMA, 3,4-methylenedioxymethampheamine.

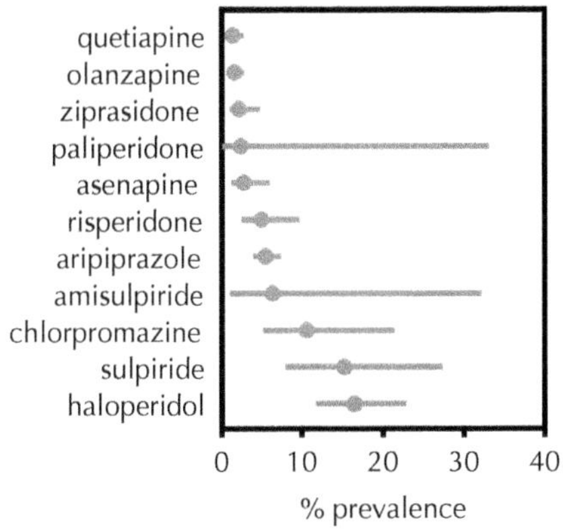

Figure 19.1. Risk of acute dystonic reactions with different drugs. This diagram shows a modified Forest plot derived from a meta-analysis of side effects summarized in 37 systematic Cochrane reviews spanning 316 randomized controlled trials of different antipsychotics.[73] The mean estimated risk for each drug is shown as solid circle symbols with error bars showing confidence intervals.

also seems to be higher if the initial dose is given in the evening compared to the morning.[74] Some studies have also suggested that these reactions are more common in males than females.

Clinical Features

In the study of 1,152 individuals described above, multiple body regions were affected with dystonia, often in combination; most commonly the neck (30%), tongue (17%), jaw (15%), eyes (6%), and trunk (3%).[114] Other large series have described the commonly affected regions to include the neck (41%), jaw (38%), pharynx (18%), lower limb (18%), tongue (17%), upper limb (17%), eyes (14%), and trunk (12%).[74] Cervical dystonia frequently involves retrocollis, which may be fixed or marked by repetitive jerking, often combined with torticollis or laterocollis.[80] Involvement of the throat and tongue can lead to life-threatening respiratory distress.[21,59,82] Trunk and limb spasms can be severe enough to cause rhabdomyolysis and death.[20,90] Involvement of the eyes is described as *oculogyric crisis*, characterized by involuntary, sustained, and conjugate deviations of the eyes, most often in an upward and oblique direction.[6,111] The eyes may remain in a fixed position for many minutes, or they may intermittently return to normal control. The oculogyric crisis is a particularly useful sign because it is relatively specific to disorders of dopamine transmission.

Differential Diagnosis

The clinical picture of sudden onset of tonic posturing combined with jerking movements and tonic deviation of the eyes often raises concern for seizures. However, consciousness is preserved in acute dystonic reactions, and the electroencephalogram (EEG) does not usually disclose epileptic activity. A history of recent exposure to a drug can be very helpful in making the diagnosis, or a toxicology screen may be performed.

More challenging to diagnose is an acute dystonic reaction in an actively psychotic individual who has recently received an antipsychotic. Tonic posturing and jerking movements may be interpreted as agitation, and complaints of muscle tightness or respiratory distress may be interpreted as anxiety or part of a thought disorder. Also challenging to diagnose is an acute dystonic reaction caused by an antipsychotic used to suppress agitation during emergency care or in the intensive care unit.[31] Abnormal movements may be interpreted as continued agitation due to failure of the initial dose, or to seizures.[33] Sometimes, the abnormal movements are partly masked by an altered sensorium, other psychoactive substances, or physical restraints.

Treatment

Acute dystonic reactions are normally self-limited, and they may resolve spontaneously within minutes or hours. However, immediate treatment is warranted because the attacks are often associated with stress and pain and occasionally more serious consequences. Attacks usually can be terminated within 10–20 minutes following intravenous administration of an anticholinergic (e.g., benztropine), antihistamine (e.g., diphenhydramine), or benzodiazepine (e.g., diazepam or lorazepam). A second dose or an alternative agent may be given if the attack does not resolve within 30 minutes. Failure of the initial attack to resolve after a second dose should raise suspicion for phencyclidine (PCP) intoxication, which can produce a syndrome that mimics acute dystonic reactions.

An attack that initially resolves with treatment may recur because many medications used for treatment have short half-lives. In addition, recurrent acute dystonic reactions lasting for nearly 2 months have been reported.[69] Continued treatment with an oral dose for a few days following the acute dystonic reaction with a slow taper may be useful to avoid recurrence.

TARDIVE DYSTONIA

Definition

A variety of abnormal movements known collectively as *tardive syndromes* can also emerge following chronic treatment with dopamine receptor blockers (Table 19.2).[41,101] The term "tardive" distinguishes these side effects from the more acute dystonic reactions described above. Formal diagnostic criteria for a tardive syndrome require several months of exposure with abnormal movements persisting for more than a month following discontinuation. In practice, tardive syndromes may occur following much shorter exposures, and they may not last a month.

The term "tardive dyskinesia" is employed in two different ways in the literature. It is sometimes used as a non-specific umbrella term encompassing all tardive syndromes. Alternatively, it is used to refer more specifically to the most common tardive syndrome, which involves repetitive stereotypical movements of the tongue, lips, and mouth. This chapter uses the more specific meaning of tardive dyskinesia to distinguish it from the other syndromes. The other tardive syndromes include tardive dystonia, tardive tics, tardive stereotypy, tardive myoclonus, and others (Table 19.2). Oculogyric crises typically occur during acute dystonic reactions, but recurrent oculogyric crises may occur during chronic treatment with stable doses, and they may persist following discontinuation, as a tardive syndrome.[98,102] Tardive tremor has been described, too, although its existence as a distinct entity has been questioned because tremor is common and tremors may arise spontaneously at any age. Tardive parkinsonism is another uncertain entity because parkinsonism is a common acute side effect of exposure to dopamine receptor antagonists, and it can take many months to resolve. Alternatively, neuroleptics may unmask latent Parkinson disease. Mixed tardive syndromes are common, and the presence of a mixed movement disorder provides a useful clue for diagnosis, but there is often a single dominant problem.

Most studies of tardive syndromes group cases of tardive dystonia together with the more common cases of tardive dyskinesia, but it is useful to distinguish them because their clinical manifestations and treatment are distinct. For example, tardive dyskinesia occurs more commonly in older women while tardive dystonia seems to occur

Table 19.2 **Tardive syndromes**

Tardive syndrome	Description
Tardive akathisia	Persistent inner sense of restlessness, which may occur in isolation but often accompanied by pacing or other stereotypical movements to relieve the discomfort
Tardive chorea	Random dance-like or jerky movements that flow from one body region to another, or very varied movements in one body region
Tardive dyskinesia	Repetitive stereotypical movements of the lips, tongue and mouth; sometimes described as choreoathetoid, but often patterned
Tardive dystonia	Persistent dystonic movements
Tardive myoclonus	Recurrent myoclonic jerks, usually involving the upper limbs
Tardive oculogyric crisis	Recurrent oculogyric crises, which may occur in isolation, but often accompany dystonic movements in other body regions
Tardive respiratory dyskinesia	Frequent irregular breathing, sometimes with dyspnea
Tardive sensory syndrome	Persistent abnormal sensory symptoms (often pain in the mouth or pelvic region) that may occur in isolation but usually co-exist with other tardive movements
Tardive stereotypy	Repetitive and purposeless movements such as rubbing hands together, rocking, crossing legs, pelvic thrusting
Tardive tics or tourettism	Recurrent motor or vocal tics in isolation or in various combinations, sometimes resembling Tourette syndrome

More information can be found in prior reviews.[41,101]

more often in younger men.[133] Tardive dyskinesia is often restricted to the oromandibular region. In contrast, tardive dystonia more commonly involves the neck, and it often spreads to segmental or generalized patterns.[12,55,58] Tardive dystonia may respond to anticholinergics, botulinum toxins, or deep brain stimulation.[119] In comparison, these therapies are rarely useful for tardive dyskinesia.

Epidemiology

A meta-analysis that involved all tardive syndromes with a total of 11,493 subjects recruited to 41 independent randomized controlled trials of different antipsychotics reported from 2000 to 2015 revealed an overall prevalence of 25%.[17] There was a lower prevalence among individuals taking second-generation antipsychotics (21%) compared to first-generation antipsychotics (30%), but these differences are difficult to interpret because many subjects receiving second-generation drugs were previously exposed to multiple different antipsychotics over many years. The risk of tardive syndromes among individuals exposed only to second-generation antipsychotics is 7%.[17] The risk for clozapine seems to be very low, although a few isolated cases have been reported.[100,112,123] Although the risk of tardive dyskinesia is lower with second- or third-generation antipsychotics, all antipsychotics can cause it.

Smaller studies more specifically focusing on tardive dystonia rather than combining all tardive syndromes together have revealed widely varying prevalence rates.[24,42,58,108,125,132] The wide variation reflects how tardive dystonia is defined and ascertained, and whether combinations with other tardive syndromes were included. Studies summarizing all types of tardive syndromes often report a low prevalence for tardive dystonia (<2.0%), while those that more methodically evaluated cases for dystonia report a higher prevalence of 13–22%.[108,125]

Clinical Features

The clinical manifestations of tardive dystonia have been described in three large series (Table 19.3).[12,55,58] In all these series, males were more

Table 19.3 **Large series of cases with tardive dystonia**

	Burke 1982 (*n* = 42)	**Kang 1986 (*n* = 67)**	**Kiriakis 1998 (*n* = 107)**
Age at onset			
mean (yrs)	34	39	38
range (yrs)	13–60	13–73	13–68
Sex			
Males (N)	26	35	57
Females (N)	16	32	50
M:F ratio	1.6	1.1	1.1
Duration of exposure			
mean	3.7 yrs	7.3 yrs	6.2 yrs
range	3 days–20 yrs	3 weeks–38 yrs	4 days–23 yrs
Dystonia pattern (%)			
segmental	64.3	61.0	61.7
focal	21.4	38.0	15.9
generalized	11.9	1.6	23.3
Dystonia regions (%)			
neck	78.6	NR	66.3
face	54.8	NR	59.8
arms	54.8	NR	62.6
trunk	50.0	NR	43.4
legs	23.8	NR	26.1

The study by Kang et al.[55] included 16 individuals previously reported by Burke et al., while the study by Kiriakis et al. included 17 individuals previously reported by Burke et al.[12] The study by Kiriakis includes one individual described as having multifocal dystonia that was included in the segmental group in this table. Similar results were described in smaller series of 32 cases,[130] 30 cases,[78] 26 cases,[125] and 20 cases.[65]

frequently affected than females. The mean age at onset was 30–40 years, with a range of 13–70 years. It usually developed insidiously, but sometimes developed in a stepwise fashion. Most cases were identified following several years of drug exposure, but durations of exposures ranged from 3 days to nearly 40 years. Early symptoms are especially challenging to detect in individuals receiving dopamine receptor blockers for psychosis because complaints may be mistaken as a part of a thought disorder.

Tardive dystonia may begin in any body region. The most common manifestations are segmental dystonia involving the neck, craniofacial regions, and pharynx (Table 19.3). However, focal limb dystonia or progression to generalized dystonia are not uncommon. The most mildly affected cases have imperceptible abnormal movements but they describe sensations of pulling, tightness, or muscle soreness. More significantly affected cases may resemble idiopathic focal dystonias. However, careful comparisons of tardive and idiopathic dystonia have shown some differences. For example, prominent retrocollis with coarse jerky movements and additional involvement outside the neck is more common in tardive cervical dystonia than in idiopathic cervical dystonia.[80] Similarly, tardive oromandibular dystonia is more likely to be focal with additional stereotypical mouth movements when compared with idiopathic oromandibular dystonia.[116] Tardive dystonia also can be severely disabling or even life-threatening with reported examples of severe tardive cervical dystonia leading to myelopathy or fracture of the cervical spine,[61,62] oromandibular dystonia leading to inability to speak or malnutrition, dystonia of the larynx and pharynx leading to respiratory distress,[129] progression to incapacitating generalized dystonia or status dystonicus,[120] and sometimes rhabdomyolysis and renal failure.[66]

Treatment

The initial step in treatment involves identifying and weaning the offending medication (Figure 19.2).[119] Abrupt discontinuation is discouraged because of the risk of withdrawal-emergent dyskinesias, and complete discontinuation may not be feasible for individuals with severe psychiatric disorders. In these cases, it may be possible to cross-wean to a dopamine receptor antagonist

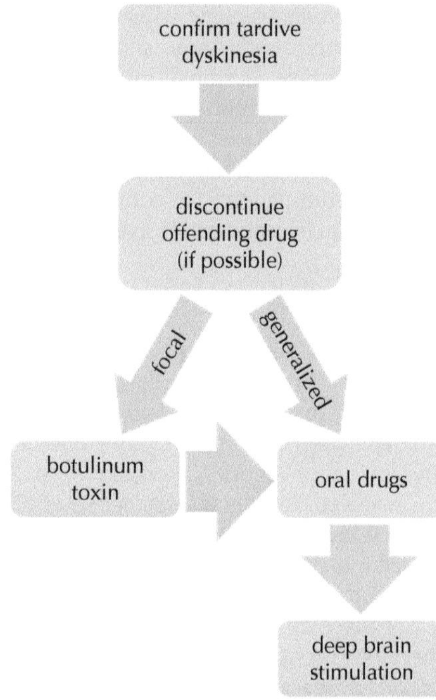

Figure 19.2. Treatment algorithm for tardive syndromes.[119] The first step is to confirm the diagnosis of a tardive syndrome caused by a specific medication, rather than some other condition. The next step is to discontinue the medication, if possible. If discontinuation is not possible, substitute clozapine. Generalized syndromes are generally treated with oral medications, such as VMAT2 inhibitors, anticholinergics, clonazepam, or baclofen. If these options prove inadequate, deep brain stimulation can be useful. Focal and segmental dystonias can be treated with botulinum toxins instead, with oral medications and/or surgery if needed.

with lower risk of tardive dyskinesia, such as clozapine.

Even following withdrawal of the offending medication, tardive dystonia frequently is permanent. In one large longitudinal observational study of 107 cases, 50% had no change or worsened following discontinuation of the drug, 39% showed partial improvements, and only 14% had a complete remission.[58] Remissions occurred on average 2.6 years following discontinuation, with a range of 1 month to 9 years. Complete remission was more likely with shorter durations of drug exposure, and remission was unlikely with more than 10 years of exposure. Similar findings were reported in another study of 67 individuals with tardive dystonia.[55] It has been suggested that these early estimates may have provided an unusually pessimistic view of recovery due to a referral bias toward more severe cases with longer durations of drug exposure. Other series that included less severely affected cases with prompt intervention reported complete remission in 64% with only 20% being permanent.[55,126] These findings imply that early recognition is important.

Although numerous reviews address the treatment of tardive dyskinesia, few specifically address tardive dystonia.[119] Early observational studies suggested at least partial benefits from medications commonly used to treat other forms of dystonia such as anticholinergics, benzodiazepines, or baclofen (Figure 19.2).[12,55,58] Clozapine also has been identified as a promising candidate in numerous subsequent case reports and small series.[119,131] Benefits with clozapine may vary from nil to marked, sometimes without return of tardive dystonia after clozapine is discontinued.

Medications that inhibit uptake of monoamines into presynaptic vesicles (VMAT2 inhibitors) deserve special attention. Early studies reported tetrabenazine to be at least partly helpful for tardive dystonia in multiple unblinded reports.[12,54,55,58] The value of newer-generation VMAT2 inhibitors is less clear. Valbenazine is a derivative of tetrabenazine in which the (+)alpha isomer is linked to valine. Following administration, the valine is cleaved, leaving the (+)alpha isomer, which is more specific than the normal racemic mixture of tetrabenazine. The overall consequence is a longer half-life of the more specific isomer, with presumably fewer side effects. Valbenazine proved to be efficacious in two independent, double-blind, placebo-controlled trials that recruited a mixed population of individuals with all tardive syndromes.[48,83] However, the Abnormal Involuntary Movement Scale used as the primary outcome measure does not discriminate tardive dystonia from the far more common stereotypical orobuccolingual syndrome. Furthermore, individuals with severe truncal dystonia were excluded. Because individuals with tardive dystonia were not discriminated from the larger group and severe dystonia cases were excluded, the specific value of valbenazine for tardive dystonia remains to be established.

Deutetrabenazine is another modification of tetrabenazine in which certain hydrogen atoms are replaced with deuterium. This substitution increases the half-life of the drug and allows for less frequent dosing. Deutetrabenazine was also efficacious in two independent, double-blind, placebo-controlled trials for individuals with all types of tardive syndromes,[5,37] with sustained benefits.[38,47] The Abnormal Involuntary Movement Scale was again used to address efficacy for deutetrabenazine, so the specific value of this drug for tardive dystonia also remains to be established.

Focal and segmental tardive dystonia may be treated with botulinum toxins, with responses similar to treatment of idiopathic cases (Figure 19.2).[11,80,104,117] The condition may remit following a few injection cycles or a few years. Tardive dystonia often responds well to deep brain stimulation surgery. A meta-analysis of deep brain stimulation studies that included 117 cases of tardive dystonia described across 35 different reports yielded an overall result of 62±15% improvement in the Abnormal Involuntary Movement Scale and 76±21% improvement in the Burke-Fahn-Marsden dystonia rating scale.[72] Benefits appear to be sustained for many years, with side effects similar to other types of dystonia treated with the same approach (see Chapter 31, "Surgical Treatments for Dystonia").

OTHER MEDICATIONS IMPACTING MONOAMINERGIC TRANSMISSION

Levodopa

Individuals with Parkinson disease or related parkinsonian disorders may also have dystonia (see Chapter 13, "Dystonia and Parkinsonism"). Dystonia may occur early in the course of the illness, prior to any treatment. In some cases, dystonia is provoked by medications used for treatment, such as levodopa.[14,109] Levodopa-induced dystonia is most common during end-of-dose wearing-off periods, but it may occur as part of peak-dose dyskinesias or diphasic dyskinesias as well. It typically affects one arm or leg, but it may also affect the neck or face. Off-period dystonia can be addressed by increasing the dose or by adding medications to mitigate against wearing off.

Dopamine Receptor Agonists

While dopamine receptor antagonists can cause either acute or tardive dystonia in individuals with presumably normal basal ganglia dopamine function, dystonia can be also sometimes triggered by dopamine receptor agonists in

Parkinson disease or related parkinsonian disorders. Pramipexole has been most commonly implicated,[53,85–88,113,121] but there are reports for other dopamine agonists including pergolide,[16] ropinirole,[4,43] and rotigotine.[32] Dystonia usually begins within days or weeks of starting the medication or following a dose change. The dystonia often develops quickly, over a period of days or weeks. The most common manifestations are axial, with cervical dystonia (particularly anterocollis) or truncal dystonia (camptocormia or Pisa syndrome). However, limb dystonia may occur, too. Following discontinuation (or reversal of the change that provoked the problem), dystonia may resolve, but it persists in some cases.

Psychostimulants

Medications that stimulate the release of monoamines, also known as psychostimulants or sympathomimetics, may occasionally provoke acute or chronic dystonia.[44,46,77,84,118,122,128] They include amphetamine, methamphetamine, methylphenidate, and atomoxetine. These medications are often used for attention-deficit hyperactivity disorder in children, sometimes in combination with dopamine receptor antagonists, so establishing a causal relationship is sometimes complicated by use of multiple medications. Dystonia usually resolves following withdrawal of the psychostimulant.

ILLICIT DRUGS

A number of illicit drugs may provoke dystonia, either acutely or after chronic exposure, so a history of potential exposure to such drugs or a toxicology screen may be helpful. Numerous different "street drugs" have been associated with acute dystonic reactions. These reactions often are not caused by the street drug, but by additives. Many illicit drugs are sold as white powders; they are mixed with other less expensive psychoactive medications that are also white powders, most notably haloperidol and phenothiazines. As a result, the toxicology screen may reveal a drug different from the one the affected individual thought they had taken.

Prescription medications may be abused or synthesized and sold as recreational drugs. The psychostimulants (amphetamine, methamphetamine, atomoxetine) may cause acute or chronic dystonia as described above. Another psychostimulant is cocaine. Crack cocaine (also known as *crack* or *rock*) is a crystalized form of the free base of cocaine that can be smoked. The effects are more rapid and intense than those obtained with other methods of cocaine use. Active use or withdrawal both have been linked with acute dystonic reactions in multiple independent reports.[19,27,36,39,64,76] There also is evidence that users of crack cocaine have a higher risk of acute dystonic reactions when later exposed to dopamine receptor inhibitors. The recreational drug methylenedioxymethamphetamine (MDMA or *ecstasy*) has occasionally be reported to cause acute dystonic reactions, too.[1]

Phencyclidine (PCP) used to be a very commonly abused street drug, although its popularity has declined in recent years. It is a white powder that may be consumed directly, snorted, or dissolved and injected. Most commonly, it is smoked following sprinkling of a powder form on cigarettes or soaking cigarettes in PCP-laden liquids. One series of 1,000 cases found the most common features of PCP intoxication to be nystagmus (57%), hypertension (57%), and changes in sensorium (54%), often with bizarre or agitated and violent behavior.[75] A smaller proportion (<5% each) had changes in autonomic signs or neurological features such as seizures or other motor behavior interpreted by emergency room personnel as dystonic. The motor manifestations may closely resemble acute dystonic reactions seen with other drugs,[89] but may also include isolated oculogyric crises[114] or rigidity of the trunk or limbs, sometimes with dynamic twisting or jerking movements and rhabdomyolysis.[29,75] PCP intoxication may also occur in young children or even infants, with the usual route of exposure being passive inhalation of smoke from adults smoking nearby, eating or smoking butts of cigarettes laced with PCP, or access to the drug itself.[103] Treatment is largely supportive until the drug washes out.

Ephedrone (methcathinone, or *cat*) has been repeatedly linked with relatively abrupt onset of a syndrome that combines dystonia with parkinsonism.[34,60,97,99,106,107,110] The syndrome may be permanent or even progressive, with evidence for neuropathological damage in the pallidum. In most cases, the culprit is not ephedrine, but manganese: potassium permanganate is used as a catalyst during the synthesis of ephedrone, and incomplete purification may leave substantial amounts of manganese in the final product.

ENVIRONMENTAL TOXINS

Delayed-Onset Dystonia

Dystonia may emerge weeks or even years following nervous system damage of many different types including hypoxia-ischemia, stroke, or toxic exposures.[10] The reasons for the delay are unknown, but there often is evidence for damage in the basal ganglia, particularly the putamen and pallidum. These regions of the brain appear to be particularly vulnerable to insults that challenge energy production.

Carbon monoxide is a colorless and odorless gas by-product of combustion, especially petroleum products. Toxicity results from exposure to fumes with inadequate ventilation. Individuals present with an acute encephalopathy followed by resolution of most or all symptoms over a period of a few days or a week. A movement disorder emerges weeks later, often in association with neuroimaging evidence of damage to the basal ganglia and deep white matter.[51] In one large study of 242 individuals with carbon monoxide poisoning, 32 developed a movement disorder, most commonly parkinsonism and/or dystonia.[26] The delay to onset of parkinsonism ranged from 2 to 26 weeks, while the delay to onset of dystonia ranged from 4 to 77 weeks. In early stages following exposure, hyperbaric oxygen may be useful as a treatment.

Methanol is an alcohol that is used as a solvent in many household cleaning products. Toxicity may result from consuming these items, but more commonly results from consuming homemade alcohols, such as "moonshine." Occasionally toxicity results in individuals who mistake methanol as a consumable alcohol. Methanol causes an acute encephalopathy with visual loss because of a high predilection for damaging the optic nerves.[93] Some individuals develop a delayed syndrome of parkinsonism often with dystonia in association with neuroimaging evidence of putaminal necrosis.[40,70,92,93,96]

Cyanide is a metabolic by-product of ingredients in certain foods, such as the cassava plant. Most reported toxic exposures, however, result from intentional consumption during attempted suicide. Following recovery from encephalopathy in the acute phase, some individuals develop delayed parkinsonism and/or dystonia, often with neuroimaging evidence of pallidal necrosis.[10,18,45,124]

Disulfiram is a prescription medication used to suppress alcohol consumption. Normal doses do not cause neurological impairments, but toxic overdoses have been reported to cause an acute encephalopathy followed by severe dystonia, often combined with parkinsonism.[25,63] Similar to other toxins in this category, there is usually neuroimaging evidence of basal ganglia damage.

Manganese

There is a well-known relationship between manganese toxicity and movement disorders. Dystonia combined with parkinsonism may be caused by inherited disorders of manganese transport that lead to manganese accumulation in the brain (see Chapter 13 and Chapter 22, "Dystonia Genetics"). Dystonia and parkinsonism also may be provoked in normal individuals exposed to toxic doses of manganese.[7,13,15,23,35,52,60] Toxic exposure may occur in miners who inhale dust laden with manganese, welders who inhale fumes that contain vaporized manganese, chronic liver disease where dietary manganese is not eliminated from the body, and illicit ephedrone that is contaminated with potassium permanganate.

Mycotoxin

Athrinium is a fungus found worldwide that can produce the mycotoxin 3-nitropropionic acid. The toxin inhibits succinate dehydrogenase, an enzyme essential for energy production.[28] Accidental ingestion of foods contaminated with this mycotoxin can cause an acute encephalopathy with striatal necrosis. Cases who survive the acute phase may develop permanent dystonia and parkinsonism, usually with a delay of a few days or weeks. Many cases have been reported from Asia,[71] although a few have been reported from Africa and Europe. Identified sources have included moldy sugar cane[49,71,79] or stale coconut water,[9] but exposures with no identifiable source have also been reported.[8]

SYNOPSIS AND FUTURE PROSPECTS

The dystonias have many potential etiologies which include prescription medications, drugs of abuse, and environmental toxins. The most common among these potential etiologies is exposure to drugs that block dopamine receptors. Acute dystonic reactions and tardive dystonia are both relatively well-recognized side effects of antipsychotics, but dopamine receptor drugs used for other indications are readily missed, most notably metoclopramide and prochlorperazine.

Acute dystonic reactions often lead to emergency evaluation because they are very stressful and may be life-threatening. They are readily mistaken for seizures but respond well to reassurance, withholding further exposures to the offending drug, and specific medications. Tardive dystonia has a more insidious onset but may become severely disabling or life-threatening. Early identification of tardive dystonia is important because early discontinuation of the offending medication may speed resolution. Both acute and tardive dystonia are not uncommon. In both cases, pathogenesis is not well understood. Further studies of pathogenesis could be valuable for developing preventative strategies, especially for tardive dystonia where existing treatments are not always satisfactory.

Illicit drugs and environmental toxins are less common causes for dystonia, but they are important to recognize so that further exposures can be prevented. A precise exposure can be difficult to identify because the history may be misleading or even unknown. A further challenge in recognizing these causes is that dystonia may be delayed by weeks or even years following exposure. However, these source for dystonia can usually be identified by a careful history, toxicology screens, and sometimes characteristic neuroimaging features. The pathogenesis of these conditions varies, although several share the common problem of energy limitation leading to striatal necrosis. Further understanding of these mechanisms is needed to develop better treatment strategies.

REFERENCES

1. Achiron A, Melamed E. Tardive eating dystonia. Mov Disord 1990;5:331–333.
2. Aguilar EJ, Keshavan MS, Martinez-Quiles MD, Hernandez J, Gomez-Beneyto M, Schooler NR. Predictors of acute dystonia in first-episode psychotic patients. Am J Psychiatry 1994;151:1819–1821.
3. Albin RL. Basal ganglia neurotoxins. Neurol Clin 2000;18:665–680.
4. Ameghino L, Rossi M, Cammarota A, Merello M. Ropinirole-induced anterocollis in Parkinson's disease. Mov Disord Clin Pract 2016;3:91–92.
5. Anderson KE, Stamler D, Davis MD, Factor SA, Hauser RA, Isojarvi J, et al. Deutetrabenazine for treatment of involuntary movements in patients with tardive dyskinesia (AIM-TD): A double-blind, randomised, placebo-controlled, phase 3 trial. Lancet Psychiatry 2017;4:595–604.
6. Barow E, Schneider SA, Bhatia KP, Ganos C. Oculogyric crises: Etiology, pathophysiology and therapeutic approaches. Parkinsonism Relat Disord 2017;36:3–9.
7. Barron TF, Devenyi AG, Mamourian AC. Symptomatic manganese neurotoxicity in a patient with chronic liver disease: Correlation of clinical symptoms with MRI findings. Pediatr Neurol 1994;10:145–148.
8. Bendiksen Skogvold H, Yazdani M, Sandas EM, Osteby Vassli A, Kristensen E, et al. A pioneer study on human 3-nitropropionic acid intoxication: Contributions from metabolomics. J Appl Toxicol 2022;42:818–829.
9. Birkelund T, Johansen RF, Illum DG, Dyrskog SE, Ostergaard JA, Falconer TM, et al. Fatal 3-nitropropionic acid poisoning after consuming coconut water. Emerg Infect Dis 2021;27:278–280.
10. Borgohain R, Singh AK, Radhakrishna H, Rao VC, Mohandas S. Delayed onset generalised dystonia after cyanide poisoning. Clin Neurol Neurosurg 1995;97:213–215.
11. Brashear A, Ambrosius WT, Eckert GJ, Siemers ER. Comparison of treatment of tardive dystonia and idiopathic cervical dystonia with botulinum toxin type A. Mov Disord 1998;13:158–161.
12. Burke RE, Fahn S, Jankovic J, Marsden CD, Lang AE, Gollomp S, Ilson J. Tardive dystonia: Late-onset and persistent dystonia caused by antipsychotic drugs. Neurology 1982;32:1335–1346.
13. Burkhard PR, Delavelle J, Du Pasquier R, Spahr L. Chronic parkinsonism associated with cirrhosis: A distinct subset of acquired hepatocerebral degeneration. Arch Neurol 2003;60:521–528.
14. Calabresi P, Standaert DG. Dystonia and levodopa-induced dyskinesias in Parkinson's disease: Is there a connection? Neurobiol Dis 2019;132:104579.
15. Calne DB, Chu NS, Huang CC, Lu CS, Olanow W. Manganism and idiopathic parkinsonism: Similarities and differences. Neurology 1994;44:1583–1586.
16. Cannas A, Solla P, Floris G, Tacconi P, Serra A, Piga M, et al. Reversible Pisa syndrome in patients with Parkinson's disease on dopaminergic therapy. J Neurol 2009;256:390–395.
17. Carbon M, Hsieh CH, Kane JM, Correll CU. Tardive dyskinesia prevalence in the period of second-generation antipsychotic use: A meta-analysis. J Clin Psychiatry 2017;78:e264–e278.

18. Carella F, Grassi MP, Savoiardo M, Contri P, Rapuzzi B, Mangoni A. Dystonic-parkinsonian syndrome after cyanide poisoning: Clinical and MRI findings. J Neurol Neurosurg Psychiatry 1988;51:1345–1348.
19. Catalano G, Catalano MC, Rodriguez R. Dystonia associated with crack cocaine use. South Med J 1997;90:1050–1052.
20. Cavanaugh JJ, Finlayson RE. Rhabdomyolysis due to acute dystonic reaction to antipsychotic drugs. J Clin Psychiatry 1984;45:356–357.
21. Centen LM, van Egmond ME, Tijssen MAJ. New developments in diagnosis and treament of adult-onset focal dystonia. Curr Opin Neurol 2023;36:317–323.
22. Chakos MH, Mayerhoff DI, Loebel AD, Alvir JM, Lieberman JA. Incidence and correlates of acute extrapyramidal symptoms in first episode of schizophrenia. Psychopharmacol Bull 1992;28:81–86.
23. Chen P, Bornhorst J, Aschner M. Manganese metabolism in humans. Front Biosci 2018;23:1655–1679.
24. Chiu H, Shum P, Lau J, Lam L, Lee S. Prevalence of tardive dyskinesia, tardive dystonia, and respiratory dyskinesia among Chinese psychiatric patients in Hong Kong. Am J Psychiatry 1992;149:1081–1085.
25. Cho YN, Lyoo CH, Lee MS. Imaging evidence of nigral damage in dystonia secondary to disulfiram intoxication. Mov Disord 2011;26:763–764.
26. Choi IS, Cheon HY. Delayed movement disorders after carbon monoxide poisoning. Eur Neurol 1999;42:141–144.
27. Choy-Kwong M, Lipton RB. Dystonia related to cocaine withdrawal: A case report and pathogenic hypothesis. Neurology 1989;39:996–997.
28. Chu NS, Huang CC, Lu CS, Calne DB. Toxin-induced dystonia. In: Tsui JKC, Calne DB, eds. *Handbook of Dystonia*. Marcel Dekker; 1995: 241–265.
29. Cogen FC, Rigg G, Simmons JL, Domino EF. Phencyclidine-associated acute rhabdomyolysis. Ann Intern Med 1978;88:210–212.
30. Dhakal OP, Dhakal M, Bhandari D. Domperidone-induced dystonia: A rare and troublesome complication. BMJ Case Rep 2014:bcr2013200282.
31. Digby G, Jalini S, Taylor S. Medication-induced acute dystonic reaction: The challenge of diagnosing movement disorders in the intensive care unit. BMJ Case Rep 2015; bcr2014207215.
32. Dohm CP, Groschel S, Liman J, Bahr M, Kermer P. Dropped head sign induced by transdermal application of the dopamine agonist rotigotine in parkinsonian syndrome: A case report. J Med Case Rep 2013;7:174.
33. Emorinken A, Agbadaola OR. Metoclopramide-induced acute dystonia misdiagnosed as an epileptic seizure in a lupus patient. J Epilepsy Res 2021;11:156–158.
34. Ennok M, Sikk K, Haldre S, Taba P. Cognitive profile of patients with manganese-methcathinone encephalopathy. Neurotoxicology 2020;76:138–143.
35. Fang JY, Phibbs FT, Davis TL. Spectrum of movement disorders in professional welders. Bratisl Lek Listy 2009;110:358–360.
36. Farrell PE, Diehl AK. Acute dystonic reaction to crack cocaine. Ann Emerg Med 1991;20:322.
37. Fernandez HH, Factor SA, Hauser RA, Jimenez-Shahed J, Ondo WG, Jarskog LF, et al. Randomized controlled trial of deutetrabenazine for tardive dyskinesia: The ARM-TD study. Neurology 2017;88:2003–2010.
38. Fernandez HH, Stamler D, Davis MD, Factor SA, Hauser RA, Jimenez-Shahed J, et al. Long-term safety and efficacy of deutetrabenazine for the treatment of tardive dyskinesia. J Neurol Neurosurg Psychiatry 2019;90:1317–1323.
39. Fines RE, Brady WJ, DeBehnke DJ. Cocaine-associated dystonic reaction. Am J Emerg Med 1997;15:513–515.
40. Franquet E, Salvado-Figueres M, Lorenzo-Bosquet C, Cuberas-Borros G, Rovira A, Castell-Conesa J, Hernandez-Vara J. Nigrostriatal pathway dysfunction in a methanol-induced delayed dystonia-parkinsonism. Mov Disord 2012;27:1220–1221.
41. Friedman JH. Tardive syndromes. Continuum 2019;25:1081–1098.
42. Friedman JH, Kucharski LT, Wagner RL. Tardive dystonia in a psychiatric hospital. J Neurol Neurosurg Psychiatry 1987;50:801–803.
43. Galati S, Moller JC, Stadler C. Ropinirole-induced Pisa syndrome in Parkinson disease. Clin Neuropharmacol 2014;37:58–59.
44. Gay CT, Ryan SG. Paroxysmal kinesigenic dystonia after methylphenidate administration. J Child Neurol 1994;9:45–46.
45. Grandas F, Artieda J, Obeso JA. Clinical and CT scan findings in a case of cyanide intoxication. Mov Disord 1989;4:188–193.
46. Grau-Lopez L, Daigre C, Mercado N, Casas M, Roncero C. Dystonia in methylphenidate withdrawal: A case report. J Addict Med 2017;11:154–156.
47. Hauser RA, Barkay H, Fernandez HH, Factor SA, Jimenez-Shahed J, Gross N, et al. Long-term deutetrabenazine treatment for tardive dyskinesia Is associated with sustained benefits and safety: A 3-year, open-label extension study. Front Neurol 2022;13:773999.
48. Hauser RA, Factor SA, Marder SR, Knesevich MA, Ramirez PM, Jimenez R, et al. KINECT 3: A phase 3 randomized, double-blind, placebo-controlled trial of valbenazine for tardive dyskinesia. Am J Psychiatry 2017;174:476–484.
49. He F, Zhang S, Qian G, Zhang C. Delayed dystonia with striatal CT lucencies induced by a mycotoxin (3-nitropropionic acid). Neurology 1995;45:2178–2183.
50. Hegarty AM, Lipton RB, Merriam AE, Freeman K. Cocaine as a risk factor for acute dystonic reactions. Neurology 1991;41:1670–1672.
51. Hsiao CL, Kuo HC, Huang CC. Delayed encephalopathy after carbon monoxide intoxication: Long-term prognosis and correlation of clinical manifestations and neuroimages. Acta Neurol Taiwan 2004;13:64–70.
52. Huang CC, Chu NS, Lu CS, Chen RS, Schulzer M, Calne DB. The natural history of neurological manganism over 18 years. Parkinsonism Relat Disord 2007;13:143–145.
53. Iijima M, Osawa M, Uchiyama S, Kitagawa K. Pramipexole-induced antecollis in patients with Parkinson's disease: Two cases and literature review. eNeurologicalSci 2015;1:21–23.
54. Jankovic J, Beach J. Long-term effects of tetrabenazine in hyperkinetic movement disorders. Neurology 1997;48:358–362.
55. Kang UJ, Burke RE, Fahn S. Natural history and treatment of tardive dystonia. Mov Disord 1986;1:193–208.
56. Kaplan AM, Pitts WB, Ahmed I. An unexpected circumstance: Acute dystonic reaction in the setting of clozapine administration. J Pharm Pract 2019;32:103–105.

57. Keepers GA, Casey DE. Prediction of neuroleptic-induced dystonia. J Clin Psychopharmacol 1987;7:342–345.
58. Kiriakakis V, Bhatia KP, Quinn NP, Marsden CD. The natural history of tardive dystonia. A long-term follow-up study of 107 cases. Brain 1998;121:2053–2066.
59. Koek RJ, Pi EH. Acute laryngeal dystonic reactions to neuroleptics. Psychosomatics 1989;30:359–364.
60. Koksal A, Baybas S, Sozmen V, Koksal NS, Altunkaynak Y, Dirican A, et al. Chronic manganese toxicity due to substance abuse in Turkish patients. Neurol India 2012;60:224–227.
61. Konrad C, Vollmer-Haase J, Anneken K, Knecht S. Orthopedic and neurological complications of cervical dystonia: Review of the literature. Acta Neurol Scand 2004;109:369–373.
62. Konrad C, Vollmer-Haase J, Gaubitz M, Nabavi DG, Reilmann R, Knecht S. Fracture of the odontoid process complicating tardive dystonia. Mov Disord 2004;8:983–985.
63. Krauss JK, Mohadjer M, Wakhloo AK, Mundinger F. Dystonia and akinesia due to pallidoputaminal lesions after disulfiram intoxication. Mov Disord 1991;6:166–170.
64. Kumor K. Cocaine withdrawal dystonia. Neurology 1990;40:863–864.
65. Lang AE. Clinical differences between metoclopramide- and antipsychotic-induced tardive dyskinesias. Can J Neurol Sci 1990;17:137–139.
66. Lazarus AL, Toglia JU. Fatal myoglobinuric renal failure in a patient with tardive dyskinesia. Neurology 1985;35:1055–1057.
67. Leo RJ. Clinical manifestations of dystonia and dyskinesia after SSRI administration. J Clin Psychiatry 1996;58:403–404.
68. Leo RJ. Movement disorders associated with the serotonin selective reuptake inhibitors. J Clin Psychiatry 1996;57:449–454.
69. Leopold NA. Prolonged metoclopramide-induced dyskinetic reaction. Neurology 1984;34:238–239.
70. LeWitt PA, Martin SD. Dystonia and hypokinesis with putaminal necrosis after methanol intoxication. Clin Neuropharmacol 1988;11:161–167.
71. Liu X, Luo X, Hu W. Studies on the epidemiology and etiology of moldy sugarcane poisoning in China. Biomed Environ Sci 1992;5:161–177.
72. Macerollo A, Deuschl G. Deep brain stimulation for tardive syndromes: Systematic review and meta-analysis. J Neurol Sci 2018;389:55–60.
73. Martino D, Karnik V, Osland S, Barnes TRE, Pringsheim TM. Movement disorders associated with antipsychotic medication in people with schizophrenia: An overview of Cochrane reviews and meta-analysis. Can J Psychiatry 2018;63:706743718777392.
74. Mazurek MF, Rosebush PI. Acute drug-induced dystonia. In: Factor SA, Lang AE, Weiner WJ, eds. *Drug-Induced Movement Disorders*, 2nd ed. Blackwell; 2005: 72–102.
75. McCarron MM, Schulze BW, Thompson GA, Conder MC, Goetz WA. Acute phencyclidine intoxication: Incidence of clinical findings in 1,000 cases. Ann Emerg Med 1981;10:237–242.
76. Merab J. Acute dystonic reaction to cocaine. Am J Med 1988;84:564.
77. Meyers KJ, Upadhyaya HP, Goodloe R, Kryzhanovskaya LA, Liles-Burden MA, Kellier-Steele NA, Mancini M. Evaluation of dystonia in children and adolescents treated with atomoxetine within the Truven MarketScan database: A retrospective cohort study. Expert Opin Drug Saf 2018;17:467–473.
78. Miller LG, Jankovic J. Neurologic approach to drug-induced movement disorders: A study of 125 patients. South Med J 1990;83:525–532.
79. Ming L. Moldy sugarcane poisoning: A case report with a brief review. J Toxicol Clin Toxicol 1995;33:363–367.
80. Molho ES, Feustel PJ, Factor SA. Clinical comparison of tardive and idiopathic cervical dystonia. Mov Disord 1998;13:486–489.
81. Nebhinani N, Avasthi A, Modi M. Oculogyric crisis with clozapine: A case report and review of similar case reports in the literature. Indian J Psychol Med 2015;37:342–344.
82. Newton-John H. Acute upper airway obstruction due to supraglottic dystonia induced by a neuroleptic. BMJ 1988;297:964–965.
83. O'Brien CF, Jimenez R, Hauser RA, Factor SA, Burke J, Mandri D, Castro-Gayol JC. NBI-98854, a selective monoamine transport inhibitor for the treatment of tardive dyskinesia: A randomized, double-blind, placebo-controlled study. Mov Disord 2015;30:1681–1687.
84. Pagliaro A, Mattio B, Paulson N, Fromm C, Vidal J. Unprovoked dystonic reaction in a child taking long-term methylphenidate. J Pharm Pract 2022;35:796–799.
85. Pandey S, Jain S. Pramipexole-associated fixed limb dystonia in Parkinson's disease. Parkinsonism Relat Disord 2016;31:159–160.
86. Pandey S, Sarma N, Jain S. Pramipexole associated dystonia. Parkinsonism Relat Disord 2017;38:104–105.
87. Park D. Pramipexole-induced limb dystonia and its associated complex regional pain syndrome in idiopathic Parkinson's disease: A case report. Medicine 2017;96:e7530.
88. Pellene A, Saenz-Farret M, Micheli F. Recurrent and alternating Pisa syndrome. Clin Neuropharmacol 2015;38:252–254.
89. Piecuch S, Thomas U, Shah BR. Acute dystonic reactions that fail to respond to diphenhydramine: Think of PCP. J Emerg Med 1999;17:527.
90. Pollera CF, Cognetli F, Nardi M, Mozza D. Sudden death after acute dystonic reaction to high-dose metoclopramide. Lancet 1984;2:460–461.
91. Priori A, Bertolasi L, Berardelli A, Manfredi M. Acute dystonic reaction to ecstasy. Mov Disord 1995;10:353.
92. Quartarone A, Girlanda P, Vita G, Battaglia F, Majorana G, Monici M, Messina C. Oromandibular dystonia in a patient with bilateral putaminal necrosis after methanol poisoning: An electrophysiological study. Eur Neurol 2000;44:127–128.
93. Reddy NJ, Sudini M, Lewis LD. Delayed neurological sequelae from ethylene glycol, diethylene glycol and methanol poisonings. Clin Toxicol (Phila) 2010;48:967–973.
94. Remington GJ, Voineskos G, Pollock B, Reed K, Coulter K. Prevalence of neuroleptic-induced dystonia in mania and schizophrenia. Am J Psychiatry 1990;147:1231–1233.
95. Revet A, Montastruc F, Roussin A, Raynaud JP, Lapeyre-Mestre M, Nguyen TTH. Antidepressants and movement disorders: A postmarketing study in the world pharmacovigilance database. BMC Psychiatry 2020;20:308.

96. Rohani M, Munhoz RP, Haeri G. Abnormal movements induced by methanol toxicity. Postgrad Med J 2017;93:1.
97. Rusz J, Megrelishvili M, Bonnet C, Okujava M, Brozova H, Khatiashvili I, et al. A distinct variant of mixed dysarthria reflects parkinsonism and dystonia due to ephedrone abuse. J Neural Transm 2014;121:655–664.
98. Sachdev P. Tardive and chronically recurrent oculogyric crises. Mov Disord 1993;8:93–97.
99. Sanotsky Y, Selikhova M, Fedoryshyn L, Kuzyk P, Matviyenko Y, Semeryak O, et al. Neuropathological rindings in ephedrone encephalopathy. Mov Disord 2020;35:1858–1863.
100. Santos HC, Oliveira J, Vieira AS, Pereira J. Clozapine-associated Pisa syndrome: A case report of an acute reaction in a bipolar patient. Clin Neuropharmacol 2021;44:222–224.
101. Savitt D, Jankovic J. Tardive syndromes. J Neurol Sci 2018;389:35–42.
102. Schneider SA, Udani V, Sankhla CS, Bhatia KP. Recurrent acute dystonic reaction and oculogyric crisis despite withdrawal of dopamine receptor blocking drugs. Mov Disord 2009;24:1226–1229.
103. Schwartz RH, Einhorn A. PCP intoxication in seven young children. Pediatr Emerg Care 1986;2:238–241.
104. Scorr LM, Factor SA, Perez-Parra S, Kaye R, Paniello RC, Norris SA, et al. Oromandibular dystonia: A clinical examination of 2,020 cases. Front Neurol 2021;12:700714.
105. Scott BL, Jankovic J. Delayed-onset progressive movement disorders after static brain lesions. Neurology 1996;46:68–74.
106. Selikhova M, Fedoryshyn L, Matviyenko Y, Komnatska I, Kyrylchuk M, Krolicki L, et al. Parkinsonism and dystonia caused by the illicit use of ephedrone: A longitudinal study. Mov Disord 2008;23:2224–2231.
107. Selikhova M, Tripoliti E, Fedoryshyn L, Matvienko Y, Stanetska H, Boychuk M, et al. Analysis of a distinct speech disorder seen in chronic manganese toxicity following Ephedrone abuse. Clin Neurol Neurosurg 2016;147:71–77.
108. Sethi KD, Hess DC, Harp RJ. Prevalence of dystonia in veterans on chronic antipsychotic therapy. Mov Disord 1990;5:319–321.
109. Shetty AS, Bhatia KP, Lang AE. Dystonia and Parkinson's disease: What is the relationship? Neurobiol Dis 2019;132:104462.
110. Sikk K, Haldre S, Aquilonius SM, Taba P. Manganese-Induced parkinsonism due to ephedrone abuse. Parkinsons Dis 2011;2011:865319.
111. Slow EJ, Lang AE. Oculogyric crises: A review of phenomenology, etiology, pathogenesis, and treatment. Mov Disord 2017;32:193–202.
112. Suresh Kumar PN, Gopalakrishnan A. Clozapine-associated Pisa syndrome: A rare type of tardive dystonia. Indian J Psychiatry 2017;59:390–391.
113. Suzuki M, Hirai T, Ito Y, Sakamoto T, Oka H, Kurita A, Inoue K. Pramipexole-induced antecollis in Parkinson's disease. J Neurol Sci 2008;264:195–197.
114. Swett C, Jr. Drug-induced dystonia. Am J Psychiatry 1975;132:532–534.
115. Tahir H, Daruwalla V. Phencyclidine induced oculogyric crisis responding well to conventional treatment. Case Rep Emerg Med 2015;2015:506301.
116. Tan EK, Jankovic J. Tardive and idiopathic oromandibular dystonia: A clinical comparison. J Neurol Neurosurg Psychiatry 2000;68:186–190.
117. Tarsy D, Kaufman D, Sethi KD, Rivner MH, Molho E, Factor S. An open-label study of botulinum toxin A for treatment of tardive dystonia. Clin Neuropharmacol 1997;20:90–93.
118. Tekin U, Soyata AZ, Oflaz S. Acute focal dystonic reaction after acute methylphenidate treatment in an adolescent patient. J Clin Psychopharmacol 2015;35:209–211.
119. Testini P, Factor SA. Treatment of tardive dystonia: A review. Dystonia 2023;2:10957.
120. Trezza A, Antonini A, Sganzerla EP, Landi A. Globus pallidus internus deep brain stimulation for the treatment of status dystonicus in tardive dystonia. Acta Neurochir 2016;158:1789–1791.
121. Uzawa A, Mori M, Kojima S, Mitsuma S, Sekiguchi Y, Kanesaka T, Kuwabara S. Dopamine agonist-induced antecollis in Parkinson's disease. Mov Disord 2009;24:2408–2411.
122. Uzun ME, Korkmaz MF, Ekici A, Kaymaz N. Methylphenidate induced acute dystonic reaction. Indian J Pediatr 2018;85:577.
123. Uzun O, Doruk A. Tardive oculogyric crisis during treatment with clozapine: Report of three cases. Clin Drug Investig 2007;27:861–864.
124. Valenzuela R, Court J, Godoy J. Delayed cyanide induced dystonia. J Neurol Neurosurg Psychiatry 1992;55:198–199.
125. van Harten PN, Matroos GE, Hoek HW, Kahn RS. The prevalence of tardive dystonia, tardive dyskinesia, parkinsonism and akathisia The Curacao Extrapyramidal Syndromes Study: I. Schizophr Res 1996;19:195–203.
126. van Harten PN, Matroos GE, Van Os J. The course of tardive dystonia in Afro Caribbean patients, a population-based study: The Curacao extrapyramidal syndromes study: VII. Schizophr Res 2008;98:79–83.
127. van Harten PN, van Trier JC, Horwitz EH, Matroos GE, Hoek HW. Cocaine as a risk factor for neuroleptic-induced acute dystonia. J Clin Psychiatry 1998;59:128–130.
128. Waugh JL. Acute dyskinetic reaction in a healthy toddler following methylphenidate ingestion. Pediatr Neurol 2013;49:58–60.
129. Weiner WJ, Goetz CG, Nausieda PA, Klawans HL. Respiratory dyskinesias: Extrapyramidal dysfunction and dyspnea. Ann Intern Med 1978;88:327–331.
130. Wojcik JD, Falk WE, Fink JS, Cole JO, Gelenberg AJ. A review of 32 cases of tardive dystonia. Am J Psychiatry 1991;148:1055–1059.
131. Wong J, Pang T, Cheuk NKW, Liao Y, Bastiampillai T, Chan SKW. A systematic review on the use of clozapine in treatment of tardive dyskinesia and tardive dystonia in patients with psychiatric disorders. Psychopharmacology 2022;239:3393–3420.
132. Yassa R, Nair V, Dimitry R. Prevalence of tardive dystonia. Acta Psychiatr Scand 1986;73:629–633.
133. Yassa R, Nair V, Iskandar H. A comparison of severe tardive dystonia and severe tardive dyskinesia. Acta Psychiatr Scand 1989;80:155–159.

Chapter 20

Dystonia and Trauma

INTRODUCTION

The relationship between trauma and dystonia is complex. In some cases, a clear and well-recognized relationship exists. In other cases, the nature of the relationship is controversial. This chapter summarizes the spectrum of all types of trauma-related dystonia, noting also the controversial relationships.

There are several circumstances in which trauma is clearly linked with dystonia. Dystonia may occur following a penetrating head injury with associated brain damage. Dystonia has also been described with closed-head injuries, where there is neuroimaging evidence for encephalomalacia, white matter changes, or hematoma. However, dystonia has also been described for closed-head injuries where there are no obvious neuroimaging correlates. Severe traumatic brain injury may also be associated with dystonic posturing in the syndrome of paroxysmal sympathetic hyperactivity.

Trauma to peripheral sites has also been reported to cause dystonia. Peripheral traumas may be severe, with obvious soft tissue injury, nerve damage, or fracture of underlying bone. In other cases, peripheral trauma may appear minor, such as an ankle sprain, with no detectable tissue injury. Dystonia has even been reported following recovery from uncomplicated surgical procedures or lengthy casting following a surgical procedure. Dystonia associated with peripheral trauma shares some features with complex regional pain syndrome (CRPS), where dystonic posturing also is common.

A clear and consistent relationship between trauma and dystonia has also been established for certain genetic disorders, where dystonia occurs alongside other neurological problems. In these cases, a central or peripheral trauma may trigger relatively abrupt onset of dystonia, often with neuroimaging evidence for striatal necrosis. For many of the more common adult-onset focal dystonias, there also are reported links with trauma,[19,21] but the most methodical studies have failed to confirm a causal relationship.[6]

In some cases of trauma-related dystonia, there is a plausible causal association between the trauma and subsequent dystonia, such as a penetrating head injury caused by a bullet, with obvious damage to components of the sensorimotor network implicated in dystonia. In other cases, such as peripherally induced trauma, a causal association between the trauma and dystonia is less clear, and the link may occasionally be ascribed to psychological factors (see Chapter 25, "Psychogenic [Functional] Dystonia").

DYSTONIA FOLLOWING BRAIN INJURY

Head Injury with Delayed-Onset Dystonia

There are many reports of dystonia caused by head trauma. In one comprehensive review focusing mainly on adults, hemidystonia and hand dystonia were the most common manifestations.[8] Less common were focal cervical dystonia, blepharospasm, oromandibular dystonia, laryngeal dystonia, lower limb dystonia, and generalized dystonia. Dystonia tended to develop in a region that was first affected by sensorimotor abnormalities. As weakness or sensory anomalies abated, dystonia emerged. As a result, dystonia usually emerged after a delay of several weeks or months. However, it may emerge immediately or after several years.[8] In another large study of 379 children with traumatic brain injury, dystonia occurred in 12 cases (3.2%), usually within a month of injury.[25]

Neuroimaging studies often disclose evidence of brain injury, but sometimes overt structural lesions are lacking.[8] Lesions are most often in or near the basal ganglia or thalamus, but may occur in other regions including the midbrain or brainstem, cerebellum, cerebral cortex, or even the cervical spinal cord.

The treatment of dystonia related to head trauma follows the same approach as other forms of dystonia. Oral medications may be at least partially useful, but they often have undesirable side effects (see Chapter 28, "Symptom-Targeted Oral Medications for Dystonia"). The botulinum toxins may also be used, but success rates appear to be lower than in idiopathic and inherited forms of dystonia. Deep brain stimulation and pallidotomy may also be offered, but success rates are again lower than for other forms of dystonia (see Chapter 31, "Surgical Treatments for Dystonia").

Head Injury with Paroxysmal Sympathetic Hyperactivity

Severe head trauma can be also associated with recurrent episodes of severe autonomic instability with abnormal posturing. The syndrome has been called *paroxysmal autonomic instability with dystonia* in the neurological literature,[2,3] but more than 30 alternative names have been used. An international consensus group has recommended using *paroxysmal sympathetic hyperactivity* for consistency.[1] The syndrome is not uncommon, occurring in 8–33% of head trauma cases.[18] Episodes of autonomic instability with dystonic posturing may occur shortly after head trauma or even during the convalescent period. They can occur one or many times per day, and they typically last minutes to hours. They tend to be triggered by sensory stimuli that are not normally noxious.

Key clinical features include transient episodes of posturing movements combined with signs of sympathetic nervous system overactivity. Autonomic signs include sinus tachycardia, tachypnea, hypertension, hyperpyrexia, and sweating. These signs occur simultaneously with abnormal movements that range from mild to severe, sometimes severe enough to cause rhabdomyolysis. Movements may affect axial structures and/or limbs. These movements have been described in varying ways including *dystonia, extensor or flexor posturing, opisthotonos,* and *decerebrate* or *decorticate* posturing resembling brain herniation syndromes (but without actual herniation). The relationship between these movements and other forms of dystonia is not clear, so some have suggested the movements be listed among the pseudodystonias (see Chapter 26, "Pseudodystonia and Differential Diagnosis").[10]

Although this syndrome is most often reported following traumatic brain injury, it can occur in other settings. In a large review of 349 cases, 80% occurred following trauma, 10% following anoxic brain injury due to cardiac arrest or drowning, 5% following ischemic or hemorrhagic stroke, and a smaller percentage due to tumors, infections, hydrocephalus, and other disorders.[26] A clinically similar syndrome can be seen with autoimmune conditions such as encephalitis associated with antibodies to N-methyl-D-aspartic acid (NMDA) receptors or progressive encephalomyelitis with rigidity.[39] It has also been reported to occur spontaneously in some inherited dystonic disorders, such as Lesch-Nyhan disease[22,28] or neuronal ceroid lipofuscinosis.[24]

Whether all of these syndromes share the same pathogenesis is unknown. They are thought to reflect disconnection of brainstem autonomic centers from higher-level inhibitory controls. The syndrome must be distinguished from several similar conditions including the neuroleptic malignant syndrome, malignant hyperthermia associated with anesthetics, cerebral herniation, and pain in an inadequately anesthetized patient. Treatments include opiates, adrenergic antagonists (beta blockers and beta-2-blockers), benzodiazepines, bromocriptine, gabapentin, and baclofen.

PERIPHERAL TRAUMA

Dystonia Following Peripheral Injury

There are numerous reports of movement disorders caused by trauma to peripheral body regions. A systematic review of 133 reports that included a total of 713 cases found dystonia to be the most common of all peripherally induced movement disorders, accounting for 72% of the total.[36] The types of trauma were varied and included soft tissue injuries, fractures, surgical procedures, nerve injuries, and others. However, these cases exhibited some clinical features not typical for other types of dystonia, questioning whether the abnormal movements should be classified along with other types of dystonia (Table 20.1).[11]

Dystonia does not usually emerge immediately following peripheral trauma, but after a delay of weeks or months. In the review of movement disorders following peripheral trauma noted above, the median delay was 21 days, although the delay was sometimes more than a year.[36] The delays often lead to questions regarding a causal role of the injury. However, similar delays (sometimes extending for many years) are also seen in cases where etiologies for dystonia are more clearly established.[5,12,15,27,30,32] Therefore, the temporal dissociation between peripheral trauma and dystonia does not provide strong evidence for or against a causal role of the trauma.

The most common regions reported to be affected with dystonia include the head/neck following a whiplash injury, or an upper or lower limb.[8] There also are reports of oromandibular dystonia following jaw trauma or uncomplicated dental procedures. Laryngeal dystonia has been reported following neck injury, uncomplicated intubation, and laryngitis. Several studies have compared cervical dystonia occurring shortly after peripheral trauma with other types of cervical dystonia. Cervical dystonia following peripheral trauma is more likely to be fixed with limited mobility, with prominent laterocollis rather than torticollis. Cervical dystonia following peripheral trauma is more likely to be associated with severe pain, less likely to have a *geste antagoniste*, and less likely to be responsive to botulinum toxin therapy.[23,33] Cases of cervical dystonia following peripheral trauma also have a high frequency of features associated with psychogenic movement disorders.[7,29] Similarly, large studies of individuals with psychogenic dystonia have identified peripheral trauma as a common feature.[4,9] These features have suggested that some cases may be psychogenic, questioning a causal relationship between peripheral trauma and cervical dystonia for all cases.

Dystonia of a limb following peripheral injury may also differ from other causes of limb dystonia. Limb dystonia following peripheral injury is more likely to have abrupt onset and is more likely to be fixed rather than mobile, with characteristic postures.[20] The characteristic posture of the lower limb is intorsion and plantar flexion of the foot, sometimes with

Table 20.1 **Comparison of dystonia following peripheral trauma with other conditions**

Characteristic	Dystonia after peripheral trauma	CRPS with dystonia	Psychogenic dystonia	Typical dystonias
Pain	Common	Always	Sometimes	Sometimes
Fixed postures	Common	Common	Common	Uncommon
Onset	Days to months	Days to months	Often sudden	Weeks to months
Geste antagoniste	Uncommon	Uncommon	Uncommon	Common
Muscle hypertrophy	Uncommon	Uncommon	Uncommon	Common
Response to BoNT	Often poor	Often poor	Often poor	Usually good
Response to DBS	Often poor	Often poor	Unpredictable	Often good

Abbreviations: BoNT, botulinum toxin; CRPS, complex regional pain syndrome; DBS, deep brain stimulation.

flexion of the knee (Figure 20.1A). The characteristic posture of the upper limb involves flexion of the fingers and wrist, often with flexion and internal rotation of the upper arm (Figure 20.1B). Dystonia of a limb following peripheral trauma is more likely than other causes of limb dystonia to be associated with severe pain, less likely to have a *geste antagoniste*, less likely to be responsive to therapy including botulinum toxins, and more likely to have features suggestive of psychogenic dystonia.[14,17,31]

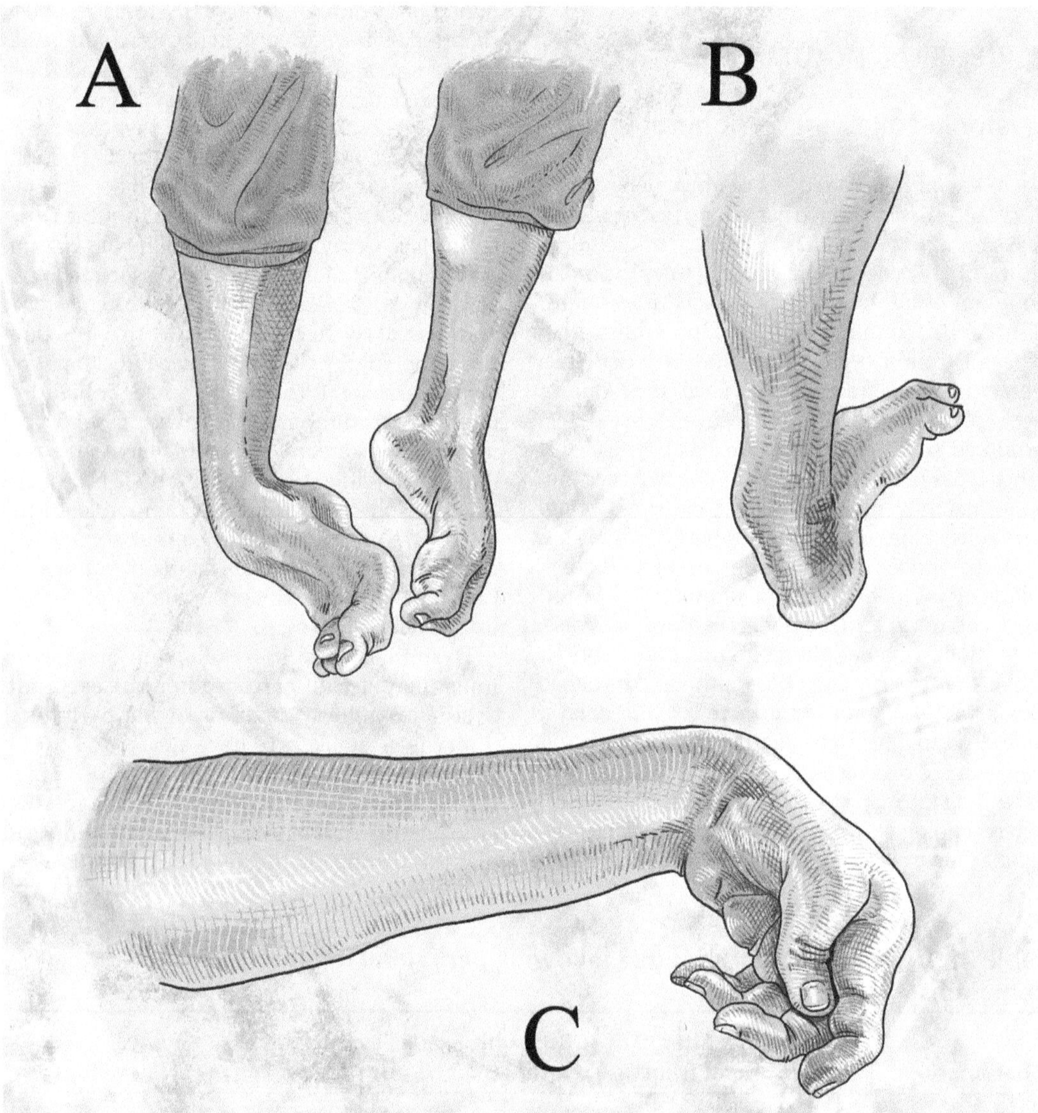

Figure 20.1. Peripherally induced dystonia. While many postures are possible, the most characteristic is intorsion with plantar flexion of the foot, usually with flexion (curling) of the toes. Panel A shows an example with this posture on one side, with a variant where the toes are extended on the other side. These postures remain relatively fixed at rest and with walking, in contrast with other types of foot dystonia which are often more varied and dynamic depending on task. Panel B shows an example for the hand, where the most characteristic posture is flexion of the wrist, flexion of the fingers and/or thumb at the metacarpophalangeal joints, with either hyperextension or flexion of interphalangeal joints. The hand is often combined with abduction and internal rotation of the arm. The postures are relatively immobile, unlike other types of dystonia where the posture changes with task.

Illustration by Loren Bergantini.

The majority of cases are young, otherwise healthy women. Dystonia usually first emerges at the site of injury, but spread beyond the site of injury is common. This spread may occur over a period of weeks or even years. For example, foot intorsion may begin several weeks after an ankle sprain. Months later, it may spread to the whole leg or even the contralateral leg. Alternatively, ulnar nerve injury may lead to the expected pattern of sensorimotor loss, followed by dystonia in the same distribution, and then spread of dystonia outside the ulnar distribution to the upper arm and shoulder. These patterns of spread also lead to questions regarding a causal role for the trauma because they defy obvious biological mechanisms. However, such patterns of spread sometimes occur in inherited forms of dystonia, even without any trauma. Therefore, these apparently unusual patterns of spread do not provide definitive evidence for or against a cause role of the trauma.

Overall, the idea that dystonia can be triggered by peripheral trauma remains controversial. While some cases have clinical features typical of other forms of dystonia, many have atypical features. The delay between trauma and onset of dystonia often leads to questions about any potential etiological relationship, but such delays may occur in other types of dystonia with an established biological cause. The apparently non-anatomical distribution of spread in some cases of peripherally induced dystonia also leads to questions about etiology, but such spread may be seen in other forms of dystonia, too. An etiological relationship between peripheral trauma and dystonia may be further questioned by coexisting psychological factors, ongoing litigation, additional non-organic neurological features, the lack of any definitive diagnostic test, and an apparent lack of plausible biological mechanisms. In view of these considerations, some experts view peripherally induced dystonia as primarily psychogenic. However, it is feasible that this is a mixed population where peripheral trauma plays a more direct causal biology role in some cases but a more indirect psychogenic role in many others.

Complex Regional Pain Syndrome and Dystonia

There are many parallels between dystonia induced by peripheral trauma and CRPS, a syndrome that has also been called reflex sympathetic dystrophy, causalgia, or Sudeck syndrome.[8,11] Peripheral trauma usually precedes CRPS. The trauma may be mild or severe, or it may involve an uncomplicated surgery. Pain is severe, often out of proportion to the trauma. Dystonia and pain may spread from the original site of injury to nearby sites. Affected individuals also develop local autonomic signs such as swelling, red or purple discoloration of the skin, changes in skin temperature or abnormal sweating, or trophic changes of the hair or nails. Many have a reduction in underlying bone mineralization that can be measured with bone density scans.

In one large series of 829 cases with CRPS, approximately half had some type of movement disorder.[37] A methodical survey of the type of movement disorder revealed dystonia to be the most common, affecting 91% of the total.[35] Therefore, dystonia is common in CRPS. One study suggested that dystonia occurred in CRPS without accompanying neuropathy (CRPS type 1) and not in CRPS with accompanying nerve damage (CRPS type 2).[38] Among cases with CRPS, the clinical features of the dystonia are quite similar to those of non-painful dystonia following peripheral injury (Table 20.1), with similar fixed postures (Figure 20.1).

In other words, many cases of CRPS have dystonia, and many cases of dystonia following peripheral trauma have pain. However, CRPS may occur without dystonia. Similarly, dystonia following peripheral trauma may be painless, and there are not usually accompanying local autonomic signs.

INHERITED DYSTONIAS TRIGGERED BY TRAUMA

There are several rare inherited disorders in which dystonia is consistently associated with trauma. Trauma-induced dystonia is best described for rapid-onset dystonia-parkinsonism associated with the *ATP1A3* gene.[13] The syndrome most commonly emerges in late childhood or adolescence but may emerge in adulthood as well. Affected individuals are often clinically normal until the trauma. Trauma may involve the head or another body region, or it may involve an uncomplicated surgical procedure. Following trauma, a syndrome of encephalopathy and dystonia evolves over a period of hours or days. The syndrome may last for days or weeks. Encephalopathy usually resolves, but dystonia may be permanent, or it may only partially remit. The dystonia may be generalized, often with prominent involvement of the oromandibular region. The pathogenesis of dystonia associated with *ATP1A3* is only partly understood (see Chapter 14, "Dystonia and Ataxia"), and brain MRI usually shows no apparent abnormality.

There are other inherited disorders in which trauma can trigger dystonia, along with obvious neuroimaging signs of injury to the basal ganglia and sometimes frank striatal necrosis.[34] These disorders include glutaric aciduria type 1 (*GCDH*), methylmalonic aciduria (*MUT*), propionic acidemia (*PCCA* and *PCCB*), biotin-thiamin-responsive basal ganglia disease (*SL319A3*), and others. Onset is usually in early childhood, prior to 2 years of age. Trauma may involve the head, another body region, or an uncomplicated surgery. Similar to rapid-onset dystonia-parkinsonism syndrome, trauma with these other disorders is followed by relatively abrupt development of encephalopathy with dystonia. Encephalopathy may resolve, but dystonia is often permanent. The pathogenesis most likely involves metabolic stress that leads to injury to energetically demanding cells in the striatum.

There also are reports of dystonia following trauma for genetic isolated dystonias, such as dystonia associated with *TOR1A*, but the most methodical studies have found no clear relationship.[16]

SYNOPSIS AND FUTURE PROSPECTS

The dystonias have many potential etiologies, including trauma to the head or peripheral body sites. The assessment of an individual with trauma-induced dystonia can be challenging. For some cases, a clear etiological relationship between the trauma and the dystonia seems plausible. Examples include severe head trauma with evidence for brain injury, the syndrome of paroxysmal sympathetic hyperactivity, and certain rare inherited disorders in which trauma triggers striatal necrosis with dystonia. The mechanisms responsible for trauma-induced dystonia in these inherited disorders are unknown, but they provide a biological precedent and a potentially valuable window for further studies regarding how trauma can produce dystonia.

In other cases, an etiological relationship between trauma and dystonia is less clear, especially in cases of dystonia following peripheral trauma or dystonia associated with CRPS. It seems likely that the group of individuals with dystonia induced by peripheral trauma is heterogeneous, with some reflecting an unusual maladaptive response of the nervous system to abnormal sensory feedback and others reflecting psychological or other factors. Tools for discriminating trauma-related dystonia from psychogenic processes would be very valuable to develop. In the meantime, the approach to trauma-induced dystonia must be considered on a case-by-case basis.

REFERENCES

1. Baguley IJ, Perkes IE, Fernandez-Ortega JF, Rabinstein AA, Dolce G, Hendricks HT, Consensus Working Group. Paroxysmal sympathetic hyperactivity after acquired brain injury: Consensus on conceptual definition, nomenclature, and diagnostic criteria. J Neurotrauma 2014;31:1515–1520.
2. Blackman JA, Patrick PD, Buck ML, Rust RS, Jr. Paroxysmal autonomic instability with dystonia after brain injury. Arch Neurol 2004;61:321–328.
3. Cardoso Vale T, Echenique L, Barsottini OGP, Pedroso JL. Paroxysmal autonomic instability with dystonia after severe traumatic brain injury. Tremor Other Hyperkinet Mov 2020;10:12.
4. Centen LM, van Egmond ME, Tijssen MAJ. New developments in diagnosis and treament of adult-onset focal dystonia. Curr Opin Neurol 2023;36:317–323.
5. Corp DT, Greenwood C, Morrison-Ham J, Pullinen J, McDowall G, Younger E, et al. Clinical and structural findings in patients with lesion-induced dystonia: Descriptive and quantitative analysis of published cases. Neurology 2022;99:e1957–e1967.
6. Defazio G, Fabbrini G, Erro R, Albanese A, Barone P, Zibetti M, et al. Does acute peripheral trauma contribute to idiopathic adult-onset dystonia? Parkinsonism Relat Disord 2020;71:40–43.
7. Ercoli T, Defazio G, Geroin C, Marcuzzo E, Fabbrini G, Bono F, et al. Sudden onset, fixed dystonia and acute peripheral trauma as diagnostic clues for functional dystonia. Mov Disord Clin Pract 2021;8:1107–1111.
8. Frei K. Posttraumatic dystonia. J Neurol Sci 2017;379:183–191.
9. Garcin B, Villain N, Mesrati F, Naccache L, Roze E, Degos B. A single-center series of 482 patients with functional motor disorders. J Psychosom Res 2021;148:110565.
10. Gupta HV, Sharma VD, Espay AJ. The pseudodystonia of paroxysmal sympathetic hyperactivity: A reversible post-anoxic complication. Mov Disord Clin Pract 2020;7:987–989.

11. Hawley JS, Weiner WJ. Psychogenic dystonia and peripheral trauma. Neurology 2011;77:496–502.
12. He F, Zhang S, Qian G, Zhang C. Delayed dystonia with striatal CT lucencies induced by a mycotoxin (3-nitropropionic acid). Neurology 1995;45:2178–2183.
13. Heinzen EL, Arzimanoglou A, Brashear A, Clapcote SJ, Gurrieri F, Goldstein DB, et al. Distinct neurological disorders with ATP1A3 mutations. Lancet Neurol 2014;13:503–514.
14. Ibrahim NM, Martino D, van de Warrenburg BP, Quinn NP, Bhatia KP, Brown RJ, et al. The prognosis of fixed dystonia: A follow-up study. Parkinsonism Relat Disord 2009;15:592–597.
15. Kim JS. Delayed onset mixed involuntary movements after thalamic stroke. Brain 2001;124:299–309.
16. Martino D, Gajos A, Gallo V, Cif L, Coubes P, Tinazzi M, et al. Extragenetic factors and clinical penetrance of DYT1 dystonia: An exploratory study. J Neurol 2013;260:1081–1086.
17. McKeon A, Matsumoto JY, Bower JH, Ahlskog JE. The spectrum of disorders presenting as adult-onset focal lower extremity dystonia. Parkinsonism Relat Disord 2008;14:613–619.
18. Meyfroidt G, Baguley IJ, Menon DK. Paroxysmal sympathetic hyperactivity: The storm after acute brain injury. Lancet Neurol 2017;16:721–729.
19. Molloy A, Kimmich O, Williams L, Butler JS, Byrne N, Molloy F, et al. An evaluation of the role of environmental factors in the disease penetrance of cervical dystonia. J Neurol Neurosurg Psychiatry 2015;86:331–335.
20. Munts AG, Mugge W, Meurs TS, Schouten AC, Marinus J, Moseley GL, et al. Fixed dystonia in complex regional pain syndrome: A descriptive and computational modeling approach. BMC Neurol 2011;11:53.
21. Newman JR, Boyle RS, O'Sullivan JD, Silburn PA, Mellick GD. Risk factors for idiopathic dystonia in Queensland, Australia. J Clin Neurosci 2014;21:2145–2149.
22. Nyhan W, Lucas M. Malignant hyperthermia in Lesch-Nyhan disease. Arch Clin Nephrol 2019:1–2.
23. O'Riordan S, Hutchinson M. Cervical dystonia following peripheral trauma: A case-control study. J Neurol 2004;251:150–155.
24. Ostergaard JR. Paroxysmal sympathetic hyperactivity in juvenile neuronal ceroid lipofuscinosis (Batten disease). Auton Neurosci 2018;214:15–18.
25. Pentony M, Featherstone M, Sheikh Y, Stroiescu A, Bruell H, Gill I, Gorman KM. Dystonia in children with acquired brain injury. Eur J Paediatric Neurol 2022;41:41–47.
26. Perkes I, Baguley IJ, Nott MT, Menon DK. A review of paroxysmal sympathetic hyperactivity after acquired brain injury. Ann Neurol 2010;68:126–135.
27. Pettigrew LC, Jankovic J. Hemidystonia: A report of 22 patients and a review of the literature. J Neurol Neurosurg Psychiatry 1985;48:650–657.
28. Rana M, Cuttin K, Berry GT, Torres A. Paroxysmal hyperthermia, dysautonomia and rhabdomyolysis in a patient with Lesch-Nyhan syndrome. JIMD Rep 2021;62:30–34.
29. Sa DS, Mailis-Gagnon A, Nicholson K, Lang AE. Posttraumatic painful torticollis. Mov Disord 2003;18: 1482–1491.
30. Saint Hilaire MH, Burke RE, Bressman SB, Brin MF, Fahn S. Delayed-onset dystonia due to perinatal or early childhood asphyxia. Neurology 1991;41:216–222.
31. Schrag A, Trimble M, Quinn N, Bhatia K. The syndrome of fixed dystonia: An evaluation of 103 patients. Brain 2004;127:2360–2372.
32. Scott BL, Jankovic J. Delayed-onset progressive movement disorders after static brain lesions. Neurology 1996;46:68–74.
33. Tarsy D. Comparison of acute- and delayed-onset posttraumatic cervical dystonia. Mov Disord 1998; 13:481–485.
34. Tonduti D, Chiapparini L, Moroni I, Ardissone A, Zorzi G, Zibordi F, et al. Neurological disorders associated with striatal lesions: Classification and diagnostic approach. Curr Neurol Neurosci Rep 2016;16:54.
35. van Rijn MA, Marinus J, Putter H, van Hilten JJ. Onset and progression of dystonia in complex regional pain syndrome. Pain 2007;130:287–293.
36. van Rooijen DE, Geraedts EJ, Marinus J, Jankovic J, van Hilten JJ. Peripheral trauma and movement disorders: A systematic review of reported cases. J Neurol Neurosurg Psychiatry 2011;82:892–898.
37. Veldman PH, Reynen HM, Arntz IE, Goris RJ. Signs and symptoms of reflex sympathetic dystrophy: Prospective study of 829 patients. Lancet 1993;342: 1012–1016.
38. Verdugo RJ, Ochoa JL. Abnormal movements in complex regional pain syndrome: Assessment of their nature. Muscle Nerve 2000;23:198–205.
39. Wang D, Su S, Tan M, Wu Y, Wang S. Paroxysmal sympathetic hyperactivity in severe anti-N-methyl-d-aspartate receptor encephalitis: A single center retrospective observational study. Front Immunol 2021;12:665183.

Chapter 21

Dystonia and Autoimmunity

INTRODUCTION

Dystonia can be a manifestation of autoimmune disease. Autoimmune dystonia only rarely resembles the commonly recognized patterns of isolated idiopathic or genetic dystonias. Instead, dystonia is usually found mixed with other clinical manifestations. Dystonia can be associated with specific neuronal autoantibodies, usually in the context of a more complex neurological syndrome, often with encephalopathy. Alternatively, dystonia can occur in the context of a systemic autoimmune rheumatological disease, when it is more often associated with systemic signs or symptoms.

The term *pseudodystonia* indicates abnormal postures or movements that have a pathogenesis different from most forms of dystonia (see Chapter 26, "Pseudodystonia and Differential Diagnosis"). For some autoimmune diseases, the term *pseudodystonia* may be more appropriate for the abnormal movements because the pathobiological mechanisms may be unique. These pathobiological mechanisms vary widely. Here, the term *dystonia* is used to encompass all dystonia-like movements, regardless of pathogenesis.

BASIC PRINCIPLES OF NEURONAL AUTOANTIBODIES

Movement disorders may be the first or most prominent presentation of autoimmune disease associated with a wide variety of autoantibodies. These autoantibodies are listed in Tables 21.1 and 21.2, which also serve as a reference and glossary of terms. There are several biological mechanisms by which autoimmune disease can trigger movement disorders. Autoantibodies may affect neuronal function directly by blocking or activating the target antigen (e.g., a neurotransmitter receptor or ion channel), downregulating the target antigen, activating complement at the cell surface, or triggering cell death and neurodegeneration. Cytotoxic T cells may also target neurons or glia directly. There are also indirect mechanisms involving inflammatory lesions that can be seen on a macroscopic level, or tissue ischemia at the microscopic level.

Neuronal autoantibodies can be divided into three groups, based on the location of their antigen and their presumed pathologic relevance (Table 21.1). These three groups differ also with regards to their associations with neoplasm, best type of treatment, treatment response, and

Table 21.1 **Neuronal surface autoantibodies associated with dystonia-like movements**

Antibody	Relative frequency	Antigen	Malignancy association	Typical malignancy	Movement disorder	Other clinical features
Anti-CASPR1	+	Contactin-associated protein 1	–		Dystonia-like movements, tremor	Chronic inflammatory demyelinating polyradiculoneuropathy
Anti-CASPR2	++	Contactin-associated protein 2	+/–	Thymoma	Ataxia, chorea, neuromyotonia, myokymia	Morvan syndrome, limbic encephalitis, neuropathic pain, reflex loss
Anti-CNTN1	+	Contactin-1	–		Dystonia-like movements, tremor	Chronic inflammatory demyelinating polyradiculoneuropathy
Anti-DPPX	++	Dipeptidyl peptidase-like protein 6	+/–	B-cell lymphoma	Dystonia-like movements, myoclonus, startle, ataxia, tremor, parkinsonism, Opsoclonus-myoclonus Stiff person spectrum disorder	Multifocal encephalitis or brainstem encephalitis with prominent gastrointestinal symptoms (prolonged diarrhoea, constipation), other dysautonomic signs (urinary or erectile dysfunction, cardiac arrhythmia, thermodysregulation, Raynaud´s phenomenon), somatosensory disturbance (allodynia or neurogenic pruritus)
Anti-D2R	(+)	Dopamine 2 receptor	–		Dystonia-like movements, chorea, parkinsonism; Sydenham´s chorea	Basal ganglia encephalitis, psychiatric and sleep disturbance
Anti-$GABA_A$R	++	Gamma-aminobutyric acid A receptor	(+)/–	Thymoma	Stiff-person spectrum disorder (opsoclonus-myoclonus, chorea, dystonia)	Limbic encephalitis with prominent seizures
Anti-GlyR	+++	Glycine receptor	+/–	Thymoma, small cell lung cancer, breast cancer, Hodgkin lymphoma, chronic lymphocytic leukaemia	Stiff person spectrum disorder (myoclonus, hyperekplexia, ataxia, dystonia)	Brainstem encephalitis; optic neuritis; limbic/epileptic encephalopathy; steroid-responsive deafness
Anti-IgLON5	+	IgLON family member 5	–		Chorea, parkinsonism, ataxia, dystonia, myoclonus, myorhythmia	REM and non-REM sleep behaviour disorder; oculomotor disturbance, dementia
Anti-LGI1	+++	Leucine-rich glioma inactivated protein 1	(+)/–		Faciobrachial dystonic seizures, Chorea,	Limbic encephalitis; hyponatraemia, bradycardia
Anti-NMDAR	++++	N-methyl-D-aspartate receptor	+/–	Ovarian teratoma >> extraovarian teratomas, ovarian carcinomas; lung, breast, testicular and pancreatic tumors	Rofacial and limb dyskinesia, Dystonia-like movements, myoclonus, ataxia, parkinsonism, paroxysmal dyskinesias	Encephalitis with prodromal symptoms like headache or, fever and subacute onset of neuropsychiatric disturbance and subsequent development of movement disorders, epilepsy, dysautonomia and central hypoventilation
Anti-NF155 Anti-NF140/186	+	Neurofascin 155, Neurofascin 140/186	–		Dystonia-like movements, tremor	Chronic inflammatory demyelinating polyradiculoneuropathy

Some antibodies have more than one name. Exact prevalences are unknown, and relative frequencies are based on the literature and personal experience. The term *dystonia* is used here even though some of the dystonia-like movements may be classified as pseudodystonia.

Table 21.2 **Antibodies targeting intracellular cytosolic, synaptic, or nuclear antigens**

Antibody	Relative frequency	Antigen	Malignancy association	Typical malignancy	Movement disorder	Other clinical features
Anti-amphiphysin	+	Amphiphysin	+++	Breast cancer, Small cell lung cancer	Stiff person spectrum disorder	Sensory ganglionopathy
Anti-GAD	+++	Glutamic acid decarboxylase	+/–		Stiff person spectrum disorder, ataxia	Limbic encephalitis; focal epilepsy; often concomitant autoimmunity (e.g. diabetes type 1, thyroid disease, vitiligo, pernicious anaemia)
Anti-CRMP5 Anti-CV2	++	Collapsin response mediator protein 5	+++	Small cell lung cancer, thymoma	Chorea	Optic neuritis, myelitis (can mimic neuromyelitis optica), cognitive decline, neuropathy
Anti-Hu ANNA-1	++	Hu proteins (hud, huc)	+++	Small cell lung cancer>> neuroblastoma or intestinal, prostate, breast, bladder, and ovary carcinoma	Chorea, ataxia, opsoclonus-myoclonus	Encephalomyelitis; limbic encephalitis; brainstem encephalitis, sensory neuropathy, gastrointestinal pseudo-obstruction
Anti-Ma2 Anti-Ta	++	Paraneoplastic Ma antigen 2	+++ (rarely none)	Testis >> lung cancer	Parkinsonism	Limbic encephalitis; hypothalamic involvement; eye movement abnormalities (opsoclonus, supranuclear gaze palsy); dysphagia; muscular atrophy; fasciculations
Anti-Ri ANNA-2	++	Nova-1, nova-2	+++	Gynecological tumours, mainly breast cancer, and lung cancer	Dystonia (jaw, laryngospasm), opsoclonus-myoclonus, ataxia, oculopalatal myoclonus, stiff person spectrum disorder,	Brainstem encephalitis with cranial nerve palsies, ataxia, nystagmus, dysarthria, rigidity, trismus, pyramidal signs
Anti-Yo PCA1	++	Cdr62, cdr2, cdr34, cdr1	+++	Gynecological tumours	Ataxia	Rhombencephalitis

Some antibodies have more than one name. Exact prevalences are unknown, and relative frequencies are based on the literature and personal experience. The term "dystonia" is used here even though some of the dystonia- like movements may be classified as pseudodystonia.

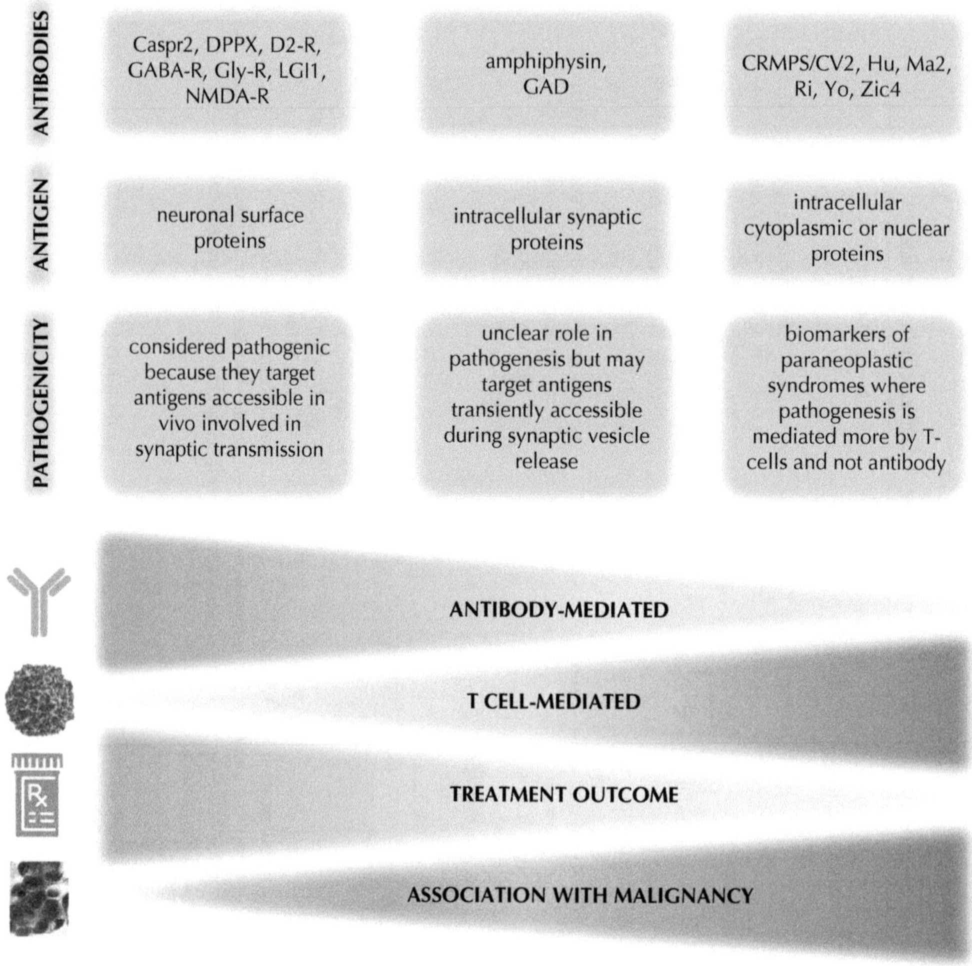

Figure 21.1. Immune mechanisms in autoimmune dystonias. This schematic shows the relationship between antibodies, antigens, T cells, treatment response, and tumor association. Some autoantibodies are thought to be pathogenic, with good treatment response. Other autoantibodies are thought to be biomarkers, where T cells play a more relevant role in pathogenesis, and there is greater risk of associated tumor and poorer treatment response.

prognosis (Figure 21.1). While the classic paraneoplastic antibodies are indicative of an underlying neoplasm, neuronal surface antibodies associate less frequently with malignancy and have an overall better response to immunotherapy and outcome. Cytotoxic T cells associated with tumors cause irreversible neuronal damage, while surface antibodies are typically less destructive.

Nonetheless, even within the group of neuronal surface antibodies, there are differences with regard to pathologic mechanisms.[1,4] No matter the underlying immunopathology, prompt initiation of immunotherapy is the most important prognostic factor across all of these conditions. To facilitate prompt immunotherapy, it is of great importance to recognize characteristic phenotypes and/or associated red flags.

ABNORMAL MOVEMENTS AND NEURONAL AUTOANTIBODIES

The Clinical Spectrum

Dystonia associated with autoantibodies is usually combined with other neurological problems, most often an encephalopathic syndrome.[6,48] The phenotypic spectrum depends on the autoantibody as well as on the age and sex of the affected individual. Some of the classic syndromes are described below, and a more complete list is provided in Tables 21.1 and 21.2.

Anti-NMDAR Encephalitis

In children and adolescents, the classic picture is dystonia in the context of antibodies targeting the glutamatergic N-methyl-D-aspartate receptor (NMDAR), where dystonia is combined with encephalopathy and other movement disorders, mostly chorea and stereotypies. Unlike many other types of isolated dystonia, the dystonia in anti-NMDA encephalitis often occurs at rest, albeit with spontaneous exacerbations and severe spasms.

There often is a reduced level of consciousness. The associated encephalopathy may include seizures, aphasia, and other cognitive or psychiatric problems.[6,50] Children with NMDAR antibodies can have oculogyric crises or seizures with tonic upgaze. These abnormal eye movements may resemble genetic disorders with dystonia, such as mitochondrial or metabolic disease, biotin-thiamine-responsive basal ganglia disease, or disorders of dopamine synthesis and metabolism.

While neuronal autoantibody-associated dystonia only rarely mimics isolated idiopathic or genetic dystonia, there are a few reports of children and young adults who harbored NMDAR antibodies and had hemidystonia or craniocervical dystonia as the sole or most prominent feature.[2,34,42] However, the significance of the antibodies in these cases is still a matter of debate.[4]

Anti-Ri Encephalitis

In adults, the phenotypic and serological spectrum is different. Cranio-cervical dystonia including jaw closing or jaw opening dystonia is seen with Ri antibodies, a paraneoplastic antibody occurring predominantly in women (~80%) in their sixties (range: 47–87 years) and often associated with breast cancer.[46] Jaw closing dystonia with recurrent episodes of laryngospasm is nearly pathognomonic for anti-Ri encephalitis.[38] The symptoms can be severe enough to impair nutrition or require tracheostomy. Apart from dystonia, the anti-Ri syndrome is broad, the most frequent sign being ataxia, but also encompassing oculomotor disturbances, encephalopathy, and other movement disorders. The MRI may be unrevealing in some cases, or it may display T2-hyperintensities mainly in the brainstem and temporal lobes.

Anti-IgLON5 Encephalopathy

Antibodies to IgLON5, an immunoglobulin-like cell adhesion molecule expressed on the surface of neurons, are associated with characteristic sleep–wake rhythm disorders and particularly sleep behavior disorders. The antibody was identified in individuals who shared a characteristic non–rapid eye movement (REM) parasomnia with fine distal movements, resembling manipulating an object or preparing food. These movements are different from the thrashing, violent movements more typical of REM sleep behavior disorders.[16,44] The spectrum of sleep disorders in anti-IgLON5 disease is, however, much broader, encompassing also REM behavior disorders, periodic leg movements of sleep, sleep apnea, and excessive sleepiness.

Anti-IgLON5 disease occurs later in life, typically in the seventh decade (range fifth to eighth decade), and equally in men and women.[16] Clues to diagnosis are the sleep disorders, prominent bulbar symptoms, vocal cord paralysis, and breathing difficulties that can be severe enough to require tracheostomy. Other frequent features are gaze palsies and ptosis. Apart from these core features, the movement disorder spectrum is very broad, consisting mainly of chorea and parkinsonism with early postural instability, but featuring sometimes also dystonia or myoclonus. Additional features seen with IgLON5 antibodies are ataxia, myorhythmia, cognitive decline including executive dysfunction, apraxia or hallucinations, or motoneuron signs. Dystonia is rarely the most prominent feature, but may be part of a syndrome where some of the above features point to the diagnosis. Unlike most other antibody-mediated movement disorders, anti-IgLON5 disease often has a slowly progressive course, and affected indivdiuals may manifest symptoms for a decade prior to diagnosis.

Stiff Person Syndrome

Defining features of stiff person spectrum disorders include muscle stiffness and spasms, sometimes with abnormal postures or movements resembling dystonia. Abnormal postures may include lumbar hyperlordosis, truncal scoliosis, or plantar flexion of the foot. A useful diagnostic clue is excessive startle (hyperekplexia). The abnormal postures or spasms are often tonic or sustained rather than mobile, and they are often painful. Although abnormal movements or postures may resemble dystonia, abnormal movements are usually considered among the "pseudodystonias" because of their unique pathogenesis that presumably relates to disruption of spinal cord inhibitory neurons (see Chapter 26).

When accompanied by antibodies to glutamic acid decarboxylase (GAD), there may be additional signs such as ataxia or epilepsy. In the related variant of progressive encephalomyelitis with rigidity and myoclonus (often with antibodies to glycine receptors [GlyR]), there may be additional brainstem signs that include oculomotor abnormalities, facial sensory changes, bulbar disturbances, and corticospinal signs. Antibodies to GlyR can also be associated with "lockjaw," resembling tetanus and an important differential diagnosis to anti-Ri encephalitis. Long-lasting diarrhea points to antibodies to dipeptidyl peptidase-like protein 6 (DPPX) and sensory ataxia to amphiphysin antibodies. However, the clinical spectrum is broad, and the phenotype does not necessarily predict the underlying antibody. Nevertheless, identification of the underlying antibody is important because of the implications of underlying neoplasia and comorbidities (Table 21.1).[5] Very rarely, the stiff person spectrum phenotype has been reported with antibodies to Ri or $GABA_AR$.

Other Antibodies

Dystonia as a feature in a broader encephalopathic syndrome has been described with a variety of additional autoantibodies (Table 21.2). Dystonia in children has also been reported in the context of an epileptic encephalopathy with antibodies targeting gamma-amino butyric acid receptors ($GABA_AR$). While brain MRI in anti-$GABA_AR$ encephalitis can show characteristic T2 hyperintensities, it is typically unremarkable in anti-NMDAR encephalitis.

Dystonia has also been associated with the paraneoplastic Ma antigen 2 (Ma2). Dystonia is rarely the most prominent feature, and a relatively rapid disease progression and combination with other signs and symptoms should point to the diagnosis. For example, the classic anti-Ma syndrome includes dystonia-parkinsonism with vertical gaze palsy, often also with blepharospasm, sleep–wake rhythm disturbance and change of appetite. It occurs mostly in young men with testicular tumors.

Dystonia has also been associated with dopamine D_2 receptor (D_2R) antibodies, although these appear to be extremely rare. Associated parkinsonism with akinesia and tremor are present more commonly than in other autoimmune encephalopathies.[34] Brain MRI in cases with D_2R antibodies can show basal ganglia or brainstem hyperintensities, or it can be normal.

PAROXYSMAL DYSKINESIAS

The paroxysmal dyskinesias are a group of disorders characterized by transient attacks of involuntary movements without impaired consciousness. Although the movements can be quite varied, dystonia is a common feature and sometimes the sole feature (see Chapter 17, "Dystonia and the Paroxysmal Dyskinesias"). They can occur at any age. In children they are often inherited. In adults, acquired causes must be considered, including autoimmune causes.

The classic antibody-related paroxysmal movement disorder is the *faciobrachial dystonic seizure* associated with antibodies to leucine-rich glioma inactivated protein 1 (LGI1).[7,22,25] Faciobrachial dystonic seizures are characteristically brief (<3 seconds) and frequent (hundreds/day) episodes of abnormal posturing, typically the ipsilateral face and arm. They have an abrupt onset and termination, often with concurrent facial grimacing. Characteristic limb posturing involves recurrent elevation of the shoulder along with flexion of the elbow, wrist, and metacarpophalangeal joints. More distally the fingers may be flexed or extended. Usually only one side is affected, although the affected side may switch. Involvement of the legs can cause drop attacks, and various combinations of affected body parts including bilateral involvement can occur.

The electroencephalogram (EEG) may show associated ictal epileptiform discharges, but it is more often normal. Some individuals may have additional features often associated with seizures including automatisms, sensory aura, postictal fear, or speech arrest. The MRI may show basal ganglia hyperintensities on T1- or T2-weighted sequences.[14] In this regard, faciobrachial dystonic seizures may represent an interphase between basal ganglia and epileptic disorders. They may precede the development of more severe limbic encephalitis with cognitive impairment, hence early recognition and timely initiation of immunotherapy are of paramount importance. Anti-LGI1 disease responds particularly well to corticosteroids.

While LGI1 antibodies predominantly occur in older men, younger women with a paroxysmal movement disorder are more likely to have tonic spasms related to demyelinating disease. Tonic spasms occur more frequently in neuromyelitis optica spectrum disorders with antibodies to aquaporin 4 (AQP4 than in multiple sclerosis).[26] However, these tonic spasms have also been reported to be one of the most frequent movement disorders in multiple sclerosis.[49] Tonic spasms in neuromyelitis optica spectrum disorders and multiple sclerosis resemble classic paroxysmal dyskinesias because episodes are short and frequent. Like paroxysmal dyskinesias, tonic spasms in multiple sclerosis can be triggered by voluntary movement. Unlike paroxysmal dyskinesias, tonic spasms in multiple sclerosis are also triggered by sensory stimulation or hyperventilation. Spasms may rarely occur spontaneously. Tonic spasms are often quite painful, a telltale feature lacking in most other paroxysmal movement disorders. Spasms typically last only seconds, but may rarely last 1–2 minutes. The underlying demyelinating lesions can be in the motor pathway from the level of the posterior limb of the internal capsule to the spinal cord. An important underlying anatomic factor is how close the demyelinating lesion is to motor fibers, where a high proportion of axons can be affected by spread of ephaptic activation. The preservation of the underlying corticospinal fibers makes it easier for pathologic discharges to reach the peripheral effectors. Episodes may respond to medications that suppress ephaptic transmission from demyelination, such as carbamazepine or oxcarbazepine.

The treatment response to carbamazepine or related drugs is usually good, but it is important not to miss the underlying cause. Painful tonic spasms might be the first manifestation of a demyelinating disease requiring immunotherapy. Knowledge of these spasms being more often associated with AQP4-related neuromyelitis optica rather than multiple sclerosis can aid further management, in particular the choice of the immunomodulator. For example, interferon beta can be used in multiple sclerosis, but should not be used in neuromyelitis optica. Rarely, brief dystonic posturing in young women can be seen with NMDAR antibodies.

WORKUP

Antibody Testing: Patient Characteristics

Autoantibody-related dystonia (or pseudodystonia) is overall rare but not to be missed as it is potentially treatable. Missing the diagnosis can lead to delayed treatment, but overdiagnosis also has negative consequences. Overdiagnosis can lead to potentially harmful immunosuppression, unnecessary tumor screening, and a delay in a more appropriate treatment. Therefore, basic knowledge of the role and limitations of antibody testing is crucial.

Antibody testing should be undertaken when there is a clinical suspicion of an autoimmune etiology because of a characteristic phenotype and/or relatively rapid clinical course. Autoantibody tests should not be used as a screening tool when clinical suspicion is low because of the high risk of false positives or antibodies of unknown significance.[4,15] Screening also cannot rely on brain MRI or CSF as both have a high risk of being normal or having non-specific abnormalities.[1] The likelihood of obtaining a normal or non-specific test result with either MRI or CSF depends on the particular underlying autoimmune etiology. Non-diagnostic tests are less likely in anti-NMDAR encephalitis but very likely in anti-IgLON5 disease.[9,21] Hence, clinical suspicion and awareness of clues for an autoimmune etiology are of paramount importance (Table 21.3).

Antibody Testing: Specimen

When testing for antibodies, the gold standard is pairing of serum and CSF samples to achieve highest sensitivity and specificity.[10,18,19,30] The presence of autoantibodies in CSF as well as serum increases specificity and suggests CNS

Table 21.3 **Clues raising suspicion for autoimmune dystonia**

Clue	Example
Suggestive clinical features	Rapid progression Coexisting encephalopathy Painful tonic spasms Faciobrachial dystonic seizures Adult-onset paroxysmal dyskinesia Excessive startle Hemi-syndrome without MRI lesion
Coexisting conditions	Other autoimmune disorder History of malignancy Features suggestive of unrecognized malignancy
Laboratory findings	Inflammatory cerebrospinal fluid Evidence for inflammatory changes on MRI

autoimmunity.[19,30,41] The presence of serum antibodies without CSF antibodies in an autoimmune CNS disease seems mechanistically not intuitive but may occur. Potential mechanisms may relate to methodological issues of antibody testing, a primarily peripherally driven immunopathophysiology where breakdown of the CSF–blood barrier is enough, or "brain as sink" hypothesis, where antibodies bound to brain antigens are no longer detectable. In cases of peripheral syndromes (e.g., peripheral nerve hyperexcitability with Caspr2-antibodies), CSF antibodies seem not to be a prerequisite,[24] and, for AQP4 antibodies, serum suffices as well.

If present, CSF antibodies enable calculation of the antibody index to identify intrathecal synthesis, rather than passive diffusion over the blood–CSF barrier. This antibody index can be a strong predictor of CNS autoimmunity.[8,23,41] This index can be particularly relevant for antibodies occasionally found in healthy subjects or non-neurological disease, such as anti-GAD.[23,31] Last, in some cases, there are only CSF but no serum antibodies, thus highlighting further the importance of testing the CSF.

Antibody Testing: Methodology

There are various methods of antibody detection, such as tissue-based immunohistochemistry, cell-based assay, radio immunoprecipitation assay, Western blot, or enzyme-linked immunosorbent assay (ELISA).[40] Neuronal cell surface antibodies, for example, are often screened using cell-based assays, where the antigen is expressed, in a conformation akin to that in vivo, on the cell surface. Such cell-based assays are designed to detect antibodies that are pathogenic, but they have some limitations (both live and fixed cell-based assays). However, some laboratories offer other test methods that are not designed to detect such pathogenic antibodies against conformational epitopes. For example, antibodies against the dopamine D_2 receptor were originally described and detected by tissue-based immunohistochemistry and cell-based assays,[13] but ambiguous (and false-positive) findings resulted from testing by ELISA, a test detecting peptides or linear epitopes.[7,11] Similarly, testing laboratories may offer tests for D_2R-like antibodies or "basal ganglia antibodies" that are not useful in the diagnosis of autoimmune movement disorders.[3] Some laboratories may also offer testing for IgM or IgA antibodies,[12] but pathogenic relevance has been questioned.[20,36]

There is good evidence for an overall correlation between neuronal surface antibody titers and clinical symptoms and course, although titers between patients may differ greatly, so strict cutoff values are hard to define.[19] While future studies will hopefully allow the generation of generally accepted values to define a clinically relevant range for the various antibodies in specific tests, low serum titers are sometimes unspecific for some antibodies (e.g., Caspr2, $GABA_A$R, GlyR).[37] On the other hand, titers might be low early in the disease, and repeated testing is sometimes warranted.

Overall, replication of test results with a different methodology (e.g., combining cell-based assays with tissue immunohistochemistry) or referral to a reference laboratory are recommended, particularly if results are ambiguous.[18,19,27,29] For example, a recent study has shown that the predictive value of onconeuronal antibodies positive in line blot assays is low and that positive results must be confirmed by immunohistochemistry.[43] The same observations apply to neuronal surface antibodies. In short, it is important to ensure that the appropriate test has been selected in the first place and that results can be replicated in a second, confirmatory test.

TREATMENT

Immunotherapy and the treatment of any underlying tumor should be initiated promptly. The optimal immunotherapy varies according to the antibody and phenotype. Treatment is started with first-line immunotherapy (corticosteroids, intravenous immunoglobulins, or plasma exchange) and escalated to second-line immunotherapy (e.g., rituximab, cyclophosphamide) if required. The decision to escalate immunotherapy, as well as the approach to maintenance therapy, is based on the particular underlying antibody and its implications as delineated mainly by retrospective, observational cohort studies or case series; meta-analysis case and cohort studies; and expert consensus.[35,47] The selection of a particular therapy will also be based on availability, cost of treatments, and practical considerations. For example, plasma exchange may be difficult for patients who have severe autonomic instability or marked agitation.

A better understanding of the underlying immunological mechanisms may lead to more precisely tailored immunotherapy in the future. An example is neuromyelitis optica with AQP4 antibodies, where the complement inhibitor eculizumab has been shown to be very efficacious in otherwise treatment-refractory cases.[39] Indeed, there are single case reports and studies investigating the use of other, less commonly used immunotherapies, such as bortezomib, a proteasome inhibitor.[51] Nonetheless, the more potent immunotherapies often come at the cost of a higher risk of infections, which may be serious.[45] Therapy must balance these risks against any possible benefit.

Apart from immunotherapy, often there is also a need for symptom-based and often empirical treatment. This type of treatment does not differ from symptomatic treatment of other types of dystonia and may include benzodiazepines, anticholinergics, muscle relaxants, and/or botulinum toxin injections (see Chapter 28, "Symptom-Targeted Oral Medications for Dystonia"). Caution is warranted with regards to the application of dopamine receptor blockers in individuals with NMDAR antibodies. Although they are often used because of the high rate of psychiatric symptoms and the frequent need to suppress chorea, there is an increased sensitivity with a higher risk of adverse events, including rhabdomyolysis, most likely due to the interaction of the NMDAR with the dopamine D_1 receptor.[28]

DYSTONIA IN SYSTEMIC AUTOIMMUNE DISEASE

Systemic autoimmune diseases are a heterogenous group of disorders characterized by immunological loss of self-tolerance that induces pathological changes in many different organ systems such as kidneys, joints, or skin. Classic examples include systemic lupus erythematosus, Sjögren syndrome, or Behcet disease. If the nervous system is affected, the neurological manifestations may involve movement disorders.[32,33] Typically, the systemic symptoms and signs lead to the diagnosis of an autoimmune disorder before the movement disorder emerges. Sometimes, however, movement disorders may be one of the presenting signs, or they may precede diagnosis of an autoimmune disorder.

Dystonia is the least common movement disorder described in systemic autoimmune diseases, the main one being Sjögren syndrome, albeit only very infrequently. Dry mouth and dry eyes are the most common symptoms of Sjögren syndrome, but dryness can also occur in the nose, sinuses, ears, throat, skin, and, in women, the vagina. Sjögren syndrome can also affect the joints, muscles, nervous system (central nervous system and peripheral nervous system, including the autonomic nervous system), gastrointestinal tract (including the pancreas and liver), skin, blood vessels, lungs, and kidneys. Joint pain and stiffness with mild swelling are common, even in those without rheumatoid arthritis. Rashes may occur, including inflammation of small blood vessels (vasculitis), most commonly on the lower legs. Sun-sensitive rash is more common on the back, chest, face, and arms. While subjective symptoms of dry eyes and dry mouth can be assessed by tests detecting decreased lacrimal or saliva production, antibody tests typically include antibodies to SSA/Ro, SSB/La, and rheumatoid factor. There are also seronegative forms of Sjögren syndrome, where the diagnosis is secured by biopsy of the minor salivary glands.

There are three potential connections between Sjögren syndrome and dystonia. The first is that dry and scratchy eyes are very common in blepharospasm, and many patients with blepharospasm may be initially diagnosed with Sjögren syndrome. However, most patients with blepharospasm do not have the other systemic features of Sjögren syndrome, so this diagnosis may be questioned. The second is craniocervical dystonia in older women. It could be argued that craniocervical dystonia and autoimmune disease are coincidental, except that some individuals appear to have relevant brain MRI lesions, or the movement disorder may respond to immunotherapy. The third connection is that of paroxysmal dystonic attacks involving one or both limbs on one side of the body. The attacks are painful, last less than 2 minutes, occur several times per day, and are related to inflammatory and/or ischemic lesions in the brain or spinal cord. Thus, it is most likely that they are related to the painful tonic spasms of demyelinating disorders and, in particular, neuromyelitis optica with AQP4 antibodies, a syndrome which also has a strong association with Sjögren syndrome.

Immunotherapy for Sjögren syndrome involves typically hydroxychloroquine, corticosteroids, or other immunosuppressants (methotrexate, azathioprine mycophenolate mofetil, leflunomide, cyclophosphamide) or biologicals (rituximab), depending on the severity.

SUMMARY AND FUTURE PROSPECTS

In summary, autoimmune dystonia (or pseudodystonia) is rare, but, given its treatment implications, it should not be missed. For both neuronal autoantibody or systemic autoimmune diseases, there often are characteristic phenotypes and sometimes additional tell-tale signs and symptoms that facilitate making the diagnosis.

Antibody testing should be applied only in cases where clinical suspicion is high, and clinicians should be aware of some of the intricacies and pitfalls of antibody testing regarding false-negative or false-positive results. Nonetheless, antibody testing can facilitate a more precise diagnosis, and knowledge of the exact underlying immunopathology is crucial to tailor the treatment and monitor for associated diseases.

New autoantibody-associated neurological disorders continue to be discovered, and it is likely that the full spectrum of autoimmune dystonia will expand in the future. There is a clear need for better understanding of the mechanisms responsible for disease so that therapies can be more precisely targeted. There also is a clear need for improving and standardizing the clinical tests used to identify these conditions.

REFERENCES

1. Balint B. Are antibody panels under-utilized in movement disorders diagnosis? Yes. Mov Disord Clin Pract 2021;8:341–346.
2. Balint B. Isolated dystonia with NMDAR antibodies: Expanding the phenotype or illustrating the intricacies of antibody testing? Movement Disorders Clinical Practice 2023;27:677–670.
3. Balint B, Bhatia K. Reopening the case for anti-basal ganglia antibodies (ABGAs): Identification of dopamine-2 receptor antibodies associated with movement disorders. Mov Disord 2013;28:733.
4. Balint B, Bhatia KP, Dalmau J. "Antibody of unknown significance" (AUS): The issue of interpreting antibody test results. Mov Disord 2021;36:1543–1547.
5. Balint B, Meinck HM. Pragmatic treatment of stiff person spectrum disorders. Mov Disord Clin Pract 2018;5:394–401.
6. Balint B, Vincent A, Meinck HM, Irani SR, Bhatia KP. Movement disorders with neuronal antibodies: Syndromic approach, genetic parallels and pathophysiology. Brain 2018;141:13–36.
7. Ben-Pazi H, Stoner JA, Cunningham MW. Dopamine receptor autoantibodies correlate with symptoms in Sydenham's chorea. PLoS One 2013;8:e73516.
8. Bien CG, Mirzadjanova Z, Baumgartner C, Onugoren MD, Grunwald T, Holtkamp M, et al. Anti-contactin-associated protein-2 encephalitis: Relevance of antibody titres, presentation and outcome. Eur J Neurol 2017;24:175–186.
9. Blinder T, Lewerenz J. Cerebrospinal fluid findings in patients with autoimmune encephalitis: A systematic analysis. Front Neurol 2019;10:804.
10. Budhram A, Dubey D, Sechi E, Flanagan EP, Yang L, Bhayana V, et al. Neural antibody testing in patients with suspected autoimmune encephalitis. Clin Chem 2020;60:1496–1509.
11. Chain JL, Alvarez K, Mascaro-Blanco A, Reim S, Bentley R, Hommer R, et al. Autoantibody biomarkers for basal ganglia encephalitis in Sydenham chorea and pediatric

autoimmune neuropsychiatric disorder associated with streptococcal infections. Front Psychiatry 2020;11:564.
12. Dahm L, Ott C, Steiner J, Stepniak B, Teegen B, Saschenbrecker S, et al. Seroprevalence of autoantibodies against brain antigens in health and disease. Ann Neurol 2014;76:82–94.
13. Dale RC, Merheb V, Pillai S, Wang D, Cantrill L, Murphy TK, et al. Antibodies to surface dopamine-2 receptor in autoimmune movement and psychiatric disorders. Brain 2012;135:3453–3468.
14. Flanagan EP, Geschwind MD, Lopez-Chiriboga AS, Blackburn KM, Turaga S, Binks S, et al. Autoimmune encephalitis misdiagnosis in adults. JAMA Neurol 2023;80:30–39.
15. Flanagan EP, Kotsenas AL, Britton JW, McKeon A, Watson RE, Klein CJ, et al. Basal ganglia T1 hyperintensity in LGI1-autoantibody faciobrachial dystonic seizures. Neurol Neuroimmunol Neuroinflamm 2015;2:e161.
16. Gaig C, Graus F, Compta Y, Hogl B, Bataller L, Bruggemann N, et al. Clinical manifestations of the anti-IgLON5 disease. Neurology 2017;88:1736–1743.
17. Govert F, Abrante L, Becktepe J, Balint B, Ganos C, Hofstadt-van Oy U, et al. Distinct movement disorders in contactin-associated-protein-like-2 antibody-associated autoimmune encephalitis. Brain 2023;146:657–667.
18. Graus F, Titulaer MJ, Balu R, Benseler S, Bien CG, Cellucci T, et al. A clinical approach to diagnosis of autoimmune encephalitis. Lancet Neurol 2016;15:391–404.
19. Gresa-Arribas N, Titulaer MJ, Torrents A, Aguilar E, McCracken L, Leypoldt F, et al. Antibody titres at diagnosis and during follow-up of anti-NMDA receptor encephalitis: A retrospective study. Lancet Neurol 2014;13:167–177.
20. Hara M, Martinez-Hernandez E, Ariño H, Armangué T, Spatola M, Petit-Pedrol M, et al. Clinical and pathogenic significance of IgG, IgA, and IgM antibodies against the NMDA receptor. Neurology 2018;90:e1386–e1394.
21. Hermetter C, Fazekas F, Hochmeister S. Systematic review: Syndromes, early diagnosis, and treatment in autoimmune encephalitis. Front Neurol 2018;9:706.
22. Irani SR, Stagg CJ, Schott JM, Rosenthal CR, Schneider SA, Pettingill P, et al. Faciobrachial dystonic seizures: The influence of immunotherapy on seizure control and prevention of cognitive impairment in a broadening phenotype. Brain 2013;136:3151–3162.
23. Jarius S, Stich O, Speck J, Rasiah C, Wildemann B, Meinck HM, Rauer S. Qualitative and quantitative evidence of anti-glutamic acid decarboxylase-specific intrathecal antibody synthesis in patients with stiff person syndrome. J Neuroimmunol 2010;229:219–224.
24. Joubert B, Saint-Martin M, Noraz N, Picard G, Rogemond V, Ducray F, et al. Characterization of a subtype of autoimmune encephalitis with anti-contactin-associated protein-like 2 antibodies in the cerebrospinal fluid, prominent limbic symptoms, and seizures. JAMA Neurol 2016;73:1115–1124.
25. Kaaden T, Madlener M, Angstwurm K, Bien CG, Bogarin Y, Doppler K, et al. Seizure semiology in antibody-associated autoimmune encephalitis. Neurol Neuroimmunol Neuroinflamm 2022;9(6):e200034. doi:10.1212/NXI.0000000000200034.
26. Kim SM, Waters P, Woodhall M, Kim JY, Kim JE, Yang JW, et al. Utility of aquaporin-4 antibody assay in patients with neuromyelitis optica spectrum disorders. Mult Scler 2013;19:1060–1067.
27. Kunchok A, Zekeridou A, McKeon A. Autoimmune glial fibrillary acidic protein astrocytopathy. Curr Opin Neurol 2019;32:452–458.
28. Lejuste F, Thomas L, Picard G, Desestret V, Ducray F, Rogemond V, et al. Neuroleptic intolerance in patients with anti-NMDAR encephalitis. Neurol Neuroimmunol Neuroinflamm 2016;3:e280.
29. McCracken L, Zhang J, Greene M, Crivaro A, Gonzalez J, Kamoun M, Lancaster E. Improving the antibody-based evaluation of autoimmune encephalitis. Neurol Neuroimmunol Neuroinflamm 2017;4:e404.
30. McKeon A, Lennon VA. NMDAR encephalitis: Which specimens, and the value of values. Lancet Neurol 2014;13:133–135.
31. Meinck HM, Faber L, Morgenthaler N, Seissler J, Maile S, Butler M, et al. Antibodies against glutamic acid decarboxylase: Prevalence in neurological diseases. J Neurol Neurosurg Psychiatry 2001;71:100–103.
32. Menezes R, Pantelyat A, Izbudak I, Birnbaum J. Movement and other neurodegenerative syndromes in patients with systemic rheumatic diseases: A case series of 8 patients and review of the literature. Medicine 2015;94:e0971.
33. Menozzi E, Mulroy E, Akbarian-Tefaghi L, Bhatia KP, Balint B. Movement disorders in systemic autoimmune diseases: Clinical spectrum, ancillary investigations, pathophysiological considerations. Parkinsonism Relat Disord 2021;88:116–128.
34. Mohammad SS, Fung VS, Grattan-Smith P, Gill D, Pillai S, Ramanathan S, et al. Movement disorders in children with anti-NMDAR encephalitis and other autoimmune encephalopathies. Mov Disord 2014;29:1539–1542.
35. Nosadini M, Mohammad SS, Ramanathan S, Brilot F, Dale RC. Immune therapy in autoimmune encephalitis: A systematic review. Expert Rev Neurother 2015;15:1391–1419.
36. Pedreño M, Sepúlveda M, Armangué T, Sabater L, Martínez-Hernandez E, Arrambide G, et al. Frequency and relevance of IgM, and IgA antibodies against MOG in MOG-IgG-associated disease. Mult Scler Relat Disord 2019;28:230–234.
37. Petit-Pedrol M, Armangue T, Peng X, Bataller L, Cellucci T, Davis R, et al. Encephalitis with refractory seizures, status epilepticus, and antibodies to the GABAA receptor: A case series, characterisation of the antigen, and analysis of the effects of antibodies. Lancet Neurol 2014;13:276–286.
38. Pittock SJ, Parisi JE, McKeon A, Roemer SF, Lucchinetti CF, Tan KM, et al. Paraneoplastic jaw dystonia and laryngospasm with antineuronal nuclear autoantibody type 2 (anti-Ri). Arch Neurol 2010;67:1109–1115.
39. Pittock SJ, Berthele A, Fujihara K, Kim HJ, Levy M, Palace J, et al. Eculizumab in aquaporin-4–positive neuromyelitis optica spectrum disorder. N Engl J Med 2019;381:614–625.
40. Probst C, Saschenbrecker S, Stoecker W, Komorowski L. Anti-neuronal autoantibodies: Current diagnostic challenges. Mult Scler Relat Disord 2014;3:303–320.
41. Reiber H, Peter JB. Cerebrospinal fluid analysis: Disease-related data patterns and evaluation programs. J Neurol Sci 2001;184:101–122.
42. Rubio-Agustí I, Dalmau J, Sevilla T, Burgal M, Beltrán E, Bataller L. Isolated hemidystonia associated with

NMDA receptor antibodies. Movement Disorders 2011;26:351–352.
43. Ruiz-García R, Martínez-Hernández E, Saiz A, Dalmau J, Graus F. The diagnostic value of onconeural antibodies depends on how they are tested. Front Immunol 2020;11:1482.
44. Sabater L, Gaig C, Gelpi E, Bataller L, Lewerenz J, Torres-Vega E, et al. A novel non-rapid-eye movement and rapid-eye-movement parasomnia with sleep breathing disorder associated with antibodies to IgLON5: A case series, characterisation of the antigen, and post-mortem study. Lancet Neurol 2014;13:575–586.
45. Scheibe F, Ostendorf L, Reincke SM, Prüss H, von Brünneck AC, Köhnlein M, et al. Daratumumab treatment for therapy-refractory anti-CASPR2 encephalitis. J Neurol 2020;267:317–323.
46. Simard C, Vogrig A, Joubert B, Muñiz-Castrillo S, Picard G, Rogemond V, et al. Clinical spectrum and diagnostic pitfalls of neurologic syndromes with Ri antibodies. Neurol Neuroimmunol Neuroinflamm 2020;7(3):e699. doi:10.1212/NXI.0000000000000699.
47. Siriratnam P, McArthur L, Chen Z, Kempster P, Monif M. Movement disorders in cell surface antibody mediated autoimmune encephalitis: A meta-analysis. Front Neurol 2023;14:1225223.
48. Sturchio A, Dwivedi AK, Gastaldi M, Grimberg MB, Businaro P, Duque KR,et al. Movement disorders associated with neuronal antibodies: A data-driven approach. J Neurol 2022;269:3511–3521.
49. Tranchant C, Bhatia KP, Marsden CD. Movement disorders in multiple sclerosis. Mov Disord 1995;10:418–423.
50. Varley JA, Webb AJS, Balint B, Fung VSC, Sethi KD, Tijssen MAJ, et al. The movement disorder associated with NMDAR antibody-encephalitis is complex and characteristic: An expert video-rating study. J Neurol Neurosurg Psychiatry 2019;90:724–726.
51. Wickel J, Chung HY, Platzer S, Lehmann T, Prüss H, Leypoldt F, et al. Generate-Boost: Study protocol for a prospective, multicenter, randomized controlled, double-blinded phase II trial to evaluate efficacy and safety of bortezomib in patients with severe autoimmune encephalitis. Trials 2020;21:625.

Chapter 22

Dystonia Genetics

INTRODUCTION

The majority of cases of dystonia, especially those arising in adults, are idiopathic. A cause cannot be found even after extensive workup. For some cases, however, a cause can be identified. There are many potential causes, both acquired and genetic. This chapter addresses genetic etiologies.

The field of genetics has undergone dramatic changes in the past decades, driven in large part by rapid advances in technology that have enabled analysis of the human genome with increasing precision and speed. These advances have led to a rapid growth in the number of genes linked with dystonia, and new genes are being described every year. The technological advances have also led to a shift in the clinical approach to genetic disorders. The traditional strategy relied on delineating syndromic patterns to guide selection of individual genes to test one at a time. The modern approach involves simultaneously testing many genes at once. The advances have also produced a new language to describe new genetic methods and findings (Table 22.1).

The genetics of dystonia has been rapidly evolving, with numerous reviews describing new genes every year.[5,14,15,18,20,22,35,36,45,51,55,56] This chapter takes a pragmatic approach to this topic. Rather than provide a catalog of the many genes and associated clinical phenotypes, it addresses core conceptual issues in genetics that drive clinical application. Lists of genes for more specific dystonia syndromes can be found in chapters addressing dystonia with parkinsonism, ataxia, myoclonus, paroxysmal dyskinesia, and others.

DYSTONIA GENES

Many genes are linked with dystonia. A precise number of "dystonia genes" is difficult to ascertain because the number depends on which genes are included. Only six genes have been linked with disorders where dystonia is consistently the sole problem (Table 22.2). Among these genes, *CIZ1* appears to be so rare that its status as a dystonia gene has been questioned. Two other genes (*ANO3* and *COL6A3*) have been linked with dystonia in many unrelated cases, but causal links have proved challenging in some cases because of difficulties distinguishing pathological from non-pathological variants.[25,39]

Several other genes are sometimes included among lists of those causing isolated dystonia, but the spectrum of disease is not yet fully known because the number of cases reported is very small. While each of these genes can indeed cause isolated dystonia, some proportion of

Table 22.1 **Glossary of genetic lingo**

Term	Explanation
Aneuploidy	Too many or too few chromosomes
Clinical exome sequencing	Sequencing all exons for all genes known to be associated with human disease
Codon	Series of 3 nucleotides that code for a specific amino acid
Copy number variant (CNV)	Insertion or deletion of a piece of DNA
Exome	The gene sequences of all exons
Exon	Part of a gene that is transcribed into mRNA
Frame shift	A genetic change that shifts the protein reading sequence
Genetic variant	A change in the normal gene sequence that may be benign or pathological
Genome	The entire genetic constitution
Indel	Insertion or deletion of a piece of DNA
Intron	DNA that falls between exons of a gene
Karyotype	A method for visualizing chromosomes
Massively parallel sequencing	A method for measuring many genes at one time
Microarray	Many small pieces of DNA arranged separately in a grid as a reference to compare test samples
Monosomy	A karyotype with a missing chromosome
Mutation	Historical term for a pathological change in the normal gene sequence, no longer recommended in clinical medicine
Next generation sequencing (NGS)	Method for simultaneous sequencing of many genes (tens to thousands) at once
Nonsense variant	Introduction of a stop codon, usually pathogenic
Non-synonymous variant	A genetic change that alters the amino acid coded, may be pathogenic or benign
Pleiotropy	Phenomenon in which a single gene may cause multiple different phenotypes
Sanger sequencing	Method for assessing the sequence of individual nucleotides in a specific piece of DNA; also called "targeted sequencing"
Segregation	Phenomenon where a genetic variant correlates with disease among several members of a family
Short tandem repeat	Repeated sequences of 3, 4, or more nucleotides
Single nucleotide polymorphism (SNP)	Change of a single nucleotide in a sequence of DNA
Splicing variant	A genetic change that may alter the splicing of introns and exons
Stop codon	Three nucleotides that signal the stop of protein translation
Synonymous variant	A genetic change that does not alter the amino acid coded, usually benign unless it alters splicing
Translocation	A piece of a chromosome has moved to a different chromosome
Triplet repeat	A short tandem repeat of 3 nucleotides
Trisomy	A karyotype with an extra chromosome
Variant of unknown significance (VUS or VOUS)	A genetic change that may be benign or pathological
Whole exome sequencing	Sequencing all exons for all known genes
Whole genome sequencing	Sequencing the entire genome, including exons, introns and non-coding DNA between genes

cases also develop additional clinical problems. For example, *EIF2AK2* is often associated with early-onset generalized dystonia, but many cases also have developmental delay, intellectual disability, and corticospinal signs. *AOPEP* has also been reported to cause isolated dystonia, but several cases have also developed parkinsonism[13,62] or chorea.[32] *VPS16* also is linked with isolated dystonia, but some individuals have intellectual disability[40,49] or myoclonus[16,41] These examples demonstrate that the distinction between genes for isolated or combined dystonia is not always clear and depends on how frequently an associated disorder occurs.

A much larger number of genes has been linked to syndromes where dystonia is a consistent and prominent part of a syndrome that usually includes additional clinical features

Table 22.2 **Genes linked with isolated dystonia syndromes**

Gene	Inheritance	Gene product	Usual age at onset	Usual body distribution
ANO3	Autosomal dominant	Anoctamin-3	Adulthood	Neck, with prominent tremor
CIZ1	Autosomal dominant	Cip1-interacting zinc finger protein 1	Adulthood	Neck
COL6A3	Autosomal recessive	α3 subunit of type VI collagen	Early childhood	Neck, arms, often generalized
GNAL	Autosomal dominant	G-protein subunit alpha l	Adult	Head, neck, arms
THAP1	Autosomal dominant	Thanatos-associated domain-containing apoptosis protein 1	Adolescence	Head, neck, arms
TOR1A	Autosomal dominant	TorsinA	Childhood	Arms, legs, often generalized

This table includes genes associated with the clinical phenotype of isolated dystonia only. Isolated dystonia may be focal, segmental, multifocal or generalized. Many other genes may be associated with isolated dystonia phenotypes, but they are not included here because they are frequently associated with additional clinical features such as cognitive impairment, parkinsonism, or other problems.

(Table 22.3).[11] The most common additional features include parkinsonism, ataxia, myoclonus, developmental delay, spasticity, and cognitive impairments. These conditions are addressed in Chapter 13, "Dystonia and Parkinsonism," Chapter 14, "Dystonia and Ataxia," Chapter 15, "Dystonia and Myoclonus," and Chapter 18, "Dystonia Combined with Other Features." More than 300 genes have been linked with disorders where dystonia may be a relatively minor aspect of a syndrome in which other clinical features are more severe.[11]

Table 22.3 **Genes linked with selected combined dystonia syndromes**

Syndrome	Combined phenotype	Usual age at onset	Example genes	Notes
Dystonia-myoclonus	Dystonia plus myoclonus	Childhood to adolescence	*SGCE, KCTD17, RELN, VPS16, YY1*	Myoclonus or dystonia may predominate; frequent involvement of neck
Dystonia-parkinsonism	Dystonia plus parkinsonism	Childhood to young adulthood	*AOPEP, ATP1A3, ATP7B, GCH1, PINK1, PRKN, PTS, SLC30A10, SLC39A14, SPR, TH*	Includes dopa-responsive dystonias and neurodegeneration with brain iron accumulation
Dystonia-ataxia	Dystonia plus ataxia	Childhood to older adulthood	*ATM, CTX, NPC1, NPC2, POLG*, many spinocerebellar ataxias	Ataxia predominates in most cases, but dystonia may predominate in others
Rapid-onset dystonia	Acute onset of dystonia, usually with parkinsonism	Childhood to adolescence	*ATP1A3, GCHD, MUT, PCCA, PCCB, SLC19A3*	Often involves oromandibular region and often triggered by stress
Paroxysmal dyskinesias	Intermittent episodes of dystonia often with other abnormal movements	Childhood to adolescence	*PRRT2, MR1, SLC2A1*	Often mistaken for epilepsy

This is a partial list of some syndromes where dystonia is frequently combined with other problems.

Because there are so many potential dystonia genes, published reviews can be confusing because they often focus on selected subgroups of the genes. Some reviews limit discussion to genes linked with isolated dystonia.[15,22,55] Other reviews focus on genes where dystonia is combined with a specific problem, such as parkinsonism[35,56] or ataxia.[36,45] Other reviews select genes that can be grouped into shared biological pathways,[5,14,18,51] and some cover only the most recently described genes.[20] These reviews often provide a narrow representation of the full spectrum of potential genes.

Another area of confusion relates to the way genes are named. Many prior articles and reviews of dystonia genetics are based on a nomenclature recommended by the Human Genome Organization for genetic loci.[31] This approach uses the prefix DYT, followed by a number that was given according to historical order of discovery. This approach to nomenclature was developed to describe genetic loci (genomic locations of genes), not the actual gene. This approach has many flaws and is no longer recommended.[29,31] A new approach to nomenclature has been proposed in which the number is replaced by the gene name, and multiple prefixes may be combined according to the dominant phenotype, such as DYT/PARK-*GCH1* for dystonia combined with parkinsonism caused by pathogenic variants in *GCH1*.[28] However, this approach is cumbersome to use, especially for practicing clinicians who are not expert in genetics.[31] As a result, the nomenclature strategy used in this chapter refers only to the name of the disorder and/or its relevant gene.

IDENTIFYING PATIENTS WHO MAY BENEFIT FROM GENETIC TESTING

Overview

When considering all types of dystonia, most are idiopathic, and some are acquired. A genetic etiology accounts for only a small fraction of cases. As a result, it is not useful to conduct genetic testing in all individuals who have dystonia. However, several clinical clues make a genetic etiology more likely. These include a family history of dystonia, early onset of symptoms, and combinations of clinical problems that point to specific genetic syndromes.[21,60] These clues increase the value of genetic testing. Each of these clues is helpful, but each also has some limitations.

Family History

A strong family history of dystonia provides an obvious clue for a heritable cause, and it can be even more useful when the family tree suggests dominant, recessive, or another pattern of inheritance. However, the lack of a family history does not exclude a genetic cause for several reasons. First, modern families are now much smaller than in the past. Smaller families make it harder to recognize patterns of inheritance.

Second, several genes responsible for dystonia are only partly penetrant, a phenomenon in which individuals carrying a pathogenic gene never develop symptoms. For example, pathogenic variants in *THAP1* cause symptoms in 50% of carriers, while pathogenic variants in *TOR1A* cause symptoms in only 30%.[22] For pathogenic variants in *SGCE*, penetrance is determined by the parent of origin: paternal inheritance nearly always produces symptoms (100% penetrance), while maternal inheritance usually does not (0% penetrance).[43] The transmitting father might not have any symptoms, depending on whether he inherited his pathogenic variant from his mother or father. This phenomenon is caused by imprinting of the maternal *SGCE* gene, which involves its deactivation by methylation. These phenomena related to penetrance can make it difficult to recognize familial patterns of inheritance.

The final reason that family history of dystonia may be absent relates to the occurrence of sporadic cases where neither parent carries the defect, but a pathogenic variant arises de novo during development.[54] When this phenomenon occurs during gametogenesis or early in development at the level of a single cell shortly after fertilization, all cells of the individual carry the genetic variant. When a genetic variant emerges later in development, only some tissues and cells are affected, a phenomenon known as *mosaicism*.[3] The frequencies of these mechanisms that produce sporadic cases are not well understood. For some genes, there is nearly always a family history, and sporadic cases are uncommon. For other genes, many cases are sporadic and familial cases are less common, such as *KMT2B*. Therefore, a family history can be very useful when present, but absence of a family history does not rule out a genetic etiology. In these cases, other clues may point to a genetic etiology.

Syndromic Pattern

Recognizing a syndromic pattern also provides a useful clue for a potential genetic cause. For isolated dystonias, generalized dystonias are more likely to be inherited than focal dystonias. The combination of dystonia with other problems that point to a known syndromic pattern can be even more useful (Table 22.3). For example, dystonia may be combined with another movement disorder such as parkinsonism (see Chapter 13), ataxia (see Chapter 14), or myoclonus (see Chapter 15). Dystonia may also be combined with other neurological problems such as spasticity, intellectual disability or dementia, seizures, or retinopathy (see Chapter 18). Alternatively, dystonia may be combined with medical problems such as liver disease, hematological abnormalities, or dermatologic findings.

A basic laboratory workup can add useful information to identify syndromic patterns. Brain MRI, in particular, can be helpful for pointing toward an underlying genetic defect. For example, abnormalities in the basal ganglia can provide valuable clues for a genetic disorder, many of which have highly characteristic involvement of specific subregions.[34,52] A few have nearly pathognomonic patterns, such as the "eye of the tiger" sign related to *PANK2*.[7] Similarly, white matter disease can point to the leukoencephalopathies, with characteristic patterns of involvement pointing to specific genetic disorders.[26]

The combination of dystonia with additional problems can help to narrow the list of potential genes to consider. In some cases, syndromic patterns are specific enough to suggest a single gene. For example, Wilson disease caused by pathogenic variants in *ATP7B* becomes the top suspicion for an individual who has dystonia with parkinsonism, a corneal Kaiser-Fleischer ring, and lab testing suggestive of liver disease.[1] Lesch-Nyhan disease, caused by defects in *HPRT1*, is another disorder with a specific syndromic pattern that combines dystonia, self-injurious behavior, cognitive impairment, and elevated serum uric acid.[10] Some clinical features are sufficiently characteristic to serve as a "red flag" for a specific genetic disorder.[17] Good examples of red flags are the tendon xanthomas in cerebrotendinous xanthomatosis[7] or the visibly tortuous blood vessels of ataxia-telangiectasia.[24] There are many such red flags, and they can be very helpful if found. For most inherited dystonias, however, highly specific red flags or syndromic patterns are lacking. As a result, a syndromic pattern can be very useful if found, but relying on red flags and syndromic patterns is not sufficient to identify many genetic dystonias.

Age at Onset

The third useful clue for a potential genetic cause is the age at which dystonia first emerges. A discoverable genetic cause is uncommon for most focal dystonias that emerge after 40 years of age. On the other hand, a genetic cause is more likely in younger individuals, and the age at onset provides a clue for specific subtypes. For example, dystonia in the first year of life is suspicious for an inherited metabolic disorder. Dystonia that begins in early childhood is often linked with *TOR1A* (DYT1 dystonia) or *GCH1* (dopa-responsive dystonia), while dystonia that begins in adolescents or young adults can often be linked with *ANO3*, *GNAL*, or *THAP1*. Thus, early onset of dystonia provides a clue for a potential genetic cause, although the precise gene involved cannot be precisely predicted because of substantial overlap in the ages of onset for many genes.[15,22,56]

A precise age that distinguishes "late onset" from "early onset" is hard to define. Although there is no precise age cutoff that discriminates these two groups, the suspicion for a genetic etiology generally increases with decreasing age. Early studies suggested an age cutoff of younger than 27 years.[2] However, these studies were based on individuals with dystonia caused by *TOR1A*, and the results do not apply to other genetic dystonias. For example, the median age at onset for dystonia associated with *THAP1* is 28 years.[58] A cutoff at age 27 would miss half the cases. A strict age cutoff is even more challenging to define for treatable inherited dystonias, such as Wilson disease. Although the vast majority of cases develop symptoms before 20 years of age, exceptional cases have presented after 60 years of age.[1] When life-saving treatments are available, specific age cutoffs for genetic testing are inappropriate (see Chapter 28, "Symptom-Targeted Oral Medications for Dystonia").

Putting It All Together

In short, the most useful clues for a genetic etiology include family history, a syndromic pattern, and age at onset. Each of these clues has limitations, so they must be considered together. In general, a genetic cause is not usually suspected for sporadic dystonias that arise in older adults. However, a genetic etiology might be considered in older adults who have a family history or a suspicious syndromic pattern. In contrast, a genetic etiology should be suspected for all early-onset dystonias unless there is good documentation for an acquired cause.

The most common acquired etiology for early-onset dystonia is dyskinetic cerebral palsy (see Chapter 16, "Dystonia and Cerebral Palsy"). Historically, this diagnostic label was most often associated with acquired brain injury from perinatal stroke or asphyxia. Such cases may have a clear history of birth injury or hypoxia or MRI evidence of brain injury. However, this diagnosis is also applied in cases without definitive evidence for perinatal brain injury, even when the cause is unknown. Recent studies have shown that approximately 30% of all cases with the diagnosis of cerebral palsy have a genetic etiology.[9] Genetic testing in this population should be considered when there is a family history with multiple individuals affected. Genetic testing might also be considered when the clinical syndrome does not fit acquired cerebral palsy, such as the coexistence of additional unexplained clinical features or progressive worsening over time. Genetic testing might also be considered when there are MRI abnormalities pointing to an alternative diagnosis or even lack of MRI evidence consistent with perinatal brain injury.

SELECTING GENETIC TESTS

Overview

Many different methods are available for genetic testing (Table 22.4). Some of these tests are most suitable for specific genes. Other tests are more suitable for testing large groups of genes. This section provides a brief summary of these methods, along with their advantages and disadvantages and strategies for using them in different situations. More detailed information on these tests can be found elsewhere.[38,47]

Types of Tests

A *karyotype* involves the visualization of chromosomes by staining DNA. It is most useful for detecting large chromosomal anomalies, such as an extra chromosome (*trisomy*), a missing chromosome (*monosomy*), large stretches of DNA that are flipped within a chromosome (*inversion*),

Table 22.4 **Genetic tests**

	Advantages	Disadvantages	Utility in dystonia
Karyotype	Inexpensive, widely available	Detects only large chromosomal defects > 5mb	Syndromic pattern points to a large chromosomal defect
Chromosomal microarray	Inexpensive, widely available	Detects defects only down to 100 kb	Syndromic pattern includes intellectual disability or seizures
Sanger sequencing	Moderately expensive, highly specific, widely available	Feasible for targeting only a few genes	Syndromic pattern points to one (or a few) genes
Southern blot	Moderately, widely available	Feasible for targeting only a few genes	Syndromic pattern suspicious for a tandem repeat disorder
NGS gene panel	Expensive, not widely available	Panels often incomplete	Non-specific dystonia syndrome
Clinical exome	Very expensive, not widely available	May miss large insertions or deletions, repeat expansion disorders, and genes with GC rich regions	Non-specific dystonia syndrome

or errors in which a piece of one chromosome is connected to another chromosome (*translocation*). To detect a defect in a karyotype, its size must be large, usually more than 5 million bases (megabases, or Mb). This method is most useful when there is a syndromic pattern suggestive of a chromosomal defect, such as trisomy 21 (Down syndrome).

Smaller defects, down to about 100 kilobases (kb), can be detected by *chromosomal microarray*.[4,48] With this method, a test sample is compared against a reference sample in which many separate pieces of DNA spanning the entire human genome are methodically and individually arrayed. Even smaller defects, down to the level of single exons, require a method known as *multiplex ligation-dependent probe amplification*. This method targets a finite number of genes, which must be selected in advance. Chromosomal microarray and multiplex ligation-dependent probe amplification are methods that are most suitable for phenotypes frequently associated with deletion or duplication events, sometimes called *copy number variants*.

Other methods can detect smaller genetic changes, even down to a single nucleotide. *Sanger sequencing*, named after its inventor, is a method that reads the precise sequence of nucleotides in a piece of DNA. Its main strength is precision, but its application involves focusing on one gene (or one part of a gene) at a time. It is labor-intensive and its utility for multiple genes, especially long ones, is limited by cost.

Next-generation sequencing (NGS), also known as *massively parallel sequencing*, is the most recently developed method, and it is suitable for determining the sequences of many (hundreds to thousands) of genes at one time. Its power lies in its ability to simultaneously assess many genes down to the single nucleotide level. The main criticism of this method is that it provides an enormous amount of genetic information, some of which is hard to interpret. This technology has been clinically implemented in several ways. The first is *whole-genome sequencing*, in which the entire genome is sequenced.[21] This strategy is rarely used clinically because it is expensive, only a small fraction of the genome contains regions of interest linked with human disease, and most data from other regions cannot be interpreted. Second is *whole-exome sequencing*, in which all exons known to encode proteins are sequenced. This method also generates a substantial amount of unusable data because not all proteins have been linked with human disease. Third is *clinical exome sequencing*, where exome sequencing is limited to proteins already associated with human disease. Finally, there are NGS panels, which typically focus on exons for genes known to be associated with a specific phenotype, such as dystonia. While clinical exomes and panels mitigate the problem of uninterpretable data, they still suffer some limitations. They are not suitable for detection of certain types of genetic changes including large chromosomal defects, large deletions or insertions, most repeat expansions, genes which may have multiple homologs or pseudogenes, and genes with regions that have a high content of guanidine (G) and cytidine (C) bases (*GC-rich* regions).

Alternative genetic tests may be required in special circumstances. For example, the methods described above are not suitable for detection of abnormal expansion of short tandem repeats associated with many diseases, such as the trinucleotide repeat associated with Huntington disease and other repeats linked with many spinocerebellar ataxias. Such cases may occasionally present with dystonia. Detection of these repeats requires a Southern blot, where the number of repeats can be measured. Additionally, many genetic tests focus on the nuclear genome so they cannot detect pathogenic changes in DNA encoded by the mitochondrial genome, where many genes have been associated with dystonia.[14,30] Finally, some genes may be abnormally activated or silenced by epigenetic mechanisms, and detection of these mechanisms requires methylation-sensitive assays.

Strategies for Selecting Tests

No single genetic test can capture all dystonia genes. In view of the constant discovery of new genes and the rapid evolution of methods to detect them, choosing the best test can be challenging, and recommendations may vary even among experts. As a result, consultation with a clinical geneticist is recommended. However, all clinicians can benefit from a working knowledge of these tests and especially their limitations. The situation for genetic testing is similar to the situation for radiology, where the clinician can greatly aid in the selection of the best tests and the interpretation of findings by the consulting radiologist.

The most appropriate initial test depends on the condition being evaluated. For example, a chromosomal microarray may be the best initial test for intellectual disability or seizures because a large proportion of such cases have small deletions or insertions. In contrast, most genetic dystonias are caused by smaller defects such as single nucleotide polymorphisms, so a sequencing-based method is preferable.

The best initial test is also influenced by the dystonia syndrome. Historically, many experts in clinical genetics recommended an approach that started with a detailed clinical exam focusing on careful delineation of specific syndromic patterns that could guide the selection of the most appropriate gene for testing.[6] Several developments have questioned the application of this strategy in many circumstances. First, a number of studies have revealed that phenotype–genotype correlations are not as specific as originally believed.[8,12,27] When relying on these correlations as a guide for genetic testing, the wrong genes are often selected in a substantial proportion of cases. Second, the incorrect selection of initial candidate genes often leads to serial testing of multiple genes until the answer is found, a strategy that is both expensive and time-consuming. The process is frustrating to families, who lose faith in the diagnostic process and move from one clinician to the next, a phenomenon that has become known as the *diagnostic odyssey*.[19] Third, technological advances have increased the efficiency of gene tests so that the cost of testing one or a few genes sequentially is marginally less expensive than testing many genes at the same time. The syndromic approach for selecting genes may still be useful in circumstances where there are highly specific red flags or a strong phenotype–genotype correlation, but it is not ideal for most cases.

In the absence of diagnostic red flags or highly specific syndromic patterns, screening multiple genes at the same time is more efficient. Since a high proportion of genetic variants causing both isolated and combined dystonia syndromes are small (single nucleotide polymorphisms, or small insertions or deletions), sequencing-based methods provide a valuable place to start. A NGS gene panel that focuses more precisely on the phenotype provides a convenient solution to this problem. For example, it is possible to request gene panels that focus only on genes for isolated dystonias. The main weakness of these panels is that genes responsible for combined dystonia syndromes sometimes present with a phenotype of isolated dystonia. A compromise might be NGS gene panels that span all dystonia genes. The limitation here is that the phenotype of isolated dystonia may be caused by genes more commonly associated with ataxia, parkinsonism, epilepsy, and other phenotypes.[8] A major problem with all NGS gene panels is that they are not standardized across test labs. Some laboratories offer dystonia gene panels with 20 genes, while other laboratories offer panels with more than 200 genes. In one large study of 1,100 cases of mixed types of dystonia, a genetic diagnosis could be established in 220 cases. However, 71% of the genes were not found in common dystonia panels but in panels for ataxia, parkinsonism, hereditary spastic paraparesis, and others.[8] Therefore, panels that are labeled as "comprehensive" can be misleading.

In view of these limitations of gene panels, a clinical exome may be preferable, even if it generates unexpected results that were not intended or results that are difficult to interpret. When sequencing methods with broad coverage of many genes are applied to large cohorts of individuals with dystonia, the diagnostic yield for a definite or probable pathogenic variant varies from 11% to 20%, depending on the characteristics of the cohort (Table 22.5). The diagnostic yield depends on several factors including family history, age at onset, and features of the dystonia syndrome, such as whether it was isolated or combined with other problems. Even when the clinical exome is negative, it is important to recognize that few clinical tests have 100% sensitivity. As noted above, the clinical exome will not identify most large chromosomal defects, repeat expansion disorders, mitochondrial disorders, and genes with GC-rich regions or pseudogenes. If the clinical syndrome is suspicious for a condition that falls into one of these categories, alternative tests may be required.

INTERPRETING GENETIC TESTS

The outcome of genetic testing can fall into one of three categories: a pathogenic genetic variant is found, no pathogenic variant is found, or a variant is found but its pathogenicity is unknown. The latter is called a *variant of uncertain significance* (VUS). The American College of Medical Genetics has recommendations for

Table 22.5 **Diagnostic yield for broad sequencing methods**

Study	Method	Total probands	Isolated dystonias	Other dystonias	Diagnostic yield
Van Egmond, 2017[53]	94-gene panel	61	21.3	78.7	14.8
Kumar, 2019[21]	Genome sequencing	111	67.6	32.4	11.7
Powis, 2019[42]	Exome sequencing	189	30.7	69.3	20.2
Zech, 2020[60]	Exome sequencing	728	54.8	45.2	18.5
Wu, 2022[57]	72-gene panel	318	80.5	19.5	12.6

Exome sequencing included whole exome and clinical exome sequencing. One article (*) included cases previously reported,[59,61] and only the final cohort is shown here.

classifying all variants into five groups: pathogenic, likely pathogenic, uncertain significance, likely benign, and benign.[44] When a pathogenic or likely pathogenic variant is found, genetic counseling is important. The patient should be informed of the implications of the result as well as the significance for other family members.

When a pathogenic variant is not found or any variants found are benign, the possibility of a non-genetic etiology should be reconsidered. However, it also is important to consider the potential limitations of the test performed. Like all other laboratory tests in clinical medicine, the sensitivity of genetic testing is not 100%. There are many dystonia genes yet to be discovered, and all available genetic tests have some limitations. If a genetic etiology is strongly suspected despite a negative test result, other types of tests may have to be considered. For example, if a clinical exome returns normal, it may be necessary to consider tests that address the types of variants not detected by this method, such as large insertions or deletions, or repeat expansion disorders. It is also valuable to follow the patient over time because the evolution of the clinical condition may make the diagnosis more obvious.

When genetic testing discloses a VUS, interpretation requires a bit more effort. This result is not uncommon because all normal individuals carry thousands of genetic variants, most of which are benign. A VUS means that the test lab has found something in the genetic code of an individual that varies from most other normal individuals. However, the lab cannot assess pathogenicity because the variant is novel and not previously been linked with disease. A VUS should not be dismissed as irrelevant without further clinical, genetic, and sometimes additional laboratory tests.

One important action to take when a VUS is found involves careful clinical "reverse phenotyping" by comparing the clinical features of the individual's phenotype with other individuals who have pathogenic variants in the same gene. It is often necessary to reevaluate the individual, looking for subtle or unusual clinical features that may have been missed in initial evaluations. If the gene is associated with specific laboratory abnormalities, then these should be tested, too. If the genotype–phenotype correlation is strong, this increases the likelihood that the VUS may be pathogenic. However, a lack of close correlation does not exclude pathogenicity because some phenotypic variation occurs with all genes.

Another action to take when assessing a VUS is to determine whether the genetic variant is predicted to alter function using computational tools or "in silico" analyses. Such analyses are often provided by the testing lab, but they can be conducted by any physician using freely available online tools such as the Combined Annotation Dependent Depletion (CADD; http://cadd.gs.washington.edu/). For some genes, such as those encoding enzymes, functional assays can be conducted, too.

Another useful step to take in addressing a VUS is to determine whether the variant correlates with disease in other family members, a phenomenon called *segregation*. This step may involve clinical evaluation and genetic testing of additional family members. If two different variants are detected in a gene that is associated with recessive inheritance, trio analysis of the parents with the proband can determine whether the variants lie on the same (*cis*) or different (*trans*) gene copies in the patient. Trio analysis can also help to determine if the variant is carried by the parents or if it is de novo. To aid in assessing family members, many test labs that report a VUS will evaluate other family members at no cost. Finding the same variant in an unaffected parent argues against pathogenicity, although the phenomenon of partial penetrance also needs to be considered.

Sometimes, undertaking all the above steps is either not possible or results in ongoing uncertainty about the VUS. In this situation, especially if the genotype–phenotype correlation is strong, the status of the VUS should be reassessed every few years to determine if it has been updated to being pathogenic or benign. The original exome sequencing findings can be reassessed every few years. Most clinical testing labs collect NGS results into shared databases, and knowledge grows as more cases with more variants are added every year. New pathogenic variants are added routinely, variants previously classified as VUS may be reclassified as benign or pathogenic, and sometimes the original assignment of a variant as either benign or pathogenic can be reversed.

SUMMARY AND FUTURE PROSPECTS

Some patients with dystonia have a discoverable genetic etiology. The likelihood of a genetic etiology is increased when dystonia occurs at a young age, when there is a family history, and/or when there a recognizable syndromic pattern. There are many different types of genetic tests, each with different strengths and limitations. It is useful for clinicians who care for individuals with dystonia to have a working knowledge of options for genetic testing and the interpretation of test results, although consultation with a geneticist is advisable.

A definitive genetic diagnosis has become increasingly valuable over the years. For many years, its main value has been in counseling to aid in expectations for the future and to identify potentially affected family members. A genetic diagnosis also has become increasingly important because of the growing list of disorders where specific treatments are available (see Chapter 28). Although these disorders are rare, they should not be missed because treatments can be life-changing. In recent years, a genetic diagnosis has also become a requirement to enter certain clinical trials that target specific mechanisms in dystonia.[33,50] Finally, there has been growing awareness of a frequent phenomenon, known as the *diagnostic odyssey*, in which patients and families with undiagnosed disorders move from clinician to clinician until they find an answer. This process is time-consuming, frustrating to patients and their clinicians, and expensive because individuals often repeat the same basic laboratory tests with each new clinician. Multiple studies of individuals experiencing the diagnostic odyssey have concluded that early application of broad genetic tests is useful because these tests provide a definitive answer for a large percentage of these cases, saving time, money, and frustration.[19,23,46]

Technological advances in genetics have come at a very rapid rate, and they continue to come. In the near future, it is likely that the clinical workflow for selecting and interpreting tests will become simpler as new test strategies are developed. For example, novel bioinformatics tools are now being applied to NGS data so that detection of copy number variants becomes feasible, and some clinical labs have begun to offer this service. Other labs have begun to offer "reflex" testing, wherein a negative result from the requested genetic test automatically triggers the next most appropriate test. There are also ongoing studies addressing the potential value of NGS testing for all neonates, analogous to mandatory neonatal testing for several treatable metabolic disorders. Most importantly, as more and more test results accumulate in large databanks, the frequency of VUS will continue to decrease.

REFERENCES

1. Bandmann O, Weiss KH, Kaler SG. Wilson's disease and other neurological copper disorders. Lancet Neurol 2015;14:103–113.
2. Bressman SB, Sabatti C, Raymond D, de Leon D, Klein C, Kramer PL, et al. The DYT1 phenotype and guidelines for diagnostic testing. Neurology 2000;54:1746–1752.
3. D'Gama AM, Walsh CA. Somatic mosaicism and neurodevelopmental disease. Nat Neurosci 2018;21:1504–1514.
4. Dale RC, Grattan-Smith P, Nicholson M, Peters GB. Microdeletions detected using chromosome microarray in children with suspected genetic movement disorders: A single-centre study. Dev Med Child Neurol 2012;54:618–623.
5. Di Fonzo A, Albanese A, Jinnah HA. The apparent paradox of phenotypic diversity and shared mechanisms across dystonia syndromes. Curr Opin Neurol 2022;35:502–509.
6. Di Fonzo A, Monfrini E, Erro R. Genetics of movement disorders and the practicing clinician: Who and what to test for? Curr Neurol Neurosci Rep 2018;18:37.

7. Di Meo I, Tiranti V. Classification and molecular pathogenesis of NBIA syndromes. Eur J Paediatr Neurol 2018;22:272–284.
8. Dzinovic I, Boesch S, Skorvanek M, Necpal J, Svantnerova J, Pavelekova P, et al. Genetic overlap between dystonia and other neurologic disorders: A study of 1,100 exomes. Parkinsonism Relat Disord 2022;102:1–6.
9. Fahey MC, Maclennan AH, Kretzschmar D, Gecz J, Kruer MC. The genetic basis of cerebral palsy. Dev Med Child Neurol 2017;59:462–469.
10. Fu R, Ceballos-Picot I, Torres RJ, Larovere LE, Yamada Y, Nguyen KV, et al. Genotype-phenotype correlations in neurogenetics: Lesch-Nyhan disease as a model disorder. Brain 2014;137:1282–1303.
11. Fung VS, Jinnah HA, Bhatia K, Vidailhet M. Assessment of the patient with dystonia: An update on dystonia syndromes. Mov Disord 2013;28:889–898.
12. Gannamani R, van der Veen S, van Egmond M, de Koning TJ, Tijssen MAJ. Challenges in clinicogenetic correlations: One phenotype – many genes. Mov Disord Clin Pract 2021;8:311–321.
13. Garavaglia B, Vallian S, Romito LM, Straccia G, Capecci M, Invernizzi F, et al. AOPEP variants as a novel cause of recessive dystonia: Generalized dystonia and dystonia-parkinsonism. Parkinsonism Relat Disord 2022;97:52–56.
14. Ghaoui R, Sue CM. Movement disorders in mitochondrial disease. J Neurol 2018;265:1230–1240.
15. Gomez-Garre P, Jesus S, Perinan MT, Adarmes A, Alonso-Canovas A, Blanco-Ollero A, et al. Mutational spectrum of GNAL, THAP1 and TOR1A genes in isolated dystonia: Study in a population from Spain and systematic literature review. Eur J Neurol 2021;28:1188–1197.
16. Gu X, Lin J, Hou Y, Zhang L, Shang H. De novo missense mutation of VPS16 in a Chinese patient with generalized dystonia with myoclonus. Mov Disord Clin Pract 2022;9:551–552.
17. Herzog R, Weissbach A, Baumer T, Munchau A. Complex dystonias: An update on diagnosis and care. J Neural Transm 2020;128:431–455.
18. Jinnah HA, Sun YV. Dystonia genes and their biological pathways. Neurobiol Dis 2019;129:159–168.
19. Johnson NE. Whole-exome sequencing in neurologic practice: Reducing the diagnostic odyssey. Neurol Genet 2015;1:e37.
20. Keller Sarmiento IJ, Mencacci NE. Genetic dystonias: Update on classification and new genetic discoveries. Curr Neurol Neurosci Rep 2021;21:8.
21. Kumar KR, Davis RL, Tchan MC, Wali GM, Mahant N, Ng K, et al. Whole genome sequencing for the genetic diagnosis of heterogenous dystonia phenotypes. Parkinsonism Relat Disord 2019;69:111–118.
22. Lange LM, Junker J, Loens S, Baumann H, Olschewski L, Schaake S, et al. Genotype-phenotype relations for isolated dystonia genes: MDSGene systematic review. Mov Disord 2021;36:1086–1103.
23. Lazaridis KN, Schahl KA, Cousin MA, Babovic-Vuksanovic D, Riegert-Johnson DL, Gavrilova RH, et al. Outcome of whole exome sequencing for diagnostic odyssey cases of an individualized medicine clinic: The Mayo Clinic experience. Mayo Clin Proc 2016;91:297–307.
24. Levy A, Lang AE. Ataxia-telangiectasia: A review of movement disorders, clinical features and genotype correlations – Addendum. Mov Disord 2018;33:1238–1247.
25. Lohmann K, Schlicht F, Svetel M, Hinrichs F, Zittel S, Graf J, et al. The role of mutations in COL6A3 in isolated dystonia. J Neurol 2016;263:730–734.
26. Lynch DS, Wade C, Paiva ARB, John N, Kinsella JA, Merwick A, et al. Practical approach to the diagnosis of adult-onset leukodystrophies: An updated guide in the genomic era. J Neurol Neurosurg Psychiatry 2019;90:543–554.
27. Magrinelli F, Balint B, Bhatia KP. Challenges in clinicogenetic correlations: One gene - many phenotypes. Mov Disord Clin Pract 2021;8:299–310.
28. Marras C, Lang A, van de Warrenburg BP, Sue CM, Tabrizi SJ, Bertram L, Mercimek-Mahmutoglu S, et al. Nomenclature of genetic movement disorders: Recommendations of the international Parkinson and movement disorder society task force. Mov Disord 2016;31:436–457.
29. Marras C, Lohmann K, Lang A, Klein C. Fixing the broken system of genetic locus symbols: Parkinson disease and dystonia as examples. Neurology 2012;78:1016–1024.
30. Martikainen MH, Ng YS, Gorman GS, Alston CL, Blakely EL, Schaefer AM, et al. Clinical, genetic, and radiological features of extrapyramidal movement disorders in mitochondrial disease. JAMA Neurol 2016;73:668–674.
31. Mencacci NE, Jinnah HA. Naming genes for dystonia: DYT-z or Ditzy? Tremor Other Hyperkinet Mov 2019;9. doi:10.7916/tohm.v0.710.
32. Menden B, Gutschalk A, Wunderlich G, Haack TB. Expanded genetic spectrum and variable disease onset in AOPEP-associated dystonia. Mov Disord 2022;37:1113–1115.
33. Mochel F, Hainque E, Gras D, Adanyeguh IM, Caillet S, Heron B, et al. Triheptanoin dramatically reduces paroxysmal motor disorder in patients with GLUT1 deficiency. J Neurol Neurosurg Psychiatry 2016;87:550–553.
34. Mohammad SS, Angiti RR, Biggin A, Morales-Briceno H, Goetti R, Perez-Duenas B, et al. Magnetic resonance imaging pattern recognition in childhood bilateral basal ganglia disorders. Brain Commun 2020;2:fcaa178.
35. Morales-Briceno H, Fung VSC, Bhatia KP, Balint B. Parkinsonism and dystonia: Clinical spectrum and diagnostic clues. J Neurol Sci 2022;433:120016.
36. Nibbeling EA, Delnooz CC, de Koning TJ, Sinke RJ, Jinnah HA, Tijssen MA, Verbeek DS. Using the shared genetics of dystonia and ataxia to unravel their pathogenesis. Neurosci Biobehav Rev 2017;75:22–39.
37. Nie S, Chen G, Cao X, Zhang Y. Cerebrotendinous xanthomatosis: A comprehensive review of pathogenesis, clinical manifestations, diagnosis, and management. Orphanet J Rare Dis 2014;9:179.
38. Olgiati S, Quadri M, Bonifati V. Genetics of movement disorders in the next-generation sequencing era. Mov Disord 2016;31:458–470.
39. Olschewski L, Jesus S, Kim HJ, Tunc S, Lons S, Junker J, et al. Role of ANO3 mutations in dystonia: A large-scale mutational screening study. Parkinsonism Relat Disord 2019;62:196–200.
40. Ostrozovicova M, Jech R, Steel D, Pavelekova P, Han V, Gdovinova Z, et al. A recurrent VPS16 p.Arg187* nonsense variant in early-onset generalized dystonia. Mov Disord 2021;36:1984–1985.
41. Park J, Reilaender A, Petry-Schmelzer JN, Stobe P, Cordts I, Harmuth F, Rautenberg M, et al. Transcript-specific loss-of-function variants in VPS16 are enriched in patients with dystonia. Neurol Genet 2022;8:e644.

42. Powis Z, Towne MC, Hagman KDF, Blanco K, Palmaer E, Castro A, et al. Clinical diagnostic exome sequencing in dystonia: Genetic testing challenges for complex conditions. Clin Genet 2019;97:305–307.
43. Raymond D, Saunders-Pullman R, de Carvalho Aguiar P, Schule B, Kock N, Friedman J, et al. Phenotypic spectrum and sex effects in eleven myoclonus-dystonia families with epsilon-sarcoglycan mutations. Mov Disord 2008;23:588–592.
44. Richards S, Aziz N, Bale S, Bick D, Das S, Gastier-Foster J, et al. Standards and guidelines for the interpretation of sequence variants: A joint consensus recommendation of the American College of Medical Genetics and Genomics and the Association for Molecular Pathology. Genet Med 2015;17:405–424.
45. Rossi M, Balint B, Millar Vernetti P, Bhatia KP, Merello M. Genetic dystonia-ataxia syndromes: Clinical spectrum, diagnostic approach, and treatment options. Mov Disord Clin Pract 2018;5:373–382.
46. Sawyer SL, Hartley T, Dyment DA, Beaulieu CL, Schwartzentruber J, Smith A, et al. Utility of whole-exome sequencing for those near the end of the diagnostic odyssey: Time to address gaps in care. Clin Genet 2016;89:275–284.
47. Silveira-Moriyama L, Paciorkowski AR. Genetic diagnostics for neurologists. Continuum (Minneap Minn) 2018;24:18–36.
48. Soliani L, Alcala San Martin A, Balsells S, Hernando-Davalillo C, Ortigoza-Escobar JD. Chromosome microarray analysis for the investigation of deletions in pediatric movement disorders: A systematic review of the literature. Mov Disord Clin Pract 2023;10:547–557.
49. Steel D, Zech M, Zhao C, Barwick KES, Burke D, Demailly D, et al. Loss-of-function variants in HOPS complex genes VPS16 and VPS41 cause early onset dystonia associated with lysosomal abnormalities. Ann Neurol 2020;88:867–877.
50. Thakur N, Klopstock T, Jackowski S, Kuscer E, Tricta F, Videnovic A, Jinnah HA. Rational design of novel therapies for pantothenate kinase-associated neurodegeneration. Mov Disord 2021;36.
51. Thomsen M, Lange LM, Zech M, Lohmann K. Genetics and pathogenesis of dystonia. Annu Rev Pathol 2023;19:99–131.
52. Tonduti D, Chiapparini L, Moroni I, Ardissone A, Zorzi G, Zibordi F, et al. Neurological disorders associated with striatal lesions: Classification and diagnostic approach. Curr Neurol Neurosci Rep 2016;16:54.
53. van Egmond ME, Lugtenberg CHA, Brouwer OF, Contarino MF, Fung VSC, Heiner-Fokkema MR, et al. A post hoc study on gene panel analysis for the diagnosis of dystonia. Mov Disord 2017;32:569–575.
54. Veltman JA, Brunner HG. De novo mutations in human genetic disease. Nat Rev Genet 2012;13:565–575.
55. Weisheit CE, Pappas SS, Dauer WT. Inherited dystonias: Clinical features and molecular pathways. Handb Clin Neurol 2018;147:241–254.
56. Weissbach A, Pauly MG, Herzog R, Hahn L, Halmans S, Hamami F, et al. Relationship of genotype, phenotype, and treatment in dopa-responsive dystonia: MDSGene review. Mov Disord 2021;2022:237–252.
57. Wu MC, Chang YY, Lan MY, Chen YF, Tai CH, Lin YF, et al. A clinical and integrated genetic study of isolated and combined dystonia in Taiwan. J Mol Diagn 2022;24:262–273.
58. Xiromerisiou G, Houlden H, Scarmeas N, Stamelou M, Kara E, Hardy J, et al. THAP1 mutations and dystonia phenotypes: Genotype phenotype correlations. Mov Disord 2012;27:1290–1294.
59. Zech M, Boesch S, Jochim A, Weber S, Meindl T, Schormair B, et al. Clinical exome sequencing in early-onset generalized dystonia and large-scale resequencing follow-up. Mov Disord 2016;32:549–559.
60. Zech M, Jech R, Boesch S, Skorvanek M, Weber S, Wagner M, et al. Monogenic variants in dystonia: An exome-wide sequencing study. Lancet Neurol 2020;19:908–918.
61. Zech M, Jech R, Wagner M, Mantel T, Boesch S, Nocker M, et al. Molecular diversity of combined and complex dystonia: Insights from diagnostic exome sequencing. Neurogenetics 2017;18:195–205.
62. Zech M, Kumar KR, Reining S, Reunert J, Tchan M, Riley LG, et al. Biallelic AOPEP loss-of-function variants cause progressive dystonia with prominent limb involvement. Mov Disord 2022;37:137–147.

Chapter 23

The Neuroanatomical Substrates of Dystonia

INTRODUCTION

The control of movement is mediated by three main pathways in the human brain. They include the corticospinal (pyramidal) pathways, the basal ganglia (extrapyramidal) pathways, and cerebellar pathways. Multiple areas of the cerebral cortex play different roles, with the primary motor cortex being most directly responsible for activating motor neurons of the brainstem and spinal cord to produce movement. The basal ganglia are thought to play a role in reinforcing intended movements and suppressing extraneous movements. The cerebellum is thought to be responsible for the timing and coordination of ongoing movements. All three regions play a role in motor learning. Although these three regions are often described as distinct pathways with distinct functions, they are highly interconnected. These connections mean that the activity of one region influences other regions, and dysfunction of one region may disrupt other regions.

Historically, the anatomical substrates for many neurological disorders were often inferred from surveys of focal lesions of the nervous system.[9] The value of the lesion method for localization of brain function and dysfunction is well-established. Early application of the lesion method in cases of hemidystonia pointed to the basal ganglia, and dystonia therefore was initially considered a basal ganglia disorder.[69,83] However, subsequent studies revealed that lesions for other types of dystonia were not always in the basal ganglia (Table 23.1).[36,71] In addition, limitations of the lesion method were increasingly recognized, so the modern approach to localization of function incorporates data obtained from many sources including lesion studies, histopathology of autopsy material, clinical neuroimaging studies, more advanced neuroimaging techniques, physiological studies, observations from genetics, animal models, and other methods.[21,78]

These many converging sources of information have implicated several regions of the nervous system in dystonia. As a result, the current view is that dystonia is a network disorder that involves multiple regions.[43] This chapter focuses on anatomical evidence for involvement of different brain regions in dystonia and how the network model integrates the many sources of information into a single cohesive paradigm for understanding the neuroanatomical substrates of dystonia. Chapter 24, "Dystonia Physiology"

Table 23.1 **Locations of lesions in acquired dystonia**

Type of dystonia	Study	New cases	Cases from literature	Location of lesions: Basal ganglia	Cerebellum	Cortex	Thalamus	Other
Hemidystonia	Marsden 1985[69]	28	21	45	0	1	7	Internal capsule (13)
Hemidystonia	Pettigrew 1985[83]	22	52	11	0	0	1	Internal capsule (13)
Mixed	Obeso 1988[80]	39	32	68	6	8	16	Brainstem (1)
Mixed	Lee 1994[61]	0	62	0	1		22	Midbrain (4)
Mixed	Kostic 1996[54]	16	0	11	0	4	5	Brainstem (1)
Hemidystonia	Nardocci 1996[75]	13	0	10	0	4	0	NR
Upper limb or hemidystonia	Kim 2001[50]	31	0	0	0	7	31	NR
Hemidystonia	Chuang 2002[15]	33	157	12	0	8	7	Midbrain (1)
Cervical	LeDoux 2003[58]	4	21	6	11	0	0	Spinal cord (7)
Mixed	LeBer 2006[57]	12	0	0	12	0	0	NR
Mixed	Strader 2011[103]	32	0	4	0	12	1	NR
Blepharospasm	Khooshnoodi 2013[49]	18	30	9	9	1	12	Brainstem (11) Midbrain (7)
Cervical	Fafara-Les 2014[26]	12	0	0	5	0	0	Brainstem (6) Spinal cord (2)
Cervical/segmental	Batla 2015[3]	26	0	0	26	0	0	NR
Upper limb	Liuzzi 2016[64]	4	72	17	1	4	39	Spinal cord (7) Brainstem (4)
Lingual	Pandey 2018[81]	11	4	10	2	9	4	Brainstem (1)

This table summarizes reports that included least 10 cases where focal lesions were thought to be responsible for dystonia. For studies reporting different movement disorders occurring after focal lesions, only those with dystonia are included. Some cases had lesions spanning more than one region, so the numbers of lesions may exceed the total number of cases. Some cases may be reported more than once, because several studies included a literature review. A more exhaustive summary of all lesions has also been reported.[19]

Abbreviation: NR, not reported.

addresses the evidence for functional disturbances in the network.

NERVOUS SYSTEM REGIONS INVOLVED IN DYSTONIA

Basal Ganglia

The role of the basal ganglia in dystonia has been summarized many times over the years.[2,4,10] Some of the earliest and most methodical studies linking dystonia with the basal ganglia came from autopsy studies.[37] Most cases with dystonia had no obvious brain lesions. Only a minority had lesions, but these lesions tended to cluster in the putamen, caudate, and pallidum. These early lesion studies were later corroborated by additional autopsy and structural imaging studies such as brain CT and MRI (Table 23.1).

Although overt lesions are only apparent in a small fraction of cases, more subtle abnormalities in the basal ganglia often can be found using advanced imaging methods.[63,78,112] For example, abnormalities of the size of basal ganglia subregions can be measured by voxel-based morphometry (VBM), an MRI-based method that precisely quantifies volumes of individual brain regions. Functional abnormalities of the basal ganglia can also be disclosed by techniques that measure regional brain glucose utilization with fluorodeoxyglucose positron-emission tomography (FDG-PET) or regional brain blood flow with [^{15}O]-labeled H_2O PET, single-photon emission tomography (SPECT), or blood-oxygen level dependent functional MRI (fMRI). Finally, numerous other subtle abnormalities of the basal ganglia can be found in various types of dystonia using other advanced fMRI methods such as resting state fMRI or diffusion tensor imaging and tractography.

There also is a strong link between dystonia and dopamine, an important neurotransmitter of the basal ganglia.[2,44,92] Dystonia is a common feature of multiple genetic disorders affecting dopamine pathways including defects in dopamine synthesis (*GCH1, PTS, SPR, TH*), dopamine reuptake at the plasma membrane (*SLC6A3*), intracellular vesicular storage of dopamine (*SLC18A2*), and dopamine receptor signaling (*GNAL, GNAO1*).[44] Dystonia also is frequent in Parkinson disease, which is associated with degeneration of dopaminergic neurons (see Chapter 13, "Dystonia and Parkinsonism").[101] Dopamine receptor antagonists can cause both acute transient dystonic reactions and more persistent tardive syndromes in which dystonia is a major feature (see Chapter 19, "Dystonia Induced by Medications, Illicit Drugs, and Environmental Exposures).[25] Imaging studies have also suggested abnormalities in dopamine transporters in nigrostriatal pathways,[40] and reduced dopamine release in idiopathic writer's cramp and laryngeal dystonia.[6,102] Some post-mortem histopathological studies also have suggested subtle loss of substantia nigra dopamine neurons.[39]

The basal ganglia have also been implicated in numerous physiological studies in humans with dystonia using non-invasive methods such as transcranial magnetic stimulation[66] or direct recording of basal ganglia neurons during deep brain stimulation surgery (see Chapter 24).[76] Genetic studies have also contributed to the idea that the basal ganglia are important for dystonia because many dystonia genes are expressed in the basal ganglia, where they frequently cause syndromes that combine dystonia with parkinsonism, often with overt pathology (see Chapter 13).[44]

Numerous animal studies have also linked dystonia with basal ganglia dysfunction.[35,42,110] Experimental lesions or pharmacological manipulations of the basal ganglia induces dystonia in both rodents and non-human primates.[12,23] Dystonia also occurs in non-human primates treated with the dopamine neuron toxin, MPTP (1-methyl-4-phenyl-1,2,3,6-tetrahydropyridine).[67,111] Dystonia and other abnormal movements also occur after administration of levodopa to rodents in which dopaminergic neurons have been damaged with the neurotoxin, 6-hydoxydopamine.[82,104] Altogether, these many sources of information provide strong evidence that the basal ganglia play an important role in dystonia.

Cerebellum

A role for the cerebellum in dystonia also has been highlighted in several prior reviews.[1,30,63,78,87,96,100] The literature suggests that overt lesions of the basal ganglia may be more often associated with hemidystonia, while lesions of the cerebellum are more often associated with cervical dystonia. One study of 25 cases of cervical dystonia summarized lesions that appeared to be scattered in

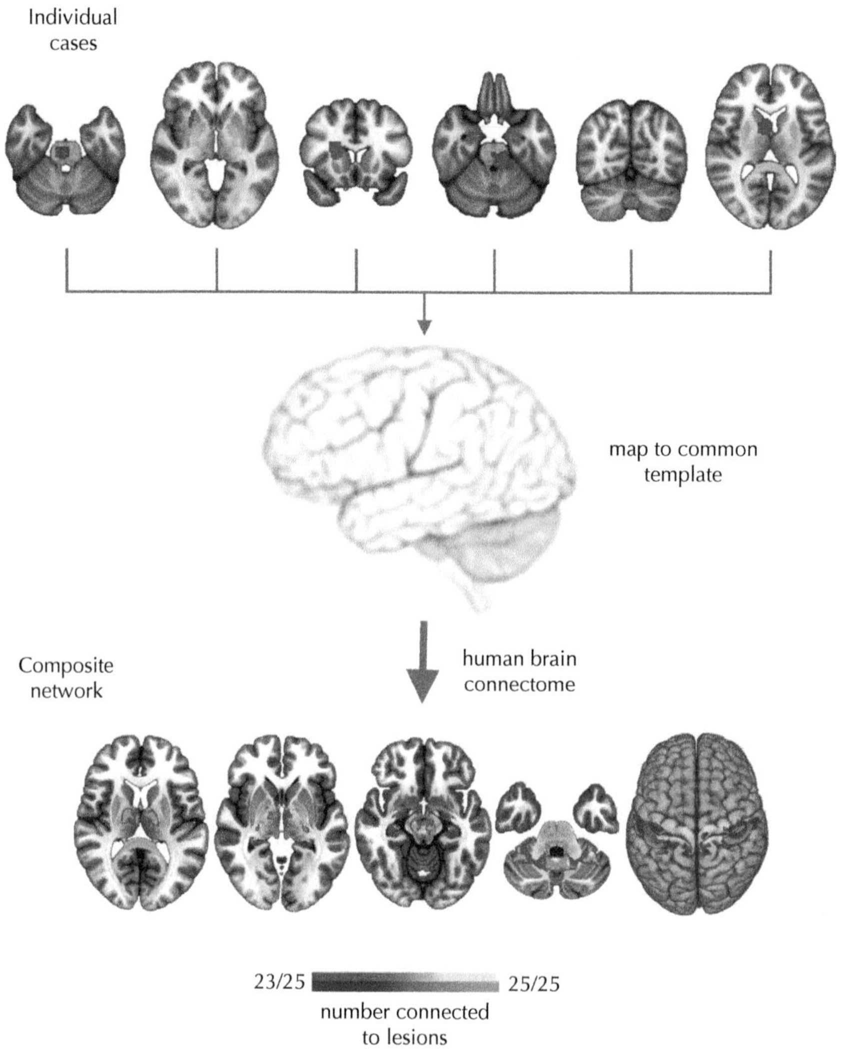

Figure 23.1. Lesion network mapping for cervical dystonia. The top row shows representative lesions from different brain regions causing cervical dystonia in 25 different cases taken from a prior report.[20] To determine if these lesions share connections to a shared network, each individual lesion is mapped to a single template of the human brain connectome, and all connections from each lesion are traced. Despite the heterogenous starting locations, the vast majority of lesions for cervical dystonia were linked with a shared network that involves the sensorimotor cortex and cerebellum, shown in the bottom row.

many brain regions.[20] However, mapping the individual lesions to the human brain connectome identified a shared functional circuit involving the cerebellum and sensorimotor cortex (Figure 23.1). A subtle loss of cerebellar Purkinje neurons has been described in two studies of cervical dystonia,[68,88] one of blepharospasm,[27] and another of mixed dystonias.[65]

Overt lesions disclosed by clinical imaging studies may be found in the cerebellum of individuals with dystonia, but they are uncommon (Table 23.1). The same regions identified in cases of cervical dystonia caused by discrete lesions also showed abnormal connectivity in fMRI studies of idiopathic cervical dystonia, where overt lesions were absent.[20] In fact, advanced imaging methods have also revealed abnormalities of the cerebellum for many other types of dystonia, too. Cerebellar abnormalities have been demonstrated using VBM, PET studies of blood flow or glucose utilization, SPECT, and various fMRI methods.[63,78]

Similar to the case for the basal ganglia, studies of genetic disorders have also revealed a strong link between genes that cause dystonia and those that cause cerebellar ataxia.[79] Physiological studies involving transcranial magnetic stimulation and direct neuronal recordings have also pointed to abnormalities of the cerebellum,[66,73,94,98] and some investigators have begun to target cerebellar structures via deep brain stimulation or transcranial methods for treatment of dystonia (see Chapter 24).[31,73,100]

Also, as with the basal ganglia, numerous animal studies have linked dystonia with cerebellar dysfunction.[11,42,43,110] These models have suggested that dystonia may be more likely to arise from physiological changes in cerebellar activity rather than destructive lesions that cause loss of activity.[11,43,99] For example, genetic models of dystonia in rodents have pointed to a common abnormality that involves abnormal burst-firing of cerebellar Purkinje neurons.[11,59,60,77,90] Removal of this abnormal activity eliminates dystonia. In keeping with this concept, pharmacological stimulation of the cerebellar cortex with glutamatergic drugs can induce dystonia in normal animals.[28,84,89]

Thalamus

Multiple reports have linked focal lesions of the thalamus with dystonia. One of the largest studies of hand dystonia secondary to focal lesions summarized 72 cases, and the thalamus was the most frequently affected region.[64] Although hand dystonia may be particularly common with thalamic lesions, other types of dystonia may also occur with thalamic lesions (Table 23.1).[61] Lesions in different regions of the thalamus have been reported to produce different qualities in dystonia. Lesions that occur in thalamic subnuclei related to the basal ganglia have been reported to produce dystonia with a twisting and writhing quality, while lesions in thalamic subnuclei related to the cerebellum have been linked dystonia that has a more tremulous or jerky quality.[62] Further studies are needed to corroborate these suggestions.

Although thalamic lesions have been linked with dystonia, small lesions that selectively affect only a single thalamic nucleus are uncommon. Most thalamic lesions involve multiple subnuclei, fibers of passage to and from cortex, and often the nearby basal ganglia. Despite the limitations of the lesion method, abnormalities of the thalamus are also frequent findings in other types of imaging studies including VBM, PET, and fMRI.[63,78] The involvement of the thalamus in dystonia may be related to its role as an important relay station of the motor network for the cerebral cortex, the basal ganglia, and the cerebellum.

Cerebral Cortex

Although destructive lesions of the primary motor cortex typically cause weakness and not dystonia, abnormal function of the motor cortex is often suggested by VBM and functional imaging studies of dystonia.[63,78] These findings are not surprising because the motor cortex provides a major final pathway for motor processing in basal ganglia or cerebellum. However, many additional cortical regions are also implicated using advanced imaging methods including premotor cortex, supplementary motor area, cingulate gyrus, and primary somatosensory regions.[63,78] Whether these abnormalities are a cause or consequence of dystonia is not entirely clear.

The parietal cortex is one cortical region where dystonia has repeatedly been linked with focal lesions such as strokes,[13,41,47,49,103] compressive lesions,[17,46,48,55] or focal trauma.[51] Lesions in this region typically cause hemidystonia or dystonia of one upper limb,[13,17,46,47,55,103] but craniofacial,[41,49] and cervical dystonia[51] have also been reported. In a systematic survey of neurological problems in 32 individuals with isolated parietal strokes, dystonia occurred in 84%.[33] These observations may reflect the role of the parietal cortex in processing of sensory feedback for perception and internal representations of movement.[7,72] If this sensory input is misinterpreted, the brain's interpretation of movement will be faulty, potentially leading to abnormal motor responses.

Midbrain and Brainstem

Lesions of the midbrain and brainstem are sometimes also implicated in dystonia in humans.[24,93] However, lesions in these areas often affect multiple nuclei and fibers of passage so findings may reflect distant changes in the basal ganglia or cerebellum.[108] Despite the limitations of information from human studies, these regions have been more clearly implicated in animal studies, where dystonic movements can be induced by precise experimental manipulations of the substantia nigra, red nucleus, interstitial nucleus of Cajal, superior colliculus, and other regions.[18,32,38,53,70,74]

Spinal Cord

There are multiple reports linking focal lesions of the cervical spinal cord with cervical or limb dystonia.[26,52,56,58,86,106] The lesions are usually compressive (e.g., tumor) or demyelinating (e.g., multiple sclerosis), rather than destructive (e.g., stroke). The mechanism is thought to involve disruption of sensory feedback from muscles, leading to distorted perception of movement by the brain. Animal studies have also linked dystonia with spinal cord defects.[85]

Some authors describe abnormal movements and postures resulting from spinal cord dysfunction as *pseudodystonia* because they do not involve the brain's motor network, although consensus on the meaning of this term is lacking (see Chapter 26, "Pseudodystonia and Differential Diagnosis").

THE NETWORK MODEL

Motor Network and Pathogenesis

It is clear that multiple regions of the nervous system are implicated in dystonia. The motor network model provides a broad conceptual framework that explains the involvement of these many regions.[21,43,78] In this model, different regions of the nervous system serve as nodes which communicate with each other to produce normal motor output (Figure 23.2). For dystonia, the nodes include all the major motor pathways of the brain including the basal ganglia, cerebellum, and cerebral cortex. The network model suggests that dystonia may arise from three different mechanisms: (1) dysfunction of a single node, (2) simultaneous dysfunction of multiple nodes, or (3) abnormal communication between nodes. There is evidence supporting each of these mechanisms as well as evidence that suggests different mechanisms may apply to different types of dystonia.

For example, many studies that link dystonia with focal lesions in both humans and animals imply that dysfunction of a single node may

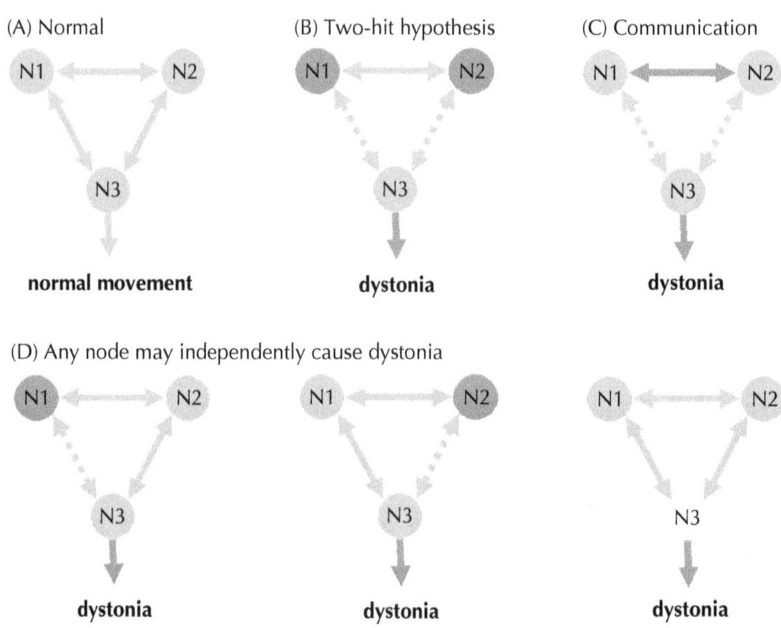

Figure 23.2. Motor network model for dystonia. This schematic depicts a normal motor network (Panel A) with three hypothetical nodes (N1, N2, N3). Abnormalities may arise when two nodes are simultaneously abnormal (Panel B), from abnormal communication between two nodes (Panel C), or dysfunction of any one node (Panel D). For dystonia, the main nodes of the network are thought to include the basal ganglia, cerebellum, and motor cortex.

provide the initial trigger for dystonia (Table 23.1). A comprehensive summary of all studies of lesion-induced dystonia suggested that basal ganglia lesions are most likely to cause dystonia of the limbs, lesions of the thalamus tend instead to cause dystonia of the hand, while lesions of the cerebellum are more likely to cause cervical dystonia.[19] Whether these lesions are a direct cause of dystonia remains unclear because lesion-induced dystonia almost always occurs after a delay of several weeks and sometimes years.[19] This delay suggests some secondary process is also required. A second process may involve communication with another node or maladaptive plastic changes in other portions of the network. For most imaging studies, it is not feasible to distinguish abnormalities that may cause dystonia from abnormalities that are the consequence of sensory feedback or adaptive changes.[109] For hemidystonia due to focal lesions of the basal ganglia, efforts to identify these secondary abnormalities have reported functional changes in many regions including cortex and cerebellum, and these changes vary among individuals.[34]

There is also evidence that simultaneous dysfunction of multiple nodes may be important in dystonia. In rodents, it is feasible to experimentally produce partial lesions of nigrostriatal dopamine pathways or mild injuries of the nerve to the orbicularis oculi that have no obvious consequences.[97] However, when the two subclinical lesions are combined, animals develop blepharospasm. This "two-hit model" for blepharospasm has been implied by other animal models of dystonia, too.[77,91]

There also is strong evidence that the nodes of the motor network communicate directly with each other and that dysfunction of one node can affect another. The basal ganglia and cerebellum communicate with each other via the thalamus so evidence implicating the thalamus in dystonia provides a potential mechanism that involves aberrant communication between nodes. Numerous modern imaging studies of different types of dystonia have demonstrated abnormal functional connectivity between cortex, basal ganglia, and cerebellum.[8,22,29,45,95] It is also important to acknowledge that an overt lesion often causes negative effects that may suggest the function of the region, but positive effects of a lesion may arise from adaptive changes in remaining structures in the network. Whether these abnormalities reflect downstream defects starting in one node or abnormal communication between nodes remains to be determined.

Clinical Relevance of the Motor Network

Many years ago, attempts were made to treat individuals with dystonia by making focal ablative lesions of various regions of the brain, most notably the thalamus.[16,107] Some individuals responded very well to thalamic lesions, while others did not respond or they got worse. The lesion approach was ultimately abandoned because outcomes were unreliable. Nowadays the reasons for varied outcomes following lesions to a single brain region are better understood. Dystonia is not a single disorder resulting from dysfunction of a single brain region, but a heterogenous group of disorders that may have different underling neuroanatomical substrates. A better understanding of the brain regions responsible for different types of dystonia is likely to result in better surgical targeting.

By the same token, deep brain stimulation targeting the main outflow pathways of the basal ganglia provides an effective treatment for certain types of dystonia, but not others (see Chapter 31, "Surgical Treatment for Dystonia"). The motor network model suggests that the optimal brain targets may not be the same for all types of dystonia. Indeed, recent efforts have begun to target the cerebellum for certain types of dystonia.[14,73,105] A better understanding of the contributions of the motor network in different types of dystonia is very likely to improve these strategies for treatment.

SUMMARY AND FUTURE PROSPECTS

There is strong evidence from both humans and animals that dystonia may be triggered by dysfunction in different regions of the nervous system including the basal ganglia, cerebellum, sensorimotor cortex, thalamus, midbrain, brainstem, and even the spinal cord. Lesions visible in routine clinical imaging studies such as CT or MRI may occur in any of these regions, but they are uncommon in most cases of dystonia. Even when overt lesions are absent, abnormal function of these regions is readily detectable in many different types of human dystonia by advanced imaging methods such as VBM, PET, SPECT, and fMRI. In addition, dystonia can be induced by selective experimental manipulations of each of these regions in experimental animals.

The motor network model provides an overall paradigm that explains how these different regions may be involved in dystonia. In this model, dystonia can arise from dysfunction of a single node of the network, simultaneous dysfunction of multiple nodes, or abnormal communication between nodes. Further elucidating the anatomical substrates for different types dystonia is important for guiding therapies that target underlying abnormalities.

REFERENCES

1. Avanzino L, Abbruzzese G. How does the cerebellum contribute to the pathophysiology of dystonia. Basal Ganglia 2012;2:231–235.
2. Balint B, Mencacci NE, Valente EM, Pisani A, Rothwell J, Jankovic J, et al. Dystonia. Nat Rev Dis Primers 2018;4:25.
3. Batla A, Sanchez MC, Erro R, Ganos C, Stamelou M, Balint B, et al. The role of cerebellum in patients with late onset cervical/segmental dystonia? Evidence from the clinic. Parkinsonism Relat Disord 2015;21:1317–1322.
4. Berardelli A, Rothwell JC, Hallett M, Thompson PD, Manfredi M, Marsden CD. The pathophysiology of primary dystonia. Brain 1998;121:1195–1212.
5. Berlot R, Bhatia KP, Kojovic M. Pseudodystonia: A new perspective on an old phenomenon. Parkinsonism Relat Disord 2019;62:44–50.
6. Berman BD, Hallett M, Herscovitch P, Simonyan K. Striatal dopaminergic dysfunction at rest and during task performance in writer's cramp. Brain 2013;136:3645–3658.
7. Bianchi S, Fuertinger S, Huddleston H, Frucht SJ, Simonyan K. Functional and structural neural bases of task specificity in isolated focal dystonia. Mov Disord 2019;34:555–563.
8. Blood AJ, Kuster JK, Woodman SC, Kirlic N, Makhlouf ML, Multhaupt-Buell TJ, et al. Evidence for altered basal ganglia-brainstem connections in cervical dystonia. PLoS One 2012;7:e31654.
9. Brazis PW, Masdeu JC, Biller J. *Localization in Clinical Neurology*, 7th ed. Wolters Kluwer; 2017.
10. Breakefield XO, Blood AJ, Li Y, Hallett M, Hanson PI, Standaert DG. The pathophysiological basis of dystonias. Nat Rev Neurosci 2008;9:222–234.
11. Brown AM, van der Heijden ME, Jinnah HA, Sillitoe RV. Cerebellar dysfunction as a source of dystonic phenotypes in mice. Cerebellum 2023;22:719–729.
12. Burbaud P, Bonnet B, Guehl D, Lagueny A, Bioulac B. Movement disorders induced by gamma-aminobutyric agonist and antagonist injections into the internal globus pallidus and substantia nigra pars reticulata of the monkey. Brain Res 1998;780:102–107.
13. Burguera JA, Bataller L, Valero C. Action hand dystonia after cortical parietal infarction. Mov Disord 2001;16:1183–1185.
14. Cajigas I, Morrison MA, Luciano MS, Starr PA. Cerebellar deep brain stimulation for the treatment of movement disorders in cerebral palsy. J Neurosurg 2023;139:605–614.
15. Chuang C, Fahn S, Frucht SJ. The natural history and treatment of acquired hemidystonia: Report of 33 cases and review of the literature. J Neurol Neurosurg Psychiatry 2002;72:59–67.
16. Cooper IS. 20-year followup study of the neurosurgical treatment of dystonia musculorum deformans. Adv Neurol 1976;14:423–452.
17. Coria F, Blanco Martin AI, Rivas Vilas MD. Pseudodystonic hand posturing contralateral to a metastasis of the parietal association cortex. Neurologia 2000;15:362–365.
18. Corneil BD, Olivier E, Munoz DP. Neck muscle responses to stimulation of monkey superior colliculus. II. Gaze shift initiation and volitional head movements. J Neurophysiol 2002;88:2000–2018.
19. Corp DT, Greenwood C, Morrison-Ham J, Pullinen J, McDowall G, Younger E, et al. Clinical and structural findings in patients with lesion-induced dystonia: Descriptive and quantitative analysis of published cases. Neurology 2022;99:e1957–e1967.
20. Corp DT, Joutsa J, Darby RR, Delnooz CCS, van de Warrenburg BPC, Cooke D, et al. Network localization of cervical dystonia based on causal brain lesions. Brain 2019;2019:1660–1674.
21. Corp DT, Morrison-Ham J, Jinnah HA, Joutsa J. The functional anatomy of dystonia: Recent developments. Int Rev Neurobiol 2023;169:105–136.
22. DeSimone JC, Archer DB, Vaillancourt DE, Wagle Shukla A. Network-level connectivity is a critical feature distinguishing dystonic tremor and essential tremor. Brain 2019;142:1644–1659.
23. Dybdal D, Forcelli PA, Dubach M, Oppedisano M, Holmes A, Malkova L, Gale K. Topography of dyskinesias and torticollis evoked by inhibition of substantia nigra pars reticulata. Mov Disord 2013;28:460–468.
24. Esteban Munoz J, Tolosa E, Saiz A, Vila N, Marti MJ, Blesa R. Upper limb dystonia secondary to a midbrain hemorrhage. Mov Disord 1996;11:96–99.
25. Factor SA, Burkhard PR, Caroff S, Friedman JH, Marras C, Tinazzi M, Comella C. Recent developments in drug-induced movement disorders: A mixed picture. Lancet Neurol 2019;18:880–890.
26. Fafara-Les A, Kwiatkowski S, Marynczak L, Kawecki Z, Adamek D, Herman-Sucharska I, Kobylarz K. Torticollis as a first sign of posterior fossa and cervical spinal cord tumors in children. Childs Nerv Syst 2014;30:425–430.
27. Fagan M, Scorr L, Bernhardt D, Hess EJ, Perlmutter JS, Pardo CA, Jinnah HA. Neuropathology of blepharospasm. Exp Neurol 2021;346:113855.
28. Fan X, Hughes KE, Jinnah HA, Hess EJ. Selective and sustained AMPA receptor activation in cerebellum induces dystonia in mice. J Pharmacol Exp Ther 2012;340:733–741.
29. Filip P, Gallea C, Lehericy S, Bertasi E, Popa T, Marecek R, et al. Disruption in cerebellar and basal ganglia networks during a visuospatial task in cervical dystonia. Mov Disord 2017;32:757–768.
30. Filip P, Lungu OV, Bares M. Dystonia and the cerebellum: A new field of interest in movement disorders? Clin Neurophysiol 2013;124:1269–1274.
31. Franca C, de Andrade DC, Teixeira MJ, Galhardoni R, Silva V, Barbosa ER, Cury RG. Effects of cerebellar

neuromodulation in movement disorders: A systematic review. Brain Stimul 2018;11:249–260.
32. Fukushima K. The interstitial nucleus of Cajal and its role in the control of movements of the head and eyes. Prog Neurobiol 1987;29:107–192.
33. Ghika J, Ghika-Schmid F, Bogousslasvky J. Parietal motor syndrome: A clinical description in 32 patients in the acute phase of pure parietal strokes studied prospectively. Clin Neurol Neurosurg 1998;100:271–282.
34. Gonzalez V, Le Bars E, Cif L, van Dokkum LE, Laffont I, Bonafe A, et al. The reorganization of motor network in hemidystonia from the perspective of deep brain stimulation. Brain Imaging Behav 2015;9:223–235.
35. Guehl D, Cuny E, Ghorayeb I, Michelet T, Bioulac B, Burbaud P. Primate models of dystonia. Prog Neurobiol 2009;87:118–131.
36. Hedreen JC, Zweig RM, DeLong MR, Whitehouse PJ, Price DL. Primary dystonias: A review of the pathology and suggestions for new directions of study. In Fahn S, Marsden DC, Calne DB, eds. Adv Neurol 1988;50:123–132.
37. Herz E. Dystonias, part 3: Pathology and conclusions. Arch Neurol Psychiatr 1944;52:20.
38. Holmes AL, Forcelli PA, Desjardin JT, Decker AL, Teferra M, West EA, et al. Superior colliculus mediates cervical dystonia evoked by inhibition of the substantia nigra pars reticulata. J Neurosci 2012;32:13326–13332.
39. Iacono D, Geraci-Erck M, Peng H, Rabin ML, Kurlan R. Reduced number of pigmented neurons in the substantia nigra of dystonia patients? Findings from extensive neuropathologic, immunohistochemistry, and quantitative analyses. Tremor Other Hyperkinet Mov 2015;5. tre-5-301. doi:10.7916/D8T72G9G.
40. Ikezawa J, Yokochi F, Okiyama R, Kumada S, Tojima M, Kamiyama T, et al. Is generalized and segmental dystonia accompanied by impairments in the dopaminergic system? Front Neurol 2021;12:751434.
41. Jacob PC, Chand RP. Blepharospasm and jaw closing dystonia after parietal infarcts. Mov Disord 1995;10:794–795.
42. Jinnah HA, Hess EJ, LeDoux MS, Sharma N, Baxter MG, DeLong MR. Rodent models for dystonia research: Characteristics, evaluation, and utility. Mov Disord 2005;20:283–292.
43. Jinnah HA, Neychev V, Hess EJ. The anatomical basis for dystonia: The motor network model. Tremor Other Hyperkinet Mov 2017;7:506.
44. Jinnah HA, Sun YV. Dystonia genes and their biological pathways. Neurobiol Dis 2019;129:159–168.
45. Jochim A, Li Y, Gora-Stahlberg G, Mantel T, Berndt M, Castrop F, et al. Altered functional connectivity in blepharospasm/orofacial dystonia. Brain Behav 2018;8:e00894.
46. Jung HJ, Choi SM, Kim BC. Hemidystonia as an initial manifestation of leptomeningeal metastasis. J Mov Disord 2009;2:82–85.
47. Karsidag S, Ozer F, Sen A, Arpaci B. Lesion localization in developing poststroke hand dystonia. Eur Neurol 1998;40:99–104.
48. Khan AA, Sussman JD. Focal dystonia after removal of a parietal meningioma. Mov Disord 2004;19:714–716.
49. Khooshnoodi MA, Factor SA, Jinnah HA. Secondary blepharospasm associated with structural lesions of the brain. J Neurol Sci 2013;331:98–101.
50. Kim JS. Delayed onset mixed involuntary movements after thalamic stroke. Brain 2001;124:299–309.
51. Kim JW, Lee PH. Dystonic head tremor associated with a parietal lesion. Eur J Neurol 2007;14:e32–33.
52. Kiwak KJ, Deray MJ, Shields WD. Torticollis in three children with syringomyelia and spinal cord tumor. Neurology 1983;33:946–948.
53. Klier EM, Wang H, Constantin AG, Crawford JD. Midbrain control of three-dimensional head orientation. Science 2002;295:1314–1316.
54. Kostic VS, Stojanovic-Svetel M, Kacar A. The symptomatic dystonias associated with structural lesions: Report of 16 cases. Can J Neurol Sci 1996;23:53–56.
55. Krauss JK, Mohadjer M, Nobbe F, Scheremet R. Hemidystonia due to a contralateral parieto-occipital metastasis: Disappearance after removal of the mass lesion. Neurology 1991;41:1519–1520.
56. Kumandas S, Per H, Gumus H, Tucer B, Yikilmaz A, Kontas O, et al. Torticollis secondary to posterior fossa and cervical spinal cord tumors: Report of five cases and literature review. Neurosurg Rev 2006;29:333–338.
57. Le Ber I, Clot F, Vercueil L, Camzuat A, Viemont M, Benamar N, et al. Predominant dystonia with marked cerebellar atrophy: A rare phenotype in familial dystonia. Neurology 2006;67:1769–1773.
58. LeDoux MS, Brady KA. Secondary cervical dystonia associated with structural lesions of the central nervous system. Mov Disord 2003;18:60–69.
59. LeDoux MS, Lorden JF, Ervin JM. Cerebellectomy eliminates the motor syndrome of the genetically dystonic rat. Exp Neurol 1993;120:302–310.
60. LeDoux MS, Lorden JF, Meinzen-Derr J. Selective elimination of cerebellar output in the genetically dystonic rat. Brain Res 1995;697:91–103.
61. Lee MS, Marsden CD. Movement disorders following lesions of the thalamus or subthalamic region. Mov Disord 1994;9:493–507.
62. Lehericy S, Grand S, Pollak P, Poupon F, LeBas JF, Limousin P, et al. Clinical characteristics and topography of lesion in movement disorders due to thalamic lesions. Neurology 2001;57:1055–1066.
63. Lehericy S, Tijssen MA, Vidailhet M, Kaji R, Meunier S. The anatomical basis of dystonia: Current view using neuroimaging. Mov Disord 2013;28:944–957.
64. Liuzzi D, Gigante AF, Leo A, Defazio G. The anatomical basis of upper limb dystonia: Lesson from secondary cases. Neurol Sci 2016;37:1393–1398.
65. Louis ED, Kerridge CA, Chatterjee D, Martuscello RT, Diaz DT, Koeppen AH, et al. Contextualizing the pathology in the essential tremor cerebellar cortex: A patholog-omics approach. Acta Neuropathol 2019;138:859–876.
66. Lozeron P, Poujois A, Richard A, Masmoudi S, Meppiel E, Woimant F, Kubis N. Contribution of TMS and rTMS in the understanding of the pathophysiology and in the treatment of dystonia. Front Neural Circuits 2016;10:90.
67. Lundblad M, Picconi B, Lindgren H, Cenci MA. A model of L-DOPA-induced dyskinesia in 6-hydroxydopamine lesioned mice: Relation to motor and cellular parameters of nigrostriatal function. Neurobiol Dis 2004;16:110–123.
68. Ma K, Babij R, Cortes E, Vonsattel JP, Louis ED. Cerebellar pathology of a dual clinical diagnosis: Patients with essential tremor and dystonia. Tremor Other Hyperkinet Mov 2012;2:1–6.
69. Marsden CD, Obeso JA, Zarranz JJ. The anatomical basis of symptomatic hemidystonia. Brain 1985;108:463–483.

70. Matsumoto RR, Pouw B. Correlation between neuroleptic binding to sigma(1) and sigma(2) receptors and acute dystonic reactions. Eur J Pharmacol 2000;401:155–160.
71. McGeer EG, McGeer PL. The dystonias. Can J Neurol Sci 1988;15:447–483.
72. Merchant SHI, Frangos E, Parker J, Bradson M, Wu T, Vial-Undurraga F, et al. The role of the inferior parietal lobule in writer's cramp. Brain 2020;143:1766–1779.
73. Miterko LN, Baker KB, Beckinghausen J, Bradnam LV, Cheng MY, Cooperrider J, et al. Consensus paper: Experimental neurostimulation of the cerebellum. Cerebellum 2019;18:1064–1097.
74. Nakazawa M, Kobayashi T, Matsuno K, Mita S. Possible involvement of a o- receptor subtype in the neck dystonia in rats. Pharmacol Biochem Behav 1999;62:123–126.
75. Nardocci N, Zorzi G, Grisoli M, Rumi V, Broggi G, Angelini L. Acquired hemidystonia in childhood: A clinical and neuroradiological study of thirteen patients. Pediatr Neurol 1996;15:108–113.
76. Neumann WJ, Horn A, Ewert S, Huebl J, Brucke C, Slentz C, et al. A localized pallidal physiomarker in cervical dystonia. Ann Neurol 2017;82:912–924.
77. Neychev V, Fan X, Mitev VI, Hess EJ, Jinnah HA. The basal ganglia and cerebellum interact in the expression of dystonic movement. Brain 2008;131:2499–2509.
78. Neychev VK, Gross R, Lehericy S, Hess EJ, Jinnah HA. The functional neuroanatomy of dystonia. Neurobiol Dis 2011;42:185–201.
79. Nibbeling EA, Delnooz CC, de Koning TJ, Sinke RJ, Jinnah HA, Tijssen MA, Verbeek DS. Using the shared genetics of dystonia and ataxia to unravel their pathogenesis. Neurosci Biobehav Rev 2017;75:22–39.
80. Obeso JA, Gimenez-Roldan S. Clinicopathologic correlation in symptomatic dystonia. Adv Neurol 1988;50:113–122.
81. Pandey S, Tater P. Post-stroke lingual dystonia: Clinical description and neuroimaging findings. Tremor Other Hyperkinet Mov 2018;8:610.
82. Pearce RK, Jackson M, Smith L, Jenner P, Marsden CD. Chronic L-DOPA administration induces dyskinesias in the 1-methyl-4- phenyl-1,2,3,6-tetrahydropyridine-treated common marmoset (Callithrix Jacchus). Mov Disord 1995;10:731–740.
83. Pettigrew LC, Jankovic J. Hemidystonia: A report of 22 patients and a review of the literature. J Neurol Neurosurg Psychiatry 1985;48:650–657.
84. Pizoli CE, Jinnah HA, Billingsley ML, Hess EJ. Abnormal cerebellar signaling induces dystonia in mice. J Neurosci 2002;22:7825–7833.
85. Pocratsky AM, Nascimento F, Ozyurt MG, White IJ, Sullivan R, O'Callaghan BJ, et al. Pathophysiology of Dyt1-Tor1a dystonia in mice is mediated by spinal neural circuit dysfunction. Sci Transl Med 2023;15:eadg3904.
86. Previdi P, Buzzi P. Paroxysmal dystonia due to a lesion of the cervical cord, case report. Ital J Neurol Sci 1992;13:521–523.
87. Prudente CN, Hess EJ, Jinnah HA. Dystonia as a network disorder: What is the role of the cerebellum? Neuroscience 2014;260:23–35.
88. Prudente CN, Pardo CA, Xiao J, Hanfelt J, Hess EJ, LeDoux MS, Jinnah HA. Neuropathology of cervical dystonia. Exp Neurol 2012;241:95–104.
89. Raike RS, Pizoli CE, Weisz C, van den Maagdenberg AM, Jinnah HA, Hess EJ. Limited regional cerebellar dysfunction induces focal dystonia in mice. Neurobiol Dis 2012;49:200–210.
90. Raike RS, Weisz C, Hoebeek FE, Terzi MC, De Zeeuw CI, van den Maagdenberg AM, et al. Stress, caffeine and ethanol trigger transient neurological dysfunction through shared mechanisms in a mouse calcium channelopathy. Neurobiol Dis 2013;50:151–159.
91. Rauschenberger L, Knorr S, Pisani A, Hallett M, Volkmann J, Ip CW. Second hit hypothesis in dystonia: Dysfunctional cross talk between neuroplasticity and environment? Neurobiol Dis 2021;159:105511.
92. Ribot B, Aupy J, Vidailhet M, Mazere J, Pisani A, Bezard E, et al. Dystonia and dopamine: From phenomenology to pathophysiology. Prog Neurobiol 2019;182:101678.
93. Rondot P, Bathien N, de Recondo J, Gueguen B, Fredy D, de Recondo A, Samson Y. Dystonia-parkinsonism syndrome resulting from a bullet injury in the midbrain. J Neurol Neurosurg Psychiatry. 1994;57(5):658.
94. Rossi M, Balint B, Millar Vernetti P, Bhatia KP, Merello M. Genetic dystonia-ataxia syndromes: Clinical spectrum, diagnostic approach, and treatment options. Mov Disord Clin Pract 2018;5:373–382.
95. Rothkirch I, Granert O, Knutzen A, Wolff S, Govert F, Pedersen A, et al. Dynamic causal modeling revealed dysfunctional effective connectivity in both, the cortico-basal-ganglia and the cerebello-cortical motor network in writers' cramp. Neuroimage Clin 2018;18:149–159.
96. Sadnicka A, Hoffland BS, Bhatia KP, van de Warrenburg BP, Edwards MJ. The cerebellum in dystonia - Help or hindrance? Clin Neurophysiol 2012;123:65–70.
97. Schicatano EJ, Basso MA, Evinger C. Animal model explains the origins of the cranial dystonia benign essential blepharospasm. J Neurophysiol 1997;77:2842–2846.
98. Semenova U, Medvednik R, Popov V, Jinnah HA, Shaikh AG, Sedov A. Neuronal activity of pallidal versus cerebellar receiving thalamus in patients with cervical dystonia. Cerebellum 2021;20:151–155.
99. Shakkottai VG. Physiologic changes associated with cerebellar dystonia. Cerebellum 2014;13:637–644.
100. Shakkottai VG, Batla A, Bhatia K, Dauer WT, Dresel C, Niethammer M, et al. Current opinions and areas of consensus on the role of the cerebellum in dystonia. Cerebellum 2017;16:577–594.
101. Shetty AS, Bhatia KP, Lang AE. Dystonia and Parkinson's disease: What is the relationship? Neurobiol Dis 2019;132:104462.
102. Simonyan K, Berman BD, Herscovitch P, Hallett M. Abnormal striatal dopaminergic neurotransmission during rest and task production in spasmodic dysphonia. J Neurosci 2013;33:14705–14714.
103. Strader S, Rodnitzky RL, Gonzalez-Alegre P. Secondary dystonia in a botulinum toxin clinic: Clinical characteristics, neuroanatomical substrate and comparison with idiopathic dystonia. Parkinsonism Relat Disord 2011;17:749–752.
104. Tabbal SD, Mink JW, Antenor JAV, Carl JL, Moerlein SM, Perlmutter JS. 1-methyl-4-phenyl-1,2,3,6-tetrahydropyridine-induced acute transient dystonia in monkeys with low striatal dopamine. Neurosci 2006;141:1281–1287.

105. Tai CH, Tseng SH. Cerebellar deep brain stimulation for movement disorders. Neurobiolo Dis 2022;175:105899.
106. Uncini A, Di Muzio A, Thomas A, Lugaresi A, Gambi D. Hand dystonia secondary to cervical demyelinating lesion. Mov Disord 1996;11:96–99.
107. Vercueil L. Fifty years of brain surgery for dystonia: Revisiting the Irving S. Cooper's legacy, and looking forward. Acta Neurol Belg 2003;103:125–128.
108. Vidailhet M, Dupel C, Lehericy S, Remy P, Dormont D, Serdaru M, et al. Dopaminergic dysfunction in midbrain dystonia. Arch Neurol 1999;56:982–989.
109. Vo A, Nguyen N, Fujita K, Schindlbeck KA, Rommal A, Bressman SB, et al. Disordered network structure and function in dystonia: Pathological connectivity vs. adaptive responses. Cereb Cortex 2023;33:6943–6958.
110. Wilson B, Hess EJ. Animal models for dystonia. Mov Disord 2013;28:982–989.
111. Winkler C, Kirik D, Bjorklund A, Cenci MA. L-DOPA-induced dyskinesias in the intrastriatal 6-hydroxydopamine model of Parkinson's disease: Relation to motor and cellular parameters of nigrostriatal function. Neurobiol Dis 2002;10:165–186.
112. Zoons E, Booij J, Nederveen AJ, Dijk JM, Tijssen MA. Structural, functional and molecular imaging of the brain in primary focal dystonia: A review. Neuroimage 2011;56:1011–1020.

Chapter 24

Dystonia Physiology

INTRODUCTION

Dystonia may sometimes result from visible focal lesions or more extensive developmental or degenerative changes in a sensorimotor network responsible for dystonia (see Chapter 23, "The Neuroanatomical Substrates of Dystonia"). However, cases with overt anatomical abnormalities are not common. As a result, the more common types of dystonia are thought to result from changes in the function, rather than the structure of the network. Such physiological changes might reflect differences in neuronal firing rates or patterns, or differences in the types or strengths of synaptic activity.

This chapter focuses on the physiological underpinnings of the dystonias. The first part describes findings from standard clinical neurophysiological methods, such as electromyography (EMG) or electroencephalography (EEG). The second part focuses on physiological changes in the central nervous system of individuals with dystonia obtained from non-invasive methods such as transcranial magnetic stimulation (TMS). The third part covers more direct changes in brain activity recorded during surgical procedures for dystonia such as deep brain stimulation (DBS). The last part briefly summarizes key findings from animal studies that have clinical relevance.

ROUTINE CLINICAL NEUROPHYSIOLOGICAL STUDIES

The dystonias are characterized by abnormal muscle contractions. Abnormalities typically include overcontraction of muscles leading to excessive force, excessively long-duration or repetitive muscle contractions, overflow of contractions to nearby muscles, and/or co-contraction of muscles that normally function as antagonists. In many cases with dystonia, these abnormal muscle contractions can be detected by EMG.[12,14,21,71] Another frequent EMG finding in dystonia is repetitive 4–7 Hz activity even when repetitive activity is not apparent by clinical examination of movements.

These EMG findings are not specific for dystonia. Many of the EMG abnormalities found in dystonia are seen with other movements, such as a voluntary isometric contraction. Some of the EMG findings can be seen in other disorders, such as tonic epilepsy or stiff person syndrome. Because the EMG features are not specific for dystonia, routine clinical EMG is not particularly useful as a diagnostic tool. However, EMG can be helpful to rule out disorders that may mimic dystonia such as myotonia (disorders intrinsic to muscle that produce abnormal contractions) or neurotonia (disorders of motor neuron excitability leading to abnormal muscle contractions). Excessive muscle contractions in these disorders can be mistaken for dystonia, but there are usually distinct EMG characteristics (see Chapter 26, "Pseudodystonia and Differential Diagnosis"). EMG can also be useful for identification of abnormal muscles for injection of botulinum toxin treatments.[14,43]

The physiological origins of dystonia lie within the central nervous system, but they are not detectable using standard clinical EEG. Therefore, EEG is not often useful in the diagnosis of dystonia. However, EEG can be useful when there is concern that dystonic posturing has an epileptic basis, such as seizures associated with intermittent tonic or twisting movements. EEG can also be useful to exclude epilepsy when dystonia appears in intermittent episodes, such as the paroxysmal dyskinesias (see Chapter 17, "Dystonia and the Paroxysmal Dyskinesias").

NON-INVASIVE PHYSIOLOGICAL STUDIES IN HUMANS

Non-Invasive Techniques

The physiological functioning of the human nervous system has been probed with a number of non-invasive techniques. Application of these methods to subjects with dystonia has led to three conceptual models that could account for the physiological basis for dystonia. These include loss of inhibition, abnormal sensorimotor integration, and maladaptive plasticity. Each of these models is outlined below.

Loss of Inhibition

Proper function of the nervous system requires a balance between inhibitory and excitatory activity. One early model for the pathophysiology of dystonia focused on an imbalance between these processes, with a loss of inhibition. Because excessive muscle activity is a defining feature of dystonia, this model is intuitively attractive. The concept of "surround inhibition" is also important for functional specificity in the nervous system. It was originally described for the sensory system, but a loss of this type of inhibition in motor pathways also provides a potential explanation for unintentional spread of dystonic muscle activity to nearby muscles.[60]

At the spinal cord level, the H-reflex (Hoffman's reflex) is the physiological equivalent of a tendon jerk. By stimulating a sensory nerve containing muscle spindle afferents, it is possible to measure a response at the muscle by EMG. The H-reflex is modulated by the excitability of local spinal circuits and by descending inputs so it can be used to infer the excitability of these circuits. The blink reflex serves a similar purpose for probing the excitability of brainstem circuits. The excitability of the cerebral cortex also can be probed via TMS. A brief TMS pulse on the surface of the skull over the motor cortex produces a motor evoked potential (MEP) at the muscle. By adjusting the strength of the pulse, it is possible to infer excitability of circuits originating from the motor cortex. This is followed by a period of reduced excitability, known as the *silent period*. A weaker, conditioning TMS pulse can also cause transient short-interval intracortical inhibition (SICI) or long-interval intracortical inhibition (LICI) of the ipsilateral motor cortex, another probe of cortical excitability. A TMS pulse to the cortex also produces transcallosal inhibition of the opposite side of the brain (TCI).

All of these methods have been used to probe the physiology of subjects with many different types of dystonia. Multiple studies have revealed a loss of inhibition at multiple levels of the neuraxis including the cerebral cortex,[52] midbrain/brainstem,[6] and even the spinal cord.[40,46] This loss of inhibition has been described for many different types of dystonia including adult-onset idiopathic focal dystonias and inherited childhood-onset generalized dystonias. The frequent finding of loss of inhibition across multiple levels of the nervous system in many different types of dystonia has led to proposals that it could be a central neurophysiological defect underlying dystonia.

While loss of inhibition is a common finding in dystonia and is an intuitively attractive explanation for its pathophysiology, it has never been shown to play a causal role in the pathogenesis of dystonic movement. Recent studies have pointed out that it is not a universal finding in dystonia, questioning whether it could be the fundamental shared defect.[13] In addition, the magnitudes of the experimentally measured effects are often small, with large experimental variance, and many studies have included only small numbers of cases that could produce conclusions that cannot be generalized to broader dystonia populations.[13,18,31] Furthermore, loss of inhibition is not specific for dystonia. It has been reported for other disorders where abnormal movements occur such as stroke, Parkinson disease, and even psychiatric conversion disorders.[5,17,50] These findings have raised questions regarding whether loss of inhibition is a cause or a consequence of motor dysfunction.

Abnormal Sensorimotor Integration

During movement, concurrent sensory feedback is needed to guide speed, strength, and accuracy. After a movement, sensory feedback is important to verify that the movement was executed properly. Without feedback, errors cannot be identified and corrected during execution, and improvement in movement (motor learning) is impossible.

Sensory feedback for movement comes from several sources, most notably muscle spindles. Muscle spindles are specialized sensory receptors, ontogenically evolved from muscle fibers. They are embedded within muscles where they can sense muscle stretch and tension. They are actively contracted by gamma motor neurons to maintain a length for optimal sensing even when muscles shorten during contraction. Feedback from muscle spindles is handled subconsciously by the motor network. Abnormalities of this type of sensory feedback provide an intuitively attractive explanation for abnormal muscle contractions in dystonia. For example, abnormalities in the gain of sensory feedback could lead to contractions with excessive agonist strength and/or excessive antagonist braking. Distorted feedback may cause abnormal movements because the motor network may try to make corrections that are not appropriate. In fact, there are multiple reports suggesting abnormal sensory feedback from muscle spindle proprioceptors.[7,19,29,58] Some studies suggest abnormalities of sensory feedback may be related to the phenomenon of the *geste antagoniste*.[9] Whether these abnormalities play a causal role in dystonia remains undetermined.

In addition to the abnormalities of muscle spindle feedback, there is evidence that sensory perception may be abnormal. The neurological exam does not typically reveal overt defects in conscious sensory perception for most individuals with dystonia, but there are multiple reports of abnormal temporal discrimination, the ability to perceive two distinct stimuli occurring very close in time.[13,45,66] Spatial discrimination, the ability to perceive two simultaneous stimuli that are physically very close to each other, may also be abnormal in dystonia.[38] Sensorimotor representations in the cerebral cortex that can be mapped by TMS are often reported to be enlarged or distorted.[30,41] Such findings can be present even over the sensorimotor cortex contralateral to the unaffected limb among individuals with unilateral limb dystonia. Individuals with dystonia also show distorted perception of body parts in space.[2,3] Altogether, these observations provide important evidence for subclinical defects in sensory perception in dystonia.

Despite these many observations and the intuitively attractive concept that defective sensorimotor integration might be responsible for the pathogenesis of dystonia, it is not clear if the abnormalities of sensory perception play a causal role in pathogenesis. Changes in sensory discrimination and cortical sensorimotor maps occur in other disorders of movement. Such changes can also be seen following motor training in normal individuals.[15,72,73] These observations have raised questions regarding whether abnormalities of sensory functions in dystonia are a cause or a consequence of motor dysfunction.

Maladaptive Plasticity

Neural *plasticity* refers to the ability of the nervous system to adapt to change. Plasticity is mediated at the cellular level by changes in the strengths of existing synapses or changes in the excitability of postsynaptic targets. It may also involve pruning synapses or forming new synapses. In some cases, plasticity may involve remodeling of axonal or dendritic arbors or even neurogenesis. Adaptive plasticity is essential for normal learning and memory, including motor learning. However, defects in these mechanisms may also occur, leading to dysfunctional changes known as *maladaptive plasticity*. Maladaptive plasticity is an intuitively attractive explanation for dystonia because many types of dystonia are task-specific and emerge after intensive training to refine a motor skill.[48]

Plasticity can be probed in humans using a number of non-invasive methods. Low-frequency repetitive TMS (rTMS) produces MEPs with a progressively decrementing response in normal individuals. This decrement reflects adaptability (plasticity) of the nervous system over time. In writer's cramp, rTMS produces the opposite effect, with increasing MEPs, suggesting an abnormality in nervous system plasticity.[59] Another method has involved measuring MEPs following pairing of median nerve stimulation with TMS over the motor cortex, a technique called "paired associative stimulation" (PAS). Pairing of stimuli results in an increase in MEP amplitude in normal individuals, a phenomenon exaggerated in writer's cramp.[47] Using the PAS method, many subsequent studies revealed similar abnormalities in different types of dystonia. However, more recent studies have shown normal plasticity in certain types of dystonia, questioning whether it is relevant to all types of dystonia.[33,34] The same methods also reveal abnormal plasticity for other disorders such as Alzheimer disease, thus questioning its specificity. Recent studies also have revealed large individual variations of responses with these measures, cautioning against overgeneralization of results obtained from small numbers of subjects.[18,53]

The regions of the nervous system that may mediate abnormalities of plasticity cannot be definitively identified using these methods because plasticity is known to occur at all levels of the motor network involved in dystonia, including the sensorimotor cortex, basal ganglia, cerebellum, and brainstem or spinal circuits. Some studies have attempted to define anatomic sources of abnormal plasticity in dystonia. One method involves the conditioned eye blink reflex, which is mediated by the cerebellum.[24,65] In normal individuals, directing a brief puff of air to the cornea stimulates a reflexive eye blink. If the puff is repeatedly preceded by a sound, the blink begins to occur with the sound alone. This reflex is abnormal in subjects with some types of dystonia including sporadic adult-onset focal dystonias[22,64] or the inherited myoclonus-dystonia syndrome.[26,33] However, this abnormality is not universal in dystonia since it is absent among individuals with acquired dystonia or in those with inherited generalized dystonia related to *TOR1A* or *THAP1* genes.[33,56,57] Dystonia and tremor are frequently combined in the same individual, and some have argued that abnormalities of the conditioned eyeblink reflexes are linked with coexisting tremor and not related to dystonia.[4]

Other types of motor plasticity are also thought to be mediated by the cerebellum, such as the adaptation of ocular saccades to a changing visual target. Saccadic adaptation is abnormal in subjects with the myoclonus-dystonia syndrome[26] and tremor-dominant cervical dystonia.[35] Tasks that involve adaptation of hand movements are abnormal in writer's cramp[25] and dystonia associated with pathogenic variants in *TOR1A*.[55] Tasks that involve gait adaptations are abnormal in writer's cramp and blepharospasm.[23] However, most individuals with cervical dystonia have normal adaptive responses for saccades, hand, and gait.[23,32,54]

Overall, the available results seem to suggest that plasticity of the nervous system may be abnormal in some types of dystonia but not in others. Similar to concepts relating to loss of inhibition or abnormalities of sensorimotor integration, it remains unclear if abnormalities related to plasticity play a causal role.

Treatment Using Non-Invasive Physiological Methods

Numerous studies have attempted to determine if non-invasive physiological methods such as TMS or transcranial direct current stimulation (TDCS) could be exploited to reverse symptoms.[39,49] A meta-analysis of 27 of these studies concluded there may be a small beneficial effect.[39] However, effects are often short-lived, and many of the studies were not entirely blinded so exclusion of a placebo effect is challenging.

DIRECT NEUROPHYSIOLOGICAL RECORDINGS IN HUMANS

More direct recordings of neurophysiological activity have been obtained during surgical procedures for dystonia.[67] Most studies have focused on the internal segment of the globus pallidus (GPi) because this region has been the most common target for both ablation and DBS. However, some studies have addressed other regions including the subthalamic nucleus and thalamus. Two main strategies for recording neuronal activity have been used. They include single-neuron (single-unit) recordings and local field potentials that measure the aggregate activity of many neurons near an electrode.

Single-unit studies of the GPi in different types of dystonia have revealed irregular grouped discharges separated by silent pauses. Since such recordings are not available for normal control individuals, findings have been compared to individuals with Parkinson disease undergoing similar surgeries. Compared to Parkinson disease, single-unit grouped discharges in dystonia occur more frequently but at a lower rate and with more irregularity. Some of these grouped discharges correlate with the severity of dystonia.

Most studies of local field potentials in dystonia have also focused on the GPi. Compared to Parkinson disease, studies in dystonia have revealed increased power of low-frequency oscillations in the 4–12 Hz range. One study combined local field potential recordings with magnetoencephalography to demonstrate three relevant circuits in dystonia. They included cortico-pallidal activity with coherence at 13–30 Hz, pallido-temporal activity with 4–8 Hz coherence, and pallido-cerebellar activity with 7–13 Hz coherence.[42] Among these circuits, pallido-cerebellar activity correlated with dystonia severity. Whether these changes in single-unit or local field potentials play a causal role in dystonia remains to be established.

PHYSIOLOGICAL STUDIES OF ANIMALS

The Value of Animal Models

There are clear limitations in the types of studies that can be conducted with human volunteers, and neurophysiological studies using autopsy material are not feasible. In this setting, animal models can be useful. There are two different categories of animal models.[27] The first group of animal models includes those where a biological insult known to cause dystonia is reproduced in an animal. Such insults may include focal lesions, drugs or toxins, or a gene defect known to cause dystonia in humans. These *etiological* models are valuable for studying how these insults affect the brain. The second group of animal models includes those that have abnormal movements that meet clinical criteria used to define dystonia. These *phenotypic* models are useful for understanding the origins of dystonic movement. Animal models for dystonia have been reviewed numerous times,[20,28,37,44,51,70] so only a few examples that illustrate key lessons are summarized here.

Anatomical Versus Functional Abnormalities

Different types of human dystonia are often classified into separate groups thought to have primarily physiological abnormalities without clear anatomical pathology versus those with overt structural defects such as focal lesions.[1] However, precise anatomical studies of different types of human dystonias often reveal subtle (microanatomical) structural changes that would not be detectable with routine clinical neuroimaging or neuropathological studies. These findings suggest that the dichotomy between human dystonias with or without anatomical abnormalities is oversimplified.

For example, anatomical studies of dystonia associated with *TOR1A* do not reveal obvious structural abnormalities in routine clinical imaging or postmortem histopathological studies of humans, although advanced neuroimaging studies have implied microanatomical abnormalities may exist.[10,11,69] Indeed, studies of animal models based on *TOR1A* have confirmed the existence of microanatomical abnormalities in several brain regions, such as subtle changes in neuronal density, neuronal size, lengths or complexity of dendrites or axons.[36,61–63,68,74] These microanatomical abnormalities are not detectable with most of the imaging or even autopsy methods used in human studies. Similar findings have been reported for numerous other animal models where the human counterpart has no known anatomical correlate. These results from animals indicate that distinctions between structural and functional causes reflect the anatomical resolution of the structural methods used.

Physiological Abnormalities in Animal Models

Numerous studies of different types of animal models have confirmed that physiological abnormalities can be detected even when anatomical abnormalities are not obvious. For example, several mouse models of dystonia associated with *TOR1A* have revealed abnormal activity or plasticity in basal ganglia circuitry including nigrostriatal dopamine pathways, corticostriatal pathways, and cholinergic interneurons.[16,37,51] These findings are consistent with numerous human studies implying basal ganglia dysfunction in several types of dystonia. It remains to be determined if these findings are causally related to dystonic movement.

Studies of other rodent models of dystonia have revealed abnormal activity in cerebellar circuitry. A common finding is that the regular firing of cerebellar Purkinje neurons is replaced with a pattern characterized by frequent rapid bursts and intervening silent periods.[8,51] These bursts correlate with dystonic movement. These findings in animals are consistent with other studies indicating abnormal cerebellar function in some types of human dystonia. Once again, a causal role for abnormal burst-firing of Purkinje neurons has yet to be established.

SUMMARY AND FUTURE PROSPECTS

Although rare cases of dystonia may be caused by overt anatomic lesions of the nervous system, most cases are thought to arise from abnormalities of brain function rather than brain structure. Across many different types of dystonia, there is ample evidence from non-invasive studies for physiological changes such as loss of inhibition, abnormal sensorimotor integration, and maladaptive plasticity. There also is more direct evidence for changes in neuronal activity in the brains of people with dystonia. However, it remains unclear if these physiological changes are a cause or a consequence of dystonia.

One very important lesson from these studies is that dystonias are a heterogeneous group of disorders, with varied etiologies and varied pathophysiologies. Although the final outcome of abnormal physiology in dystonia may share many similarities when looking at the EMG level, the physiological changes in the central motor network may not be identical for all types of dystonia. Therefore, studies of one type of dystonia should not be overgeneralized as if they apply to all types of dystonia. Dissecting the physiological changes in dystonia must be done with close attention to the type of dystonia being studied.

A better understanding of the physiology of dystonia is important because the information may be exploited to develop strategies for novel treatments. Numerous studies have attempted to manipulate the physiology of different brain regions as a treatment for dystonia using non-invasive methods such as transcranial magnetic or electrical current stimulation. More direct physiological stimulation is currently used as a therapy for some types of dystonia (see Chapter 31, "Surgical Treatments for Dystonia"), although its mechanisms of action are not fully understood. Improving the invasive and non-invasive strategies for treatment will require a better understanding of the physiological abnormalities in different parts of the motor network responsible for dystonia.

REFERENCES

1. Albanese A, Bhatia K, Bressman SB, DeLong MR, Fahn S, Fung VSC, et al. Phenomenology and classification of dystonia: A consensus update. Mov Disord 2013;28:863–873.
2. Anastasopoulos D, Bhatia K, Bisdorff A, Bronstein AM, Gresty MA, Marsden CD. Perception of spatial orientation in spasmodic torticollis. Part I: The postural vertical. Mov Disord 1997;12:561–569.
3. Anastasopoulos D, Nasios G, Psilas K, Mergner T, Maurer C, Lucking CH. What is straight ahead to a patient with torticollis? Brain 1998;121:91–101.
4. Antelmi E, Di Stasio F, Rocchi L, Erro R, Liguori R, Ganos C, et al. Impaired eye blink classical conditioning distinguishes dystonic patients with and without tremor. Parkinsonism Relat Disord 2016;31:23–27.
5. Avanzino L, Martino D, van de Warrenburg BP, Schneider SA, Abbruzzese G, Defazio G, et al. Cortical excitability is abnormal in patients with the "fixed dystonia" syndrome. Mov Disord 2008;23:646–652.
6. Berardelli A, Rothwell JC, Day BL, Marsden CD. Pathophysiology of blepharospasm and oromandibular dystonia. Brain 1985;108:593–608.
7. Bove M, Brichetto G, Abbruzzese G, Marchese R, Schieppati M. Neck proprioception and spatial orientation in cervical dystonia. Brain 2004;127:2764–2778.
8. Brown AM, van der Heijden ME, Jinnah HA, Sillitoe RV. Cerebellar dysfunction as a source of dystonic phenotypes in mice. Cerebellum 2022;22:719–729.
9. Brugger F, Peters A, Georgiev D, Kagi G, Balint B, Bhatia KP, Day BL. Sensory trick efficacy in cervical dystonia is linked to processing of neck proprioception. Parkinsonism Relat Disord 2019;61:50–56.
10. Carbon M, Kingsley PB, Su S, Smith GW, Spetsieris P, Bressman SB, Eidelberg D. Microstructural white matter changes in carriers of the DYT1 gene mutation. Ann Neurol 2004;56:283–286.
11. Carbon M, Kingsley PB, Tang C, Bressman S, Eidelberg D. Microstructural white matter changes in primary torsion dystonia. Mov Disord 2008;23:234–239.

12. Cohen LG, Hallett M. Hand cramps: Clinical features and electromyographic patterns in a focal dystonia. Neurology 1988;38:1005–1012.
13. Conte A, Rocchi L, Latorre A, Belvisi D, Rothwell JC, Berardelli A. Ten-year reflections on the neurophysiological abnormalities of focal dystonias in humans. Mov Disord 2019;34:1616–1628.
14. Deuschl G, Heinen F, Kleedorfer B, Wagner M, Lucking CH, Poewe W. Clinical and polymyographic investigation of spasmodic torticollis. J Neurol 1992;239:9–15.
15. Draganski B, May A. Training-induced structural changes in the adult human brain. Behav Brain Res 2008;192:137–142.
16. Eskow-Jaunarajs KL, Bonsi P, Chesselet MF, Standaert DG, Pisani A. Striatal cholinergic dysfunction as a unifying theme in the pathophysiology of dystonia. Prog Neurobiol 2015;127-128:91–107.
17. Espay AJ, Morgante F, Purzner J, Gunraj CA, Lang AE, Chen R. Cortical and spinal abnormalities in psychogenic dystonia. Ann Neurol 2006;59:825–834.
18. Fischer P, Pina-Fuentes D, Kassavetis P, Sadnicka A. Physiology of dystonia: Human studies. Int Rev Neurobiol 2023;169:137–162.
19. Grunewald RA, Yoneda Y, Shipman JM, Sagar HJ. Idiopathic focal dystonia: A disorder of muscle spindle afferent processing? Brain 1997;120:2179–2185.
20. Guehl D, Cuny E, Ghorayeb I, Michelet T, Bioulac B, Burbaud P. Primate models of dystonia. Prog Neurobiol 2009;87:118–131.
21. Herz E. Dystonia. I. Historical review; analysis of dystonic symptoms and physiologic mechanisms involved. Arch Neurol Psychiat 1944;51:305–318.
22. Hoffland BS, Kassavetis P, Bologna M, Teo JT, Bhatia KP, Rothwell JC, et al. Cerebellum-dependent associative learning deficits in primary dystonia are normalized by rTMS and practice. Eur J Neurosci 2013;38:2166–2177.
23. Hoffland BS, Veugen LC, Janssen MM, Pasman JW, Weerdesteyn V, van de Warrenburg BP. A gait paradigm reveals different patterns of abnormal cerebellar motor learning in primary focal dystonias. Cerebellum 2014;13:760–766.
24. Hopp JJ, Fuchs AF. The characteristics and neuronal substrate of saccadic eye movement plasticity. Prog Neurobiol 2004;72:27–53.
25. Hubsch C, Roze E, Popa T, Russo M, Balachandran A, Pradeep S, et al. Defective cerebellar control of cortical plasticity in writer's cramp. Brain 2013;136:2050–2062.
26. Hubsch C, Vidailhet M, Rivaud-Pechoux S, Pouget P, Brochard V, Degos B, et al. Impaired saccadic adaptation in DYT11 dystonia. J Neurol Neurosurg Psychiatry 2011;82:1103–1106.
27. Jinnah HA, Hess EJ, LeDoux MS, Sharma N, Baxter MG, DeLong MR. Rodent models for dystonia research: Characteristics, evaluation, and utility. Mov Disord 2005;20:283–292.
28. Jinnah HA, Richter A, Mink JW, Caldwell GA, Caldwell KA, Gonzalez-Alegre P, et al. Animal models for drug discovery in dystonia. Expert Opin Drug Discovery 2008;3:83–97.
29. Kaji R, Rothwell JC, Katayama M, Ikeda T, Kubori T, Kohara N, et al. Tonic vibration reflex and muscle afferent block in writer's cramp. Ann Neurol 1995;38:155–162.
30. Kanovsky P, Bares M, Streitova H, Klajblova H, Daniel P, Rektor I. Abnormalities of cortical excitability and cortical inhibition in cervical dystonia Evidence from somatosensory evoked potentials and paired transcranial magnetic stimulation recordings. J Neurol 2003;250:42–50.
31. Kassavetis P, Sadnicka A, Saifee TA, Parees I, Kojovic M, Bhatia KP, et al. Reappraising the role of motor surround inhibition in dystonia. J Neurol Sci 2018;390:178–183.
32. Katschnig-Winter P, Schwingenschuh P, Davare M, Sadnicka A, Schmidt R, Rothwell JC, et al. Motor sequence learning and motor adaptation in primary cervical dystonia. J Clin Neurosci 2014;21:934–938.
33. Kojovic M, Parees I, Kassavetis P, Palomar FJ, Mir P, Teo JT, et al. Secondary and primary dystonia: Pathophysiological differences. Brain 2013;136:2038–2049.
34. Latorre A, Cocco A, Bhatia KP, Erro R, Antelmi E, Conte A, et al. Defective somatosensory inhibition and plasticity are not required to develop dystonia. Mov Disord 2021;36:1015–1021.
35. Mahajan A, Gupta P, Jacobs J, Marsili L, Sturchio A, Jinnah HA, et al. Impaired saccade adaptation in tremor-dominant cervical dystonia: Evidence for maladaptive cerebellum. Cerebellum 2020;20:678–686.
36. McCarthy DM, Gioioso V, Zhang X, Sharma N, Bhide PG. Neurogenesis and neuronal migration in the forebrain of the TorsinA knockout mouse embryo. Dev Neurosci 2012;34:366–378.
37. Meringolo M, Tassone A, Imbriani P, Ponterio G, Pisani A. Dystonia: Are animal models relevant in therapeutics? Rev Neurol (Paris) 2018;174:608–614.
38. Molloy FM, Carr TD, Zeuner KE, Dambrosia JM, Hallett M. Abnormalities of spatial discrimination in focal and generalized dystonia. Brain 2003;126:2175–2182.
39. Morrison-Ham J, Clark GM, Ellis EG, Cerins A, Joutsa J, Enticott PG, Corp DT. Effects of non-invasive brain stimulation in dystonia: A systematic review and meta-analysis. Ther Adv Neurol Disord 2022;15:17562864221138144.
40. Nakashima K, Rothwell JC, Day BL, Thompson PD, Shannon K, Marsden CD. Reciprocal inhibition between forearm muscles in patients with writer's cramp and other occupational cramps, symptomatic hemidystonia and hemiparesis due to stroke. Brain 1989;112:681–697.
41. Nelson AJ, Blake DT, Chen R. Digit-specific aberrations in the primary somatosensory cortex in Writer's cramp. Ann Neurol 2009;66:146–154.
42. Neumann WJ, Jha A, Bock A, Huebl J, Horn A, Schneider GH, et al. Cortico-pallidal oscillatory connectivity in patients with dystonia. Brain 2015;138:1894–1906.
43. Nijmeijer SW, Koelman JH, Standaar TS, Postma M, Tijssen MA. Cervical dystonia: Improved treatment response to botulinum toxin after referral to a tertiary centre and the use of polymyography. Parkinsonism Relat Disord 2013;19:533–538.
44. Oleas J, Yokoi F, M.P. D, Pisani A, Li Y. Engineering animal models for dystonia: What have we learned? Mov Disord 2013;28:990–1000.
45. Patel N, Jankovic J, Hallett M. Sensory aspects of movement disorders. Lancet Neurol 2014;13:100–112.
46. Priori A, Berardelli A, Mercuri B, Manfredi M. Physiological effects produced by botulinum toxin treatment of upper limb dystonia. Changes in reciprocal inhibition between forearm muscles. Brain 1995;118:801–807.
47. Quartarone A, Bagnato S, Rizzo V, Siebner HR, Dattola V, Scalfari A, et al. Abnormal associative

plasticity of the human motor cortex in writer's cramp. Brain 2003;126:2586–2596.
48. Quartarone A, Pisani A. Abnormal plasticity in dystonia: Disruption of synaptic homeostasis. Neurobiol Dis 2011;42:162–170.
49. Quartarone A, Rizzo V, Terranova C, Cacciola A, Milardi D, Calamuneri A, et al. Therapeutic use of non-invasive brain stimulation in dystonia. Front Neurosci 2017;11:423.
50. Quartarone A, Rizzo V, Terranova C, Morgante F, Schneider S, Ibrahim N, et al. Abnormal sensorimotor plasticity in organic but not in psychogenic dystonia. Brain 2009;132:2871–2877.
51. Rey Hipolito AG, van der Heijden ME, Sillitoe RV. Physiology of dystonia: Animal studies. Int Rev Neurobiol 2023;169:163–215.
52. Ridding MC, Sheean G, Rothwell JC, Inzelberg R, Kujirai T. Changes in the balance between motor cortical excitation and inhibition in focal, task specific dystonia. J Neurol Neurosurg Psychiatry 1995;59:493–498.
53. Sadnicka A, Hamada M. Plasticity and dystonia: A hypothesis shrouded in variability. Exp Brain Res 2020;238:1611–1617.
54. Sadnicka A, Patani B, Saifee TA, Kassavetis P, Parees I, Korlipara P, et al. Normal motor adaptation in cervical dystonia: A fundamental cerebellar computation is intact. Cerebellum 2014;13:558–567.
55. Sadnicka A, Stevenson A, Bhatia KP, Rothwell JC, Edwards MJ, Galea JM. High motor variability in DYT1 dystonia is associated with impaired visuomotor adaptation. Sci Rep 2018;8:3653.
56. Sadnicka A, Teo J, Kojovic M, Kassavetis P, Saifee T, Isabel P, et al. Genotype specific cerebellar involvement in dyt1 and dyt6 dystonia? J Neurol Neurosurg Psychiatry 2013;84:e2.
57. Sadnicka A, Teo JT, Kojovic M, Parees I, Saifee TA, Kassavetis P, et al. All in the blink of an eye: New insight into cerebellar and brainstem function in DYT1 and DYT6 dystonia. Eur J Neurol 2015;22:762–767.
58. Shaikh AG, Wong AL, Zee DS, Jinnah HA. Keeping your head on target. J Neurosci 2013;33:11281–11295.
59. Siebner HR, Tormos JM, Ceballos-Baumann AO, Auer C, Catala MD, Conrad B, Pascual-Leone A. Low-frequency repetitive transcranial magnetic stimulation of the motor cortex in writer's cramp. Neurology 1999;52:529–537.
60. Sohn YH, Hallett M. Disturbed surround inhibition in focal hand dystonia. Ann Neurol 2004;56:595–599.
61. Song CH, Bernhard D, Bolarinwa C, Hess EJ, Smith Y, Jinnah HA. Subtle microstructural changes of the striatum in a DYT1 knock-in mouse model of dystonia. Neurobiol Dis 2013;54:362–371.
62. Song CH, Bernhard D, Hess EJ, Jinnah HA. Subtle microstructural changes of the cerebellum in a knock-in mouse model of DYT1 dystonia. Neurobiol Dis 2013;62C:372–380.
63. Song CH, Fan X, Exeter CJ, Hess EJ, Jinnah HA. Functional analysis of dopaminergic systems in a DYT1 knock-in mouse model of dystonia. Neurobiol Dis 2012;48:66–78.
64. Teo JT, van de Warrenburg BP, Schneider SA, Rothwell JC, Bhatia KP. Neurophysiological evidence for cerebellar dysfunction in primary focal dystonia. J Neurol Neurosurg Psychiatry 2009;80:80–83.
65. Thompson RF, Steinmetz JE. The role of the cerebellum in classical conditioning of discrete behavioral responses. Neuroscience 2009;162:732–755.
66. Tinazzi M, Fiorio M, Fiaschi A, Rothwell JC, Bhatia KP. Sensory functions in dystonia: Insights from behavioral studies. Mov Disord 2009;24:1427–1436.
67. Tisch S, Limousin P. Neurophysiological insights in dystonia and its response to deep brain stimulation treatment. Exp Brain Res 2020;238:1645–1657.
68. Vanni V, Puglisi F, Bonsi P, Ponterio G, Maltese M, Pisani A, Mandolesi G. Cerebellar synaptogenesis is compromised in mouse models of DYT1 dystonia. Exp Neurol 2015;271:457–467.
69. Vo A, Nguyen N, Fujita K, Schindlbeck KA, Rommal A, Bressman SB, et al. Disordered network structure and function in dystonia: Pathological connectivity vs. adaptive responses. Cereb Cortex 2023;33:6943–6958.
70. Wilson B, Hess EJ. Animal models for dystonia. Mov Disord 2013;28:982–989.
71. Yanagisawa N, Goto A. Dystonia musculorum deformans. Analysis with electromyography. J Neurol Sci 1971;13:39–65.
72. Zatorre RJ, Fields RD, Johansen-Berg H. Plasticity in gray and white: Neuroimaging changes in brain structure during learning. Nat Neurosci 2012;15:528–536.
73. Zeuner KE, Bara-Jimenez W, Noguchi PS, Goldstein SR, Dambrosia JM, Hallett M. Sensory training for patients with focal hand dystonia. Ann Neurol 2002;51:593–598.
74. Zhang L, Yokoi F, Jin YH, DeAndrade MP, Hashimoto K, Standaert DG, Li Y. Altered dendritic morphology of Purkinje cells in Dyt1 DeltaGAG knock-in and purkinje cell-specific Dyt1 conditional knockout mice. PLoS One 2011;6:e18357.

Chapter 25

Psychogenic (Functional) Dystonia

INTRODUCTION

The dystonias are defined by their overt clinical manifestations, which typically include abnormal postures and/or movements (see Chapter 2, "Defining the Clinical Features of Dystonia"). There are many known etiologies, which cause dystonia by disrupting the control of movement by the central nervous system. However, abnormal postures and/or movements may sometimes occur for other reasons (see Chapter 26, "Pseudodystonia and Differential Diagnosis"). The term *psychogenic dystonia* refers to individuals who have abnormal postures and/or movements that are thought to differ from classic forms of dystonia because they reflect important contributions from psychological, psychiatric, or behavioral processes. This condition has been given many different labels in the literature, including *functional dystonia*, but the term *psychogenic dystonia* is retained here for reasons outlined below.

Some obvious examples of normal behaviors associated with apparently abnormal movements and postures that may resemble dystonia include dancing and yoga. In these examples, the movements and postures are not abnormal but reflect intentional and learned behaviors. In other cases, physical or emotional stresses may cause apparently abnormal movements or postures that are not necessarily intentional. In psychiatry, these conditions are referred to as *conversion disorders* or *somatization disorders*, in which a stressful event is thought to be converted into a somatic manifestation.[30,46,48] In still other cases, abnormal movements and/or postures may emerge with no obvious cause yet the clinical features resemble those of conversion or somatization disorders more than they resemble classic types of dystonia with established biological etiologies.

In the 2013 Consensus Group Classification of Dystonia,[1] there was uncertainty regarding how psychogenic or functional dystonias should be classified. Some experts felt they should be grouped with other acquired forms of dystonia with a known etiology because of their known or presumed psychological or psychiatric etiology. Others felt psychogenic dystonias should be grouped among the *pseudodystonias*, as conditions that may mimic dystonia (see Chapter 26). Ultimately, the 2013 group placed psychogenic dystonias with other acquired dystonias. However, psychogenic dystonias differ from other acquired forms of dystonia in their phenomenological characteristics, natural history and prognosis, recommended investigations and treatments, and underlying pathophysiology. For these reasons, psychogenic dystonia has been reclassified as a pseudodystonia in the

2025 revision of the Consensus Update on the Classification of Dystonia.[2]

TERMINOLOGY

Historical Perspective

In the first half of the nineteenth century, the terms *functional nervous disorder* and *neurosis* were both used to refer to neurological rather than psychiatric disorders. They encompassed conditions in which there was no obvious pathological correlate, in contrast to *organic* diseases, where a visible lesion or pathological abnormality could be identified, such as stroke or multiple sclerosis.[34,46] Examples of functional nervous disorders and neuroses according to these early definitions included migraine, epilepsy, and Parkinson disease. At that time, there was no apparent neuropathological correlate for any of these disorders. Hysteria was also classified as a functional nervous disorder or neurosis, but, even then, it was recognized that it had signs clearly distinctive from other neurological disorders.[34]

In the second half of the nineteenth and early twentieth centuries, Briquet proposed that hysteria was a psychiatric rather than neurological disorder, the role of dissociation was emphasized by Janet, and the term *conversion disorder* was coined by Breur and Freud to reflect a proposed pathophysiological mechanism of conversion of an underlying psychological problem into a neurological symptom or sign.[34] The term *neurosis* also underwent an evolution in meaning so that the terms *neurosis*, *hysteria*, and *conversion disorder* took on connotations of illnesses with an underlying psychiatric basis.[34] In this setting, dystonia has vacillated between being a psychiatric or neurological disorder for a long time, with early reports of focal dystonias being grouped among the hysterias (Figure 25.1).

The history of dystonia is reviewed in the Chapter 1, "A Brief History of the Concept of Dystonia and Its Evolution." The term *dystonia* was coined by Oppenheim in 1901, to describe a neurological condition characterized by the combination of hypotonia and action-induced hypertonia. Oppenheim considered dystonia to be a "functional nervous disorder or . . . a neurosis" and favored the former possibility: "I therefore believe that the affliction we are dealing with today is not a neurosis but rather originates from subtle changes in the central nervous system, in special areas that control or influence the muscle tone and that it will be possible sooner or later to discover the pathological-anatomical cause."[27] Oppenheim stated that dystonia was *not* "something factitious, psychogenic, hysterical," concluding that "the affection does not have anything to do with hysteria."[27] Subsequent reports emphasized the organic nature of dystonia. The existence of cases with psychogenic dystonia as an entity distinct from classical dystonia was delineated some time later.[17,29]

In contrast to neurosis, hysteria, and conversion disorder, the term "functional" continued to be used for most of the nineteenth and twentieth centuries exclusively to describe *neurological* diseases without obvious structural pathology,

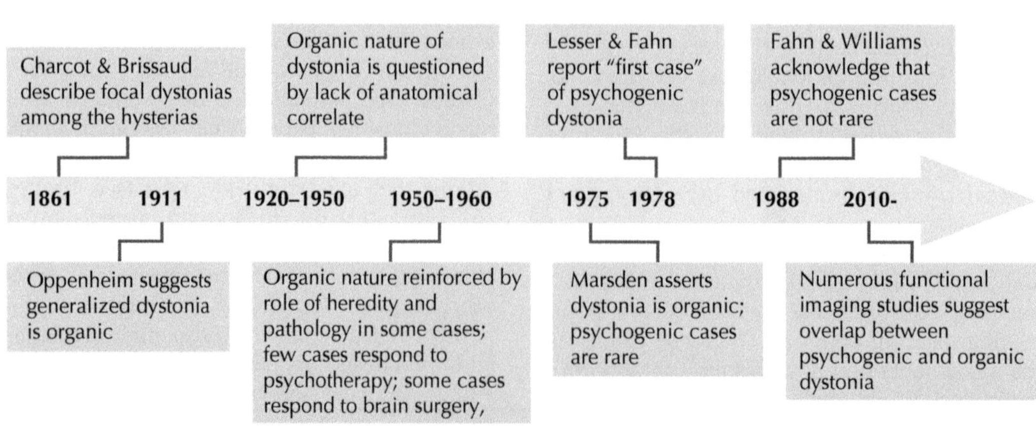

Figure 25.1. Historical views of dystonia as a psychiatric or neurological disorder.

not psychiatric illness. This meaning remains in contemporary use.[6] More recently, the term *functional neurological disorder* has been recommended as a replacement for psychogenic neurological disorders.[12] Thus, the term "functional" can have ambiguous meanings for neurological disorders.

Subspecialty Differences

In addition to the evolution of terminology over time, there are significant differences in terminology among different medical specialists. In neurology, psychogenic dystonia is currently considered a manifestation of a *functional neurological disorder*.[3,23] Experts in neurology have recommended that the term "functional neurological disorder" should include hysteria, conversion, and psychogenic disorders.[53] There also has been a trend to rename *psychogenic* movement disorders as *functional* movement disorders.[12] While *functional movement disorder* is now favored by more than 80% of experienced clinicians, *psychogenic movement disorder* remains in use by more than 60%.[28] However, for individuals who are not experts in neurology, including primary care providers and affected individuals, the term *functional neurological disorder* can be misleading. It implies the disorder is neurological despite widespread recognition that psychological or psychiatric factors play a critical role.[13,23] The term *functional* also conflicts with historical uses of the term as it referred to neurological disorders, not psychiatric disorders.

In psychiatry, the most recent compendium of psychiatric disorders (the *Diagnostic and Statistical Manual of Mental Disorders* [DSM-5-TR]) classifies Functional Neurological Symptom Disorder under Somatic Symptom and Related Disorders, a section that includes related disorders such as somatic symptom disorder, illness anxiety disorder, and factitious disorder. A subtype with dystonia is recognized. The criteria for functional neurological symptom disorder include (1) one or more symptoms that affect body movement or senses, (2) symptoms cannot be explained by a neurological or other medical condition or another mental health disorder, and (3) symptoms cause significant distress or problems in social, work, or other areas, or are significant enough that medical evaluation is recommended.[30,48]

In contrast to the DSM-5-TR, the *International Classification of Diseases* version 11 of the World Health Organization classifies psychogenic dystonia with the dissociative psychiatric disorders under the term *dissociative neurological symptom disorder, with movement disturbance* (https://icd.who.int/en).

Surgical subspecialists often do not usually use diagnostic terms such as *functional neurological disorder* or related psychiatric diagnoses such as *conversion disorder* or *dissociative disorder*. Terms such as *behavioral voice disorder* or *muscle tension dysphonia* are preferred by otolaryngologists to describe individuals with voice disorders resembling laryngeal dystonia, when there is a suspected psychological or psychiatric etiology.[8,37] The term *behavioral* is also used by ophthalmologists to describe individuals who have apparent blepharospasm when there is suspicion for a psychological or psychiatric etiology. This use of the term may include both intentional and unintentional abnormal movements and/or postures resembling dystonia.

In view of the historical and clinical ambiguities of the term *functional dystonia*, the term *psychogenic dystonia* will be retained for this chapter to denote a movement disorder that mimics dystonia but may reflect psychological, psychiatric, or behavioral influences. The term *classical dystonia* is used to denote dystonia arising primarily from a disorder of motor control networks in the nervous system. Arguments for retaining the term *psychogenic* have been made before by others.[16]

EPIDEMIOLOGY

Most epidemiological studies do not address psychogenic dystonia (see Chapter 4, "Epidemiology of the Dystonias").[42] The Hannover epidemiology study found a prevalence of psychogenic dystonia of 28.5 per million people, representing 5% of all cases of dystonia.[10] Psychogenic neurological disorders are seen around the world with similar prevalence and clinical manifestations across different geographies and socioeconomic circumstances.[5]

Psychogenic dystonia is a common manifestation of psychogenic neurological disorders. In several large series of psychogenic movement disorders from multiple different countries, psychogenic dystonia accounted for 20–30% of all cases.[7,56,57] In a meta-analysis of 4,905 cases of all types of movement disorders spanning all ages from across the world, 11.7% had psychogenic dystonia.[31] The lower percentage of psychogenic dystonia cases in the larger study reflected two factors. First, 23.0% of cases had mixed phenotypes, in many of whom dystonic-appearing movements combined with other abnormal movements. Second, inclusion criteria were broader and included functional weakness and seizures.

Psychogenic dystonia may occur at any age. In the large meta-analysis of 4,905 cases, the average age at onset was 39.7 years with a standard deviation of 16.1 years (range <5 to >80 years).[31] Psychogenic dystonia is more common in female individuals. In the same meta-analysis, female individuals accounted for 72.6% of the entire cohort and 78.4% of those with mainly dystonic features.

CLINICAL FEATURES

Features Suggestive of Psychogenic Dystonia

IMPORTANCE OF POSITIVE SIGNS

Psychogenic dystonia is not a diagnosis of exclusion. It is not necessary to conduct extensive evaluations to rule out every potential organic explanation before the diagnosis is made. In fact, there is evidence that this strategy may be counterproductive because it is associated with unnecessary delays in diagnosis, unnecessary laboratory testing, and a diagnostic odyssey that reinforces anxiety that the diagnosis defies explanation.[51,64]

The diagnosis of psychogenic dystonia, like other psychogenic movement disorders, should be anchored by positive findings. Shortly after the description of psychogenic dystonia, diagnostic criteria were proposed to discriminate it from classical dystonia.[17] In this scheme, two central features characteristic of psychogenic dystonia were *inconsistency* over time and *incongruence* of motor phenomenology with classical dystonia. Other features include the presence of additional psychogenic signs or multiple somatizations. Additional features were identified over time.[21] Later, certain combinations of these features were recognized as characteristic psychogenic syndromes.

The reliance on incongruency and inconsistency to identify psychogenic dystonia is a great clinical challenge. A high degree of clinical expertise is needed to appreciate the broad and sometimes unusual clinical manifestations of classical dystonia. Some of the unusual manifestations of classical dystonia include task-specificity, the *geste antagoniste*, worsening with stress or depression, and sometimes marked changes over time. As with any psychogenic movement disorder, no single sign is pathognomonic for psychogenic dystonia, and many exceptions exist so multiple incongruent or inconsistent features give greater certainty to the diagnosis of psychogenic dystonia. Below is a summary of specific features useful for recognizing psychogenic dystonia, followed by a description of some of the more common syndromic patterns.

PATTERNED VERSUS VARIED MOVEMENTS

One of the most characteristic features of classical dystonias is that abnormal postures or associated involuntary movements are patterned (see Chapter 2). The same abnormal movement or posture tends to recur in a relatively stereotyped fashion. In cervical dystonia, for example, the head typically moves repeatedly to the same abnormal posture. For gait dystonias, the foot may demonstrate recurrent inversion at the same phase of the gait cycle (e.g., mid-swing phase).

In contrast, abnormal movements and postures of psychogenic dystonia are often more varied, even when performing the same task. For example, the head in cervical dystonia may assume very different abnormal postures at different times, either during a single clinical visit or over a period of days and weeks. Alternatively, there may be very varied movements of the foot or leg when walking, abnormalities may abate when the gait is stressed by walking on toes or heels, or the gait may become entirely normal when the individual leaves the exam room and is not being examined directly. Additional psychogenic neurological abnormalities may come and go over time.[60] Absence of patterning is one of the major features of psychogenic dystonia that is *incongruent* with classical dystonia.

Absence of patterning is typical of psychogenic dystonia, but sometimes classical dystonias also are not clearly patterned. For example, individuals with cervical dystonia may have a very jerky mobile head movement during the history, and they may develop relatively stable right torticollis when examined at rest and given instructions to allow the head to drift. Alternatively, the abnormal posture may change after several months or years. Craniofacial dystonias may also be varied with different combinations of blinking, spasms, and apraxia of eyelid opening. Variability in these features may be exaggerated by different lighting conditions or stress, or it may be present at rest and disappear with speaking. Similarly, oromandibular dystonia is often very mobile and characterized by multiple coexisting movement patterns such as jaw opening and closing during speaking or multidirectional tongue or jaw movements at rest. Abnormal movements and postures can also vary in their morphology across individual attacks of the inherited paroxysmal dyskinesias, especially with the *ADCY5* gene. Despite these caveats, the lack of patterning of movement remains a key feature that raises suspicion that an abnormal movement is *incongruent* with classical dystonia.

ABRUPT CHANGES OVER TIME

Most classical dystonias of both children and adults begin insidiously and progress gradually over a period of weeks, months, or years. Once established, they only rarely remit. Even dystonia caused by stroke or traumatic brain injury usually evolves relatively slowly over a period of weeks or more. In contrast, a rapid onset is common in psychogenic dystonia. Abnormal movements may reach maximal severity within hours to days, sometimes immediately. A related phenomenon suggestive of psychogenic dystonia is sudden remission, either spontaneously or after psychiatric or rehabilitation therapy. A relapsing-remitting course or paroxysmal phenotype are both suspicious for psychogenic dystonia.[20] Indeed, *inconsistency over time* was one of the earliest features to be recognized as a red flag for psychogenic dystonia.[17]

Of course, abrupt changes over time do not always point to a psychogenic dystonia. Rapid onset of severe dystonia may occur with drug exposure (e.g., acute dystonic reactions associated with neuroleptics), certain genetic disorders (e.g., rapid-onset dystonia parkinsonism associated with the *ATP1A3* gene or genes that cause acute striatal necrosis), and occasionally illicit drugs or toxins (e.g., phencyclidine). Dopa-responsive dystonia associated with *GCH1* mutations frequently has a diurnal variation which may be dramatic. These individuals may have subtle or no dystonia on waking, but they may develop profound difficulty walking later in the day. Classical dystonias may also have intermittent attacks of abnormal movements superimposed on a normal baseline (see Chapter 17, "Dystonia and the Paroxysmal Dyskinesias").

Spontaneous remissions may also occur in adult-onset idiopathic dystonias[33] and occasionally in early-onset genetic dystonias such as those associated with *SGCE* or *GCH1*.[39] Such remissions occur in no more than 5–10% of cases, usually early after onset, and relapses are common. For the genetic paroxysmal dyskinesias, complete remission with age is common for some subtypes (see Chapter 17).

In short, abrupt changes over time (sudden onset, sudden remission, paroxysmal attacks) and inconsistency over time are characteristic of psychogenic dystonia. However, abrupt changes may sometimes occur in classical dystonia, too. Therefore, inconsistency over time alone is not sufficient to make a diagnosis of psychogenic dystonia.

FIXED POSTURES

Another valuable clinical sign suggesting psychogenic dystonia is postures that are relatively fixed (immobile) even at rest.[14,49] In psychogenic dystonia, postures are often near the extreme (or even beyond the range) of normal movement, and posture varies little with rest or action. An examiner usually cannot correct a psychogenic fixed posture, or the posture is altered only slightly. These postures often develop relatively quickly, over days or weeks. Attempted passive straightening of the joint, even gently and slightly, often provokes severe pain.

Fixed postures may also occur in organic dystonia, although they are uncommon, occur usually under very specific circumstances, and rarely develop quickly. They are usually preceded by a period of months or years with an initial phase that is more mobile with gradual progression to more fixed postures. Unlike psychogenic dystonia, passive attempts to correct the abnormal posture in classical dystonia are not usually painful, unless too much force is applied. Painful fixed dystonia can also develop in idiopathic Parkinson disease and especially in the closely related corticobasal syndrome. In short, fixed postures may be a useful clue for psychogenic dystonia, but they are not pathognomonic for psychogenic dystonia.

PSYCHIATRIC OR PSYCHOLOGICAL PROBLEMS

Early studies of psychogenic dystonia also emphasized other psychiatric features, such as anxiety or depression. Individuals with psychogenic dystonia have a higher rate of psychiatric comorbidity compared to those with idiopathic dystonia.[61] Almost half had a history of prior psychiatric treatment or stress preceding their illness as well as higher apathy, dissociative, and somatoform scores. Differences in emotional and social cognitive processing among individuals with psychogenic dystonia have been demonstrated in psychophysical studies.[44]

However, several studies have acknowledged that many individuals with psychogenic dystonia have no apparent psychiatric comorbidities. Also, depression and anxiety are common in many of the classic dystonias (see Chapter 11, "Non-Motor Features of Dystonia"), so their existence is not a strong argument in favor of psychogenic dystonia. Nevertheless, the resolution of abnormal movements and postures with psychotherapy is considered a key factor in establishing a diagnosis of psychogenic dystonia. While the coexistence of psychiatric factors is neither required nor pathognomonic of psychogenic dystonia, psychiatric factors are recognized to play a critical role in the biopsychosocial model of psychogenic disorders as predisposing vulnerabilities, triggers, and or perpetuating factors (Table 25.1).

OTHER ASSOCIATED FEATURES

Numerous other features have been associated with psychogenic dystonia. Perhaps the most useful is the presence of additional psychogenic neurological symptoms or signs such as false weakness or non-physiological sensory deficits.[52] These additional features may be inconsistent over time,[60] but their occurrence provides a useful diagnostic clue. However, it is important to recognize that psychogenic dystonia can

Table 25.1 **Biopsychosocial model for psychogenic dystonia**

	Biological	Psychological	Social
Predisposing vulnerabilities	Female sex Coexisting functional somatic disorders Coexisting neurological disorder Coexisting medical disorder Intellectual disability Sensory processing limitations	Coexisting mood disorder Coexisting anxiety disorder Coexisting personality disorder Maladaptive personality traits Dissociation Alexithymia	Dysfunctional family dynamics Traumatic family event Chronic family illness Physical abuse Sexual abuse Financial insecurities Inadequate social support Attitudes toward health Symptom modeling
Precipitating factors	Physical event such as accident, surgery Sleep deprivation Other physical stressor Compensatory behaviors following injury	Emotional life event Stressful event Dissociative event Panic attack	Loss of employment Marital discord Divorce Death of loved one Other stressors
Perpetuating factors	Chronic pain Chronic fatigue Physiological arousal Deconditioning Chronic medical disability Chronic neurological disability	Negative expectations Illness beliefs Fear of injury Avoidance behavior Resisting diagnosis Maladaptive behaviors	Poor family support Social benefit from illness Pending litigation Pending disability claims Ambiguous diagnosis Disorganized care Reliance on others Social stigma

Adapted from McKee et al.[35]

coexist with organic neurological disease, such as migraine headaches or tremor. Often, the neurological disorder precedes the development of psychogenic dystonia.[56]

A related problem is an increased rate of coexisting somatic complaints such as fibromyalgia, irritable bowel syndrome, chronic fatigue syndrome, and complex regional pain syndrome. There may also be autonomic symptoms including gastroparesis (even leading to gastrostomy tube placement) and postural orthostatic tachycardia syndrome (affecting 7.1% of psychogenic and no classical dystonia patients).[51]

Psychogenic dystonia is also more likely to be associated with preceding trauma. Of course, there are clear circumstances where trauma causes classical dystonia such as severe traumatic brain injury (see Chapter 20, "Dystonia and Trauma"). In contrast, trauma preceding psychogenic dystonia is often minor, such as a sprained ankle or an uncomplicated surgery.

Pain often is a prominent feature of psychogenic dystonia. It may be the most severely disabling feature, it may seem out of proportion to the abnormal movements or postures, it is often recalcitrant to botulinum toxin therapy, and it may be triggered by minor movement or even lightly touching the skin. Pain also is common in classical dystonia including cervical dystonia, writer's cramp, and generalized dystonias (see Chapter 11). However, the pain in classical dystonia often occurs under certain circumstances and typically responds well to botulinum toxins.

Typical Psychogenic Dystonia Syndromes

COMBINATIONS OF INDIVIDUAL SYMPTOMS AND SIGNS

As noted above, numerous symptoms and signs may raise suspicion for psychogenic dystonia. However, none of them is pathognomonic for psychogenic dystonia since they may sometimes occur in classical dystonia, too. As a result, most of the recommended diagnostic strategies for psychogenic dystonia focus on combinations of these features. In fact, certain syndromic phenotypes are now recognized as typical for psychogenic dystonia (Table 25.2).

One case control study compared 99 consecutive psychogenic dystonia cases with 99 classical dystonia cases matched for body regions affected.[51] Psychogenic dystonia could be predicted with high sensitivity (89%) and specificity

Table 25.2 **Well-recognized psychogenic dystonia syndromes**

Syndrome	Descriptions
Abrupt-onset fixed postures, often with pain	Typical foot posture is tonic plantar flexion with intorsion of the foot and downward curling of toes[14,38,49] Typical upper limb posture is tonic flexion of the wrist and fingers but sparing the thumb, sometimes with hyper-extension of the metacarpophalangeal joint, and sometimes with abduction of the shoulder and flexion at the elbow[14,49] Typical shoulder posture is tonic or phasic elevation of one shoulder, often with depression of opposite shoulder[47,55]
Psychogenic paroxysmal dyskinesia	Adult-onset and incongruent with classical paroxysmal dyskinesias because of variable attack frequency and duration, and atypical triggers[20]
Psychogenic craniofacial movements resembling dystonia	Lateral or downward pulling of the lower face, often combined with ipsilateral deviation of the jaw, sometimes with ipsilateral deviation of the tongue and/or ipsilateral platysma activation; movements are often paroxysmal and reflect a combination of brief and long contractions[3,18,26,52] Recurrent jaw or tongue movements incongruent with classical dystonia because of lack of patterning and significant fluctuations in severity, speed, and direction[64]
Psychogenic gaits resembling dystonia	Fixed plantar flexion and intorsion with walking on the ball of the foot or the outside edge of the foot, often with flexion of the knee and hip[25,58] Recurrent buckling of the knees without leg weakness or falling, often combined with flexion of the hip[25,58] Uneconomic abnormal postures such as walking with persistent flexion of the knees and hips or eccentric displacement of the center of gravity[25,58]

(92%), with an area under the curve of 0.95 (0.92–0.98) by including information related to abrupt onset, spontaneous resolution and/or recurrence, pain, cognitive complaints, disability claim, lifetime mood or anxiety disorder, comorbid functional somatic disorders, and having three or more medication allergies. Another case control study compared 113 psychogenic dystonia cases with 125 cases with classical dystonia and suggested that only 1 of 3 variables (sudden onset, fixed, prior trauma) may have sufficient specificity to identify psychogenic cases.[14]

ABRUPT ONSET COMBINED WITH FIXED DYSTONIA

Several studies have indicated that abrupt onset of fixed dystonia is likely to be psychogenic, especially with a history of trauma and coexisting pain.[14,49] This syndrome may occur at any age, and the majority are females. Individuals with sudden onset of fixed dystonia have a higher prevalence of associated psychiatric comorbidity than individuals with classical dystonia and can demonstrate a non-physiological rapid improvement after small doses of botulinum toxin, helping to support a psychogenic syndrome.[11]

The most common body regions affected are the limbs. The most characteristic posture of the lower limb is plantar flexion with inversion of the foot (Figure 25.2). One or both feet may be involved. The abnormal postures may be relatively fixed, occurring even at rest. The upper limb may also be affected, often with excessive flexion of the metacarpophalangeal and interphalangeal joints of the fingers (especially digits 4–5) but sparing of the thumb (Figure 25.2). The shoulder may also be involved, with a typical posture that includes marked elevation of one ipsilateral shoulder, often with depression of the contralateral shoulder, and sometimes laterocollis to the side of the raised shoulder.

ADULT-ONSET PSYCHOGENIC PAROXYSMAL DYSKINESIAS

Psychogenic syndromes are often intermittent.[20] Abnormal movements or postures may occur suddenly, lasting less than a second to several days, with variable periods of remission in between. These cases sometimes give the impression of a classical paroxysmal dyskinesia.

The classical paroxysmal phenotypes have been well-delineated and fall into distinct categories that include paroxysmal kinesigenic dyskinesia, paroxysmal non-kinesigenic dyskinesia, paroxysmal exertional dyskinesia, and paroxysmal nocturnal dyskinesia (see Chapter 17). These subgroups are delineated by the frequency and duration of attacks and the nature of the abnormal movements, as well as typical triggers. For each affected individual, the attack is often relatively stereotyped.

The psychogenic paroxysmal phenotypes often do not fit the classically recognized phenotypes (Table 25.3). One major clue is that genetic paroxysmal dyskinesias begin in childhood, while the psychogenic paroxysmal syndromes more often begin in adults.[20] Classical paroxysmal dyskinesias may emerge in adults, but they are rare. The adult-onset classic phenotypes often reflect an acquired etiology such as multiple sclerosis or endocrinopathy, which can be ascertained by appropriate neuroimaging studies or bloodwork. Another clue is that psychogenic paroxysmal phenotypes are less patterned and more varied in the quality of movements and their time course. They sometimes have triggers atypical for classical paroxysmal dyskinesias, such as lightly stroking the skin or loud noises.

PSYCHOGENIC CRANIOFACIAL DYSTONIAS

For the craniofacial region there are several well-recognized psychogenic syndromes.[3,18,26,52,64] One characteristic phenotype is lateral or downward pulling of the lower face, often combined with ipsilateral deviation of the jaw, sometimes with ipsilateral deviation of the tongue and/or ipsilateral platysma activation (Figure 25.3). Movements often reflect a combination of rapid phasic contractions combined with longer tonic contractions, sometimes lasting several minutes. These movements may resemble dystonia or hemifacial spasm.[3]

Isolated portions of this syndrome may also occur, such as isolated downward or lateral pulling of the lip, isolated deviation of the jaw, or isolated tongue or platysma activation. Another phenotype suspicious for psychogenic dystonia is downward movement of one eyebrow combined with upward movement of the contralateral eyebrow (Figure 25.3). Repetitive phasic movements

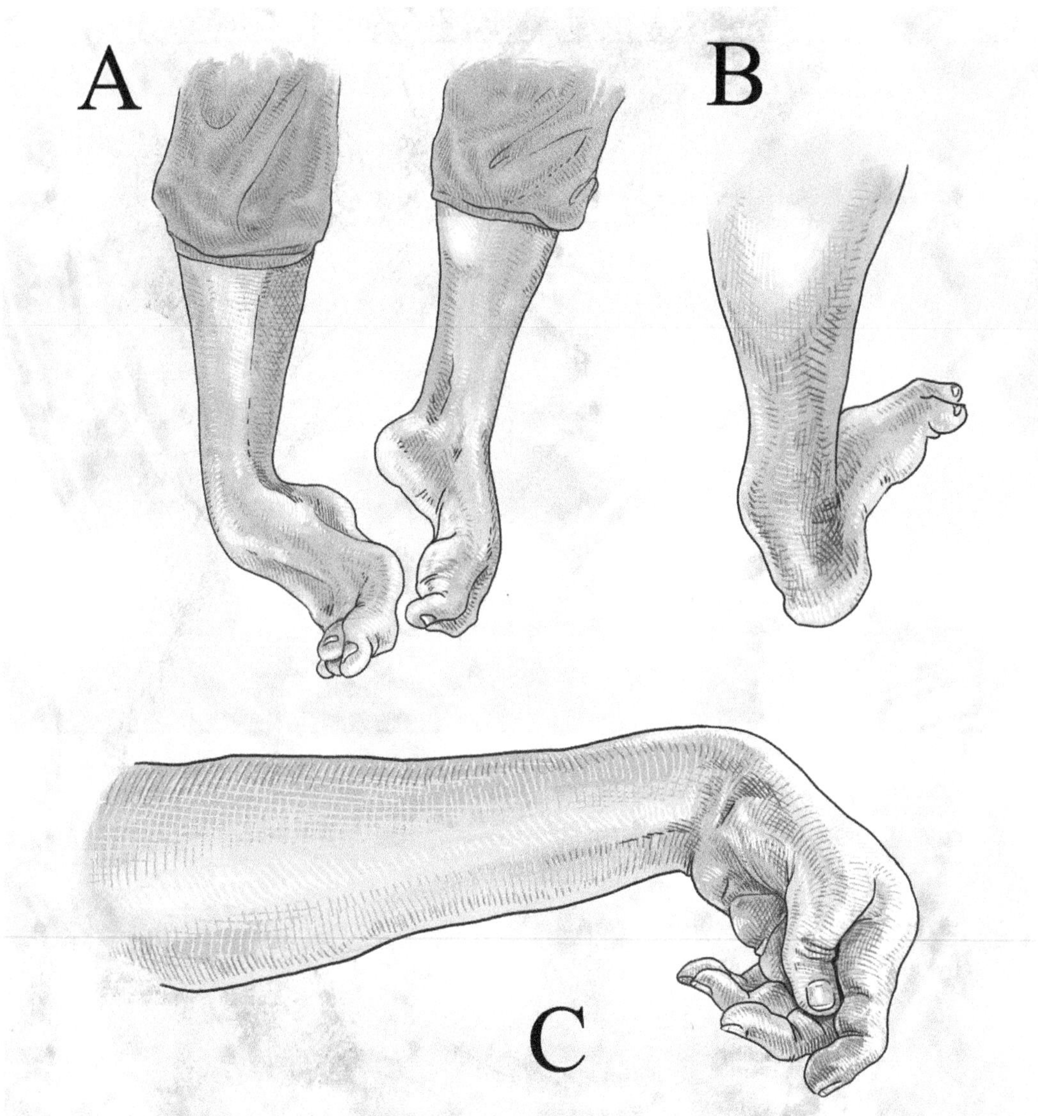

Figure 25.2. Typical psychogenic postures of the limbs. Panel A shows the most characteristic lower limb postures, which include fixed intorsion with plantar flexion of the foot, usually with flexion (curling) of the toes, although extension of the toes or foot eversion may also occur. These postures remain relatively fixed at rest and with walking, in contrast with other types of foot dystonia which are often more varied and dynamic depending on task. Panel B shows the most characteristic upper limb postures, which is flexion of the wrist and flexion of the fingers and/or thumb at the metacarpophalangeal joints, with either hyperextension or flexion of interphalangeal joints. There is often additional abduction and internal rotation of the arm.

Illustration by Loren Bergantini.

combined with longer tonic movements of the jaw and tongue may also occur.[64]

While all these abnormal movements in psychogenic craniofacial dystonia may occur in classical dystonia as well, several clues point toward a psychogenic dystonia. For example, half of the lower face is often involved in psychogenic cases. In comparison, classic craniofacial dystonias are usually bilateral. Other features more typical of psychogenic dystonia than classical dystonia

Table 25.3 **Features suggestive of psychogenic paroxysmal dyskinesia**

Feature	Psychogenic PxD	Classical PxD phenotypes	
Age at onset	Adult	PKD	1–20 years
		PED	5–30 years
		PNKD	1–10 years
		PND	1–20 years
Triggers	Atypical	PKD	Sudden movement, startle
		PED	>10 minutes of exercise
		PNKD	Fatigue, alcohol, coffee, tea
		PND	Sleepy or sleeping
Duration of attacks	Variable within an individual	PKD	<2 minutes
		PED	5–60 minutes
		PNKD	10–240 minutes
		PND	5–120 minutes
Frequency of attacks	Variable within an individual	PKD	Up to dozens per day
		PED	Depends on exertion level
		PNKD	Few per day to few per month
		PND	Few per day to few per month
Associated features	Coexisting functional features, somatizations	PKD	ICCA, episodic ataxia, migraine, hemiplegia
		PED	Epilepsy, intellectual disability, ataxia
		PNKD	Migraine
		PND	Epilepsy, intellectual disability, ataxia
Family history	Rare	PKD	Likely
		PED	Sometimes
		PNKD	Likely
		PND	Likely

Abbreviations: ICCA, infantile convulsions with choreoathetosis; PED, paroxysmal exertional dyskinesia; PKD, paroxysmal kinesigenic dyskinesia; PND, paroxysmal nocturnal dyskinesia;, PNKD, paroxysmal non-kinesigenic dyskinesia; PxD, paroxysmal dyskinesia. Modified from Ganos et al.[20]

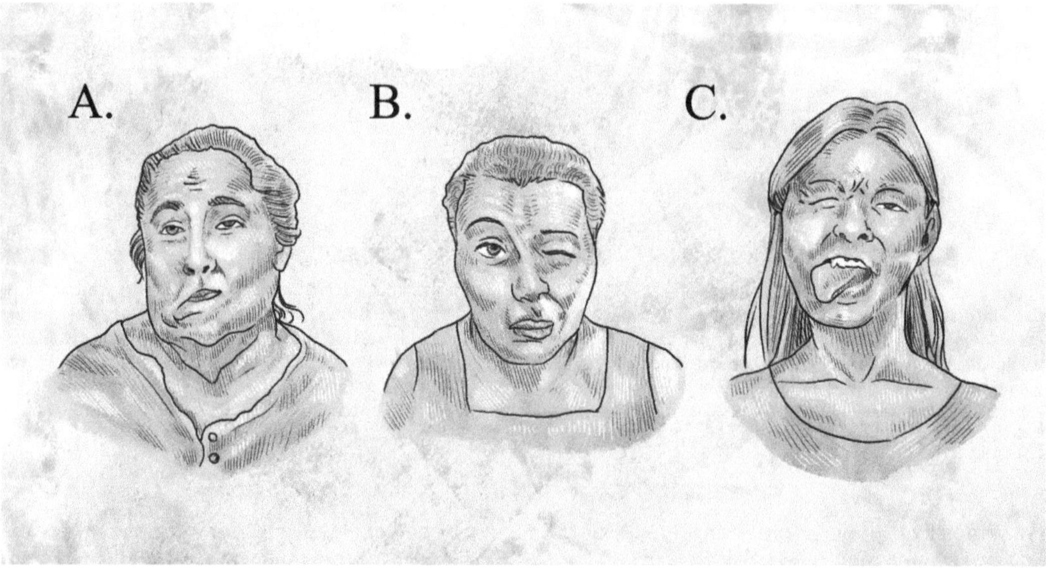

Figure 25.3. Typical psychogenic movements of the craniofacial region. Panel A shows a characteristic often tonic but variable posture that includes lateral and downward pulling of the lower face. Panel B shows a similar posture of the lower face, combined with ipsilateral eye squinting and upward movement of the contralateral eyebrow. Panel C shows prominent lateral deviation of the tongue and jaw with ipsilateral eye closures. This montage was adapted from prior publications.[3,18,26]

Illustration by Loren Bergantini.

include inconsistency of movement appearance and duration over time, paroxysmal nature, and lack of sensory tricks. Unlike classic oromandibular dystonia or tardive dystonia, the movements in psychogenic cases often fluctuate in severity, speed, and direction.

PSYCHOGENIC DYSTONIC GAITS

The most common psychogenic dystonic gait is seen among cases with acute onset of fixed dystonia described above, where the foot is usually persistently plantar flexed and inverted, even at rest. The associated gait is characterized by walking on the ball of the foot or the outside edge of the foot, with flexion of the knee and hip and an antalgic appearance.

Other psychogenic gaits that may resemble dystonia have also been described.[25,58] One involves sudden and recurrent buckling of the knees without weakness or falling. Another has been described as *uneconomic postures*, where maintenance of abnormal postures (such as walking with persistent flexion of the knees and hips or eccentric displacement of the center of gravity) require enormous strength and energy.

PATHOGENESIS

Etiology

Functional neurological disorders, including psychogenic dystonia, fall at the interface of neurology and psychiatry. A focus on purely psychiatric or neurological disease may be too reductionist. Instead, a biopsychosocial model has been proposed as a framework for understanding the more complex pathogenesis of functional movement disorders.[19,35,44] The model includes some predisposing vulnerability, precipitating factors, and perpetuating factors (Table 25.1).

The capacity for normal motor function is thought to be intact in individuals with pure functional neurological disorders.[13] This observation gives rise to two fundamental questions regarding psychogenic dystonia. The first question is why do affected individuals manifest a dystonia phenotype? In some cases, exposure to illness among family members or close friends has an impact on the expression of a psychogenic movement disorder, suggesting that the affected individual is copying or *modeling* from experience.[43] However, evidence for modeling can be found only in the minority of cases.

The second question is why do affected individuals fail to access their intact motor control networks to move normally? The answer to this question is not always clear. It has been hypothesized that subconscious mechanisms are involved and that the disorder is not voluntary, feigned, or malingering.[12] Instead, abnormal motor behavior may be reinforced by some psychosocial influence, such as *secondary gain*, where the abnormal behavior results in the return of some positive reinforcement. Alternatively, the abnormal motor behavior may permit avoidance of some negative psychological or social experience.

Neuroimaging

One small study used positron emission tomography to compare six individuals with psychogenic dystonia, five with leg dystonia associated with *TOR1A* variants, and six normal controls. The psychogenic group had increased activity in the cerebellum and basal ganglia and decreased activity in primary motor cortex. In contrast, those with *TOR1A* variants had an opposite pattern of increased activity in primary motor cortex and thalamic regions with decreased cerebellar activity compared to the controls. This study suggests differences in the function of cortical and subcortical structures in psychogenic versus classical dystonia.

Another study used functional MRI to examine connectivity of the primary motor cortex in fixed versus mobile psychogenic dystonia compared to healthy controls. For the affected groups, differences were found in areas involved in emotional processes and sense of agency.[45] The fixed psychogenic dystonia group showed functional connectivity abnormalities mainly to areas related to sense of agency, whereas the mobile psychogenic dystonia group showed reduced connectivity in areas important in sensorimotor functions and increased connectivity to areas important in emotional processing. The same study also found differences between fixed and mobile psychogenic dystonia in volumetric and tractography MRI studies. The fixed psychogenic dystonia group had global white matter disconnection affecting main sensorimotor and emotional control circuits. The mobile psychogenic dystonia group had alterations in gray matter structures crucial for sensorimotor processing and emotional and cognitive control. Fixed psychogenic dystonia showed major abnormalities of white matter tracts including the corpus callosum, corticospinal tract, and anterior thalamic radiations.[59]

Abnormalities in areas related to emotional processing have also been demonstrated in other functional imaging studies of psychogenic dystonia or functional movement disorder cohorts that included psychogenic dystonia. Unlike normal controls, the affected groups showed a lack of changes in the amygdala when exposed to fearful and happy faces, suggesting differences in processing of emotional valence. There was also greater functional connectivity between the right amygdala and the right supplementary motor area in the functional movement disorder group, providing evidence of increased linkage between psychological or physical stressors and movement.[63] A functional MRI study that compared psychogenic and classical dystonia with healthy controls showed decreased activation in response to basic emotional stimuli in selected motor and sensory areas, right middle temporal gyri, and bilateral precuneus and decreased activation following exposure to intense emotional stimuli in the left insular and left motor cortices.[15] These results further suggest abnormalities in emotional processing in psychogenic dystonia cases.

Neurophysiology

Despite the many clinical differences and etiologies between psychogenic and classical dystonia, neurophysiological studies have not been able to differentiate them.[19,54] The neurophysiological abnormalities of classical dystonia can also be found in psychogenic dystonia. There are no consistent differences between psychogenic and organic dystonias when considering cortical and spinal mechanisms of inhibition or plasticity, and even intraoperative neurophysiological recordings of globus pallidus neuronal firing patterns have not found consistent differences between the groups.[19,54]

During a voluntary reaction time task, individuals with psychogenic fixed dystonia had less co-contraction compared with those with fixed dystonia from organic disease, although there was still overlap between the two groups.[32] All together, these results may imply that the neurophysiological underpinnings of psychogenic and organic dystonia are similar. Alternatively, it is also possible that these neurophysiological measures do not differentiate the groups because they reflect the consequence of similar abnormal movements rather than their causes (see Chapter 24, "Dystonia Physiology").

MANAGEMENT

Multidisciplinary Strategy

Psychogenic disorders fall into a gray zone between medicine and psychology. Often predisposing biological vulnerabilities (either neurological or medical) combined with psychosocial factors (psychological or psychiatric) trigger and often maintain the condition (Table 25.1). A multidisciplinary management plan therefore often is needed and is best combined with physical and/or occupational therapists to reinforce normal movements.[19]

A neurologist and internist may be needed to monitor and address any underlying biological issues as best possible and to reinforce the importance of a treatment plan that is not limited to medicines and surgical procedures. Pain is a frequent complaint and must be addressed as appropriate. A psychiatrist is needed to address underlying psychiatric or social issues that contribute to the disorder, and a psychologist is useful for cognitive-behavioral therapy.

Counseling

One of the most important aspects of a successful management plan is communication of the diagnosis with the affected individual. There are many strategies for communicating the diagnosis, and some degree of skepticism from the patient is not uncommon. Nevertheless, acceptance of the diagnosis by the affected individual is a key ingredient for success. The same message must come from all members of the multidisciplinary team so that skepticism regarding the diagnosis does not undermine the treatment plan.

Following delivery of the diagnosis, ongoing counseling is often necessary. Many of the psychosocial issues that trigger or maintain psychogenic disorders are chronic or recurrent, and regular attention is therefore needed.

Physical and Occupational Therapy

Another important feature of a successful management plan involves physical forms of therapy, including physiotherapy, occupational therapy, and speech therapy.[40,41] The fundamental goal is to attenuate maladaptive motor behaviors and encourage more normal movements. Numerous methods have been recommended including demonstrating that normal movements can sometimes occur, graded task performance, distraction when abnormal movements occur, sensorimotor retraining, and others.

Botulinum Toxin Therapy

Botulinum toxin (BoNT) therapy does not appear to be useful in psychogenic dystonia. One small randomized and placebo-controlled trial showed no apparent benefit for 14 individuals with psychogenic dystonia, all of whom also received cognitive behavioral therapy.[62] Another randomized placebo-controlled trial of BoNT showed no benefit in 48 individuals with psychogenic jerks or tremor, just under half of whom also had psychogenic dystonia.[9]

Deep Brain Stimulation Surgery

A characteristic feature of psychogenic disorders is inconsistency over time with regards to both severity and qualitative features. Outcomes for all types of therapies are varied and unpredictable. In view of these observations, a diagnosis of a psychogenic movement disorder is usually considered a contraindication for brain surgery.[4] However, some experts have noted that psychogenic symptoms may coexist with classical dystonia, and therefore deep brain stimulation surgery may be warranted.[36]

Prognosis

Even with a multidisciplinary approach, the prognosis for complete and permanent recovery is poor.[19,24] Several studies of different types of psychogenic neurological disorders have suggested that significant improvement occurs less than half of all cases, and many cases relapse, sometimes with a different type of psychogenic disorder.

There are limited studies reporting on the prognosis of individuals with psychogenic dystonia. One follow-up of a cohort of 41 patients with fixed dystonia after an average of 7 years showed improvement in 23% with remission in only 6%, whereas 77% were the same or worse. [24,49] One systematic review of 14 studies addressing prognosis found highly varied methods of reporting and highly varied outcomes, although early diagnosis appeared to be a predictor of more favorable outcomes.[22]

SYNOPSIS AND FUTURE PROSPECTS

The psychogenic dystonias may be among the most difficult of all types of dystonia to recognize and diagnose with certainty because their features overlap with classical forms of dystonia. Nevertheless, it is usually possible to distinguish psychogenic and classical dystonias. The diagnosis does not require exclusion of all potential classical forms of dystonia with extensive diagnostic testing. Instead, it relies on expert recognition of positive clinical clues from both the history and exam. None of these clues is pathognomonic for psychogenic dystonia, but certain combinations can be very helpful. Despite the challenges, early clinical recognition is important to avoid a diagnostic odyssey that includes multiple unnecessary diagnostic tests and ineffective treatment strategies.

Treatment strategies for psychogenic dystonia differ from classical dystonias. Treatment responses in psychogenic dystonia are unpredictable for oral medications, BoNT, and surgical strategies such as deep brain stimulation. Best responses are achieved with a multidisciplinary team approach that emphasizes supportive neurological care along with professional counseling, behavioral interventions, and physical therapy. The prognosis is guarded. Long-term studies suggest less than a quarter achieve remission, and relapses are common, often with a different psychogenic disorder.

There is a great need for development of strategies or tools for early recognition of psychogenic dystonia that can be applied by primary care providers and general neurologists who may not be experts in recognizing the sometimes subtle differences between psychogenic and classical dystonia. There is a great need for a simple biomarker, either blood-based, imaging-based, or physiological. Of course, a better understanding of the factors that trigger and maintain psychogenic dystonia may also provide novel strategies for improving treatments.

REFERENCES

1. Albanese A, Bhatia K, Bressman SB, DeLong MR, Fahn S, Fung VSC, et al. Phenomenology and classification of dystonia: A consensus update. Mov Disord 2013;28:863–873.
2. Albanese A, Bhatia K, Fung V, Hallett M, Jankovic J, et al. Definition and Classification of Dystonia, 2025 (first presented at the International Dystonia Symposium in 2023).
3. Baizabal-Carvallo JF, Jankovic J. Distinguishing features of psychogenic (functional) versus organic hemifacial spasm. J Neurol 2017;264:359–363.
4. Bramstedt KA, Ford PJ. Protecting human subjects in neurosurgical trials: The challenge of psychogenic dystonia. Contemp Clin Trials 2006;27:161–164.
5. Carota A, Calabrese P. Hysteria around the world. Front Neurol Neurosci 2014;35:169–180.
6. Corp DT, Morrison-Ham J, Jinnah HA, Joutsa J. The functional anatomy of dystonia: Recent developments. Int Rev Neurobiol 2023;169:105–136.
7. Cubo E, Hinson VK, Goetz CG, Garcia Ruiz P, Garcia de Yebenes J, et al. Transcultural comparison of psychogenic movement disorders. Mov Disord 2005;20:1343–1345.
8. Desjardins M, Apfelbach C, Rubino M, Verdolini Abbott K. Integrative review and framework of suggested mechanisms in primary muscle tension dysphonia. J Speech Lang Hear Res 2022;65:1867–1893.
9. Dreissen YEM, Dijk JM, Gelauff JM, Zoons E, van Poppelen D, Contarino MF, et al. Botulinum neurotoxin treatment in jerky and tremulous functional movement disorders: A double-blind, randomised placebo-controlled trial with an open-label extension. J Neurol Neurosurg Psychiatry 2019;90:1244–1250.
10. Dressler D, Altenmuller E, Giess R, Krauss JK, Adib Saberi F. The epidemiology of dystonia: The Hannover epidemiology study. J Neurol 2022;269:6483–6493.
11. Edwards MJ, Bhatia KP, Cordivari C. Immediate response to botulinum toxin injections in patients with fixed dystonia. Mov Disord 2011;26:917–918.
12. Edwards MJ, Stone J, Lang AE. From psychogenic movement disorder to functional movement disorder: It's time to change the name. Mov Disord 2014;29:849–852.
13. Edwards MJ, Yogarajah M, Stone J. Why functional neurological disorder is not feigning or malingering. Nat Rev Neurol 2023;19:246–256.
14. Ercoli T, Defazio G, Geroin C, Marcuzzo E, Fabbrini G, Bono F, et al. Sudden onset, fixed dystonia and acute peripheral trauma as diagnostic clues for functional dystonia. Mov Disord Clin Pract 2021;8:1107–1111.
15. Espay AJ, Maloney T, Vannest J, Norris MM, Eliassen JC, Neefus E, et al. Dysfunction in emotion processing underlies functional (psychogenic) dystonia. Mov Disord 2018;33:136–145.
16. Fahn S, Olanow CW. "Psychogenic movement disorders": They are what they are. Mov Disord 2014;29:853–856.
17. Fahn S, Williams DT. Psychogenic dystonia. Adv Neurol 1988;50:431–455.
18. Fasano A, Valadas A, Bhatia KP, Prashanth LK, Lang AE, Munhoz RP, et al. Psychogenic facial movement disorders: Clinical features and associated conditions. Mov Disord 2012;27:1544–1551.
19. Frucht L, Perez DL, Callahan J, MacLean J, Song PC, Sharma N, Stephen CD. Functional dystonia: Differentiation from primary dystonia and multidisciplinary treatments. Front Neurol 2021;11:605262.
20. Ganos C, Aguirregomozcorta M, Batla A, Stamelou M, Schwingenschuh P, Munchau A, et al. Psychogenic paroxysmal movement disorders: Clinical features and diagnostic clues. Parkinsonism Relat Disord 2014;20:41–46.
21. Ganos C, Edwards MJ, Bhatia KP. The phenomenology of functional (psychogenic) dystonia. Mov Disord Clin Pract 2014;1:36–44.
22. Gelauff J, Stone J, Edwards M, Carson A. The prognosis of functional (psychogenic) motor symptoms: A systematic review. J Neurol Neurosurg Psychiatry 2014;85:220–226.
23. Hallett M, Aybek S, Dworetzky BA, McWhirter L, Staab JP, Stone J. Functional neurological disorder: New subtypes and shared mechanisms. Lancet Neurol 2022;21:537–550.
24. Ibrahim NM, Martino D, van de Warrenburg BP, Quinn NP, Bhatia KP, Brown RJ, et al. The prognosis of fixed dystonia: A follow-up study. Parkinsonism Relat Disord 2009;15:592–597.
25. Issak S, Kanaan R, Nielsen G, Fini NA, Williams G. Functional gait disorders: Clinical presentations, phenotypes and implications for treatment. Brain Inj 2023;37:437–445.
26. Kaski D, Bronstein AM, Edwards MJ, Stone J. Cranial functional (psychogenic) movement disorders. Lancet Neurol 2015;14:1196–1205.
27. Klein C, Fahn S. Translation of Oppenheim's 1911 paper on dystonia. Mov Disord 2013;28:851–862.
28. LaFaver K, Lang AE, Stone J, Morgante F, Edwards M, Lidstone S, et al. Opinions and clinical practices related to diagnosing and managing functional (psychogenic) movement disorders: Changes in the last decade. Eur J Neurol 2020;27:975–984.
29. Lesser RP, Fahn S. Dystonia: A disorder often misdiagnosed as a conversion reaction. Am J Psychiatry 1978;135:349–352.
30. Levenson JL, Sharpe M. The classification of conversion disorder (functional neurologic symptom disorder) in ICD and DSM. Handb Clin Neurol 2016;139:189–192.
31. Lidstone SC, Costa-Parke M, Robinson EJ, Ercoli T, Stone J, FMD GAP Study Group. Functional movement disorder gender, age and phenotype study: A systematic review and individual patient meta-analysis of 4905 cases. J Neurol Neurosurg Psychiatry 2022;93:609–616.
32. Macerollo A, Batla A, Kassavetis P, Parees I, Bhatia KP, Edwards MJ. Using reaction time and co-contraction to differentiate acquired (secondary) from functional 'fixed' dystonia. J Neurol Neurosurg Psychiatry 2015;86:933–934.

33. Mainka T, Erro R, Rothwell J, Kuhn AA, Bhatia KP, Ganos C. Remission in dystonia: Systematic review of the literature and meta-analysis. Parkinsonism Relat Disord 2019;66:9–15.
34. Marsden CD. Hysteria: A neurologist's view. Psychol Med 1986;16:277–288.
35. McKee K, Glass S, Adams C, Stephen CD, King F, Parlman K, et al. The inpatient assessment and management of motor functional neurological disorders: An interdisciplinary perspective. Psychosomatics 2018;59:358–368.
36. Morigaki R, Miyamoto R, Mure H, Fujita K, Matsuda T, Yamamoto Y, et al. Can pallidal deep brain stimulation rescue borderline dystonia? possible coexistence of functional (psychogenic) and organic components. Brain Sci 2020;10:636.
37. Morrison MD, Rammage LA, Belisle GM, Pullan CB, Nichol H. Muscular tension dysphonia. J Otolaryngol 1983;12:302–306.
38. Munts AG, Mugge W, Meurs TS, Schouten AC, Marinus J, Moseley GL, et al. Fixed dystonia in complex regional pain syndrome: A descriptive and computational modeling approach. BMC Neurol 2011;11:53.
39. Nardocci N, Zorzi G, Barzaghi C, Zibordi F, Ciano C, Ghezzi D, Garavaglia B. Myoclonus-dystonia syndrome: Clinical presentation, disease course, and genetic features in 11 families. Mov Disord 2008;23:28–34.
40. Nicholson C, Edwards MJ, Carson AJ, Gardiner P, Golder D, Hayward K, et al. Occupational therapy consensus recommendations for functional neurological disorder. J Neurol Neurosurg Psychiatry 2020;91:1037–1045.
41. Nielsen G, Stone J, Matthews A, Brown M, Sparkes C, Farmer R, et al. Physiotherapy for functional motor disorders: A consensus recommendation. J Neurol Neurosurg Psychiatry 2015;86:1113–1119.
42. Ortiz R, Scheperjans F, Mertsalmi T, Pekkonen E. The prevalence of adult-onset isolated dystonia in Finland 2007–2016. PLoS One 2018;13:e0207729.
43. Pellicciari R, Superbo M, Gigante AF, Livrea P, Defazio G. Disease modeling in functional movement disorders. Parkinsonism Relat Disord 2014;20:1287–1289.
44. Pick S, Goldstein LH, Perez DL, Nicholson TR. Emotional processing in functional neurological disorder: A review, biopsychosocial model and research agenda. J Neurol Neurosurg Psychiatry 2019;90:704–711.
45. Piramide N, Sarasso E, Tomic A, Canu E, Petrovic IN, Svetel M, et al. Functional MRI connectivity of the primary motor cortex in functional dystonia patients. J Neurol 2022;269:2961–2971.
46. Rowe JB. Conversion disorder: Understanding the pathogenic links between emotion and motor systems in the brain. Brain 2010;133:1295–1297.
47. Sa DS, Mailis-Gagnon A, Nicholson K, Lang AE. Posttraumatic painful torticollis. Mov Disord 2003;18:1482–1491.
48. Scamvougeras A, Howard A. Somatic symptom disorder, medically unexplained symptoms, somatoform disorders, functional neurological disorder: How DSM-5 got it wrong. Can J Psychiatry 2020;65:301–305.
49. Schrag A, Trimble M, Quinn N, Bhatia K. The syndrome of fixed dystonia: An evaluation of 103 patients. Brain 2004;127:2360–2372.
50. Schrag AE, Mehta AR, Bhatia KP, Brown RJ, Frackowiak RS, Trimble MR, et al. The functional neuroimaging correlates of psychogenic versus organic dystonia. Brain 2013;136:770–781.
51. Stephen CD, Perez DL, Chibnik LB, Sharma N. Functional dystonia: A case-control study and risk prediction algorithm. Ann Clin Transl Neurol 2021;8:732–748.
52. Stone J, Hoeritzauer I, Tesolin L, Carson A. Functional movement disorders of the face: A historical review and case series. J Neurol Sci 2018;395:35–40.
53. Stone J, Wojcik W, Durrance D, Carson A, Lewis S, MacKenzie L, et al. What should we say to patients with symptoms unexplained by disease? The "number needed to offend." BMJ 2002;325:1449–1450.
54. Thomsen BLC, Teodoro T, Edwards MJ. Biomarkers in functional movement disorders: A systematic review. J Neurol Neurosurg Psychiatry 2020;91:1261–1269.
55. Thyagarajan D, Kompoliti K, Ford B. Post-traumatic shoulder dystonia: Persistent abnormal postures of the shoulder after minor trauma. Neurology 1998;51:1205–1207.
56. Tinazzi M, Geroin C, Marcuzzo E, Cuoco S, Ceravolo R, Mazzucchi S, et al. Functional motor phenotypes: To lump or to split? J Neurol 2021;268:4737–4743.
57. Tinazzi M, Morgante F, Marcuzzo E, Erro R, Barone P, Ceravolo R, et al. Clinical correlates of functional motor disorders: An Italian multicenter study. Mov Disord Clin Pract 2020;7:920–929.
58. Tinazzi M, Pilotto A, Morgante F, Marcuzzo E, Cuoco S, Ceravolo R, et al. Functional gait disorders: Demographic and clinical correlations. Parkinsonism Relat Disord 2021;91:32–36.
59. Tomic A, Agosta F, Sarasso E, Petrovic I, Basaia S, Pesic D, et al. Are there two different forms of functional dystonia? A multimodal brain structural MRI study. Mol Psychiatry 2020;25:3350–3359.
60. Tomic A, Jecmenica Lukic M, Petrovic I, Svetel M, Dragasevic Miskovic N, et al. Changes of phenotypic pattern in functional movement disorders: A prospective cohort study. Front Neurol 2020;11:582215.
61. Tomic A, Petrovic I, Pesic D, Voncina MM, Svetel M, Miskovic ND, et al. Is there a specific psychiatric background or personality profile in functional dystonia? J Psychosom Res 2017;97:58–62.
62. Vizcarra JA, Lopez-Castellanos JR, Dwivedi AK, Schmerler DA, Ries S, Espay AJ. OnabotulinumtoxinA and cognitive behavioral therapy in functional dystonia: A pilot randomized clinical trial. Parkinsonism Relat Disord 2019;63:174–178.
63. Voon V, Brezing C, Gallea C, Ameli R, Roelofs K, LaFrance WC, Jr., Hallett M. Emotional stimuli and motor conversion disorder. Brain 2010;133:1526–1536.
64. Yoshida K. Clinical characteristics of functional movement disorders in the stomatognathic system. Front Neurol 2020;11:123.

Chapter 26

Pseudodystonia and Differential Diagnosis

INTRODUCTION

The term *pseudodystonia* combines the term *dystonia* with the term *pseudo*, the latter coming from the Greek word meaning *false*. The hybrid term was coined to highlight disorders that might resemble dystonia but were not considered to be true dystonia.[20]

At the time the term was introduced, dystonia was viewed as a disorder of the basal ganglia. Abnormal movements linked with other regions of the nervous system, such as those in the posterior fossa, were considered pseudodystonias. Since then, there have been significant advances in understanding dystonia as a network disorder that may involve different regions of the nervous system including regions in the posterior fossa (see Chapter 23, "The Neuroanatomical Substrates of Dystonia"). However, the extent of the network has not been fully delineated, resulting in some uncertainties regarding which disorders to label as pseudodystonia. This changing view of the neuroanatomical basis for dystonia has led to an evolution of the types of dystonias viewed as pseudodystonias.

The most recent conceptualization of the term *pseudodystonia* suggests that it be reserved for disorders that may mimic dystonia but have a known or presumed biological mechanism that differs from dystonia.[1] This concept is challenging because the anatomical network for dystonia is not yet fully elucidated, leading to some differences of opinion regarding what is *pseudo* dystonia and what is *real* dystonia. Although there are persisting ambiguities in the term pseudodystonia, its main value is to call attention to the differential diagnosis of abnormal movements that raise suspicion for dystonia. This chapter focuses on differential diagnosis rather than attempts to define or compile lists of pseudodystonias.

ORTHOPEDIC ABNORMALITIES

Rationale

Dystonia is a disorder of the nervous system, not the bones and joints. Nevertheless, disorders of the bones and joints may cause abnormal postures, sometimes accompanied by muscle spasms and abnormal movements (Table 26.1). These orthopedic disorders are often classified among the pseudodystonias. These abnormal

Table 26.1 **Orthopedic disorders that may mimic dystonia**

Orthopedic disorder	Dystonic mimic
Contractures	
Dupuytren contracture	Finger dystonia
Erb's deformity	Finger/hand dystonia
Fibrodysplasia ossificans	Neck, trunk or limb dystonia
Congenital muscular torticollis	Cervical dystonia
Volkmann contracture	Wrist dystonia
Joint abnormalities	
Arthritic destruction	Abnormal postures
Atlantoaxial dislocation	Cervical dystonia
Shoulder dislocation	Shoulder/arm dystonia
Hip dislocation	Pelvic/leg dystonia
Vertebral abnormalities	
Ankylosing spondylitis	Truncal dystonia
Compression fractures	Cervical or truncal dystonia
Klippel-Feil anomaly	Cervical dystonia
Orthopedic scoliosis	Truncal dystonia

postures and movements may mimic dystonia and should therefore be considered in the differential diagnosis of dystonia. Discriminating orthopedic problems from dystonia is important because they require different approaches to treatment.

Vertebral Abnormalities

Abnormal postures of the head/neck may result from structural defects of cervical vertebra, such as acquired compression fractures or congenital fusions of cervical vertebrae as in the Klippel-Feil anomaly.[4] These problems may be associated with pain leading to muscle spasms and abnormal movements. Therefore, cervical spine problems can mimic cervical dystonia. Structural defects of the thoracic or lumbar vertebrae may also cause the trunk or hips to bend laterally (scoliosis), mimicking truncal dystonia. Fractures and inflammatory disorders of the spine such as ankylosing spondylitis may also cause backward (extension, or lordosis) or forward (flexion) bending of the spine.

Usually, these orthopedic problems can be identified by the history and confirmed with imaging studies. When interpreting the results of imaging studies, it is important to recognize a reciprocal relationship between dystonia and orthopedic defects. Orthopedic defects can mimic dystonia, but dystonia can cause orthopedic defects. For example, chronic untreated cervical dystonia can produce early degenerative joint disease of the cervical spine, typically affecting the upper cervical spine at C2–C4.[11,38] Dystonia may also cause scoliosis when there is severe pulling of truncal muscles.[16] Orthopedic scoliosis is common in idiopathic [14]cervical dystonia and may be the presenting or sole feature of idiopathic[51] or inherited isolated dystonias.[6,23,65] In a study of 292 individuals with cerebral palsy, scoliosis occurred in 41%, usually in association with dystonia.[71] Hyperextension of the spine is typical of tardive dystonia caused by neuroleptics (see Chapter 19, "Dystonias Induced by Medications, Illicit Drugs, and Environmental Exposures"), and dystonic extensor spasms (opisthotonos) are characteristic of a number of inherited metabolic dystonias.[22,30,62] Both of these dystonic conditions may cause injury to the spine.

Joint Abnormalities

Dislocation of a joint can also produce a clinical picture resembling dystonia. Rotary subluxation of the atlantoaxial joint can produce abnormal postures of the head/neck (Grisel's syndrome).[4,27] Similar dislocations can produce abnormal postures of the shoulder or hip joints, or even a finger or toe. All can be associated with muscle spasms and pain, further mimicking dystonia. Dislocations can usually be identified by a history of trauma, but spontaneous dislocations may occur. In addition, it is useful to remember that severe dystonia can cause joint dislocation of the atlanto-axial joint, hips, and other joints.[33]

Severe arthritis can lead to substantial joint deformities, with abnormal postures of the fingers, toes, or other joints. These joint deformities are often fixed, although voluntary movements may be abnormal because of the abnormal joint. The history and exam, aided by imaging, are usually sufficient to identify abnormal postures caused by arthritic joint disease.

Contractures

Contractures consist of fibrosis and shortening of muscles and/or tendons and ligaments. Contractures may mimic dystonia because they produce abnormal postures. A relatively common example is Dupuytren's contracture, which is caused by inflammation and shortening of one or more tendons of the hand.[46] This disorder most commonly affects the third digit of one hand, with flexion at the proximal interphalangeal or metacarpophalangeal joints, but it can affect other fingers as well.

Congenital muscular torticollis is a relatively common disorder of infancy.[15,44] It can be caused by congenital fibrosis and shortening of one or more neck muscles, usually the sternocleidomastoid, leading to abnormal head posture. Abnormal head postures may resolve spontaneously during the first year of life, but some require surgical intervention. Congenital muscular torticollis can also be caused by an irritative mass in one of the neck muscles or by excessive neck muscle activity, and some cases respond to botulinum toxin treatment. Therefore, etiologies for congenital muscular torticollis are mixed, with some reflecting an orthopedic process and others potentially reflecting dystonia.

While contractures may cause abnormal postures that could be mistaken for dystonia, the converse may also occur. Contractures may result from chronic dystonia. The relationship between contractures and dystonias is complex. For example, inheritance of a pathological genetic variant on a single allele of *TOR1A* is typically associated with childhood-onset generalized dystonia, where contractures sometimes develop in cases with severe and longstanding dystonia.[43] On the other hand, inheritance of biallelic mutations of the same variant are associated with arthrogryposis multiplex congenita, a disorder in which infants are born with multiple severe contractures, and coexisting dystonia may be absent.[34,55,69]

In short, many orthopedic disorders may mimic dystonia, including structural defects in the bones, joints, and ligaments. However, chronic or severe dystonia may cause orthopedic defects. The relationships between abnormal movements and orthopedic problems are therefore bidirectional. Imaging studies with a careful history and exam are usually sufficient to discriminate the etiology.

NEUROMUSCULAR ABNORMALITIES

Rationale

Dystonia is typically viewed as a disorder of the central nervous system, not the peripheral nervous system. However, abnormalities intrinsic to muscles or neurons of the peripheral nervous system may produce abnormal postures or movements resembling dystonia (Table 26.2). Most experts agree these neuromuscular disorders should be classified as pseudodystonias because they are not caused by defects of the central nervous system. The term *myokymia* refers to subtle rippling movements of the skin caused by underling muscle contractions that are triggered by spontaneous repetitive discharges of one or a few motor units. The term *fasciculation* refers to more obvious muscle twitching, but twitches are brief and irregular, usually with no associated movement of the associated joint. *Cramps* involve more obvious and sustained muscle contractions, and they may sometimes move a joint. All of these phenomena are not considered dystonia.

Muscle Disorders

The myotonias are a group of disorders in which intrinsic muscle defects lead to sustained involuntary contractions.[59] They are divided into dystrophic or non-dystrophic subtypes, although muscle weakness may occur in both. In myotonic dystrophy, muscles often fail to release after a strong voluntary contraction, leading to transient abnormal postures or movements that may resemble dystonia. For example, hand muscles may fail to release completely after making a fist,

Table 26.2 **Neuromuscular or spinal disorders that may mimic dystonia**

Neuromuscular disorder	Dystonic mimic
Muscle disorders	
Eyelid myokymia	Blepharospasm
Head drop	Cervical dystonia
Muscle cramps	Limb dystonia
Myotonia congenita	Limb dystonia
Myotonic dystrophy	Limb dystonia
Neck extensor myopathy	Cervical dystonia
Paramyotonia congenita	Limb dystonia
Schwartz-Jampel syndrome	Generalized dystonia
Nerve disorders	
Carpopedal spasms	Limb dystonias
Focal and multifocal neuropathy	Limb dystonias
Hemi-facial spasm	Blepharospasm
Hemi-masticatory spasm	Oromandibular dystonia
Isaac syndrome	Limb dystonias
Morvan syndrome	Limb dystonias
Motor neuron disease	Dystonic anterocollis, limb dystonia
Muscle cramps	Limb dystonias
Myasthenia gravis	Dystonia anterocollis, blepharospasm
Spinal cord disorders	
Multiple sclerosis	Dystonic spasms
Stiff person syndrome	Trunk, leg, or arm dystonia
Strychnine poisoning	Craniofacial, cervical, or truncal dystonia
Tetanus	Craniofacial, cervical, or truncal dystonia

leading to transient clawing of the hand. Eyelid myotonia after forced eyelid closure may result in delayed eye-opening mimicking blepharospasm.

For the non-dystrophic myotonia known as *myotonia congenita*, symptoms may begin first in the legs and progress to other regions, similar to early-onset dystonias.[59] In *paramyotonia congenita*, symptoms are triggered by cold rather than muscle contractions. The Schwartz-Jampel syndrome emerges in infancy with non-dystrophic myotonia combined with joint contractures, bone dysplasia, and dysmorphic facies. The rigid spine syndrome is another condition associated with a number of different genetically determined myopathies and muscular dystrophies.[39,47] It is associated with progressive spinal and neck deformity that can potentially be mistaken for axial dystonia. All these muscle disorders can be identified by characteristic findings on electromyogram (EMG), and genetic testing can often confirm the diagnosis.

Head drop can also occur due to both acquired and inherited myopathies that have a propensity to affect the neck extensors. These disorders are not caused by overactivity of neck muscles but instead by weakness that leads to abnormal posture of the head. An abnormal forward posture of the head and neck is not unusual in Parkinson disease and related parkinsonian conditions, sometimes in response to dopamine-related therapy. Some of these cases reflect neck extensor weakness while others reflect dystonic anterocollis, and the delineation of the underlying cause of abnormal head posture may be challenging.[56,57,61] A useful test to determine if anterior bending of the head and neck reflects neck extensor weakness or neck flexor dystonia is to ask the affected individual to lie down in the prone position. Abnormal postures relating to neck weakness usually resolve when lying down, while abnormal postures due to sustained neck flexor contractions often do not.

Disorders of Peripheral Nerves or Motor Neurons

Muscle cramps are characterized by abrupt onset and brief duration, usually a few seconds or minutes.[63] In some individuals, recurrent muscle cramps may lead to concern for dystonia. The most commonly affected area is the calf or thigh, but cramps may occur anywhere. They are common even among normal individuals. They may be associated with exercise, certain medical illnesses, peripheral neuropathies, and motor neuron disease. Carpopedal spasms resulting from electrolyte disturbances probably fall in the same category. Historically the pathogenesis was thought to involve electrolyte disturbances leading to spontaneous muscle contraction, but recent studies have indicated that muscle cramps originate from motor neurons or spinal circuits.[26] Muscle cramps can usually be discriminated from dystonia by their sudden onset, brief duration, characteristic locations, characteristic triggers, and high-frequency discharges (50–100 Hz) on EMG.[26]

Hyperexcitability of peripheral nerves may lead to muscle cramps combined with fasciculations in a spectrum of disorders.[26] The most benign is the cramp-fasciculation syndrome. More severe is Isaac syndrome, which combines cramps, fasciculations, myokymia, and autonomic dysfunction (hyperhidrosis). Peripheral nerve hyperexcitability is also part of Morvan syndrome, which features additional abnormalities of the central nervous system, such as sleep disturbance and encephalopathy. The most commonly associated autoantibodies are directed to contactin-associated protein 2 (Caspr2) or, rarely, leucine-rich glioma-inactivated protein 1 (LGI1), two proteins linked to voltage-gated potassium channels responsible for repolarizing membranes after depolarization (see Chapter 21, "Dystonia and Autoimmunity").

Hemifacial spasm is another disorder caused by autonomous activity of the seventh cranial nerve.[19] It is characterized by twitching and tonic pulling of muscles in the face resembling dystonia. It may be caused by compressive irritation of the seventh nerve by an aberrant artery or mass lesion or by small lesions where the nerve exits the brainstem. Hemifacial spasm usually affects only one side of the face, while blepharospasm usually affects both. However, the diagnosis can be difficult in cases of bilateral hemifacial spasm[21] or asymmetrical craniofacial dystonia (see Chapter 6, "Craniofacial Dystonias").

Hemi-masticatory spasm is a similar condition caused by irritation of the fifth cranial nerve.[54] It is characterized by sudden spasms of jaw closure, jaw opening, or jaw deviation. Although both hemifacial and hemimasticatory spasm can be treated with botulinum toxins, neither is considered to be dystonia.

In addition to overactivity of peripheral nerves, neuromuscular causes of weakness may sometimes produce abnormal postures that can be mistaken for dystonia. For example, focal and multifocal neuropathies can produce asymmetric weakness with abnormal postures. One example is the claw hand deformity, characterized by tonic flexion of the proximal and distal interphalangeal joints, with hyperextension of the metacarpophalangeal joints. The posture results from asymmetric weakness of muscles controlling the hand, usually caused by motor neuron disease or disorders of peripheral nerve such as Charcot-Marie-Tooth disease or mononeuritis multiplex. The diagnosis is usually apparent from the history and coexisting weakness, and it may be confirmed with EMG or nerve conduction studies (NCS).

Defects of the neuromuscular junction can also cause weakness that may be mistaken for dystonia. For example, individuals with myasthenia gravis often suffer from head drop due to weakness of neck extensors. Head drop must be distinguished from dystonic anterocollis, where excessive activities of anterior neck muscles pull the head forward. Stridor from vocal cord weakness may mimic laryngeal dystonia. The eyelids are another area where neuromuscular causes must be discriminated from dystonia. The eyelids may droop closed or fail to open with ptosis caused by weakness of the levator palpebrae muscles. However, the craniofacial dystonias may also be associated with partial eyelid closures due to activity of the palpebral portion of the orbicularis oculi (see Chapter 6). The diagnosis of eyelid dystonia can be made because of visible spasms of the palpebral or orbital orbicularis oculi, but sometimes spasms are not obvious with visual inspection.

BEHAVIORAL PHENOMENA

Certain behavioral reactions may also mimic dystonia (Table 26.3). One example includes head tilt due to ocular misalignment from impairments of one or more nerves controlling eye movements.[4] The head tilt may be relatively fixed, or more dynamic. Presumably, the affected individual maintains an abnormal head posture to correct for visual incongruity

Table 26.3 **Behaviors that may mimic dystonia**

Behavior	Dystonic mimic
Behavioral compensations	
Cranial nerve weakness	Cervical dystonia
Vestibular abnormalities	Cervical dystonia
Weakness	Limb dystonia
Ataxia	Limb dystonia
Muscle tension dysphonia	Laryngeal dystonia
Pain behaviors	
Guarding	Any dystonia
Inflammatory torticollis	Cervical dystonia
Sandifer syndrome	Cervical and truncal dystonia
Posterior fossa lesions	Cervical dystonia
Behavior disorders	
Somatoform disorders	Any dystonia
Malingering	Any dystonia

from the eyes. This behavioral reaction may be intentional or subconscious. Head tilt may also occur with asymmetric vestibulopathy or brainstem stroke. A careful history and examination of eye movements may disclose these conditions.

Another example of a behavioral reaction resembling dystonia is pain-guarding behavior, such as pain in an upper limb that leads to holding the arm close to the body with flexion of the fingers and elbow. Similar abnormal postures and movements may occur with pain of the lower limb. Pain-guarding behavior is not limited to the limbs but may occur in the neck and shoulders due to head or neck pain. Abdominal flexion or scoliosis is associated with abdominal pain. Pain-guarding behavior is normally easy to identify by history, except in young children or cognitively disabled individuals who may not be able to verbalize a cause for their abnormal postures.

Abdominal discomfort from gastroesophageal reflux or hiatal hernia may also be the explanation for the abnormal cervical and truncal posturing seen in children with Sandifer syndrome. Acute-onset torticollis is common in young children and often triggered by an inflammatory condition such as upper respiratory or sinus infection, cervical adenitis, retropharyngeal abscess, or mastoiditis.[9] The occiput typically is tilted to the affected side with the chin rotated to the opposite side. The cause of the abnormal head position is not entirely clear but may reflect a behavioral reaction to pain.

More challenging are the behavioral reactions that often occur in other motor disorders such as ataxia or weakness. To overcome certain motor deficits, many individuals develop strategies that exploit abnormal postures or movements to stabilize a joint. The resulting movement may resemble dystonia. The same phenomenon may occur in muscle tension dysphonia, which is thought to reflect a behavioral reaction to voice strain or weakness.[13,37] In many cases, these behavioral strategies are not intentional but subconscious. Therefore, the history may not reliably discriminate these compensations, especially in young children.

Even more challenging are behavioral disorders that resemble dystonia. They have many names in the literature including functional dystonia, psychogenic dystonia, conversion disorder, somatoform disorder, hysteria, and others (see Chapter 25, "Psychogenic [Functional] Dystonia"). The biological basis for these psychological conditions is not well understood, but they are suspected to differ from classic types of dystonia.[1,5] Also potentially included in this group is malingering, which refers to intentional simulation of dystonic-like movements for secondary gain.

SENSORY PATHWAYS

Abnormal movements and postures may result from distorted sensory feedback, either unconscious feedback regarding muscle tension and stretch from muscle spindles or conscious proprioception regarding limb and joint positions. Whether these sensory disorders should be considered pseudodystonias or true dystonias is not entirely clear. Some experts view dystonia as a disorder of the brain's *motor* network, excluding defects originating with known or presumed basis in peripheral sensory feedback.[5] Others include sensory defects as an integral aspect of the biology of dystonia, noting the many sensory abnormalities that have been uncovered in many types of dystonia.[3,12] Some studies have shown that stimulation of peripheral sensory afferents with vibration may induce dystonic postures in normal individuals, or it may normalize abnormal postures in dystonic individuals.[8,32,45] Indeed, peripheral muscle spindles may play a role in the beneficial effects of botulinum toxin in dystonia.[58] In view of these observations, it is not clear whether disorders of abnormal sensory feedback should be considered pseudodystonias or true dystonias.[52] In any event, they must be considered in the differential diagnosis.

Abnormal movements may occur with defects affecting the parietal cortex including strokes, tumors, trauma, or surgical interventions (Table 26.4). A systematic study of 32 individuals with pure parietal strokes revealed abnormal movements and postures resembling dystonia in 84%.[24] These movements may be quite dynamic, and they are commonly associated with variations in muscle tone or a coarse irregular tremor typical of dystonia. Isolated parietal lesions commonly lead to abnormal hand movements,[10,24,35] but they have also been reported to cause cervical dystonia,[36] craniofacial dystonia,[28] or hemidystonia.[31,40] Since the parietal cortex is involved in sensory processing and internal representation of the body, the mechanism causing abnormal movements is thought to reflect faulty processing of sensory feedback or distortions of perception of body position. Although some experts view abnormal movements associated with parietal lesions as pseudodystonias because they do not involve the dystonia motor circuit, others consider these disorders to be true dystonias.[50]

Abnormalities of the cervical spinal cord may also cause abnormal postures and movements of the head. There are numerous underlying pathologies including syringomyelia, benign or malignant tumors, and granuloma.[42] Most of these abnormalities cause compressive injury to the spinal cord. Postures have a tonic rather than dynamic quality and may occur in any direction of movement. Although spinal cord lesions often affect the head/neck muscles, they can also affect the upper limb.[68] Lesions of the spinal cord are thought to cause abnormal postures and movements because of distortion of sensory feedback that must pass through the affected region. Alternatively, the mechanism may involve distortion of motor signals from the brain to the muscles. Whether abnormal postures and movements resulting from spinal lesions should be considered pseudodystonia or true dystonia remains unclear.

Table 26.4 **Other disorders to consider for dystonia-like movements**

Disorder	Dystonic mimic
Sensory pathway lesions	
Parietal cortex	Limb dystonia
Syringomyelia	Cervical dystonia
Arnold-Chiari malformation	Cervical dystonia
Compressive cord lesions	Cervical dystonia
Others	
Multiple sclerosis spasms	Trunk or limb dystonia
Posterior fossa lesions	Cervical dystonia
Postural defects in Parkinsonism	Truncal dystonia
Satoyoshi syndrome	Any dystonia
Stiff person syndrome	Trunk or limb dystonia
Tonic seizures	Trunk or limb dystonia
Tonic tics	Any dystonia

OTHER DISORDERS

Numerous other disorders may resemble dystonia but are thought to have a biological basis different from most other forms of dystonia. Epileptic seizures dominated by tonic movements may be mistaken for dystonia, particularly paroxysmal dystonia. They can often be identified by associated cognitive and behavioral changes and confirmed with electroencephalography (EEG). Tics can similarly have a tonic quality, sometimes persisting with abnormal postures or writhing movements. They can often be identified by suppressibility or a premonition. Although terms such as *dystonic seizure*[48,49] or *dystonic tic*[29,64] are sometimes used to describe these disorders, hybrid terms often lead to confusion among patients and primary care providers, so they should be avoided.

Abnormalities of inhibitory circuits in the spinal cord may also be associated with excessive firing of motor neurons and involuntary spasms, movements, or postures (Table 26.4). One rare but well-known example is tetanus. Tetanus is caused by exposure to tetanus toxin, which has prominent effects on inhibitory spinal and brainstem neurons. It is characterized by trismus, sometimes with spasms in other facial muscles, the neck, and the trunk.

Another disorder affecting spinal circuits is stiff person syndrome, an autoimmune disorder that targets inhibitory neurons of the spinal cord.[60] Affected individuals have characteristic overactivity of the extensor muscles of the back combined with stiffness of the legs, producing an awkward gait. However, in some cases, only the trunk or one leg or arm is involved. Overactivity of muscles begins insidiously and may be action-induced. As a result, such cases can closely resemble dystonia. The diagnosis can be suspected by clues from the history (such as associated autoimmune disorders) or the examination (such as spasms induced by touch, exaggerated startle response, and very stiff gait pattern). The diagnosis can be confirmed by specific antibody testing (mainly glutamic acid decarboxylase, glycine receptor, and/or amphiphysin) in serum and cerebrospinal fluid (see Chapter 21).

Satoyoshi syndrome is a rare disorder that may emerge in children or adults, associated with severe muscle cramps in any region of the body, hair loss, and diarrhea. The etiology is unknown, but it is suspected to be an autoimmune disorder causing a defect in spinal cord inhibitory circuits.[17]

Individuals with multiple sclerosis or neuromyelitis optica may have involuntary movements variably described as tonic spasms, tonic seizures, or paroxysmal dyskinesias (see Chapter 21). These movements are common, occurring in 83 of 149 cases in one study.[66] Attacks are usually brief (30–120 seconds), stereotyped, and often painful. They consist of tonic posturing of one limb and sometimes the face, neck or trunk. They can occur spontaneously, or they can be precipitated by movement, hyperventilation, startle, or sensory stimulation. The pathogenesis of these movements is not clear, but they are often associated with demyelinating lesions of the spinal cord or brainstem, and they may respond to carbamazepine.

Posterior fossa mass lesions may cause abnormal postures of the head/neck, especially in children.[7,25,41,42,67] Lesions are varied and include benign and malignant brain tumors, peripheral schwannomas, granulomas, arachnoid cysts, Arnold-Chiari malformation, and others. These mass lesions impinge on the cerebellum, brainstem, and sometimes upper spinal cord. The mechanism by which these tumors cause abnormal postures is not known. The mechanism may reflect a behavioral compensation to relieve pressure in the fourth ventricle, a behavioral compensation to abnormal vestibular signals, posturing due to pain from meningeal irritation, distortion of sensory feedback from the neck muscles, or impingement on cerebellar or brainstem portions of the dystonia motor network. Therefore, whether such lesions should be viewed as a pseudodystonia or true dystonia remains unclear. Regardless of their classification, they are important to recognize because removal of the mass may reverse the abnormal postures.[41,67]

Abnormal postures of the trunk may occur in Parkinson disease and related parkinsonian disorders such as progressive supranuclear palsy or corticobasal degeneration (see Chapter 13, "Dystonia and Parkinsonism").[2,18,53,70] Severe flexion of the spine is sometimes called camptocormia, and lateral bending may be called Pisa syndrome. The pathogenesis of postural problems associated with parkinsonism is complex, with different cases reflecting orthopedic defects, dystonia, myopathy with muscle weakness, or primary defects in postural control. Some of these abnormalities resemble truncal dystonia, and it is not clear if they should be given the label of pseudodystonia.

SYNOPSIS AND FUTURE PROSPECTS

Abnormal postures or movements may sometimes occur in orthopedic disorders or neuromuscular disorders, in disorders of sensory pathways, as behavioral compensations, and as disorders of mixed or unknown etiology. Although the abnormal postures or movements may closely resemble those of dystonia, they are sometimes labeled pseudodystonias because their etiologies and underlying biological mechanisms are thought to differ from those of true dystonias. Since the biological mechanisms responsible for dystonia are not fully understood, some ambiguities remain regarding which disorders should be labeled pseudodystonias versus true dystonias. In view of these ambiguities, expert opinions differ regarding the types of disorders that might be called pseudodystonia.

Despite the long historical precedent, the continued value of the term *pseudodystonia* in the future may be questioned for several reasons. One is that expert opinions on disorders to include as pseudodystonias vary, and differences of opinion are challenging to resolve without a more complete understanding of the biological basis for dystonia. In addition, the prefix *pseudo* (false) has been discouraged in other neurological disorders because patients may readily misinterpret the label. For example, the term *pseudoseizure* has been replaced by the term *non-epileptic seizures.*

In general, the main value of the term *pseudodystonia* is to call attention to the differential diagnosis of the many potential etiologies of abnormal muscle activity leading to abnormal postures and movements. Because of ambiguities among expert opinions and potential misinterpretation by patients, it may be best to avoid the term *pseudodystonia*, and focus attention instead on differential diagnosis.

REFERENCES

1. Albanese A, Bhatia K, Bressman SB, DeLong MR, Fahn S, Fung VSC, et al. Phenomenology and classification of dystonia: A consensus update. Mov Disord 2013;28:863–873.
2. Ali F, Matsumoto JY, Hassan A. Camptocormia: Etiology, diagnosis, and treatment response. Neurol Clin Pract 2018;8:240–248.
3. Avanzino L, Fiorio M. Proprioceptive dysfunction in focal dystonia: From experimental evidence to rehabilitation strategies. Front Hum Neurosci 2014;8:1000.
4. Ballock RT, Song KM. The prevalence of nonmuscular causes of torticollis in children. J Pediatr Orthop 1996;16:500–504.
5. Berlot R, Bhatia KP, Kojovic M. Pseudodystonia: A new perspective on an old phenomenon. Parkinsonism Relat Disord 2019;62:44–50.
6. Bhandutia AK, Nangunoori R, Whiting DM, Sangimino MJ. Scoliosis secondary to dystonia: A case report and review of the literature. JBJS Case Connect 2017;7:e47.
7. Boisen E. Torticollis caused by an infratentorial tumour: Three cases. Br J Psychiatry 1979;134:306–307.
8. Bove M, Brichetto G, Abbruzzese G, Marchese R, Schieppati M. Postural responses to continuous unilateral neck muscle vibration in standing patients with cervical dystonia. Mov Disord 2007;22:498–503.
9. Bredenkamp JK, Maceri DR. Inflammatory torticollis in children. Arch Otolaryngol Head Neck Surg 1990;116:310–313.
10. Burguera JA, Bataller L, Valero C. Action hand dystonia after cortical parietal infarction. Mov Disord 2001;16:1183–1185.
11. Chawda SJ, Munchau A, Johnson D, Bhatia K, Quinn NP, Stevens J, et al. Pattern of premature degenerative changes of the cervical spine in patients with spasmodic torticollis and the impact on the outcome of selective peripheral denervation. J Neurol Neurosurg Psychiatry 2000;68:465–471.
12. Conte A, Defazio G, Hallett M, Fabbrini G, Berardelli A. The role of sensory information in the pathophysiology of focal dystonias. Nat Rev Neurol 2019;15:224–233.
13. da Cunha Pereira G, de Oliveira Lemos I, Dalbosco Gadenz C, Cassol M. Effects of voice therapy on muscle tension dysphonia: A systematic literature review. J Voice 2018;32:546–552.
14. Defazio G, Abbruzzese G, Girlanda P, Buccafusca M, Curra A, Marchese R, et al. Primary cervical dystonia and scoliosis: A multicenter case-control study. Neurology 2003;60:1012–1015.
15. Do TT. Congenital muscular torticollis: Current concepts and review of treatment. Curr Opin Pediatr 2006;18:26–29.
16. Domenech J, Tormos JM, Barrios C, Pascual-Leone A. Motor cortical hyperexcitability in idiopathic scoliosis: Could focal dystonia be a subclinical etiological factor? Eur Spine J 2010;19:223–230.
17. Drost G, Verrips A, van Engelen BG, Stegeman DF, Zwarts MJ. Involuntary painful muscle contractions in Satoyoshi syndrome: A surface electromyographic study. Mov Disord 2006;21:2015–2018.
18. Du W, Bain PG, Defazio G, Jankovic J, Kim CY, Tan EK, et al. The conundrum of dystonia in essential tremor patients: How does one classify these cases? Tremor Other Hyperkinet Mov 2022;12:15.
19. Fabbrini G, Defazio G, Colosimo C, Thompson PD, Berardelli A. Cranial movement disorders: Clinical features, pathophysiology, differential diagnosis and treatment. Nat Clin Pract Neurol 2009;5:93–105.
20. Fahn S, Bressman SB, Marsden CD. Classification of dystonia. Adv Neurol 1998;78:1–10.

21. Felicio AC, Godeiro-Junior Cde O, Borges V, Silva SM, Ferraz HB. Bilateral hemifacial spasm: A series of 10 patients with literature review. Parkinsonism Relat Disord 2008;14:154–156.
22. Fricka KB, Kim C, Newton PO. Spinal lordosis with marked opisthotonus secondary to dystonia musculorum deformans: Case report with surgical management. Spine 2001;26:2283–2288.
23. Furukawa Y, Kish SJ, Lang AE. Scoliosis in a dopa-responsive dystonia family with a mutation of the GTP cyclohydrolase I gene. Neurology 2000;54:2187.
24. Ghika J, Ghika-Schmid F, Bogousslasvky J. Parietal motor syndrome: A clinical description in 32 patients in the acute phase of pure parietal strokes studied prospectively. Clin Neurol Neurosurg 1998;100:271–282.
25. Grey EG. Studies on the localization of cerebellar tumors. Ann Surg 1916;63:129–139.
26. Hutto SK, Harrison TB. Electrodiagnostic assessment of hyperexcitable nerve disorders. Neurol Clin 2021;39:1083–1096.
27. Iaccarino C, Francesca O, Piero S, Monica R, Armando R, de Bonis P, et al. Grisel's syndrome: Non-traumatic atlantoaxial totatory subluxation-report of five cases and review of the literature. Acta Neurochir Suppl 2019;125:279–288.
28. Jacob PC, Chand RP. Blepharospasm and jaw closing dystonia after parietal infarcts. Mov Disord 1995;10:794–795.
29. Jankovic J, Stone L. Dystonic tics in patients with Tourette's syndrome. Mov Disord 1991;6:248–252.
30. Jinnah HA, Visser JE, Harris JC, Verdu A, Larovere L, Ceballos-Picot I, et al. Delineation of the motor disorder of Lesch-Nyhan disease. Brain 2006;129:1201–1217.
31. Jung HJ, Choi SM, Kim BC. Hemidystonia as an initial manifestation of leptomeningeal metastasis. J Mov Disord 2009;2:82–85.
32. Kaji R, Rothwell JC, Katayama M, Ikeda T, Kubori T, Kohara N, et al. Tonic vibration reflex and muscle afferent block in writer's cramp. Ann Neurol 1995;38:155–162.
33. Kanekar S. Atlantoaxial dislocation in idiopathic cervical dystonia. Neurol India 2004;1:124–125.
34. Kariminejad A, Dahl-Halvarsson M, Ravenscroft G, Afroozan F, Keshavarz E, Goullee H, et al. TOR1A variants cause a severe arthrogryposis with developmental delay, strabismus and tremor. Brain 2017;140:2851–2859.
35. Khan AA, Sussman JD. Focal dystonia after removal of a parietal meningioma. Mov Disord 2004;19:714–716.
36. Kim JW, Lee PH. Dystonic head tremor associated with a parietal lesion. Eur J Neurol 2007;14:e32–33.
37. Kodama N, Sanuki T, Miyamoto T, Tashiro J. Effects and differences of voice therapy on spasmodic dysphonia and muscle tension dysphonia: A retrospective pilot study. J Voice 2024;38:129–135.
38. Konrad C, Vollmer-Haase J, Anneken K, Knecht S. Orthopedic and neurological complications of cervical dystonia: Review of the literature. Acta Neurol Scand 2004;109:369–373.
39. Koul R, Al-Yarubi S, Al-Kindy H, Al-Futaisi A, Al-Thihli K, Chacko PA, Sankhla D. Rigid spinal muscular dystrophy and rigid spine syndrome: Report of 7 children. J Child Neurol 2014;29:1436–1440.
40. Krauss JK, Mohadjer M, Nobbe F, Scheremet R. Hemidystonia due to a contralateral parieto-occipital metastasis: Disappearance after removal of the mass lesion. Neurology 1991;41:1519–1520.
41. Krauss JK, Seeger W, Jankovic J. Cervical dystonia associated with tumors of the posterior fossa. Mov Disord 1997;12:443–447.
42. Kumandas S, Per H, Gumus H, Tucer B, Yikilmaz A, Kontas O, et al. Torticollis secondary to posterior fossa and cervical spinal cord tumors: Report of five cases and literature review. Neurosurg Rev 2006;29:333–338.
43. Lange LM, Junker J, Loens S, Baumann H, Olschewski L, Schaake S, et al. Genotype-phenotype relations for isolated dystonia genes: MDSGene systematic review. Mov Disord 2021;36:1086–1103.
44. Lawrence WT, Azizkhan RG. Congenital muscular torticollis: A spectrum of pathology. Ann Plast Surg 1989;23:523–530.
45. Leis AA, Dimitrijevic MR, Delapasse JS, Sharkey PC. Modification of cervical dystonia by selective sensory stimulation. J Neurol Sci 1992;110:79–89.
46. Mella JR, Guo L, Hung V. Dupuytren's contracture: An evidence based review. Ann Plast Surg 2018;81:S97–S101.
47. Merlini L, Granata C, Ballestrazzi A, Marini ML. Rigid spine syndrome and rigid spine sign in myopathies. J Child Neurol 1989;4:274–282.
48. Morano A, Fanella M, Giallonardo AT, Di Bonaventura C. Faciobrachial dystonic seizures: The borderland between epilepsy and movement disorders. Mov Disord Clin Pract 2020;7:228–229.
49. Muthusamy S, Foroush NC, Seneviratne U. Faciobrachial motor seizures: A more apt description? Epilepsy Behav Rep 2021;16:100476.
50. Neychev VK, Gross R, Lehericy S, Hess EJ, Jinnah HA. The functional neuroanatomy of dystonia. Neurobiol Dis 2011;42:185–201.
51. O'Riordan S, Lynch T, Hutchinson M. Familial adolescent-onset scoliosis and later segmental dystonia in an Irish family. J Neurol 2004;251:845–848.
52. Park CW, Chung SJ, Sohn YH, Lee PH. A case of abnormal postures in the left extremities after pontine hemorrhage: Dystonia or pseudodystonia? J Mov Disord 2020;13:62–65.
53. Rabin ML, Earnhardt MC, Patel A, Ganihong I, Kurlan R. Postural, bone, and joint disorders in Parkinson's disease. Mov Disord Clin Pract 2016;3:538–547.
54. Radhakrishnan DM, Goyal V, Shukla G, Singh MB, Ramam M. Hemi masticatory spasm: Series of 7 cases and review of literature. Mov Disord Clin Pract 2019;6:316–319.
55. Reichert SC, Gonzalez-Alegre P, Scharer GH. Biallelic TOR1A variants in an infant with severe arthrogryposis. Neurol Genet 2017;3:e154.
56. Revuelta GJ, Benatar M, Freeman A, Wichmann T, Jinnah HA, Delong MR, Factor SA. Clinical subtypes of anterocollis in parkinsonian syndromes. J Neurol Sci 2011;315:100–103.
57. Revuelta GJ, Montilla J, Benatar M, Freeman A, Wichmann T, Jinnah HA, et al. An (18)F-FDG PET study of cervical muscle in parkinsonian anterocollis. J Neurol Sci 2014;340:174–177.
58. Rosales RL, Dressler D. On muscle spindles, dystonia and botulinum toxin. Eur J Neurol 2010;17 Suppl 1:71–80.
59. Sansone VA. The dystrophic and nondystrophic myotonias. Continuum (Minneap Minn) 2016;22:1889–1915.
60. Sarva H, Deik A, Ullah A, Severt WL. Clinical spectrum of stiff person syndrome: A Review of recent reports. Tremor Other Hyperkinet Mov 2016;6:340.

61. Savica R, Kumar N, Ahlskog JE, Josephs KA, Matsumoto JY, McKeon A. Parkinsonism and dropped head: Dystonia, myopathy or both? Parkinsonism Relat Disord 2012;18:30–34.
62. Stamelou M, Lai SC, Aggarwal A, Schneider SA, Houlden H, Yeh TH, et al. Dystonic opisthotonus: A "red flag" for neurodegeneration with brain iron accumulation syndromes? Mov Disord 2013;28:1325–1329.
63. Swash M, Czesnik D, de Carvalho M. Muscular cramp: Causes and management. Eur J Neurol 2019;26:214–221.
64. Szejko N, Jakubczyk A, Dunalska A, Janik P. Dystonic tics in patients with Gilles de la Tourette syndrome. Neurol Neurochir Pol 2019;53:335–340.
65. Tai CH, Lee WT, Tseng SH. DYT6 dystonia mimicking adolescent idiopathic scoliosis successfully treated by pallidal stimulation. Int Med Case Rep J 2021;14:315–321.
66. Tranchant C, Bhatia KP, Marsden CD. Movement disorders in multiple sclerosis. Mov Disord 1995;10:418–423.
67. Turgut M, Akalan N, Bertan V, Erbengi A, Eryilmaz M. Acquired torticollis as the only presenting symptom in children with posterior fossa tumors. Childs Nerv Syst 1995;11:86–88.
68. Uncini A, Di Muzio A, Thomas A, Lugaresi A, Gambi D. Hand dystonia secondary to cervical demyelinating lesion. Mov Disord 1996;11:96–99.
69. Vengoechea J, Li H, Jinnah HA. Identical twins with progressive kyphoscoliosis and opthalmoplegia: Exerpt commentary. Parkinsonis Rel Disord 2021;92: 123–124.
70. Wijemanne S, Jankovic J. Hand, foot, and spine deformities in parkinsonian disorders. J Neural Transm 2019;126:253–264.
71. Willoughby KL, Ang SG, Thomason P, Rutz E, Shore B, Buckland AJ, et al. Epidemiology of scoliosis in cerebral palsy: A population-based study at skeletal maturity. J Paediatr Child Health 2022;58:295–301.

SECTION V

Clinical Management

Chapter 27

Workup of Dystonia

INTRODUCTION

The dystonias encompass a broad group of heterogeneous conditions (see Chapter 2, "Defining the Clinical Features of Dystonia"). The clinical heterogeneity is classified according to several features including age at onset, body region affected, certain temporal and phenomenological characteristics, and any relevant associated features (see Chapter 3, "Classification and Diagnostic Strategy for Dystonia").[1] The initial diagnosis of dystonia begins with delineating these clinical features in an attempt to identify a specific clinical syndrome.

The underlying causes and biological mechanisms responsible for dystonia also are quite heterogeneous. Many cases are idiopathic, but some are inherited or acquired.[16] There are hundreds of known genes and acquired causes. As a consequence of this clinical and biological heterogeneity, it is challenging to construct simple algorithms for the diagnostic workup of all individuals with dystonia. Numerous algorithms have been published, but most of them focus on specific subgroups such as adult-onset focal dystonias,[62] early-onset inherited dystonias,[4,8,10,61] or dystonias combined with specific features such as parkinsonism,[40] myoclonus,[38] or ataxia.[50] Only one prior review has attempted to comprehensively summarize the workup for all types of dystonia.[20] Despite the marked heterogeneity, delineating the underlying biological mechanisms is important, because some dystonias have mechanism-specific treatments (see Chapter 28, "Symptom-Targeted Oral Medications for Dystonia").

This chapter first summarizes the value of common clinical diagnostic tools in the workup of different types of dystonia including routine bloodwork, genetic studies, cerebrospinal fluid (CSF) studies, neuroimaging, and neurophysiology. A general framework for the workup of all types of dystonia is then provided, along with references to other chapters where a more detailed workup for specific types of dystonia is summarized in detail.

CLINICAL DIAGNOSTIC TESTS

Routine Bloodwork

Individuals with dystonia of all ages often have routine bloodwork conducted by their primary care provider before consultation with a specialist. Typical studies might include a complete blood count or a chemistry profile that includes electrolytes and other markers of liver or kidney function. Results most often return normal, or

Table 27.1 **Routine hematology findings**

Findings	Disorders	Cause(s)
Acanthocytes	Abetalipoproteinemia	*MTTP* gene
	Chorea-acanthocytosis	*VPS13A* gene
	Huntington disease-like 2	*JPH3* gene
	Mcleod syndrome	*XK* gene
	Panthothenate-kinase associated neurodegeneration	*PANK2* gene
Anemia	Aceruloplasminemia	*CP* gene
	Autoimmune disease	Immunological
	Beta-ketothiolase deficiency	*ACAT1* gene
	Gaucher disease	*GBA* gene
	GLUT1 deficiency	*GLUT1* gene
	Lesch-Nyhan disease	*HPRT1* gene
	Mitochondrial disease	many genes
	Phosphoglycerate kinase deficiency	*PGK1* gene
	Triosephosphate isomerase deficiency	*TPI1* gene
	Wilson disease	*ATP7B* gene
Leukopenia	Ataxia telangiectasia	*ATM* gene
	Gaucher disease	*GBA* gene
	Fumarate hydratase deficiency	*FH* gene
Polycythemia	Manganese transporter deficiency	*SLC39A14, SLC30A10* genes
	Fumarate hydratase deficiency	*MTTP* gene
Thrombocytopenia	Aceruloplasminemia	*VPS13A* gene
	Aicardi-Goutieres syndrome	*JPH3* gene
	Systemic autoimmune disease	*XK* gene
	Beta-ketothiolase deficiency	*PANK2* gene
	Gaucher disease	*CP* gene
	Manganese transporter deficiency	Immunological
	Methylmalonic aciduria	*ACAT1* gene
	Niemann-Pick type C	*GBA* gene
	Wilson disease	*GLUT1* gene

Adapted from a prior review.[20]

they may disclose incidental findings not related to dystonia. Nevertheless, some findings from these routine studies may have diagnostic significance. All these findings are associated with very rare forms of dystonia, but some may have specific treatments so the bloodwork should be reviewed with these special conditions in mind.

From the complete blood count, there is often an automated blood smear that reports on acanthocytes, which may be relevant for dystonia seen in neuroacanthocytosis, panthothenate kinase-associated neurodegeneration, and a few other disorders (Table 27.1).[2,54] Automated measures of acanthocytes are subject to numerous technical difficulties, with high rates of false-positive and false-negative findings, so any suspicious findings must be verified. Other rare genetic dystonias may be associated with anemia, or there may be increases or decreases in leukocytes or platelets (Table 27.1). Therefore, any unexplained finding in the blood count may merit further attention. Additional details regarding some of these conditions can be found in the Chapter 18, "Dystonia Combined with Other Features."

A standard blood chemistry profile may also disclose relevant findings (Table 27.2). For example, some types of dystonia such as Wilson disease are associated with liver disease so abnormalities suggestive of liver disease merit attention.[3] Abnormalities suggestive of renal dysfunction can also provide a clue. An increase in creatine phosphokinase can indicate rhabdomyolysis in severe generalized dystonia, particularly with dystonic storm,[9] or with certain drug exposures, such as phencyclidine.[37] Other enzymes from muscle may also be elevated. Creatine phosphokinase and related enzymes are also variably elevated in mitochondrial disorders with dystonia and in chorea-acanthocytosis. Uric acid is often included in routine chemistry profiles, and

Table 27.2 **Routine blood chemistry findings**

Findings	Disorders	Cause(s)
Bilirubin	Kernicterus (↑)	Neonatal hemolysis
Calcium	Hypocalcemia	Many causes
	Hypoparathyroidism	Idiopathic, autoimmune
Glucose	GLUT1 deficiency (↓)	*GLUT1* gene
	Non-ketotic hyperglycemia (↑)	Diabetes mellitus
Liver enzymes (AST, ALT)	Manganese transporter deficiency (↑)	*SLC39A14* and *SLC30A10* genes
	Mitochondrial disorders (↑)	Many different genes
	Wilson disease (↑)	*ATP7B* gene
Liver function (albumin)	Ataxia with oculomotor apraxia type 1 (↓)	*APTX* gene
	Ataxia with oculomotor apraxia type 4 (↓)	*PNKP* gene
Muscle enzymes (CPK)	Ataxia with oculomotor apraxia type 2 (↑)	*SETX* gene
	Ataxia with oculomotor apraxia type 4 (↑)	*PNKP* gene
	Chorea-acanthocytosis (↑)	*VPS13A* gene
	Drug toxicity (↑)	Phencyclidine, psychostimulants, and others
	Dystonic storm or status dystonicus (↑↑)	Any cause of severe dystonia
	McLeod syndrome (↑)	*VPS13A* gene
	Mitochondrial disorders (↑)	Many different genes
	Neuroleptic malignant syndrome (↑↑)	Dopamine receptor blocking drugs
	Severe tardive dyskinesia (↑)	Dopamine receptor blocking drugs
Renal function tests (BUN, Cr)	Lesch-Nyhan disease (↑)	*HPRT1* gene
	Mitochondrial disorders (↑)	Many different genes

Adapted from prior reviews.[20,61] The arrows show the typical direction of change.

Abbreviations: ALT, alanine aminotransferase; AST, aspartate aminotransferase; BUN, blood urea nitrogen; CPK, creatine phosphokinase; Cr, creatine

increased values in adults are commonly caused by coincidental conditions. However, increased uric acid is very uncommon in children and may suggest Lesch-Nyhan disease.[27]

Special Blood Tests

A number of other widely available blood tests may also be requested when the clinical phenotype points more specifically to certain disorders (Table 27.3). For all early-onset dystonias, a serum ceruloplasmin is essential because dystonia is common in Wilson disease and it is treatable.[3] The vast majority of Wilson disease patients become symptomatic before adolescence, so a serum ceruloplasmin is not usually assessed in adults older than 50. However, certain clinical features may raise concern for this disorder even among adults, and there are rare cases reported to present as late as 50–80 years of age.[14]

Serum antibody panels may be warranted if the clinical phenotype raises suspicion for an autoimmune dystonia (see Chapter 21, "Dystonia and Autoimmunity"). Serum alfa-fetoprotein and immunoglobulin studies may be useful if clinical features suggest ataxia telangiectasia presenting with dystonia. There is a high risk of autoimmune thyroid disease among adults with cervical[29] or laryngeal dystonias,[44] so some authorities also recommend thyroid studies in all adult-onset focal dystonias.[62]

Genetic Tests

Genetic testing has been playing an increasingly important role in the diagnostic process for the dystonias, and its value depends closely on the elements of the clinical phenotype, such as age at onset, whether there are additional clinical abnormalities, and whether there is a family history (see Chapter 22, "Dystonia Genetics"). For the most common types of focal dystonia that emerge in adults, genetic testing is not typically conducted because the chance of finding an abnormal result has been estimated to be less than 5%.[62] For adults, genetic testing is considered only when there is a family history or when

Table 27.3 **Special blood chemistry tests**

Findings	Disorders	Cause(s)
Alfa fetoprotein	Ataxia telangiectasia (↑)	*ATM* gene
	Ataxia with oculomotor apraxia type 1 (↑)	*SETX* gene
	Ataxia with oculomotor apraxia type 2 (↑)	*APTX* gene
	Ataxia with oculomotor apraxia type 4 (↑)	*PNKP* gene
Amino acids	Amino acidurias and organic acidurias	Multiple genes
Antibodies	Autoimmune encephalitis associated with neuronal autoantibodies (↑)	Encephalitis associated with antibodies against aquaporin4, CASPR2, CRMP5, GABA(A)R, IGLON5, LGI1, Ma2, NMDAR, Ri
	Rheumatological disorders associated with ANA, SSA, SSB, or dsdna (↑)	Systemic lupus erythematosus, Sjögren's syndrome
Ceruloplasmin	Aceruloplasminemia (↓↓)	*CP* gene
	Wilson disease (↓)	*ATP7B* gene
Copper	Wilson disease (↑)	*ATP7B* gene
Cholestanol	Cerebrotendinous xanthomatosis (↑)	*CTX* gene
Erythrocyte or leukocyte enzyme assays	Numerous inherited metabolic disorders	Multiple genes
Ferritin	Neuroferritinopathy (↓)	*FTL1* gene
Guanidinoacetic acid	Cerebral creatine deficiency (↓)	*AGAT* gene
	Cerebral creatine deficiency (↑)	*GAMT* gene
Immunoglobulins	Ataxia telangiectasia igg and iga (↓)	*ATM* gene
Organic acids	Organic acidurias	Many genes
Lactic acid	Mitochondrial disorders (↑)	Many different genes
	Hypoxia-ischemia (↑)	Hypotension, hypoxia
Lipids	Abetalipoproteinemia (↓)	*MTTP* gene
Manganese	Environmental exposure (↑)	Welding
	Ephedrine toxicity (↑)	Drug toxicity
	Manganese transporter deficiencies (↑)	*SLC39A14* and *SLC30A10* genes
Thyroid function tests (TSH, T4)	Adult-onset cervical dystonia (↓)	Frequent coexisting autoimmune disease
	Adult-onset laryngeal dystonia (↓)	Frequent coexisting autoimmune disease
	Allan-Herndon-Dudley syndrome (↑)	*MCT8* gene
Toxicology screen	Neuroleptics, psychostimulants, other toxins (↑)	Intentional or accidental drug exposure
Vitamin E	Ataxia with vitamin E deficiency (↓)	*TTPA* gene

Adapted from prior reviews.[20,56,61]
The arrows show the typical direction of change.

additional clinical features raise suspicion for a genetic etiology.

The approach to genetic testing differs in early-onset dystonias where the chance of finding an abnormal result is 20–30% and continues to rise.[17,36,48,68] Strategies for selecting the most appropriate genetic tests have evolved considerably in recent years, due to constant advances in genetic technologies.[19,43,63] These strategies are summarized here and described in more detail in the Chapter 22. Single-gene testing may be the most efficient and cost-effective strategy for early-onset dystonias where there is a diagnostic "red flag" or syndromic pattern that points to a specific disorder. Examples of red flags include the Kaiser-Fleischer ring in Wilson disease, ocular telangiectasias in ataxia-telangiectasia, and tendon xanthomas in cerebrotendinous xanthomatosis. An example of a highly specific syndromic pattern is Lesch-Nyhan disease, where a very specific combination of clinical features (dystonia, self-injurious behavior, and high uric acid) is quite unique.[26]

Although single-gene testing may be appropriate in some situations, diagnostic red flags and syndromic patterns are lacking for many types of dystonia or they are easily overlooked. Red flags and syndromic patterns also require a high level of expertise to learn and remember, atypical presentations are common, and tell-tale features are sometimes missing where they are expected. It is important to avoid sequential testing of one gene at a time. This strategy is time-consuming, expensive, and frustrating to affected individuals and families.[28,34,53]

With constant improvements in genetic testing, there has been increasing enthusiasm for broader genetic tests. Dystonia gene panels have been recommended, but there is growing recognition that whole-exome or genome sequencing may be preferred (see Chapter 22). If a gene panel is used, it is important to know what it includes. Gene panels vary widely in their coverage, from a handful of genes to more than 100. One study of over 1,000 exomes from individuals with undiagnosed dystonia reported that many of the genes found were not included in typical dystonia panels but were found instead in panels for neurodevelopmental delay, spasticity, or ataxia.[17] If clinical exome testing is used, it may be useful to consult with an expert in neurogenetics to aid in the interpretation of results.

Urine Tests

Urine tests can also sometimes provide clues for diagnosis of a disorder that includes dystonia (Table 27.4). The standard urinalysis most often reveals incidental findings, but stones are suspicious, especially when they are found in a young child. However, there are special tests that may be requested when the clinical phenotype warrants them, such as a toxicology screen or tests for amino acids or organic acids. These specialized tests may also be useful when a variant of unknown significance in a potentially relevant gene needs to be corroborated.

Cerebrospinal Fluid

Studies of CSF are not usually a part of the routine workup for most individuals with dystonia, but they may be useful in certain circumstances. In adults, CSF studies may be warranted when there is concern for an autoimmune dystonia because findings from CSF are more specific than findings from blood (see Chapter 21).

Among children, low CSF glucose can be useful for identifying GLUT1 deficiency.[21,45] Some experts recommend CSF studies for the detection of suspected neurotransmitter disorders, most notably dopa-responsive dystonia.[7,32] However, CSF neurotransmitter studies can be technically challenging because of the need to collect and ship samples rapidly, with tubes containing special preservatives. In addition, test results can be difficult to interpret because of issues relating to sensitivity and specificity and overlap of findings among some disorders (Table 27.5). Currently, genetic testing may be the place to start for neurotransmitter disorders, with CSF studies playing a confirmatory role if needed.

Neuroimaging

The diagnostic value of neuroimaging depends on elements of the classification plan for all dystonias, most notably age at onset (see Chapter 3). For dystonia that begins at a young age, brain imaging is mandatory because it is likely to disclose relevant abnormalities that may guide further workup. MRI is the preferred imaging

Table 27.4 **Special urine chemistry tests**

Findings	Disorders	Cause(s)
Amino acids	Amino acidurias (↑)	Multiple genes
Copper, 24h	Wilson disease (↑)	*ATP7B* gene
Guanidinoacetic acid	Cerebral creatine deficiency (↓)	*AGAT* gene
	Cerebral creatine deficiency (↑)	*GAMT* gene
Organic acids	Organic acidurias (↑)	Multiple genes
Toxicology screen	Neuroleptics, psychostimulants, other toxins (↑)	Intentional or accidental exposure
Uric acid	Lesch-Nyhan disease (↑)	*HPRT1* gene

Adapted from prior reviews.[20,56,61]
The arrows show the typical direction of change.

Table 27.5 **Cerebrospinal fluid for neurotransmitter disorders**

	Neurotransmitter metabolites					Pterin metabolites				
Gene	**HVA**	**5HIAA**	**MHPG**	**3OMD**	**5HTP**	**Biop**	**BH2**	**BH4**	**Neop**	**NH2**
AADC	↓	↓	↓	↑	↑	N	N	N	N	N
DHPR	↓	↓	↓	N	N	↑	↑	↓	N	N or ↓
DNAJC	↓	↓	N	N	N	N	N	↑	↓	N
GCH1	N or ↓	N or ↓	↓	N	N	N or ↓	↑	↓	N or ↓	↓
PTPS	↓	↓	↓	N	N	↓	N	↓	↑	↑
SR	↓	↓	↓	N	N	↑	↑	↓	N	N
SLC6A3	↑	N	N	N	N	N	N	N	N	N
TH	↓	N	↓	N	N	N	N	N	N	N
VMAT2	↑	N	↑	N	N	N	N	N	N	N

Adapted from prior reviews.[7,65] Arrows show the direction of change as increased (↑) or decreased (↓) or no change (N). The left column shows the gene responsible for neurotransmitter disorders that are sometimes associated with dystonia, often with other neurological features.

Abbreviations: 3OMD, 3-O-methyl dopa; 5HIAA, 5-hydroxyindole acetic acid; 5HTP, 5-hydroxytryptophan; Biop, biopterin; BH2, dihydrobiopterin; BH4, tetrahydrobiopterin; HVA, homovanillic acid; Neop, neopterin; NH2, dihydroneopterin. Additional CSF findings for other types of dystonia may include high lactic acid (mitochondrial disease, hypoxia-ischemia), low glucose (GLUT1 deficiency), low folate (cerebral folate deficiency), low creatine and guanidinoacetate (cerebral creatine deficiency), elevated organic acids (glutaric aciduria, methylmalonic aciduria, propionic aciduria), a diffuse or more specific increase in immunoglobulins (autoimmune disorders), and others.

modality unless there is concern for brain calcium deposition, when CT may be useful. There are characteristic findings on brain MRI for individuals with dystonia related to cerebral palsy acquired from pediatric stroke, hypoxic-ischemic encephalopathy, or kernicterus (see Chapter 16, "Dystonia and Cerebral Palsy").[39] The brain MRI may alternatively show findings characteristic of dystonia resulting from one of many genetic disorders that affect the basal ganglia. One comprehensive study used cluster analysis to identify four distinct imaging patterns that were defined by involvement of mostly putamen, mostly pallidum, both putamen and pallidum together, or whether there was accompanying abnormalities in the brainstem and cerebellum (see Chapter 13, "Dystonia and Parkinsonism").[39] In addition, some findings are highly suggestive of specific disorders or groups of disorders, such as the "eye of the tiger" sign for neurodegeneration with brain iron accumulation.

For the most common types of dystonia that begin in adults (cervical dystonia, blepharospasm, laryngeal dystonia), brain imaging often reveals incidental findings of uncertain relevance. It has therefore been suggested that brain imaging is not required in the workup of these cases.[25,62] However, brain MRI is useful for adults who have hemidystonia or generalized dystonia because these patterns are more often associated with structural lesions.[41,64] Brain MRI may also be informative for adults who have unusually rapid progression of their dystonia, particularly if it is combined with other unexplained features such as parkinsonism, ataxia, or dementia.

For cervical dystonia, imaging of the cervical spine often reveals findings suggestive of degenerative joint disease of the spine.[11,30] Cervical dystonia may rarely be caused by lesions of the cervical spinal cord, especially in children. Individuals with multiple sclerosis may also develop focal dystonia or paroxysmal dystonic spasms.[18,31,49,51,57,59] For laryngeal dystonia, laryngoscopy is useful for imaging the vocal apparatus because it can disclose structural or functional anomalies that may mimic spasmodic dysphonia.[35]

Many types of dystonia in both children and adults have been linked with dysfunction of dopamine pathways, leading to questions regarding the utility of dopamine transporter imaging studies via single photon emission tomography. This clinical imaging modality is only rarely used for dystonia. However, because adult-onset limb dystonia may be a presenting feature of Parkinson disease, dopamine transporter imaging may be useful to discriminate idiopathic limb dystonia from early Parkinson disease in some cases.[33]

Neurophysiology

Electromyography (EMG) can be used to detect several physiological characteristics of dystonia including co-contraction of antagonistic muscles, excessive muscle contraction, overflow of muscle contraction to nearby regions, and repetitive bursting activity.[13,15,23,66] None of these features is specific to dystonia, so EMG does not provide a practical diagnostic tool (see Chapter 24, "Dystonia Physiology"). The main role of EMG in the workup is to rule out other disorders that sometimes mimic dystonia, such as myotonia or neuromyotonia, and stiff person syndrome (see Chapter 26, "Pseudodystonia and Differential Diagnosis").

Nerve conduction studies (NCS) often reveal coincidental findings in adults with dystonia, where neuropathy is very common. However, NCS abnormalities among children with dystonia may point to neuropathy associated with several rare conditions including mitochondrial disorders, lysosomal storage disorders, chorea-acanthocytosis, ataxia-oculomotor apraxia, or a spinocerebellar ataxia (see Chapter 18).[20]

The physiological abnormalities underlying dystonia cannot be detected with routine clinical electroencephalography (EEG), so it does not usually play a role in the diagnostic workup of most dystonias. Nevertheless, EEG may be valuable in certain circumstances. It is frequently applied in the paroxysmal dyskinesias, where discrete attacks often raise concern for epilepsy (see Chapter 17, "Dystonia and the Paroxysmal Dyskinesias"). EEG can also be useful when there is concern that intermittent tonic or twisting movements have an epileptic basis, as in faciobrachial dystonic seizures (see Chapter 21). Occasionally, EEG is useful to document dystonia coexisting with epilepsy.

SELECTING TESTS ACCORDING TO DYSTONIA SYNDROME

Adults Versus Children

Selection of the most appropriate clinical diagnostic tests varies for adults versus children. For adults older than 50 years, no clinical diagnostic tests are needed for most of the common focal dystonias, and laboratory testing is performed only in certain circumstances. For children, some workup is almost always required. The main reason for this difference is that the vast majority of individuals with adult-onset focal dystonias are idiopathic, and a cause is not often found even after extensive diagnostic testing. By comparison, children are more likely to have a discoverable cause, and some have specific treatments.

Adult-Onset Dystonias

An algorithm for the general workup for adult-onset dystonias is provided in Figure 27.1. The first step is to perform a history and examination to verify that the individual has features consistent with dystonia rather than a condition that mimics dystonia. Typical features of dystonia and its potential mimics are summarized in Chapter 2, "Defining the Clinical Features of Dystonia." The second step addresses acquired

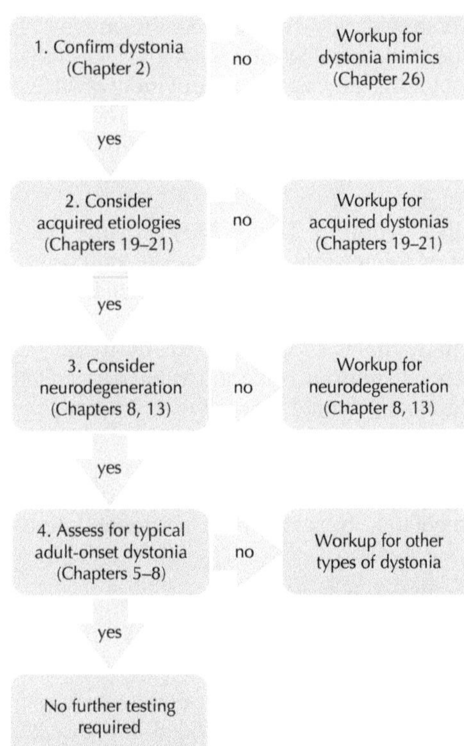

Figure 27.1. Algorithm for workup of adult-onset dystonias. This algorithm was adapted from prior work,[62] and provides only a very general overview. Further details regarding each step are indicated in detailed tables provided in other chapters noted in the diagram.

forms of dystonia such as exposure to medications or toxins, autoimmune diseases, stroke, or other space-occupying lesions. These conditions may require toxicology studies (see Chapter 19, "Dystonia Induced by Medications, Illicit Drugs, and Environmental Toxins"), antibody studies (see Chapter 21), or neuroimaging. The third step also involves considering neuroimaging studies for certain neurodegenerative disorders because they sometimes present as adult-onset focal dystonia, most often involving a limb (see Chapter 13, "Dystonia and Parkinsonism," and Chapter 8, "Limb Dystonias").

The next step is to consider whether the clinical phenotype is consistent with one of the common adult-onset focal dystonias. Details regarding each of these common forms of dystonia are summarized in Chapters 5 through 10. The assessment should address key elements from the dystonia classification system because they help to guide the diagnostic workup. These elements include age at onset, body distribution of dystonia, certain temporal and phenomenological features, and whether there are any relevant associated neurological or systemic features (see Chapter 3). The vast majority of individuals with adult-onset dystonia will fall in the group of focal or segmental dystonia with no additional clinical features, and they do not require any diagnostic testing.[62]

This algorithm (Figure 27.1) provides only a general framework for guiding the workup, and its limitations must be acknowledged. For example, adults with unusual patterns of involvement (hemidystonia or generalized dystonia) and those with unusual evolution (rapid or persistent progression) should proceed with antibody testing or neuroimaging (Step 4). Similarly, it is not necessary to consider and test for acquired etiologies (Step 2) if the clinical phenotype points immediately to a potential neurodegenerative cause (Step 3).

Childhood-Onset Dystonia

A schematic showing the general workup for early-onset dystonias is provided in Figure 27.2. The initial step for children and adolescents is similar to that for adults and involves ruling out mimics of dystonia. Later steps differ because the most common discoverable causes in children differ from those of adults. Investigations for acquired dystonia in children must include

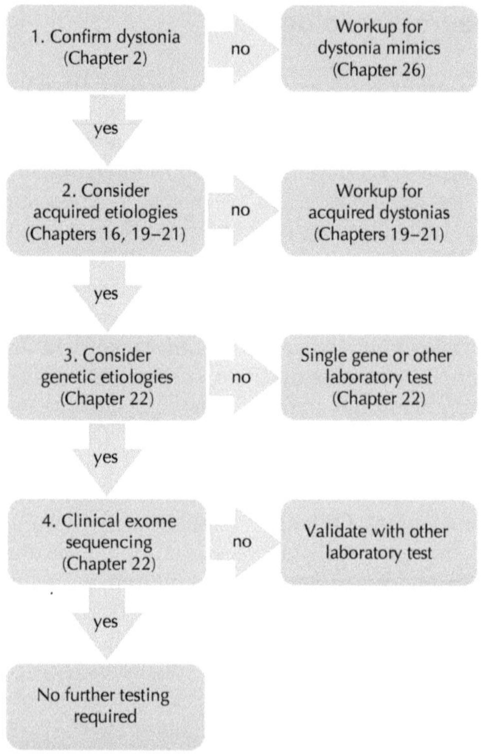

Figure 27.2. Algorithm for workup of early-onset dystonias. This algorithm was adapted from prior work,[61] and provides only a very general overview. Further details regarding each step are indicated in detailed tables provided in other chapters noted in the diagram.

brain MRI because cerebral palsy is the most common acquired dystonia, and there may be characteristic findings pointing to hypoxic-ischemic encephalopathy, stroke, or kernicterus (see Chapter 16). A trial of levodopa is mandatory because of its dramatic benefits for dopa-responsive dystonia. Following assessments for acquired dystonias and a levodopa trial, there is long list of additional genetic disorders where dystonia is usually combined with other neurological or systemic features and occasionally with isolated dystonia. A general overview of the workup for genetic dystonias is provided here, with further details summarized in Chapter 22.

Some experts advocate a strategy that begins with a careful history and exam, seeking red flags and syndromic patterns that point to a specific type of dystonia. Many of these conditions are described in Chapters 13, 14, 15, and 18. Blood tests may include organic acids, amino acids, glucose, alfa-fetoprotein, immunoglobulin or antibody studies, copper and manganese, creatine, vitamin E, uric acid, sphingomyelin, cholestanol, and biotinidase. Tests of CSF may include glucose, folate, and neurotransmitters. If a diagnosis is not forthcoming, genetic tests with broad coverage are used, such as dystonia gene panels or clinical exome sequencing.

This examination-based strategy is probably best suited for experts in neurogenetics. This strategy also has some recognized flaws. The most serious involves atypical phenotypes, which fool even experts. Other experts advocate laboratory tests that focus on types of dystonia where there are specific mechanism-based treatments (see Chapter 28). This narrower approach to diagnosis also has some flaws since there is clinical value in a definitive diagnosis even for conditions were mechanism-based treatments are lacking.

A more practical approach is to exploit exome sequencing earlier in the diagnostic workup, a strategy that often saves time and money.[63] This strategy may produce a diagnostic result, and the other laboratory tests may be used more selectively to evaluate the relevance of any variants of unknown significance. For example, a genetic variant of unknown significance in *GLUT1* may lead to a confirmatory study of CSF glucose.

Similar to the algorithmic workup of adults with dystonia (Figure 27.1), this algorithm for children (Figure 27.2) has some limitations, and exceptions must be acknowledged. For example, it is not necessary to consider and test for acquired etiologies (Step 2) if there are obvious red flags or a syndromic pattern that is suspicious for a specific genetic disorder.

SYNOPSIS AND FUTURE PROSPECTS

The dystonias are clinically and etiologically very heterogeneous. With a few exceptions where red flags or highly characteristic syndromic patterns can point to the diagnosis, there usually is no simple one-to-one correlation between the clinical phenotype of a specific syndrome and a specific cause. For most types of dystonia, the application of a methodical strategy is valuable to ensure a complete investigation of potential causes. The strategies differ for adults and children because their most common etiologies also differ. A thorough workup is valuable because some types of dystonia have life-altering therapies.

While some general algorithms may be proposed (Figure 27.1 and Figure 27.2), expert opinions vary regarding the best strategies. Recommended strategies have evolved in recent years, predominantly because of advances in clinical diagnostic methods such as clinical exome sequencing, novel neuroimaging methods, or antibody panels. These strategies will continue to evolve as diagnostic methods improve, but also as we learn more regarding the many different causes of dystonia.

Some biomarkers (blood, urine, neuroimaging) currently exist for certain very rare types of dystonia, but there are no widely available biomarkers suitable for the most common types of dystonia. The development of additional biomarkers could provide very valuable tools to aid in more rapid diagnosis. Over the years, numerous studies have attempted to measure dystonic movements using devices that detect movement.[5,6,22,24,42,46,52,55] However, these kinematic tools are cumbersome and not suitable for routine use in most clinics so they have not yet found their way into the standard clinical workup. More recently, others have proposed diagnostic tools based on digital analyses of videos taken of abnormal movements,[12,47,58] but they also are not widely available, and they have not been fully validated. Some neuroimaging biomarkers also have been proposed for the diagnosis of adult-onset focal dystonias,[60,67] but they also are not widely available and have not been independently validated. Further development of additional tools or biomarkers for diagnosis would be a great asset for future development.

REFERENCES

1. Albanese A, Bhatia K, Fung V, Hallett M, Jankovic J, et al. Definition and Classification of Dystonia, 2025 (first presented at the International Dystonia Symposium in 2023).
2. Bader B, Walker RH, Vogel M, Prosiegel M, McIntosh J, Danek A. Tongue protrusion and feeding dystonia: A hallmark of chorea-acanthocytosis. Mov Disord 2010;25:127–129.
3. Bandmann O, Weiss KH, Kaler SG. Wilson's disease and other neurological copper disorders. Lancet Neurol 2015;14:103–113.
4. Bertram KL, Williams DR. Diagnosis of dystonic syndromes-a new eight-question approach. Nat Rev Neurol 2012;8:275–283.
5. Beuter A, Legros A, Cif L, Coubes P. Quantifying motion in dystonic syndromes: The bare essentials. J Clin Neurophysiol 2004;21:209–214.

6. Boccagni C, Carpaneto J, Micera S, Bagnato S, Galardi G. Motion analysis in cervical dystonia. Neurol Sci 2008;29:375–381.
7. Boulghobra A, Bonose M. Quantification of monoamine neurotransmitter metabolites and cofactors in cerebrospinal fluid: State-of-the-art. Crit Rev Anal Chem 2022:1–16. doi:10.1080/10408347.2022.2151833.
8. Camargos S, Cardoso F. New algorithm for the diagnosis of hereditary dystonia. Arq Neuropsiquiatr 2012;70:715–717.
9. Cardoso Vale T, Echenique L, Barsottini OGP, Pedroso JL. Paroxysmal autonomic instability with dystonia after severe traumatic brain injury. Tremor Other Hyperkinet Mov 2020;10:12.
10. Charlesworth G, Bhatia KP, Wood NW. The genetics of dystonia: New twists in an old tale. Brain 2013;136:2017–2037.
11. Chawda SJ, Munchau A, Johnson D, Bhatia K, Quinn NP, Stevens J, et al. Pattern of premature degenerative changes of the cervical spine in patients with spasmodic torticollis and the impact on the outcome of selective peripheral denervation. J Neurol Neurosurg Psychiatry 2000;68:465–471.
12. Chen Q, Vu JP, Cisneros E, Benadof CN, Zhang Z, Barbano RL, et al. Postural directionality and head tremor in cervical dystonia. Tremor Other Hyperkinet Mov 2020;10. doi:10.7916/tohm.v0.745.
13. Cohen LG, Hallett M. Hand cramps: Clinical features and electromyographic patterns in a focal dystonia. Neurology 1988;38:1005–1012.
14. Członkowska A, Rodo M, Gromadzka G. Late onset Wilson's disease: Therapeutic implications. Mov Disord 2008;23:896–898.
15. Deuschl G, Heinen F, Kleedorfer B, Wagner M, Lucking CH, Poewe W. Clinical and polymyographic investigation of spasmodic torticollis. J Neurol 1992;239:9–15.
16. Di Fonzo A, Albanese A, Jinnah HA. The apparent paradox of phenotypic diversity and shared mechanisms across dystonia syndromes. Curr Opin Neurol 2022;35:502–509.
17. Dzinovic I, Boesch S, Skorvanek M, Necpal J, Svantnerova J, Pavelekova P, et al. Genetic overlap between dystonia and other neurologic disorders: A study of 1,100 exomes. Parkinsonism Relat Disord 2022;102:1–6.
18. Fafara-Les A, Kwiatkowski S, Marynczak L, Kawecki Z, Adamek D, Herman-Sucharska I, Kobylarz K. Torticollis as a first sign of posterior fossa and cervical spinal cord tumors in children. Childs Nerv Syst 2014;30:425–430.
19. Fogel BL, Satya-Murti S, Cohen BH. Clinical exome sequencing in neurologic disease. Neurol Clin Pract 2016;6:164–176.
20. Fung VS, Jinnah HA, Bhatia K, Vidailhet M. Assessment of the patient with dystonia: An update on dystonia syndromes. Mov Disord 2013;28:889–898.
21. Gras D, Roze E, Caillet S, Meneret A, Doummar D, Billette de Villemeur T, Vidailhet M, Mochel F. GLUT1 deficiency syndrome: An update. Rev Neurol 2014;170:91–99.
22. Gregori B, Agostino R, Bologna M, Dinapoli L, Colosimo C, Accornero N, Berardelli A. Fast voluntary neck movements in patients with cervical dystonia: A kinematic study before and after therapy with botulinum toxin type A. Clin Neurophysiol 2008;119:273–280.
23. Herz E. Dystonia. I. Historical review: Analysis of dystonic symptoms and physiologic mechanisms involved. Arch Neurol Psychiat 1944;51:305–318.
24. Jenkins ME, Mink JW. Kinematic analysis of a reach-grasp-drink task in children with primary dystonia and age-matched controls. Mov Disord 2004;19:S89.
25. Jinnah HA. The dystonias. Continuum 2019;25:976–1000.
26. Jinnah HA, Ceballos-Picot I, Torres RJ, Visser JE, Schretlen D, Verdu A, et al. Attenuated variants of Lesch-Nyhan disease. Brain 2010;133:671–689.
27. Jinnah HA, Visser JE, Harris JC, Verdu A, Larovere L, Ceballos-Picot I, et al. Delineation of the motor disorder of Lesch-Nyhan disease. Brain 2006;129:1201–1217.
28. Johnson NE. Whole-exome sequencing in neurologic practice: Reducing the diagnostic odyssey. Neurol Genet 2015;1:e37.
29. Kilic-Berkmen G, Scorr LM, Rosen A, Wu E, Freeman A, Silver M, Hanfelt J, Jinnah HA. Thyroid disease in cervical dystonia. Parkinsonism Relat Disord 2023;107:10524.
30. Konrad C, Vollmer-Haase J, Anneken K, Knecht S. Orthopedic and neurological complications of cervical dystonia: Review of the literature. Acta Neurol Scand 2004;109:369–373.
31. Kumandas S, Per H, Gumus H, Tucer B, Yikilmaz A, Kontas O, et al. Torticollis secondary to posterior fossa and cervical spinal cord tumors: Report of five cases and literature review. Neurosurg Rev 2006;29:333–338.
32. Kurian MA, Gissen P, Smith M, Heales S, Jr., Clayton PT. The monoamine neurotransmitter disorders: An expanding range of neurological syndromes. Lancet Neurol 2011;10:721–733.
33. Lalli S, Albanese A. The diagnostic challenge of primary dystonia: Evidence from misdiagnosis. Mov Disord 2010;25:1619–1626.
34. Lazaridis KN, Schahl KA, Cousin MA, Babovic-Vuksanovic D, Riegert-Johnson DL, Gavrilova RH, et al. Outcome of whole exome sequencing for diagnostic odyssey cases of an individualized medicine clinic: The Mayo Clinic experience. Mayo Clin Proc 2016;91:297–307.
35. Ludlow CL, Domangue R, Sharma D, Jinnah HA, Perlmutter JS, Berke G, et al. Consensus-based attributes for identifying patients with spasmodic dysphonia and other voice disorders. JAMA Otolaryngol Head Neck Surg 2018;144:657–665.
36. Ma J, Wang L, Yang YM, Wan XH. Targeted gene capture sequencing in diagnosis of dystonia patients. J Neurol Sci 2018;390:36–41.
37. McCarron MM, Schulze BW, Thompson GA, Conder MC, Goetz WA. Acute phencyclidine intoxication: Incidence of clinical findings in 1,000 cases. Ann Emerg Med 1981;10:237–242.
38. Menozzi E, Balint B, Latorre A, Valente EM, Rothwell JC, Bhatia KP. Twenty years on: Myoclonus-dystonia and epsilon-sarcoglycan: Neurodevelopment, channel, and signaling dysfunction. Mov Disord 2019;34:1588–1601.
39. Mohammad SS, Angiti RR, Biggin A, Morales-Briceno H, Goetti R, Perez-Duenas B, et al. Magnetic resonance imaging pattern recognition in childhood bilateral basal ganglia disorders. Brain Commun 2020;2:fcaa178.
40. Morales-Briceno H, Fung VSC, Bhatia KP, Balint B. Parkinsonism and dystonia: Clinical spectrum and diagnostic clues. J Neurol Sci 2022;433:120016.
41. Neychev VK, Gross R, Lehericy S, Hess EJ, Jinnah HA. The functional neuroanatomy of dystonia. Neurobiol Dis 2011;42:185–201.
42. Nowak DA, Dafotakis M, Fink GR. Kinematic analysis of grasping in focal dystonia of the face and neck. Neuroscience 2013;237:216–222.

43. Olgiati S, Quadri M, Bonifati V. Genetics of movement disorders in the next-generation sequencing era. Mov Disord 2016;31:458–470.
44. Othman S, Daggumati S, Patel R, Ross J, Sataloff RT. Laboratory evaluation of spasmodic dysphonia. J Voice 2020;34:934–939.
45. Pearson TS, Akman C, Hinton VJ, Engelstad K, De Vivo DC. Phenotypic spectrum of glucose transporter type 1 deficiency syndrome (Glut1 DS). Curr Neurol Neurosci Rep 2013;13:342.
46. Pelosin E, Bove M, Marinelli L, Abbruzzese G, Ghilardi MF. Cervical dystonia affects aimed movements of non-dystonic segments. Mov Disord 2009;24:1955–1961.
47. Peterson DA, Littlewort GC, Bartlett MS, Macerollo A, Perlmutter JS, Jinnah HA, et al. Objective, computerized video-based rating of blepharospasm severity. Neurology 2016;87:2146–2153.
48. Powis Z, Towne MC, Hagman KDF, Blanco K, Palmaer E, Castro A, et al. Clinical diagnostic exome sequencing in dystonia: Genetic testing challenges for complex conditions. Clin Genet 2019;97:305–307.
49. Previdi P, Buzzi P. Paroxysmal dystonia due to a lesion of the cervical cord, case report. Ital J Neurol Sci 1992;13:521–523.
50. Rossi M, Balint B, Millar Vernetti P, Bhatia KP, Merello M. Genetic dystonia-ataxia syndromes: Clinical spectrum, diagnostic approach, and treatment options. Mov Disord Clin Pract 2018;5:373–382.
51. Rozza L, Bortolotti P, Sica A, Weronig S, Orrico D. Kinesigenic dystonia as the first manifestation of multiple sclerosis with cervical and brainstem lesions. Eur Neurol 1993;33:331–332.
52. Samotus O, Lee J, Jog M. Personalized botulinum toxin type A therapy for cervical dystonia based on kinematic guidance. J Neurol 2018;265:1269–1278.
53. Sawyer SL, Hartley T, Dyment DA, Beaulieu CL, Schwartzentruber J, Smith A, et al. Utility of whole-exome sequencing for those near the end of the diagnostic odyssey: Time to address gaps in care. Clin Genet 2016;89:275–284.
54. Schneider SA, Aggarwal A, Bhatt MH, Dupont E, Tisch S, Limousin P, et al. Severe tongue protrusion dystonia: Clinical syndromes and possible treatment. Neurology 2006;67:940–943.
55. Shaikh AG, Zee DS, Jinnah HA. Oscillatory head movements in cervical dystonia: Dystonia, tremor, or both? Mov Disord 2015;30:834–842.
56. Sharer JD, Bodamer O, Longo N, Tortorelli S, Wamelink MM, Young S. Laboratory diagnosis of creatine deficiency syndromes: A technical standard and guideline of the American College of Medical Genetics and Genomics. Genet Med 2017;19:256–263.
57. Strader S, Rodnitzky RL, Gonzalez-Alegre P. Secondary dystonia in a botulinum toxin clinic: Clinical characteristics, neuroanatomical substrate and comparison with idiopathic dystonia. Parkinsonism Relat Disord 2011;17:749–752.
58. Trotta GF, Pellicciari R, Boccaccio A, Brunetti A, Cascarano GD, Manghisi VM, et al. A neural network-based software to recognise blepharospasm symptoms and to measure eye closure time. Comput Biol Med 2019;112:103376.
59. Uncini A, Di Muzio A, Thomas A, Lugaresi A, Gambi D. Hand dystonia secondary to cervical demyelinating lesion. Mov Disord 1996;11:96–99.
60. Valeriani D, Simonyan K. A microstructural neural network biomarker for dystonia diagnosis identified by a DystoniaNet deep learning platform. Proc Natl Acad Sci 2020;117:26398–26405.
61. van Egmond ME, Kuiper A, Eggink H, Sinke RJ, Brouwer OF, Verschuuren-Bemelmans CC, et al. Dystonia in children and adolescents: A systematic review and a new diagnostic algorithm. J Neurol Neurosurg Psychiatry 2014;86:774–781.
62. van Egmond ME, Lagrand TJ, Lizaitiene G, Smit M, Tijssen MAJ. A novel diagnostic approach for patients with adult-onset dystonia. J Neurol Neurosurg Psychiatry 2022;93:1039–1048.
63. van Egmond ME, Lugtenberg CHA, Brouwer OF, Contarino MF, Fung VSC, Heiner-Fokkema MR, et al. A post hoc study on gene panel analysis for the diagnosis of dystonia. Mov Disord 2017;32:569–575.
64. Vizcarra JA, Jinnah HA. What is hemidystonia? Movement Disord Clin Pract 2023;10:477–481.
65. Weissbach A, Pauly MG, Herzog R, Hahn L, Halmans S, Hamami F, et al. Relationship of genotype, phenotype, and treatment in dopa-responsive dystonia: MDSGene review. Mov Disord 2021;2022:237–252.
66. Yanagisawa N, Goto A. Dystonia musculorum deformans. Analysis with electromyography. J Neurol Sci 1971;13:39–65.
67. Yao D, O'Flynn LC, Simonyan K. DystoniaBoTXNet: Novel neural network biomarker of botulinum toxin efficacy in isolated dystonia. Ann Neurol 2023;93:460–471.
68. Zech M, Jech R, Boesch S, Skorvanek M, Weber S, Wagner M, et al. Monogenic variants in dystonia: An exome-wide sequencing study. Lancet Neurol 2020;19:908–918.

Chapter 28

Symptom-Targeted Oral Medications for Dystonia

INTRODUCTION

A wide variety of medications may be offered to individuals with dystonia. For most types of dystonia, there is a paucity of rigorous placebo-controlled and double-blinded clinical trials with large numbers of participants. Most of the evidence for using symptomatic oral therapy comes from small blinded or unblinded trials, case reports and anecdotal experience, expert opinion, and collective experience following years of use in the community. Several systematic evidence-based reviews have been published for both adults[1,4] and children.[6,13,35] Because rare diseases are associated with small trials that often do not meet inclusion criteria for systematic reviews, the evidence-based reviews become evidence-limited reviews, and they produce ambiguous recommendations.

Oral medications tend to be used most often in cases with broad distributions of severe dystonia, such as generalized dystonia, where local treatment with botulinum toxin injections is challenging (see Chapter 30, "Botulinum Toxin Treatment for Dystonia"). However, they are sometimes used also in focal dystonia, when the benefits of injections are incomplete or benefits wear off between doses. They may also be used in combination with surgical therapies for dystonia (see Chapter 31, "Surgical Treatments for Dystonia").

Oral medications used for dystonia can be divided into two broad categories. The first category includes drugs that target specific underlying disease mechanisms. These drugs are useful only for specific disorders, and they are summarized in Chapter 29, "Special Interventions for Certain Types of Dystonia." The second category includes drugs that suppress symptoms. These symptom-based drugs can be used for any type of dystonia, regardless of etiology. They are summarized in Table 28.1 and described further in this chapter.[21,53] The relevant drugs can be broken down into six groups as outlined below.

DRUGS INFLUENCING ACETYLCHOLINE TRANSMISSION

Antagonists of central muscarinic acetylcholine receptors are helpful in both adults and children with dystonia, regardless of the type of dystonia or its etiology.[12,16,36,37] This class of drugs

Table 28.1 **Oral medications for symptomatic treatment of dystonia**

Target	Mechanism	Examples	Typical side effects	Notes
Acetylcholine transmission	Muscarinic receptor antagonist	Benztropine, biperiden, ethopropazine, ethybenztropine, procyclidine, trihexyphenidyl	Impaired concentration, memory loss, fatigue, dry mouth and eyes, constipation, urinary retention, blurry vision	Broadly useful for many types of dystonia regardless of etiology, but use is limited by side effects
Dopamine transmission	Dopamine precursor	Levodopa	Nausea, hypotension	Not broadly useful, except for dopa-responsive dystonia and occasionally other types of dystonia
	Deplete vesicular dopamine	Deutetrabenazine, tetrabenazine, valbenazine	Parkinsonian signs, sedation, depression	Most often used in tardive dystonia
	Stimulate release	Amphetamine, methylphenidate	Insomnia, autonomic changes	Not widely used; sometimes useful in craniofacial dystonias
GABA transmission	GABA receptor activator	Benzodiazepines	Impaired concentration, sedation, impaired gait or coordination, imbalance, mood changes, withdrawal reactions	Broadly useful for many types of dystonia regardless of etiology, but use is limited by side effects
	GABA receptor agonist	Baclofen	Impaired concentration, sedation, impaired gait or coordination, imbalance, nausea, withdrawal reactions	Broadly useful for many types of dystonia regardless of etiology, but use is limited by side effects
Muscle relaxants	Varied	Carisoprodol, chlorzoxazone, clonidine, cyclobenzaprine, dantrolene, metaxalone, methocarbamol, orphenadrine, tizanidine	Varied	Broadly useful, especially for pain and phasic muscle contractions causing jerking
Others	Varied	Cannabis derivatives, carbamazepine, gabapentin, mexiletine, riluzole, sodium oxybate, zolpidem	Varied	Not widely used, but may be useful in certain circumstances

is most likely to produce some benefit for most types of dystonia. However, high doses may be required, and side effects frequently limit the dose. Therefore, despite being the most likely to be effective, only a minority of people with dystonia use these drugs long term.[42,45]

Traditionally, trihexyphenidyl and benztropine have been the most widely used anticholinergics. Others are less commonly used but may be equally effective including biperiden, ethopropazine, ethybenztropine, orphenadrine, and procyclidine. In adults, the most troublesome side effects include impaired attention and concentration, forgetfulness, sedation, and sometimes overt confusion. Other well-known side effects include urinary retention or constipation, dry mouth or dry eyes, depression, blurred vision, and worsening of narrow-angle glaucoma. Epidemiological studies also have raised concern because long-term use of anticholinergics is linked to dementia.[2,30]

It is often claimed that children tolerate anticholinergics better than adults. However, one large study revealed that 50% of children treated with trihexyphenidyl had dose-limiting side effects.[33] Even when overt side effects are not obvious, impaired attention and concentration can lead to poor scholastic performance, a problem that can be challenging to identify in young children.[13,18] The risk of late-life dementia following exposure to high doses in children is unknown.

DRUGS INFLUENCING DOPAMINE TRANSMISSION

Many sources of information have linked dystonia with abnormalities of dopamine pathways, but the mechanisms are complex, incompletely understood, and may vary among different subtypes of dystonia.[22,46] Drugs that augment or antagonize dopamine transmission can both be effective symptomatic treatments.

Drugs that augment dopamine transmission are helpful in some cases of dystonia. Levodopa is remarkably effective in dopa-responsive dystonia.[24,27,55] Although dopa-responsive dystonia is rare, a trial of levodopa is mandatory in virtually all childhood-onset cases, as described in Chapter 29. Most adult-onset idiopathic focal dystonias do not respond to levodopa,[25] although occasional individuals report positive results.[57] A good response to levodopa in an adult should raise suspicion for adult-onset dopa-responsive dystonia or Parkinson disease.[11,43,50] Levodopa also can be at least partially effective for dystonia associated with other disorders including cerebral palsy,[8,17] ataxia telangiectasia, and spinocerebellar ataxia type 3.[56] However, results are mixed, likely reflecting the varied underlying pathology in these disorders.[6]

Methylphenidate has been reported to be useful in cases of craniofacial dystonia,[10,44] but there is evidence that it can also trigger acute dystonic reactions and other dyskinetic movements. Paroxysmal non-kinesigenic dyskinesia associated with *KCNMA1* has been reported to respond to amphetamine stimulants.[23,58]

Drugs that suppress dopamine transmission can be helpful in some cases, too. Depletion of vesicular dopamine can be achieved with inhibitors of the vesicular monoamine transporter such as tetrabenazine, deutetrabenazine, and valbenazine (see Chapter 19, "Dystonia Induced by Medications, Illicit Drugs, and Environmental Toxins"). Tetrabenazine has been reported to be helpful for a variety of different types of dystonia including early-onset generalized dystonia, adult-onset focal dystonias, and tardive dystonia.[20,54] Typical side effects include sedation or reduced concentration, parkinsonism (bradykinesia, rigidity, resting tremor), depression, and hypotension. Newer drugs such as deutetrabenazine and valbenazine have not been studied for dystonia as extensively as tetrabenazine but may have similar benefits with fewer side effects.[5] This group of drugs is most commonly used in tardive dystonia.

Historically, drugs that block dopamine receptors were also recommended for dystonia. However, these drugs are no longer encouraged because they may worsen symptoms by causing acute dystonic reactions and tardive syndromes (see Chapter 19).

DRUGS INFLUENCING GABA TRANSMISSION

The benzodiazepines act at gamma aminobutyric acid (GABA) receptors to amplify GABAergic transmission. There are many benzodiazepines, including alprazolam, chlordiazepoxide, clonazepam, diazepam, lorazepam, and midazolam. Traditionally diazepam has been a favorite in children, whereas clonazepam is more often used in adults. Even though rigorous clinical trials are lacking, the benzodiazepines are among the most frequently used medications for dystonia in both children and adults.[40,42,45,57] They are most often used in children when there is dystonia combined with spasticity, as in cerebral palsy. In adults, they are used when phasic muscle contractions produce spasms, jerking movements, or tremor-like movements. Typical side effects are impaired concentration or sedation, impaired gait or coordination, and changes in mood. Abrupt discontinuation can trigger withdrawal reactions. Common but mild withdrawal symptoms include dysphoria and tremor. More severe and life-threatening withdrawal reactions may include seizures, autonomic instability, malignant hyperthermia, rhabdomyolysis, and multiorgan failure.

Baclofen is a GABA receptor agonist also sometimes used in dystonia. It is most frequently used in children with cerebral palsy where dystonia is combined with spasticity.[6,15,17,32,33] It is less commonly used in adults, although some patients report benefit.[57] Typical side effects of oral baclofen include impaired concentration, sedation, dizziness, imbalance, and nausea. Abrupt discontinuation can trigger severe withdrawal reactions that include delirium or seizures. Baclofen is most often given orally, although it can also be delivered intrathecally via an indwelling pump.[7] This strategy may mitigate some of the side effects associated with oral delivery. However, indwelling equipment may become infected, and unrecognized catheter blockages or pump failures can lead to withdrawal reactions. These reactions may be severe, causing delirium, malignant hyperthermia, rhabdomyolysis, autonomic instability, and even death.

Good responses have also been reported for zolpidem across different forms of dystonia in multiple independent reports,[3] although rigorous controlled trials are lacking. There are also several uncontrolled reports of good responses with sodium oxybate in myoclonus dystonia and laryngeal dystonia,[14,48,51] although it can be highly sedating.

MUSCLE RELAXANTS

Patients with dystonia are sometimes given muscle relaxants because they are intuitively valuable for muscle spasms and soreness.[40,42] Muscle relaxants that work by influencing GABA transmission in the brain were described above. Tizanidine is another muscle relaxant often used in spasticity. It is an agonist at central alpha-2 noradrenergic receptors, but mixed results have been reported for its use in dystonia.[26,40]

Other muscle relaxants sometimes used for dystonia have been approved only for short-term use to address muscle spasm or soreness from injury or overuse, not for chronic use in dystonia.[49] They include carisoprodol, chlorzoxazone, cyclobenzaprine, dantrolene, metaxalone, methocarbamol, and others. The mechanisms of action of these drugs are only partly understood, but they appear to act on the central nervous system not on the muscle itself. Side effects among these drugs vary. In the short term, many may cause sedation or fatigue. The long-term effects of chronic use are not well characterized. Carisoprodol may be habit-forming and must be monitored carefully.

ANALGESICS

Many individuals with dystonia also have pain and request analgesics. When considering the best treatment options, it is important to recognize the varied sources of pain in dystonia. Pain may result from chronic muscle contractions, muscle spasms, or orthopedic issues. Unexplained pain may also be related to unrecognized psychiatric problems (see Chapter 11, "Non-Motor Features of Dystonia"). These different causes for pain may respond to different treatments.

Pain from overcontraction of muscles often responds to botulinum toxin injections. Oral medications may be added as needed including muscle relaxants, benzodiazepines, or anti-spasticity drugs. Dystonia can also cause secondary orthopedic problems, and pain resulting from these orthopedic problems may respond to nonsteroidal anti-inflammatory agents or addressing the orthopedic problem more directly. Depression and anxiety can influence the way pain is perceived or reported, and these should be treated accordingly.

It is important to keep in mind that dystonia is a chronic disorder, and the treatment chosen for pain may also need to be continued for long periods. Chronic use of opiates is not usually required except in extreme circumstances.

MISCELLANEOUS DRUGS

Unblinded and often small trials have also suggested a number of other potential oral medications for dystonia. For paroxysmal kinesigenic dyskinesia, carbamazepine has been associated with a consistent and often complete suppression of dystonic attacks across numerous independent reports, often at very low doses (see Chapter 17, "Dystonia and the Paroxysmal Dyskinesias").[19] The mechanisms for its remarkable efficacy in this condition are not entirely clear.

There are also numerous reports describing the use of gabapentin in various forms of dystonia including cerebral palsy, Wilson disease, and the syndrome of paroxysmal autonomic instability with dystonia.[17,28,29,52] Gabapentin is frequently used for children with dystonia,[17,32] although evidence for its efficacy has been questioned,[35] and there are also reports of gabapentin-induced acute dystonic reactions.[41,47] Therefore, it must be used cautiously.

Two small studies described improvement of cervical dystonia with mexiletine.[31,39] One report described improvement of cervical dystonia with riluzole.[38] Mixed results have been reported for cannabis derivatives.[34]

Many other medications are described as being useful in isolated case reports or retrospective reviews of dystonia cohorts. These reports may reflect the known publication bias for positive results. However, they may also reflect the etiological heterogeneity of dystonia.

COMMUNITY-BASED STUDIES OF MEDICATION USE

In the absence of strong evidence-based studies or definitive expert guidelines for symptomatic oral therapies in dystonia, prescribing habits vary considerably. In this setting, it can be useful to consider the drugs that are most commonly used by affected individuals in the community. The trial-and-error process combined with experience over time presumably leads to the continuation of medications that are most helpful for the largest numbers of individuals.

One study from the United Kingdom explored a public database that included 4,024 individuals with cervical dystonia, and 45% were using some type of oral medication. Analgesics were used by 39% and benzodiazepines by 10%.[45] Another study evaluated medication use among 1,488 patients with predominantly adult-onset focal dystonias treated by 37 experts in North America and Europe.[42] Overall, 10–20% used some type of oral medication. The most frequently used medications were benzodiazepines, followed by muscle relaxants, baclofen, anticholinergics, and dopamine-related drugs. This study did not evaluate analgesic use. A third study in Asia addressed the preferences of 172 individuals, again with mostly adult-onset focal dystonias.[57] The most favorable responses were reported for clonazepam, baclofen, and trihexyphenidyl.

Patterns of medication use differ in children because cohorts are often dominated by cases with dystonic cerebral palsy, which is often combined with spasticity.[37] In a single-center study of 278 children in the United Kingdom, 71% were using some type of medication.[33] Among those using medications, the most common included baclofen (42%), trihexyphenidyl (35%), and levodopa (15%). In a multicenter study of 275 children in the United Kingdom, 64% used oral medications.[32] Among those using medication, the most common were baclofen (39%), trihexyphenidyl (20%), gabapentin (18%), benzodiazepines (15%), and levodopa (3%).[32] In Australia, gabapentin and baclofen are most common, with the other drugs being used far less frequently.[17] These results imply significant differences in prescribing habits, although certain trends are evident.

SYNOPSIS AND FUTURE PROSPECTS

Many drugs are used for the symptomatic relief of dystonia. Formal recommendations for using these drugs are lacking because of the paucity of definitive clinical trials. Many small trials report positive outcomes, which often cannot be replicated in subsequent trials. The challenge in confirming outcomes may reflect the known publication bias in favor of positive outcomes, but they could also reflect the often small and heterogeneous subtypes of dystonia included in the trials. Larger trials often report no overall benefit, although positive responses of individual cases with specific etiological subtypes may be obscured by group averages.

A well-known illustrative example of the relevance of etiological heterogeneity is dopa-responsive dystonia. Levodopa is not broadly useful for most patients with dystonia, but it is remarkably effective for rare cases with defects in *GCH1*. A more recently described example is the marked efficacy of amphetamine-related drugs in paroxysmal dyskinesia associated with *KCNMA1*. These drugs are not generally useful in other paroxysmal dyskinesias.[23,58] These conditions and others with special treatments are considered in more detail in Chapter 29.

Until more information becomes available about how etiological heterogeneity in dystonia influences treatment responses, evidence regarding real-world usage can be useful. For adults, most studies imply that the benzodiazepines are the most widely used, often along with analgesics. For children, baclofen is more common, although this reflects a large population with cerebral palsy, where there is often coincidental spasticity. Ultimately, the oral medication chosen must target specific symptoms, which vary among individual cases.

REFERENCES

1. Albanese A, Barnes MP, Bhatia KP, Fernandez-Alvarez E, Filippini G, Gasser T, et al. A systematic review on the diagnosis and treatment of primary (idiopathic) dystonia and dystonia plus syndromes: Report of an EFNS/MDS-ES task force. Eur J Neurol 2006;13:433–444.
2. Andre L, Gallini A, Montastruc F, Montastruc JL, Piau A, Lapeyre-Mestre M, Gardette V. Association between anticholinergic (atropinic) drug exposure and cognitive function in longitudinal studies among individuals over 50 years old: A systematic review. Eur J Clin Pharmacol 2019;75:1631–1644.
3. Badillo SPJ, Jamora RDG. Zolpidem for the treatment of dystonia. Front Neurol 2019;10:779.
4. Balash Y, Giladi N. Efficacy of pharmacological treatment of dystonia: Evidence-based review including meta-anaylsis of the effect of botulinum toxin and other cure options. Eur J Neurol 2004;11:361–370.
5. Bhidayasiri R, Jitkritsadakul O, Friedman JH, Fahn S. Updating the recommendations for treatment of tardive syndromes: A systematic review of new evidence and practical treatment algorithm. J Neurol Sci 2018;389:67–75.
6. Bohn E, Goren K, Switzer L, Falck-Ytter Y, Fehlings D. Pharmacological and neurosurgical interventions for individuals with cerebral palsy and dystonia: A systematic review update and meta-analysis. Dev Med Child Neurol 2021;63:1038–1050.
7. Bonouvrie LA, Becher JG, Vles JSH, Vermeulen RJ, Buizer AI, IDYS Group. The effect of intrathecal baclofen in dyskinetic cerebral palsy: The IDYS trial. Ann Neurol 2019;86:79–90.
8. Bradley CL, Damiano DL. Effects of dopamine on motor recovery and training in adults and children with non-progressive neurological injuries: A systematic review. Neurorehabil Neural Repair 2019;33:331–344.
9. Charlesworth G, Mohire MD, Schneider SA, Stamelou M, Wood NW, Bhatia KP. Ataxia telangiectasia presenting as dopa-responsive cervical dystonia. Neurology 2013;81:1148–1151.
10. Eftekhari K, Choe CH, Vagefi MR, Gausas RE, Eckstein LA. Oral methylphenidate for the treatment of refractory facial dystonias. Ophthalmic Plast Reconstr Surg 2015;31:e65–66.
11. Elia AE, Del Sorbo F, Romito LM, Barzaghi C, Garavaglia B, Albanese A. Isolated limb dystonia as presenting feature of Parkin disease. J Neurol Neurosurg Psychiatry 2014;85:827–828.
12. Eskow-Jaunarajs KL, Bonsi P, Chesselet MF, Standaert DG, Pisani A. Striatal cholinergic dysfunction as a unifying theme in the pathophysiology of dystonia. Prog Neurobiol 2015;127-128:91–107.
13. Fehlings D, Brown L, Harvey A, Himmelmann K, Lin JP, Macintosh A, et al. Pharmacological and neurosurgical interventions for managing dystonia in cerebral palsy: A systematic review. Dev Med Child Neurol 2018;60:356–366.
14. Frucht SJ, Bordelon Y, Houghton WH, Reardan D. A pilot tolerability and efficacy trial of sodium oxybate in ethanol-responsive movement disorders. Mov Disord 2005;20:1330–1337.
15. Greene P. Baclofen in the treatment of dystonia. Clin Neuropharmacol 1992;15:276–288.
16. Greene P, Shale H, Fahn S. Experience with high dosages of anticholinergic and other drugs in the treatment of torsion dystonia. Adv Neurol 1988;50:547–556.
17. Harvey A, Bear N, Rice J, Antolovich G, Waugh MC. National surveillance of oral medication prescription for children with dystonic cerebral palsy. J Paediatr Child Health 2021;57:1222–1227.
18. Harvey AR, Baker LB, Reddihough DS, Scheinberg A, Williams K. Trihexyphenidyl for dystonia in cerebral palsy. Cochrane Database Syst Rev 2018;5:CD012430.
19. Huang XJ, Wang T, Wang JL, Liu XL, Che XQ, Li J, et al. Paroxysmal kinesigenic dyskinesia: Clinical and genetic analyses of 110 patients. Neurology 2015;85:1546–1553.
20. Jankovic J, Beach J. Long-term effects of tetrabenazine in hyperkinetic movement disorders. Neurology 1997;48:358–362.
21. Jinnah HA. Medical and surgical treatments for dystonia. Neurol Clin 2020;38:325–348.
22. Jinnah HA, Sun YV. Dystonia genes and their biological pathways. Neurobiol Dis 2019;129:159–168.
23. Keros S, Heim J, Hakami W, Zohar-Dayan E, Ben-Zeev B, Grinspan Z, et al. Lisdexamfetamine therapy in paroxysmal non-kinesigenic dyskinesia associated with the KCNMA1-N999S variant. Mov Disord Clin Pract 2022;9:229–235.
24. Kurian MA, Gissen P, Smith M, Heales S, Jr., Clayton PT. The monoamine neurotransmitter disorders: An expanding range of neurological syndromes. Lancet Neurol 2011;10:721–733.
25. Lang AE. Dopamine agonists and antagonists in the treatment of idiopathic dystonia. Adv Neurol 1988;50:561–570.

26. Lang AE, Riley DE. Tizanidine in cranial dystonia. Clin Neuropharmacol 1992;15:142–147.
27. Lee WW, Jeon BS. Clinical spectrum of dopa-responsive dystonia and related disorders. Curr Neurol Neurosci Rep 2014;14:461.
28. Lerose M, Di Fabio R, Serrao M, Loudianos G, Pierelli F, Casali C. Gabapentin can improve dystonia in confirmed Wilson disease. Can J Neurol Sci 2014;41:284–285.
29. Liow NY, Gimeno H, Lumsden DE, Marianczak J, Kaminska M, Tomlin S, Lin JP. Gabapentin can significantly improve dystonia severity and quality of life in children. Eur J Paediatr Neurol 2016;20:100–107.
30. Lockery JE, Broder JC, Ryan J, Stewart AC, Woods RL, Chong TT, et al. A cohort study of anticholinergic medication burden and incident dementia and stroke in older adults. J Gen Intern Med 2021;36:1629–1637.
31. Lucetti C, Nuti A, Gambaccini G, Bernardini S, Brotini S, Manca ML, Bonuccelli U. Mexiletine in the treatment of torticollis and generalized dystonia. Clin Neuropharmacol 2000;23:186–189.
32. Lumsden DE, Crowe B, Basu A, Amin S, Devlin A, DeAlwis Y, et al. Pharmacological management of abnormal tone and movement in cerebral palsy. Arch Dis Child 2019;104:775–780.
33. Lumsden DE, Kaminska M, Tomlin S, Lin JP. Medication use in childhood dystonia. Eur J Paediatr Neurol 2016;20:625–629.
34. Mascia MM, Carmagnini D, Defazio G. Cannabinoids and dystonia: An issue yet to be defined. Neurol Sci 2020;41:783–787.
35. Masson R, Pagliano E, Baranello G. Efficacy of oral pharmacological treatments in dyskinetic cerebral palsy: A systematic review. Dev Med Child Neurol 2017;59:1237–1248.
36. Moehle MS, Conn PJ. Roles of the M4 acetylcholine receptor in the basal ganglia and the treatment of movement disorders. Mov Disord 2019;34:1089–1099.
37. Monbaliu E, Himmelmann K, Lin JP, Ortibus E, Bonouvrie L, Feys H, et al. Clinical presentation and management of dyskinetic cerebral palsy. Lancet Neurol 2017;16:741–749.
38. Muller J, Wenning GK, Wissel J, Baldauf A, Seppi K, Brenneis C, Poewe W. Riluzole therapy in cervical dystonia. Mov Disord 2002;17:198–200.
39. Ohara S, Hayashi R, Momoi H, Miki J, Yanagisawa N. Mexiletine in the treatment of spasmodic torticollis. Mov Disord 1998;13:934–940.
40. Peck J, Urits I, Crane J, McNally A, Noor N, Patel M, et al. Oral muscle relaxants for the treatment of chronic pain associated with cerebral palsy. Psychopharmacol Bull 2020;50:142–162.
41. Pina MA, Modrego PJ. Dystonia induced by gabapentin. Ann Pharmacother 2005;39:380–382.
42. Pirio Richardson S, Wegele AR, Skipper B, Deligtisch A, Jinnah HA. Dystonia treatment: Patterns of medication use in an international cohort. Neurology 2017;88:1–8.
43. Potulska-Chromik A, Hoffman-Zacharska D, Lukawska M, Kostera-Pruszczyk A. Dopa-responsive dystonia or early-onset Parkinson disease: Genotype-phenotype correlation. Neurol Neurochir Pol 2016;51:1–6.
44. Price KM, Ramey NA, Richard MJ, Woodward DJ, Woodward JA. Can methylphenidate objectively provide relief in patients with uncontrolled blepharospasm? A pilot study using surface electromyography. Ophthalmic Plast Reconstr Surg 2010;26:353–356.
45. Raluy-Callado M, Gabriel S, Dinet J, Wang M, Wasiak R. A retrospective study to assess resource utilization in patients with cervical dystonia in the United Kingdom. Neuropsychiatr Dis Treat 2015;11:647–655.
46. Ribot B, Aupy J, Vidailhet M, Mazere J, Pisani A, Bezard E, et al. Dystonia and dopamine: From phenomenology to pathophysiology. Prog Neurobiol 2019;182:101678.
47. Rohman L, Hebron A. Acute dystonic reaction caused by gabapentin. J Emerg Med 2014;46:e89.
48. Rumbach AF, Blitzer A, Frucht SJ, Simonyan K. An open-label study of sodium oxybate in spasmodic dysphonia. Laryngoscope 2017;127:1402–1407.
49. See S, Ginzburg R. Choosing a skeletal muscle relaxant. Am Fam Physician 2008;78:365–370.
50. Shetty AS, Bhatia KP, Lang AE. Dystonia and Parkinson's disease: What is the relationship? Neurobiol Dis 2019;132:104462.
51. Simonyan K, Frucht SJ. Long-term effect of sodium oxybate (Xyrem(R)) in spasmodic dysphonia with vocal tremor. Tremor Other Hyperkinet Mov (N Y) 2013;3. tre-03-206-4731-1.
52. Srinivasan S, Lim CC, Thirugnanam U. Paroxysmal autonomic instability with dystonia. Clin Auton Res 2007;17:378–381.
53. Sy MAC, Fernandez HH. Dystonia and leveraging oral pharmacotherapy. J Neural Transm (Vienna) 2021;128:521–529.
54. Testini P, Factor SA. Treatment of tardive dystonia: A review. Dystonia 2023;2:10957. doi:10.3389/dyst/2023.10957.
55. Wijemanne S, Jankovic J. Dopa-responsive dystonia: Clinical and genetic heterogeneity. Nat Rev Neurol 2015;11:414–424.
56. Wilder-Smith E, Tan EK, Law HY, Zhao Y, Ng I, Wong MC. Spinocerebellar ataxia type 3 presenting as an L-DOPA responsive dystonia phenotype in a Chinese family. J Neurol Sci 2003;213:25–28.
57. Woo KA, Kim HJ, Yoo D, Choi JH, Shin J, Park S, et al. Patient-reported responses to medical treatment in primary dystonia. J Clin Neurosci 2020;75:242–244.
58. Zhang G, Gibson RA, McDonald M, Liang P, Kang PW, Shi J, et al. A gain-of-function mutation in KCNMA1 causes dystonia spells controlled with stimulant therapy. Mov Disord 2020;35:1868–1873.

Chapter 29

Special Interventions for Certain Types of Dystonia

INTRODUCTION

Oral medications that suppress symptoms across many different types of dystonia are described in the Chapter 28, "Symptom-Targeted Oral Medications for Dystonia." Other interventions useful only for special circumstances are summarized here. Although all of the disorders with special treatments are rare, they should not be missed because treatment can be life-altering.

Many of these treatments are useful only for very specific populations because they target specific underlying disease mechanisms. These treatments can be conceptually grouped into three main categories.[16] These include detoxification strategies that reduce accumulation of a harmful substance, replacement strategies that restore some missing substance, and avoidance of triggers known to worsen the condition (Table 29.1). Many disorders may be treated with more than one strategy. In a few cases, effective treatments were discovered empirically to be useful for specific populations although the mechanisms may not be well understood.

Most of these disorders present at an early age, so they are most relevant for specialists in pediatrics. They also are important for adult neurologists for several reasons. First, individuals with these disorders often survive into adulthood, so adult neurologists may be asked to take over responsibility for care as affected individuals age. Second, the diagnosis of these disorders is sometimes missed during childhood. Therefore, adult neurologists may need to make the diagnosis. Third, almost all disorders that classically begin in childhood may have mild or atypical presentations that first come to attention later in life. Once again, the adult neurologist may be the first to make the diagnosis. Finally, a few of these disorders present more frequently in adults than in children. Therefore, all of these disorders are relevant for both pediatric and adult neurologists.

DISORDERS MANAGED WITH DETOXIFICATION STRATEGIES

Detoxification Mechanisms

Several types of dystonia result from accumulation of materials that cause neuronal dysfunction or degeneration. Theoretically, removing these

Table 29.1 **Treatment strategies for some rare inherited dystonias**

Strategy	Disorders
Detoxification strategies	Cerebrotendinous xanthomatosis Manganese transporter deficiencies Neurodegeneration with brain iron accumulation Niemann-Pick type C Wilson disease
Replacement strategies	Abetalipoproteinemia Aromatic amino acid decarboxylase deficiency Ataxia with vitamin E deficiency Biotin-thiamin responsive basal ganglia disease Cerebral folate deficiency Cobalamin deficiencies CoQ10 deficiency Dopa-responsive dystonias GLUT1 deficiency syndromes MOCS1 deficiency Pyruvate dehydrogenase deficiency VMAT2 deficiency
Trigger avoidance	Biotin-thiamin responsive basal ganglia disease GLUT1 deficiency syndromes Glutaric aciduria Maple syrup urine disease Methylmalonic aciduria Paroxysmal kinesigenic dyskinesias Propionic acidemia Rapid-onset dystonia-parkinsonism

Further details regarding these disorders and their specific treatments can be found in a prior review.[16]

toxic materials should be therapeutic, although therapeutic benefits are sometimes challenging to prove. For some disorders, detoxification strategies can rapidly reduce or even eliminate neurological symptoms. In other disorders, reducing the toxic materials may not produce obvious clinical benefit. The reasons for lack of benefit are not always clear. It is possible that the failure to observe a clinical benefit reflects brain damage incurred prior to starting therapy. In these cases, it is possible that the treatment may slow progression of the disorder even when it does not produce immediate benefits. It also is possible that the blood–brain barrier prevents the detoxification treatment from reaching the brain.

Because many of these disorders are rare, with slow progression over many years, longitudinal studies large enough to demonstrate clear benefit from therapy are often not feasible. In the absence of strong evidence-based medicine, treatment is often based on clinical judgment. Some illustrative examples are described below, with a more complete listing in Table 29.2.

Wilson Disease

Wilson disease results from pathogenic variants in *ATP7B*, which encodes a protein involved in the transport of copper across cell membranes.[2] Toxic levels of copper accumulate in liver and brain, and affected individuals present with hepatic dysfunction, neurological dysfunction, or both. The majority of cases become symptomatic before or during teenage years, but a minority develop symptoms as adults, with rare cases first developing symptoms their seventies. The most common neurological features include dystonia, parkinsonism, tremor, cognitive decline, and neuropsychiatric abnormalities.

Strategies aimed at reducing copper stores are required to mitigate brain injury.[29] These strategies include chelation of heavy metals with pencillamine, trientine, or tetrathiomolybdate. It can also be useful to reduce intestinal copper absorption with zinc. These strategies have proven to be effective for reversing existing symptoms in most cases, although there is sometimes a period of

Table 29.2 **Rare genetic dystonias with specific treatments**

Disease	Causative gene	Age at onset	Clinical features	Treatments
Abetalipoproteinemia (Bassen-Kornzweig syndrome)	*MTTP*	Childhood to early adulthood	Progressive ataxia, chorea, dystonia, seizures, acanthocytosis, retinitis pigmentosa, fat malabsorption syndrome	Vitamin E and reduced-fat diet can prevent or reduce symptoms
Aromatic amino acid decarboxylase deficiency	*AADC*	Infancy	Motor delay, hypotonia. dystonia, oculogyric crises, autonomic dysfunction	Dopamine agonists can partly reverse symptoms in some patients
Ataxia with vitamin E deficiency	*TTPA*	Childhood to early adulthood	Ataxia, visual loss, neuropathy (occasional patients present with dystonia)	Vitamin E can prevent or reduce symptoms
Biotin-thiamine–responsive basal ganglia disorder	*SLC19A3*	Childhood	Encephalopathic crisis followed by dystonia-parkinsonism	Biotin and thiamine can reverse or prevent symptoms
Biotinidase deficiency	*BTD*	Infancy	Encephalopathy, motor delay, dystonia, seizures, vision loss, hearing loss, skin rash	Biotin can prevent or reduce symptoms
Cerebral folate deficiency	*FLR1, SLC46A1*	Early childhood to adolescence	Developmental delay, ataxia, dystonia, seizures, neuropsychiatric disturbances	Folinic acid can prevent or reduce symptoms
Cerebrotendinous xanthomatosis	*CYP27A1*	Late childhood to adulthood	Ataxia, spasticity, dementia, myoclonus, tendon xanthomas (occasional patients present with dystonia)	Chenodeoxycholic acid may prevent progression or reverse some symptoms
Cobalamin deficiencies (inherited subtypes A through G)	Multiple	Infancy	Encephalopathy with motor delay, ataxia, spasticity, dystonia, seizures, bone marrow abnormalities	Cobalamin derivatives or protein restriction can mitigate symptoms
Coenzyme Q10 deficiency	Multiple	Any age	Varied phenotypes; progressive ataxia or encephalopathy, sometimes with dystonia	Coenzyme Q10 can mitigate symptoms
Cerebral creatine deficiency type 3	*AGAT, CRTR, GAMT*	Infancy	Developmental delay, hypotonia, dystonia, myopathy	Creatine can mitigate symptoms, in combination with specific dietary changes
Dopa-responsive dystonia, classic	*GCH1*	Early childhood to late adulthood	Dystonia, sometimes with parkinsonism	Levodopa can reverse symptoms
Dopa-responsive dystonia, complicated	*TH, PTPS, SPR*	Infancy to adolescence	Dystonia, often combined with parkinsonism, oculogyric crises, autonomic disturbances	Levodopa, 5-hydroxytryptophan, and/or tetrahydrobiopterin can completely or partly reverse symptoms

Continued

Table 29.2 **(cont.)**

Disease	Causative gene	Age at onset	Clinical features	Treatments
Dystonia with brain manganese accumulation	*SLC30A10, SLC39A14*	Childhood	Dystonia, parkinsonism, liver disease, polycythemia	Chelation therapy with EDTA can prevent or partly reverse symptoms
Galactosemia	*GALT, GALK1, GALE*	Childhood to early adulthood	Ataxia, tremor, lactose intolerance (sometimes mild dystonia)	Lactose restriction can mitigate symptoms
GLUT1 deficiency syndromes	*SLC2A1*	Childhood to adolescence	Developmental delay, seizures (sometimes paroxysmal ataxia or dystonia)	Ketogenic diet or triheptanoin can mitigate symptoms
Glutaric aciduria type 1	*GCDH*	Early childhood to early adulthood	Developmental delay, encephalopathic crisis, dystonia-parkinsonism	Treating intercurrent illness and lysine restriction can prevent encephalopathic crises
Homocystinuria	*CBS*	Childhood	Neurocognitive dysfunction, myopia, ectopic lens; stroke, sometimes generalized or paroxysmal dystonia	Methionine restriction prevents symptoms
Maple syrup urine disease	*BCKDHA, BCKDHB, DBT*	Childhood	Intermittent encephalopathy and ataxia (sometimes focal or paroxysmal dystonia)	Leucine restriction with or without thiamine mitigates symptoms
Methylmalonic aciduria	*MUT*	Childhood	Developmental delay, renal insufficiency, pancytopenia, encephalopathic crisis with dystonia-parkinsonism	Avoiding or treating intercurrent illness and protein restriction can prevent encephalopathic crises
Molybdenum cofactor deficiency	*MOCS1*	Adolescence	Developmental delay with encephalopathy and seizures (rare patients present with dystonia-parkinsonism)	Cyclic pyranopterin monophosphate can prevent symptoms
Niemann-Pick type C	*NPC1, NPC2*	Early childhood to early adulthood	Dementia, ataxia, spasticity, seizures, supranuclear gaze palsy (occasional patients present with progressive dystonia)	*N*-butyl-deoxynojirimycin can prevent or mitigate symptoms
Propionic aciduria	*PCCA, PCCB*	Early childhood to adolescence	Developmental delay, encephalopathic crisis with dystonia-parkinsonism	Avoiding or treating intercurrent illness and protein restriction can prevent encephalopathic crises
Pyruvate dehydrogenase deficiency	Multiple	Infancy	Progressive or paroxysmal dystonia	Thiamine, ketogenic diet, and dichloroacetate can mitigate symptoms
Rapid-onset dystonia-parkinsonism	*ATP1A3*	Early childhood to late adulthood	Encephalopathic crisis followed by dystonia-parkinsonism (some cases have slowly progressive phenotype)	Avoiding or treating intercurrent illness can prevent encephalopathic crises
Wilson disease	*ATP7B*	Early childhood to late adulthood	Liver disease, dystonia, cognitive and neuropsychiatric abnormalities	Zinc, tetrathiomolybdate can prevent or reduce symptoms

Modified from a prior review.[15]

worsening after they are first started. Early diagnosis and treatment are essential because treatment is less effective once brain damage has occurred. Lifelong adherence to therapy is important to maintain benefits.

Wilson disease is illustrative of the treatment challenges for many other disorders covered in this chapter. Dystonia may be a prominent feature, although it may be a minor feature of a much more complex phenotype. Therapies aimed at reducing copper are remarkably effective because they address the underlying accumulation of copper. However, large double-blind placebo-controlled trials that prove value for many available therapies are lacking and it is not likely that any such trials will ever be conducted. Copper-reducing therapies are effective for life, and many cases transition from a pediatric neurologist to an adult neurologist as they get older. Therapies work best when they are started early, before permanent brain damage occurs. If significant brain damage occurs, therapy may not reverse all symptoms, but it is still needed to prevent deterioration. Unfortunately, there are numerous reports of cases with classical childhood-onset symptoms for whom the diagnosis was missed for many years and treatment was delayed until adulthood. There are also numerous reports of cases with adult-onset symptoms. Wilson disease has been very well-studied, and many of the lessons learned are relevant for other disorders where specific treatments are available.

Manganese Transporter Deficiencies

Pathogenic variants in genes that encode proteins involved in manganese transport (*SLC30A10, SLC39A8, SLC38A14*) lead to toxic accumulation of manganese in liver and brain.[32,33,44,45] The clinical presentation can be quite similar to Wilson disease, with early onset of hepatic dysfunction, neurological dysfunction, or both. Most cases present in early childhood, although later-onset cases have been described.

These disorders can be treated via strategies that reduce tissue manganese stores, such as chelation with ethylenediaminetetraacetic acid (EDTA). Clinical benefits are obvious in some cases but not others. Early treatment is needed to prevent permanent brain damage, and lifelong therapy is needed.

Cerebrotendinous Xanthomatosis

Cerebrotendinous xanthomatosis results from pathogenic variants in *CYP27A1*, which encodes a mitochondrial enzyme involved in cholesterol metabolism (sterol 27-hydoxylase).[30,39] Common early features include diarrhea, cataracts, and xanthomas near large tendons. These xanthomas reflect accumulation of cholesterol metabolites such as cholestenol into solid deposits which are both visible and palpable on exam. Neurological symptoms typically develop in teenagers or young adults with progressive ataxia or spasticity, but a minority present with dystonia or parkinsonism. Other neurological problems may include cognitive decline, seizures, and neuropathy.

The bile acid, chenodeoxycholic acid, binds to and reduces the accumulation of cholestanol and related metabolites. Treatment is thought to prevent or reverse at least some of the clinical features if started early.[40,50]

Niemann-Pick Type C

Niemann-Pick type C is caused by pathogenic variants in *NPC1* and, less commonly, *NPC2*.[36] These genes encode proteins involved in the intracellular trafficking of cholesterol. The molecular defects lead to pathological accumulation of glycosphingolipids in lysosomes with cell death. The typical presentations include varying combinations of ataxia, spasticity, cognitive decline, seizures, and supranuclear gaze palsy. In a minority of individuals, dystonia is a prominent or presenting feature.

The synthetic glucose analog N-butyl-deoxynojirimycin inhibits glycosylceramide synthase and reduces lysosomal glycosphingolipids. Treatment may slow progression of neurological abnormalities, particularly in individuals with late-onset disease.

Neurodegeneration with Brain Iron Accumulation

Toxic accumulation of brain iron occurs with pathogenic variants in a number of different genes.[6] The most common is *PANK2*, which encodes an enzyme (pantothenate kinase) involved in the synthesis of co-enzyme A. Pantothenate kinase–associated neurodegeneration typically presents in childhood, although adult-onset cases are recognized, too. Most cases have dystonia, parkinsonism, and cognitive decline. More severely affected cases may also have retinopathy and seizures.

Brain iron stores can be reduced with deferiprone, an iron chelator.[20] However, deferiprone does not have a proven impact on clinical symptoms. Despite the lack of immediate clinical benefits, it is sometimes offered to affected individuals as it is thought to slow or stop a key aspect in the pathogenesis of the disease.[43]

DISORDERS MANAGED WITH REPLACEMENT STRATEGIES

Replacement Mechanisms

Theoretically, disorders caused by deficiency of some essential substance might be treated by replacing it. For inherited disorders caused by pathogenic gene variants leading to loss of function, gene therapy to replace the lost gene provides the most direct solution. This promising strategy is under development for individuals with inherited aromatic amino acid decarboxylase deficiency,[5] but it has not yet reached clinical application for other disorders with dystonia.

Another solution might be to replace the defective substance itself. This strategy has reached clinical application only for some cases of Gaucher disease, where replacing the defective enzyme is feasible. Instead of replacing the gene or protein, most of the treatments in this group of disorders involve providing some essential substance that bypasses the original defect. Similar to the limitations involving detoxification strategies, it has sometimes been difficult to prove the value of replacement strategies. In some cases, the benefits are immediate and obvious. In other cases, benefits are not so clear, although there are strong reasons to believe the strategies may slow progression of the disease.

Dopa-Responsive Dystonia

Dopa-responsive dystonia is most often caused by pathogenic variants in *GCH1*, which encodes GTP-cyclohydrolase.[14] This enzyme is the first and rate-limiting step in the synthesis of tetrahydrobiopterin, a cofactor required for the synthesis of dopamine. The molecular defect leads to dopamine deficiency, usually without overt neuron degeneration.

Affected individuals typically present in childhood with a combination of dystonia and sometimes mild parkinsonism.[23,47] Many are initially misdiagnosed with cerebral palsy. A minority of cases may present as adults. In adults, parkinsonism may be more prominent than dystonia. Symptoms respond dramatically to levodopa. Symptoms can also respond to dopamine agonists or to drugs that inhibit dopamine catabolism, such as monoamine oxidase inhibitors.

Dystonia can also result from pathogenic variants in other genes affecting dopamine synthesis including *TH* (tyrosine hydroxylase),[48] *SPR* (sepiapterin reductase),[10] *PTS* (6-pyruvoyl tetrahydropterin synthase),[51] QDPR (dihydropteridine reductase), and *PCBD1* (carbinolamine-4 alpha dehydratase).[14] These disorders sometimes present with dystonia only but more commonly present as dystonia combined with additional neurological features such as developmental delay, autonomic signs, and/or encephalopathy. These more complex cases may still respond to levodopa, but responses are less consistent. Additional benefits in some cases are reported for treatment with tetrahydrobiopterin and/or the serotonin precursor, 5-hydroxytryptophan.

Aromatic Amino Acid Decarboxylase Deficiency

Pathogenic variants in *AADC*, encoding aromatic amino acid decarboxylase, prevent decarboxylation of levodopa to dopamine and 5-hydroxytryptophan to serotonin.[46] They therefore produce a deficit of dopamine and serotonin. Affected individuals present with severe developmental delay, dystonia, parkinsonism, oculogyric crises, and autonomic dysfunction. Treatment with direct-acting dopamine receptor agonists can sometimes be helpful. Preliminary gene therapy trials have described promising results.[5]

Vesicular Monoamine Transporter Deficiency

Approximately 95% of brain dopamine is stored in synaptic vesicles, which release their contents into the synaptic cleft during activity-dependent neuronal depolarization. The vesicular monoamine transporter, encoded by *VMAT2*, is required for packaging dopamine into these vesicles.

Pathogenic defects in this gene impair the packaging and release of monoamines during vesicular monoamine transmitter release, and affected individuals present in early childhood with encephalopathy and a complex movement disorder that includes dystonia and other abnormal movements.[34] Levodopa may worsen symptoms, but treatment with dopamine agonists can be helpful.

GLUT1-Associated Phenotypes

The brain is a metabolically demanding organ that relies heavily on glucose. To ensure a steady supply of glucose, the brain uses a special glucose transporter (GLUT1) encoded by *SLC2A1*. Defects in this gene cause a number of different neurological phenotypes including neonatal encephalopathy with seizures and paroxysmal dyskinesia dominated by ataxia or dystonia.[11,31]

Several replacement strategies have been used to address the features observed in this disorder. One of these involves triheptanoin, a triglyceride that crosses the blood–brain barrier independently of the GLUT1 transporter and provides an alternative source for brain energy.[27] The other involves the ketogenic diet.[17] This diet results in the formation of ketones, which also cross the blood–brain barrier independently of the GLUT1 transporter to provide an alternative brain energy source. Adherence to this diet is challenging, and similar results may be obtained with a low-carbohydrate and high-fat (Atkins) diet.

Vitamin and Cofactor Deficiencies

Several other rare disorders can be treated by supplementation with natural vitamins or cofactors.[3] Pathogenic variants in *SLC19A3* disrupt brain transport of thiamine (vitamin B_1). In susceptible individuals, a minor illness during childhood can trigger a sudden encephalopathic crisis with dystonia and parkinsonism. One unusual aspect of this disorder is that it evolves rapidly, typically over a few days, with MRI evidence for acute striatal injury. Dystonia and parkinsonism may be permanent if the crisis is severe. The disorder is known as biotin-thiamine-responsive basal ganglia disease because there is evidence for acute striatal necrosis on MRI, and treatment with high doses of thiamine and/or biotin can reduce or eliminate crises.[42]

Ataxia with vitamin E deficiency results from pathogenic variants in *TTPA*, which encodes the alpha tocopherol (vitamin E) transfer protein.[37] Affected individuals usually present in childhood or as young adults with slowly progressive ataxia, neuropathy, and visual loss. Occasionally, individuals present with dystonia, either in isolation or combined with other problems. Vitamin E supplements are thought to be useful. The fat malabsorption syndrome associated with abetalipoproteinemia also leads to deficiencies of fat soluble vitamins (E and D), so supplementations with both may be helpful.[24]

Other examples include treatment of biotinidase deficiency with biotin,[49] cerebral folate deficiency with folinic acid,[28] cerebral creatine deficiency with creatine,[41] co-enzyme Q10 defects with co-enzyme Q10,[8] cobalamine-related defects with vitamin B12, and cyclic pyranopterin monophosphate for molybdenum cofactor complex deficiency (Tables 29.1 and 29.2).

DISORDERS MANAGED BY ADDRESSING TRIGGERS

Triggering Mechanisms

In several rare disorders, dystonia may be triggered by a specific environmental stimulus. Examples of such triggers are dietary changes, a minor illness such as the common cold, fever from vaccination, minor surgical procedures, or stress (either physical or psychological).[16] For some of these disorders, the trigger provokes permanent and often disabling dystonia. For other disorders, dystonia is a transient symptom that resolves when the trigger is addressed. However, in some cases, transient symptoms resolve only partially, and repeated exposure to the trigger results in progressive accumulation of permanent brain injury.

For some of these disorders, the biological mechanisms responsible for environmentally triggered dystonia are well understood. For others, the biological mechanisms are only partly understood. For all these disorders, avoidance or mitigation of the trigger can play an important role in management.

Disorders Triggered by Diet

Symptoms of GLUT1 deficiency (described briefly above) are triggered by fasting because the associated drop in blood glucose worsens the underlying impairment in transport of glucose into the brain. Avoidance of prolonged periods of fasting can reduce symptoms.

Fasting can also trigger dystonia in several metabolic disorders caused by defects in metabolic pathways responsible for producing energy in the brain. Presumably, reduced glucose associated with fasting slows metabolism enough to cause a limitation in energy production. One example is biotin-thiamin-responsive basal ganglia disease, described above. Other examples include glutaric aciduria type 1, methylmalonic aciduria, and propionic aciduria. These organic acidurias may present with a rapidly progressing encephalopathic crisis, striatal necrosis, and a permanent movement disorder dominated by dystonia. Avoidance of prolonged fasting is usually advised. A diet low in protein (especially lysine) is also recommended to reduce the burden of organic acids that are produced during amino acid metabolism.[13,21]

Maple syrup urine disease is a disorder of amino acid catabolism associated with pathogenic variants in several genes (*BCKDHA*, *BCKDHB*, or *DBT*) that encode different components of the branched-chain alpha-ketoacid dehydrogenase complex. Accumulation of branched chain amino acids typically results in neonatal encephalopathy, opisthotonus (dystonic truncal arching), and limb dyskinesia. However, late-onset cases have been described. Diets low in protein (especially leucine) provide the mainstay of treatment. Dietary non-compliance can cause recurrence of symptoms. Even with good adherence to the diet, fasting sometimes triggers symptoms because low serum glucose results in catabolism of muscle proteins to amino acids as an alternative energy source.

Fasting can also trigger symptoms in other disorders, although the responsible mechanisms are less clear. One example involves defects in *ATP1A3*, which encodes a sodium-potassium ATPase responsible for maintaining ion gradients for neuronal signaling.[12] Maintaining ion gradients is energetically very costly, so the mechanism may involve a demand for energy that exceeds capacity to produce it. The classical clinical picture evolves in children or young adults with a rapidly evolving syndrome of dystonia and parkinsonism that emerges sometimes overnight and sometimes with encephalopathy. After the neurological deficits are triggered, they may be permanent. There also are variant *ATP1A3* phenotypes that include onset in later adulthood, transient or slowly evolving dystonia-parkinsonism, or alternating hemiplegia of childhood. Although the mechanisms are not known, *ATP1A3* syndromes can also be triggered by alcohol binging, intercurrent illness, head injury, and overexertion.

The metabolism of galactose is impaired in galactosemia, which is caused by defects in several genes (*GALT*, *GALK1*, or *GALE*).[22,35] Typical clinical features begin in infancy with encephalopathy and intolerance of foods containing galactose. Galactose restriction is essential, but older children and adults may still develop dystonia, tremor, myoclonus, and/or pyramidal signs.

The metabolism of sulfur-containing amino acids is impaired in homocystinuria, which is caused by defects in *CBS*. Typical clinical features begin in infancy and include encephalopathy, seizures, ectopic lens, skeletal abnormalities, and recurrent stroke. Neurological symptoms may result from stroke, but progressive or paroxysmal dystonia without stroke may also occur.[7,18] Diets low in protein and especially in sulfur-containing amino acids are useful.

Disorders Triggered by Hyperthermia

For several rare childhood disorders, symptoms may be triggered by minor infections that produce fever, such as the common cold. They can also be triggered by fever sometimes associated with vaccination. The mechanisms by which hyperthermia triggers symptoms are not entirely understood. Presumably metabolic decompensation occurs when metabolism is accelerated by elevated temperatures.

This group of disorders contains many of the same disorders that may be triggered by fasting. Although it may be impossible to prevent infections, and vaccinations may be required, aggressive control of fever is often recommended.

Triggers of Paroxysmal Dyskinesias

The paroxysmal kinesigenic dyskinesias are a group of disorders associated with numerous different genes (see Chapter 17, "Dystonia and the Paroxysmal Dyskinesias").[9,53] The abnormal movements are varied but often include dystonic posturing. In paroxysmal kinesigenic dyskinesia, attacks can be triggered by sudden voluntary movement, startle, and sometimes other factors. Avoiding these triggers can be helpful, but avoidance is not always practical. For reasons that are not entirely understood, attacks can be eliminated with carbamazepine and related sodium channel antiseizure medications.

Paroxysmal non-kinesigenic dyskinesia is characterized by attacks of abnormal movements, often triggered by stress, caffeine, or alcohol. Avoiding these triggers may be helpful, and cases associated with *KCNMA1* may respond to amphetamine and related stimulants.[19,52]

In paroxysmal exertional dyskinesia, abnormal movements are triggered by longer periods of exercise. Avoiding extensive exercise can be helpful, and some cases respond to levodopa or dietary changes.

Pathogenic variants in *ADCY5* can cause a mixed movement disorder that may include dystonia combined with chorea, ataxia, tremor, and parkinsonism.[26] Many individuals have persistent motor abnormalities, but obvious worsening occurs with many triggers. Avoidance of triggers can be helpful, and a subgroup of individuals responds to caffeine and related drugs,[25,38] although the responsible mechanisms are not known.

SYNOPSIS AND FUTURE PROSPECTS

Dystonia may occur in several inherited disorders where specific treatments are available (Tables 29.1 and 29.2). Dystonia may be a consistent and severe aspect of the phenotype, dystonia may be an atypical manifestation of a disorder that usually presents with other features, or dystonia may only be an occasional or mild component of a multisystem disorder. All of these disorders are included in this chapter because dystonia may sometimes be the most prominent or presenting feature.

These disorders are quite rare, but they are important to recognize because specific treatments are available. For many disorders, the best results are obtained when treatment is started early, before significant brain injury or loss of function occurs. In some cases, treatment has proven value for reducing symptoms and preventing progression. In other cases, benefits are suspected from clinical experience or knowledge regarding the pathogenesis of the disorder, although large and rigorous clinical trials are lacking. When evidence-based medicine is lacking, clinical judgment is required.

This group of disorders with mechanism-specific treatments is likely to grow rapidly in the near future because the discovery of new genes is constantly revealing biological mechanisms that can then be targeted with specific interventions.[43]

REFERENCES

1. Atwal PS, Scaglia F. Molybdenum cofactor deficiency. Mol Genet Metab 2016;117:1–4.
2. Bandmann O, Weiss KH, Kaler SG. Wilson's disease and other neurological copper disorders. Lancet Neurol 2015;14:103–113.
3. Baumgartner MR. Vitamin-responsive disorders: Cobalamin, folate, biotin, vitamins B1 and E. Handb Clin Neurol 2013;113:1799–1810.
4. Carecchio M, Schneider SA, Chan H, Lachmann R, Lee PJ, Murphy E, Bhatia KP. Movement disorders in adult surviving patients with maple syrup urine disease. Mov Disord 2011;26:1324–1328.
5. Chien YH, Lee NC, Tseng SH, Tai CH, Muramatsu SI, Byrne BJ, Hwu WL. Efficacy and safety of AAV2 gene therapy in children with aromatic L-amino acid decarboxylase deficiency: An open-label, phase 1/2 trial. Lancet Child Adolesc Health 2017;1:265–273.
6. Di Meo I, Tiranti V. Classification and molecular pathogenesis of NBIA syndromes. Eur J Paediatr Neurol 2018;22:272–284.
7. Ekinci B, Apaydin H, Vural M, Ozekmekci S. Two siblings with homocystinuria presenting with dystonia and parkinsonism. Mov Disord 2004;19:962–964.
8. Emmanuele V, López LC, Berardo A, Naini A, Tadesse S, Wen B, et al. Heterogeneity of coenzyme Q10 deficiency: Patient study and literature review. Arch Neurol 2012;69:978–983.
9. Erro R, Bhatia KP. Unravelling of the paroxysmal dyskinesias. J Neurol Neurosurg Psychiatry 2019;90:227–234.
10. Friedman J, Roze E, Abdenur JE, Chang R, Gasperini S, Saletti V, et al. Sepiapterin reductase deficiency: A treatable mimic of cerebral palsy. Ann Neurol 2012;71:520–530.
11. Gras D, Roze E, Caillet S, Meneret A, Doummar D, Billette de Villemeur T, et al. GLUT1 deficiency syndrome: An update. Rev Neurol (Paris) 2014;170:91–99.
12. Heinzen EL, Arzimanoglou A, Brashear A, Clapcote SJ, Gurrieri F, Goldstein DB, et al. Distinct neurological disorders with ATP1A3 mutations. Lancet Neurol 2014;13:503–514.
13. Heringer J, Boy SP, Ensenauer R, Assmann B, Zschocke J, Harting I, et al. Use of guidelines improves the

neurological outcome in glutaric aciduria type I. Ann Neurol 2010;68:743–752.

14. Himmelreich N, Blau N, Thony B. Molecular and metabolic bases of tetrahydrobiopterin (BH4) deficiencies. Mol Genet Metab 2021;133:123–136.
15. Jinnah HA. The dystonias. Continuum 2019;25:976–1000.
16. Jinnah HA, Albanese A, Bhatia KP, Cardoso F, Da Prat G, de Koning TJ, et al. Treatable inherited rare movement disorders. Mov Disord 2018;33:21–35.
17. Kass HR, Winesett SP, Bessone SK, Turner Z, Kossoff EH. Use of dietary therapies amongst patients with GLUT1 deficiency syndrome. Seizure 2016;35:83–87.
18. Kempster PA, Brenton DP, Gale AN, Stern GM. Dystonia in homocystinuria. J Neurol Neurosurg Psychiatry 1988;51:859–862.
19. Keros S, Heim J, Hakami W, Zohar-Dayan E, Ben-Zeev B, Grinspan Z, et al. Lisdexamfetamine therapy in paroxysmal non-kinesigenic dyskinesia associated with the KCNMA1-N999S variant. Mov Disord Clin Pract 2022;9:229–235.
20. Klopstock T, Tricta F, Neumayr L, Karin I, Zorzi G, Fradette C, et al. Safety and efficacy of deferiprone for pantothenate kinase-associated neurodegeneration: A randomised, double-blind, controlled trial and an open-label extension study. Lancet Neurol 2019;18:631–642.
21. Kolker S, Christensen E, Leonard JV, Greenberg CR, Boneh A, Burlina AB, et al. Diagnosis and management of glutaric aciduria type I: Revised recommendations. J Inherit Metab Dis 2011;34:677–694.
22. Kuiper A, Grunewald S, Murphy E, Coenen MA, Eggink H, Zutt R, et al. Movement disorders and nonmotor neuropsychological symptoms in children and adults with classical galactosemia. J Inherit Metab Dis 2019;42:451–458.
23. Kurian MA, Gissen P, Smith M, Heales S, Jr., Clayton PT. The monoamine neurotransmitter disorders: An expanding range of neurological syndromes. Lancet Neurol 2011;10:721–733.
24. Lee J, Hegele RA. Abetalipoproteinemia and homozygous hypobetalipoproteinemia: A framework for diagnosis and management. J Inherit Metab Dis 2014;37:333–339.
25. Meneret A, Mohammad SS, Cif L, Doummar D, DeGusmao C, Anheim M, et al. Efficacy of caffeine in ADCY5-related dyskinesia: A retrospective study. Mov Disord 2022;37:1294–1298.
26. Menon PJ, Nilles C, Silveira-Moriyama L, Yuan R, de Gusmao CM, Munchau A, et al. Scoping review on ADCY5-related movement disorders. Mov Disord Clin Pract 2023;10:1048–1059.
27. Mochel F, Hainque E, Gras D, Adanyeguh IM, Caillet S, Heron B, et al. Triheptanoin dramatically reduces paroxysmal motor disorder in patients with GLUT1 deficiency. J Neurol Neurosurg Psychiatry 2016;87:550–553.
28. Molero-Luis M, Serrano M, O'Callaghan MM, Sierra C, Perez-Duenas B, Garcia-Cazorla A, Artuch R. Clinical, etiological and therapeutic aspects of cerebral folate deficiency. Expert Rev Neurother 2015;15:793–802.
29. Nagral A, Sarma MS, Matthai J, Kukkle PL, Devarbhavi H, Sinha S, et al. Wilson's disease: Clinical practice guidelines of the Indian National Association for Study of the Liver, the Indian Society of Pediatric Gastroenterology, Hepatology and Nutrition, and the Movement Disorders Society of India. J Clin Exp Hepatol 2019;9:74–98.
30. Nie S, Chen G, Cao X, Zhang Y. Cerebrotendinous xanthomatosis: A comprehensive review of pathogenesis, clinical manifestations, diagnosis, and management. Orphanet J Rare Dis 2014;9:179.
31. Pearson TS, Akman C, Hinton VJ, Engelstad K, De Vivo DC. Phenotypic spectrum of glucose transporter type 1 deficiency syndrome (Glut1 DS). Curr Neurol Neurosci Rep 2013;13:342.
32. Quadri M, Federico A, Zhao T, Breedveld GJ, Battisti C, Delnooz C, et al. Mutations in SLC30A10 cause parkinsonism and dystonia with hypermanganesemia, polycythemia, and chronic liver disease. Am J Hum Genet 2012;90:467–477.
33. Riley LG, Cowley MJ, Gayevskiy V, Roscioli T, Thorburn DR, Prelog K, et al. A SLC39A8 variant causes manganese deficiency, and glycosylation and mitochondrial disorders. J Inherit Metab Dis 2017;40:261–269.
34. Rilstone JJ, Alkhater RA, Minassian BA. Brain dopamine-serotonin vesicular transport disease and its treatment. N Engl J Med 2013;368:543–550.
35. Rubio-Agusti I, Carecchio M, Bhatia KP, Kojovic M, Parees I, Chandrashekar HS, et al. Movement disorders in adult patients with classical galactosemia. Mov Disord 2013;28:804–810.
36. Santos-Lozano A, Villamandos Garcia D, Sanchis-Gomar F, Fiuza-Luces C, Pareja-Galeano H, Garatachea N, et al. Niemann-Pick disease treatment: A systematic review of clinical trials. Ann Transl Med 2015;3:360.
37. Schuelke M. Ataxia with vitamin E deficiency. 2005 [Updated 2023 Mar 16]. In: Adam MP, Feldman J, Mirzaa GM, et al., eds. GeneReviews. University of Washington; 1993–2024. https://www.ncbi.nlm.nih.gov/books/
38. Shetty K, Sarma AS, Devan M, Dalal A, Dash GK, Jannabhatla A, Patil SJ. Recurrent ADCY5 mutation in mosaic form with nocturnal paroxysmal dyskinesias and video Eeectroencephalography documentation of dramatic response to caffeine treatment. J Mov Disord 2020;13:238–240.
39. Stelten BML, Dotti MT, Verrips A, Elibol B, Falik-Zaccai TC, Hanman K, et al. Expert opinion on diagnosing, treating and managing patients with cerebrotendinous xanthomatosis (CTX): A modified Delphi study. Orphanet J Rare Dis 2021;16:353.
40. Stelten BML, Huidekoper HH, van de Warrenburg BPC, Brilstra EH, Hollak CEM, Haak HR, et al. Long-term treatment effect in cerebrotendinous xanthomatosis depends on age at treatment start. Neurology 2019;92:e83–e95.
41. Stockler-Ipsiroglu S, van Karnebeek CD. Cerebral creatine deficiencies: A group of treatable intellectual developmental disorders. Semin Neurol 2014;34:350–356.
42. Tabarki B, Alfadhel M, Al Shahwan S, Hundallah K, Al Shafi S, Al Hashem A. Treatment of biotin-responsive basal ganglia disease: Open comparative study between the combination of biotin plus thiamine versus thiamine alone. Eur J Paediatr Neurol 2015;19:547–552.
43. Thakur N, Klopstock T, Jackowski S, Kuscer E, Tricta F, Videnovic A, Jinnah HA. Rational design of novel therapies for pantothenate kinase-associated neurodegeneration. Mov Disord 2021;36:2005–2016.
44. Tuschl K, Clayton PT, Gospe SM, Jr., Gulab S, Ibrahim S, Singhi P, et al. Syndrome of hepatic cirrhosis, dystonia, polycythemia, and hypermanganesemia caused by mutations in SLC30A10, a manganese transporter in man. Am J Hum Genet 2012;90:457–466.

45. Tuschl K, Meyer E, Valdivia LE, Zhao N, Dadswell C, Abdul-Sada A, et al. Mutations in SLC39A14 disrupt manganese homeostasis and cause childhood-onset parkinsonism-dystonia. Nat Commun 2016;7:11601.
46. Wassenberg T, Molero-Luis M, Jeltsch K, Hoffmann GF, Assmann B, Blau N, et al. Consensus guideline for the diagnosis and treatment of aromatic l-amino acid decarboxylase (AADC) deficiency. Orphanet J Rare Dis 2017;12:12.
47. Wijemanne S, Jankovic J. Dopa-responsive dystonia--clinical and genetic heterogeneity. Nat Rev Neurol 2015;11:414–424.
48. Willemsen MA, Verbeek MM, Kamsteeg EJ, de Rijk-van Andel JF, Aeby A, Blau N, et al. Tyrosine hydroxylase deficiency: A treatable disorder of brain catecholamine biosynthesis. Brain 2010;133:1810–1822.
49. Wolf B. Successful outcomes of older adolescents and adults with profound biotinidase deficiency identified by newborn screening. Genet Med 2017;19:396–402.
50. Yahalom G, Tsabari R, Molshatzki N, Ephraty L, Cohen H, Hassin-Baer S. Neurological outcome in cerebrotendinous xanthomatosis treated with chenodeoxycholic acid: Early versus late diagnosis. Clin Neuropharmacol 2013;36:78–83.
51. Ye J, Yang Y, Yu W, Zou H, Jiang J, Yang R, et al. Demographics, diagnosis and treatment of 256 patients with tetrahydrobiopterin deficiency in mainland China: Results of a retrospective, multicentre study. J Inherit Metab Dis 2013;36:893–901.
52. Zhang G, Gibson RA, McDonald M, Liang P, Kang PW, Shi J, et al. A gain-of-function mutation in KCNMA1 causes dystonia spells controlled with stimulant therapy. Mov Disord 2020;35:1868–1873.
53. Zima L, Ceulemans S, Reiner G, Galosi S, Chen D, Sahagian M, et al. Paroxysmal motor disorders: Expanding phenotypes lead to coalescing genotypes. Ann Clin Transl Neurol 2018;5:996–1010.

Chapter 30

Botulinum Toxin Treatment for Dystonia

INTRODUCTION

Botulinum neurotoxin (BoNT) is an extraordinarily versatile treatment for all types of dystonias. It is effective in the isolated dystonias but also in more complex disorders where dystonia is combined with other problems. It is most commonly used for focal or segmental dystonias where a relatively small number of muscles can be targeted as there are limits in the total dose that can be given and the number of injection sites that people can tolerate. However, BoNT can also be used to target the most troublesome areas in individuals with broader patterns of dystonia, such as generalized dystonia.

BoNT has been the focus of numerous reviews[1,5,12,30,53,55,84] and books.[4,57,88] These resources provide detailed information on basic mechanisms of BoNT, as well as detailed instructions for application in specific disorders. BoNT also has been the focus of numerous evidence-based and systematic reviews.[13,18,27,33,39,49,80,86,93] In these types of reviews, the criteria used to reach the highest levels of evidence regarding clinical utility require multiple independent double-blind and placebo-controlled trials with large numbers of participants, with each condition and BoNT formulation evaluated separately. Multiple studies for each product in each type of dystonia are not available because these disorders are rare. In addition, clinical benefits are obvious, thus discouraging redundant studies. As a result, several BoNT formulations do not reach the highest levels of evidence required by evidence-based criteria. Despite this limitation from evidence-based medicine, there is widespread acceptance that BoNT is the treatment of first choice for many types of dystonia.

This chapter summarizes some fundamental principles that are relevant to all applications including basic mechanism of action, timing of effects, factors that influence efficacy and side effects, and some limitations and common reasons for treatment failure. These basic principles are valuable for clinicians who may refer individuals for BoNT therapy as well as for clinicians involved in their application. Similarities among the different BoNTs are more notable than their differences,[26,33,49,60,71,86] so they are discussed as a group rather than individually. Uses of BoNT for more specific indications are further described in Chapter 5, "Cervical Dystonia," Chapter 6, "Craniofacial Dystonias," Chapter 7, "Laryngeal Dystonias," and Chapter 8, "Limb Dystonias."

BASIC MECHANISMS

Mechanism of Action

Most BoNTs originate from *Clostridium botulinum*, the bacterium responsible for botulism. There are multiple BoNT serotypes, but only serotypes A and B are available for therapeutic use (Table 30.1). Different preparations are offered in many parts of the world, and the most widely available derived from serotype A include abobotulinumtoxinA (Dysport), daxibotulinumtoxinA (Daxxify), incobotulinumtoxinA (Xeomin), onabotulinumtoxinA (Botox). Serotype B is available as rimabotulinumtoxinB (Myobloc or Neurobloc). New formulations with different properties are currently being developed.[87]

Once injected, BoNTs bind to presynaptic nerve terminals (Figure 30.1). The receptors are synaptic vesicle associated membrane glycoproteins (SV2 for serotype A and synaptotagmin for serotype B) which are transiently exposed on the external surface of the presynaptic terminals following fusion of presynaptic vesicles with the membrane during the process of exocytosis. After binding, the BoNTs are taken into the presynaptic membrane by endocytosis and then released into the cytosol. Once in the cytosol, they act as proteases to cleave specific proteins required for the release of synaptic vesicles. Serotype A cleaves a protein called synaptosomal-associated protein-25kD (SNAP-25), while serotype B cleaves vesicle-associated membrane protein (VAMP). When these proteins are cleaved, the exocytosis of synaptic vesicles containing acetylcholine becomes less efficient, and neuromuscular activity is reduced.

The most common explanation given for the mechanism of action of BoNT in dystonia involves a reduction of acetylcholine release from presynaptic alpha motor neurons leading to reduced muscle activity.[48,50,54] However, there is some evidence that other mechanisms play a role. Intramuscular injections of BoNT also reduce neural transmission from gamma motor neurons to intrafusal muscle fibers with muscle spindles. Sensory afferents innervating these spindles convey information regarding overall muscle stretch and tone. BoNT reduces intrafusal muscle contraction, relaxes the spindles, and reduces afferent spindle activity. It has been proposed that the effect of BoNT in dystonia may reflect a resetting of muscle tone, a phenomenon that could occur at the peripheral or central level.[48,58,81] This effect may explain the poor correlation between clinical efficacy and muscle weakness.[22] It may also explain why unilateral

Table 30.1 **Therapeutic botulinum toxins**

	Onabotulinum toxin A	Daxibotulinum toxin A	Abobotulinum toxin A	Incobotulinum toxin A	Rimabotulinum toxin B
Trade name	Botox	Daxxify	Dysport	Xeomin	Myobloc or Neurobloc
Receptor	SV2	SV2	SV2	SV2	synaptotagmin
Cleavage target	SNAP-25	SNAP-25	SNAP-25	SNAP-25	VAMP
Molecular weight (kD)	900	900	500-900	150	700
Preparation	Dried powder	Dried powder	Dried powder	Dried powder	Liquid
Recommended storage	<8° C	<25° C	<8° C	<25° C	<8° C
Albumen content	500 μg	none	125 μg	1,000 μg	500 μg/mL
Additional ingredients	NaCl	35 amino acid peptide, histidine, trehalaose, polysorbate	lactose	sucrose	NaCL; sodium succinate
Vial sizes (units)	50, 100, 200	50, 100	300, 500	50, 100, 200	2,500, 5,000, 10,000

Albumen is included in many preparations as a stabilizing protein. Specific activity refers to the relative amount of active botulinum toxin in relation to other added proteins.

Abbreviations: SV2, synaptic vesicle protein 2; SNAP-25, synaptosomal-associated protein-25kD; VAMP, vesicle-associated membrane protein

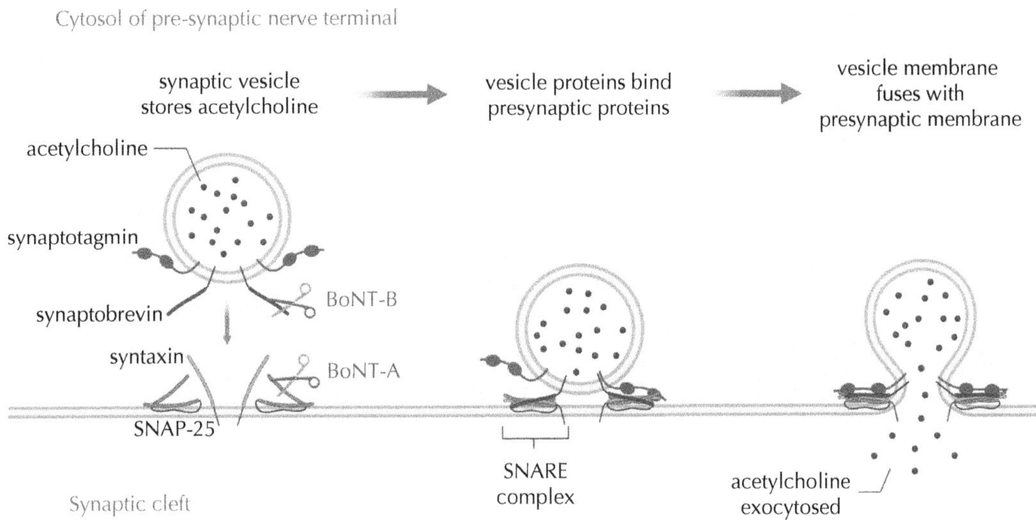

Figure 30.1. Botulinum toxin mechanism of action. This treatment targets vesicular release of acetylcholine, which is a multistep process that involves docking of the vesicle with the presynaptic cell membrane of the neuromuscular junction via SNARE complex proteins and then fusion of the vesicular and presynaptic membranes to release the acetylcholine. BoNT cleaves essential SNARE complex proteins (serotype A cleaves SNAP-25 and serotype B cleaves synaptobrevin) rendering the vesicle docking and release mechanism less efficient.

injections for blepharospasm[45] or laryngeal dystonia[11] reduce muscle activity bilaterally, or the common clinical observation that injection into one muscle seems to reduce dystonia in other muscles that are too far to reach by a spreading mechanism.

Others have proposed a central effect following migration of the toxin to the spinal cord and brain,[15,52] although definitive evidence for this mechanism is lacking. It has not been established whether the very small amounts of BoNT reaching the central nervous system have any functional effect. There are numerous functional neuroimaging studies showing changes in the activity of multiple regions of the sensorimotor cortex and other regions of the brain following BoNT,[48,52] but these changes may reflect an indirect effect of BoNT on sensorimotor feedback rather than a direct effect of BoNT on the brain.

Timing of Action

Numerous studies of many types of dystonia describe BoNT onset of action, peak effects, and overall therapeutic duration.[38,39,60,63,69,71,80,91] For the dystonias, most studies report that clinical benefits emerge in 5–15 days, although some individuals report noticing benefits almost immediately and others may not appreciate benefits for several weeks. This wide variation may be explained by the fact that most estimates of onset usually come from feedback from treated individuals, and these reports are subjective.

Peak benefits have been measured by patient-reported outcomes and quality of life measures, as well as clinician-rated outcomes. Peak benefits for dystonia usually fall between 4 and 8 weeks. The duration of benefit has been assessed by measuring the duration between injection cycles, the return of motor symptoms as assessed by clinician-rated scales, and by reports of returning symptoms in treated individuals. For cervical dystonia, a systematic review of 18 studies that included more than 1,900 individuals revealed mean durations of benefit from 63 to 143 days, with an overall average of 93 days.[69] The duration of benefit was partly dose-dependent, with higher doses giving longer durations. A similar dose effect was also described in a detailed study of the temporal profile of BoNT in blepharospasm.[71]

Many clinics routinely schedule individuals for repeat BoNT treatments every 90 days. However, it is important to recognize that estimates of duration of action reflect average values, and there are significant individual differences. A fixed 90-day retreatment interval can produce a cyclical therapeutic effect that has become known as the *yo-yo* effect or the *roller coaster* effect.[29,65,75,92] Symptoms may persist for a week or two after injection, followed by a period of relief of symptoms peaking between 4 and 6 weeks, and eventually a waning period when symptoms return after 8–12 weeks (Figure 30.2). The duration of this cycle and the amplitude of swings are not well characterized, but they vary among individuals even for the same indication. Not

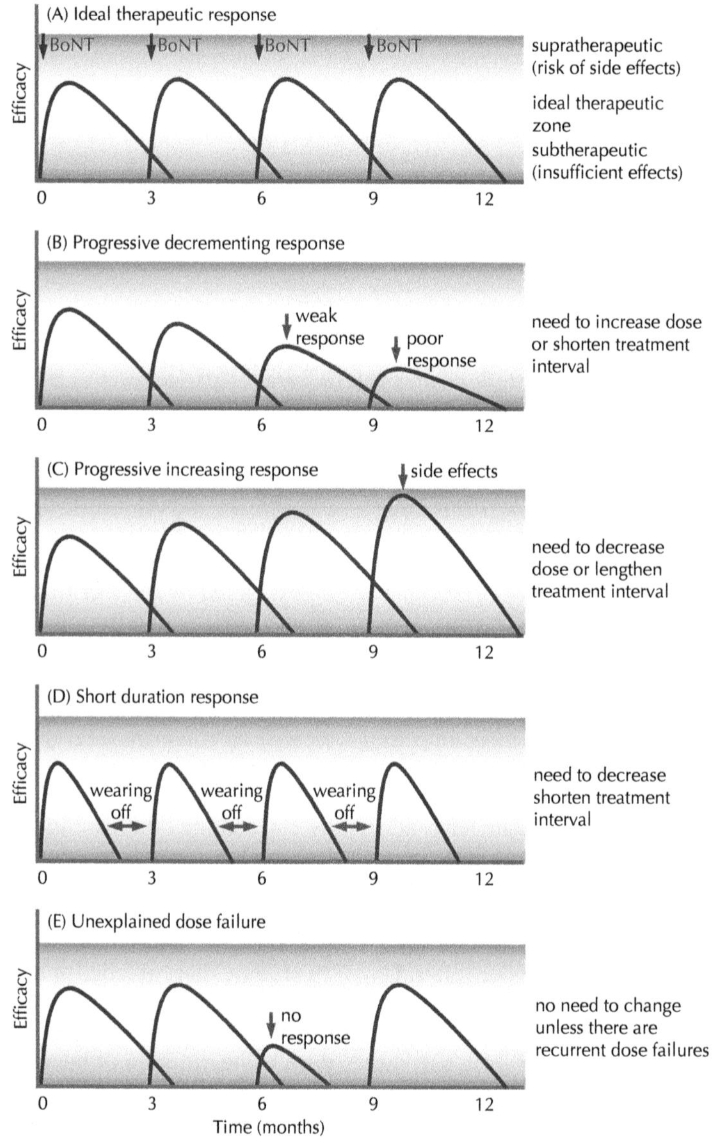

Figure 30.2. Cyclical therapeutic responses to botulinum toxin. Panel A shows the ideal therapeutic response which maximizes time in the ideal therapeutic zone. Panel B shows a progressively diminishing response, where the dose may need to be increased. Panel C shows a progressively increasing effect, where the dose may need to be decreased. Panel D shows a 3-month fixed interval for an individual who has a short-duration response, where the best approach might be to shorten the treatment interval since increasing the dose may risk side effects. Panel D shows the occasional treatment that fails even when there have been no changes in dose pattern. It is best to avoid over-reacting and increasing the dose with an unexpected dose failure because the next dose may resume its normal effects.

surprisingly, satisfaction with BoNT treatment varies according to the injection cycle, with best satisfaction at peak benefits and lower satisfaction when benefits wear off.[24,25,29,41,65,85] In view of this cyclical phenomenon, scheduling for repeat treatment must be customized according to individual needs. Scheduling should avoid waiting until benefits have entirely worn off. Some individuals may need repeat treatment every 8 weeks, while others may be able to wait for 6 months.[29,36,68,74]

Spread

The effects of BoNT are related to local actions at the site of injection. As a result, a basic understanding of mechanisms of spread of BoNT at the injection point is important for appreciating both therapeutic specificity and unwanted side effects. The term *spread* has been used in different ways in the literature,[47,78] but here is used to refer to any movement of BoNT away from the site of injection. There are four main mechanisms for spread. The most clinically relevant mechanism for spread is *convection*, which involves the immediate bulk movement of BoNT in the volume of liquid injected. The movement of injected liquid can be visualized via ultrasound. Injected liquid preferentially distributes in the direction of muscle fibers, usually the long axis of the muscle. The movement of liquid can also be seen following subcutaneous injections for blepharospasm, where a visible bleb marks the distribution of liquid as it physically dissects the virtual space between the skin and underlying tissue. Spread by convention depends on the volume of liquid injected; large volumes spread more than smaller ones. For example, a dose delivered in a small volume should have a more localized effect, while the same dose delivered in a larger volume may spread over a wider region. A larger convective spread may achieve a better outcome by distributing in a larger volume of muscle, but at the risk of increased side effects due to leakage and spread to nearby muscles (Figure 30.3).[82] Smaller muscles may require smaller volumes to limit spread, but a greater distribution of spread may be desirable in larger muscles where there is limited risk of spread to nearby muscles and spread to the endplate may be beneficial. Convection occurs almost immediately, within seconds. Further spread by convection is limited unless the site is massaged.

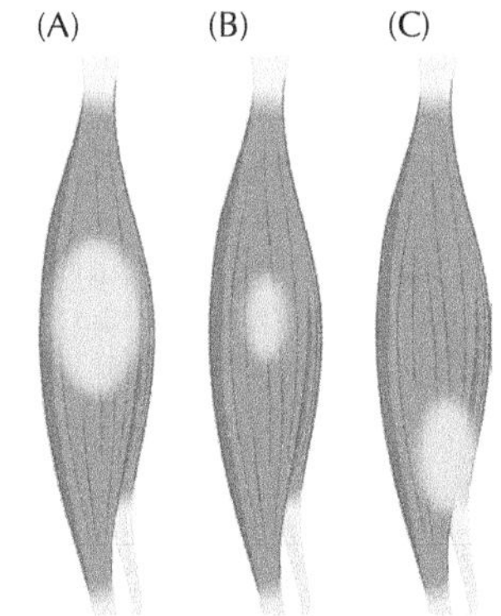

Figure 30.3. Relationship between spread and volume of injection into muscle. (A) A large volume is distributed rapidly by convection over a large area, usually in the direction of muscle fibers. (B) The same dose given in a smaller volume will spread less. (C) Care must be taken to avoid injecting too far toward the end of a muscle where muscle tissue is replaced by tendon or where bipennate muscles bifurcate into two tendinous connections, such as the biceps or sternocleidomastoid.

The relationship between dose and volume has been best studied in spasticity, where larger muscles safely permit manipulation of volumes and concentrations in relation to the known location of motor endplates.[82] These studies often report that volume of injection or proximity to motor endplates significantly impacts electrophysiological or muscle imaging characteristics, but functional outcomes often show no obvious clinical differences. The lack of impact on functional outcomes may reflect the limited ability of measurement tools to detect a meaningful change in spasticity so further studies are still needed to establish clinical relevance of these variables.

Diffusion refers to the random Brownian motion of dissolved molecules, usually following a concentration gradient. This mechanism probably contributes very little to BoNT spread, not more than a few millimeters.[47,78] *Migration* refers to the distant intracellular movement of BoNT after it is taken up by presynaptic nerve terminals. There is evidence that BoNT is transported from the axon terminal to the soma of motor neurons in the spinal cord.[6,15] From the spinal cord, it may also be transported via dendrites to higher levels of the central nervous system. The clinical relevance of migration via intracellular transport is not clear.

BoNT is also cleared from the interstitial spaces via the lymphatic system into the bloodstream, where it can have distant effects. Sensitive electrophysiological measures can detect effects in distant muscles, but these effects have limited clinical significance.[47,78] Most likely the lack of distant functional effects relates to the small amounts of BoNT reaching the bloodstream, the large volume of distribution throughout the body, and rapid clearance of the circulating proteins by the liver and other tissues.

CLINICAL APPLICATION

Targeting

Precise targeting of BoNT is important for optimizing therapeutic benefits and minimizing side effects. The muscles to treat are based on the patient's report of abnormal movements and pain, inspection to delineate areas with overt muscle spasm or hypertrophy, and palpation to identify tense or moving muscles. There are three main strategies for targeting the injection. They include clinical maneuvers, electromyography (EMG), and visually guided procedures such as ultrasound (or nasoendoscopy for laryngeal dystonia).[17,90]

The best targeting strategy is partly dependent on the condition being treated. For blepharospasm, it is often sufficient to conduct a careful visual clinical exam to delineate which portions of the orbicularis oculi or nearby muscles are most affected (see Chapter 6). Since injections targeting these thin facial muscles are often delivered subcutaneously overlying the muscles instead of intramuscularly, EMG and ultrasound are rarely used. On the other hand, targeting the muscles controlling the hand usually requires a careful clinical evaluation combined with EMG or ultrasound because the proximity of many small muscles controlling the hand makes targeting more challenging. For the small and deep muscles of the larynx, EMG or nasoendoscopy is often used. The value of targeting procedures for cervical dystonia is controversial. Many experts rely on the clinical exam alone while others advocate EMG or ultrasound for all cases (see Chapter 5).[17,73,90]

Each targeting strategy has different strengths and weaknesses (Table 30.2). The main advantage of using the clinical evaluation alone is that it keeps attention focused on the clinical problems to be addressed, including abnormal movements, muscle hypertrophy, muscle tension, and pain or pulling sensations. The obvious disadvantages include the possibility of missing the target, inadvertently injecting nearby targets, or neglecting important muscles that are active but not obvious from the clinical exam alone. Advantages of EMG include confirmation that the needle is in muscle tissue, information regarding muscle activity level, and whether the needle is close to a motor endplate where BoNT is thought to be most effective. The main disadvantage is focusing attention on the EMG signal, which sometimes does not correlate with clinical need. Additional drawbacks include the added time and cost for the EMG procedure and increased pain due to frequent manipulations of the EMG needle or equipment. The main advantage of ultrasound is visualization of the muscle being targeted. Disadvantages include the added time and cost for the procedure, the limited availability of ultrasound equipment in many clinics, and the frequent need for more than a single clinician to perform the procedure because it is technically challenging to hold the ultrasound probe and do the injection at the same time.

Table 30.2 **Botulinum toxin targeting methods**

	Main advantages	Main disadvantages
Clinical exam	Attention stays focused on exam	Potential for missing target
Electromyography	Confirmation needle is in muscle Information about activity level Information about endplate	Added expense of equipment and needles Added time for set up Increased pain from specialized needles and manipulations Sometimes poor correlation between signal and clinical need
Ultrasound	Confirmation needle is in muscle Information about location within muscle	Added expense of equipment and materials Added time for setup and clean up Frequent need for additional personnel

Dosing

Numerous resources provide guidance for BoNT doses for specific muscles.[4,57,88] These resources provide useful guides for average target doses and typical dose ranges, but doses must be customized for differences in muscle size and dystonic activity for individual patients. It is also likely that there are individual differences in sensitivity to the effects of BoNT or its duration. Finally, each muscle has a maximum dose that saturates BoNT uptake mechanisms so excessive doses will not add further benefit but may contribute to side effects.

The initial doses require careful consideration. The phrase "start low and go slow" is often applied to BoNT, but starting too low and going too slow can be frustrating to affected individuals because the typical 90-day interval between treatments combined with the need for 2–4 treatment cycles to reach optimal doses may take a year to achieve a satisfactory result. An alternative approach to selecting the initial dose is to estimate the therapeutic dose according to average target doses, modify these targets according to individual characteristics (muscle mass and dystonic activity), and apply 80% of this dose in the first visit. While this strategy leads to a therapeutic dose more quickly, it also carries a greater risk for unwanted side effects from overdosing. In view of these very different strategies, it is reasonable to engage patients in selecting the initial dosing strategy. Some individuals may prefer a more conservative approach, while others with severely discomforting dystonia may want more immediate relief regardless of risks.

Another dosing issue involves the concept of BoNT *units*. Because units are based on different standards, these units vary among products.[31,83] A basic understanding of these differences is useful when there is a need to switch products because of a medical decision, personal preference, or insurance requirements. Many studies comparing units across products define onabotulinumtoxinA as the standard because it was the first to become clinically available. A single unit of onobotulinumtoxinA is similar to 1.0 units of daxibotulinumtoxinA, 1.0–1.1 units of incobotulinum toxin, 2.5–3.0 units of abobotulinumtoxinA, and 50 units of rimabotulinumtoxinB (Table 30.1).

Some experts have argued that units are not readily converted between products and that switching to a new product should be subject to conservative first dose strategies such as "start low and go slow" described above. This strategy is likely to produce an unsatisfactory initial outcome for the second product. An alternative strategy is to estimate the equivalent dose using available information on relative units. Thus, a patient receiving 200 units of onabotulinumtoxinA would receive 200 units of daxibotulinumtoxinA, 100 units of incobotulinumtoxinA, 500–600 units of abobotulinumtoxinA, or 10,000 units of rimabotulinumtoxinB. This second strategy still carries a risk of a dose that is a bit too high or too low, but it is more likely to produce a result comparable to the first product used.

Patient Expectations

Counseling regarding expectations is an important first step in beginning therapy with BoNT.[28,70,90] The duration between symptom onset and diagnosis may span many years. Affected individuals may have seen many clinicians and may have been offered a variety of treatments with little or no benefit. As a result, they may be fearful or skeptical about BoNT, especially considering that the term "toxin" carries negative connotations in the lay community. Counseling regarding expectations of benefits and risks is therefore useful.

Other individuals may have unrealistic expectations to be completely symptom-free following BoNT so counseling is needed to set expectations. One study found that nearly two-thirds of individuals with cervical dystonia expected to be completely free of pain and/or abnormal movements following treatment.[28] Treatment may provide complete relief of symptoms, but a target of 80% relief may be a more realistic goal. There is good evidence that many patients try BoNT once or twice and then abandon treatment so they should be counseled that a period of customization of the dose and pattern may take some time.[70] It is important to be clear that BoNT is not a cure but an injectable muscle relaxant that wears off in 2–4 months. It therefore must be repeated.

Other Relevant Variables

Many individuals with dystonia ask about combining BoNT therapy with physical therapy.

Numerous small and unblinded trials have suggested potential benefits from various types of physical therapy in the dystonias (see Chapter 32, "Physiotherapy and Complementary Medicine for Dystonia").[32,76] Unfortunately, the largest and most rigorous trials of physical therapy have not demonstrated consistent benefits.[32,66,76] However, some people appear to experience at least partial or temporary relief of symptoms with physical therapy,[28,42] so it seems reasonable to offer it according to individual preferences.

For pain of musculoskeletal origin, ice packs or other cooling measures are often recommended in the acute stage to reduce inflammation, and heat is sometimes recommended in the chronic stage to speed recovery. Many individuals with dystonia therefore ask about cooling or heating sore muscles after receiving BoNT,[14] and some clinicians routinely apply cooling sprays to the skin to reduce injection site pain. There are no systematic studies addressing the impact of temperature manipulations on BoNT outcomes. In principle, low temperatures may impact the spread or uptake of BoNT, and high temperatures risk denaturing BoNT proteins. However, it is not likely that surface manipulations will change temperatures within muscle to have any significant impact on any of these processes. As a result, treated individuals may be advised to wait for 15–30 minutes following injections and then apply either cooling or heating according to personal preferences.

Many patients obtain partial relief of symptoms from massage or pressure on dystonic muscles, and they may ask about these procedures in relation to BoNT.[14] Immediately following an injection, such manipulations may encourage spread and should therefore be discouraged. However, the majority of BoNT is taken up into presynaptic terminals or eliminated from the site in a few minutes, so treated individuals may be allowed to apply muscle pressure or massage 30–60 minutes following injections.

The uptake of BoNT is partly dependent on presynaptic motor neuron activity.[34] In fact, BoNT appears to gain entry into pathologically activated motor neurons more efficiently than normal motor neurons in hemifacial spasm.[50] Therefore, it is logical to hypothesize that intentional activation of target muscles may improve the effects of BoNT. There are no large rigorous studies addressing the impact of activating target muscles on BoNT outcomes, but one unblinded study of eight individuals with writer's cramp showed that 30 minutes of writing following treatment produced slightly greater muscle weakness, but a clinical benefit for reducing dystonia was not significant.[19] Although the impact of activating pathological muscles on clinical outcomes remains to be determined, treated individuals should not be advised to try to suppress dystonic muscle activity following injections.

The protease activity of BoNT is zinc-dependent, so some have advocated zinc supplements as adjunctive therapy. One study suggested a benefit of zinc supplements when treating blepharospasm or hemifacial spasm with BoNT,[61] but the results were later called into question.[21] Since then, there have been no rigorous studies addressing the impact of zinc supplements on BoNT outcomes. Although zinc supplements are not routinely recommended, it is reasonable to provide them to individuals who are zinc-deficient.

In summary, many variables may influence efficacy and side effects of BoNT for dystonia, including concentration of BoNT, volume and number of injections, localization methods and proximity to motor endplates, muscle activity before or after injection, adjunctive use of zinc or physical therapy, and others. Many of these variables have been the target of proof-of-concept studies in animals, but translatability of the results to people with dystonia has not been established.

SIDE EFFECTS AND LIMITATIONS

Side Effects

The most common side effects of BoNT relate to excessive weakening of treated muscles and/or unwanted spread to nearby muscles. For example, excessive weakening of neck muscles in cervical dystonia may be reflected by a sensation of head heaviness, the head drooping forward when upright or leaning forward, or difficulty picking up the head when lying supine. Some individuals note worsening neck pain or headaches due to compensatory overactivity of nontreated muscles or treated muscles that have become too weak. The most common side effect of excessive weakening in blepharospasm is lagophthalmos (weak eye closure), and a period of breathiness due to weakened vocal muscles is not uncommon following treatment of laryngeal dystonia. Unwanted hand or finger weakness is the most common side effect from treating focal hand dystonia. Side effects from excessive weakening are best managed by reducing the dose.

Another category of side effects is caused by spread. Among individuals treated for cervical or laryngeal dystonia, spread of BoNT to nearby muscles of swallowing can cause dysphagia. In blepharospasm, ptosis is a common side effect related to spread of BoNT to the levator palpebrae, diplopia may result from spread to deep muscles of the orbit that control eye movements, dry eye results from spread to the nearby lacrimal glands, and watery eyes result from spread to the lacrimal pump. These side effects from spread can be managed by more precise placement of injections, reducing the volume of injection to limit spread, or reducing the dose.

Systemic effects of spread are uncommon. However, a flu-like syndrome may occur with diffuse myalgia, fatigue, and fever. This syndrome usually is mild and lasts only a few days, but it can be uncomfortable or of longer duration.[8,9] This syndrome is likely caused by activation of the immune system by BoNT or one of the complexing proteins used to stabilize it, and the problem can be managed by switching to a less immunogenic preparation.[8,43] There are also rare cases of brachial neuritis following BoNT, although a causal relationship is not clear.[16]

Treatment Failures

Treatment failures can be divided into two groups.[10] Primary resistance refers to the lack of meaningful clinical response from the start of therapy despite multiple trials. Primary resistance is rare and usually reflects inadequate dose, improper muscle targeting, or incorrect diagnosis. However, obtaining good responses is known to be difficult for certain types of dystonia.[64] For cervical dystonia, individuals with prominent head tremor or predominant anterocollis are more difficult to treat than those with torticollis or laterocollis.[40,56] Obtaining good responses for individuals with blepharospasm who have prominent apraxia of eyelid opening is more difficult than for those with excessive blinking or orbital spasms.[2,7,35,79] For laryngeal dystonia, getting reliable responses is more challenging in the abductor subtype than the adductor subtype.[91] Complex hand dystonias[59,67] or oromandibular dystonia with tongue involvement[84] can be particularly challenging. In view of these observations, failure to respond from the start of BoNT therapy may not always reflect resistance.

Several trials may be required before concluding an individual has primary resistance. In addition, clinical assessment with direct examination at the time of expected peak benefit is important to determine whether suboptimal benefit is due to an inadequate dose producing insufficient muscle weakness, targeting incorrect muscles, introduction of side effects that are wrongly interpreted by the individual as worsening of dystonia, or other reasons. For example, individuals with blepharospasm may report their eyes continue to close even after treatment, but a direct evaluation is needed to determine if this reflects residual untreated blepharospasm or ptosis from overdosing. If the individual is not examined after reporting suboptimal benefit, it can be challenging to know how to modify injection strategies to improve the outcome.

Secondary resistance refers to the loss of clinical response after a previous period of good responses. Historically, secondary resistance was ascribed to the development of neutralizing antibodies.[10] When BoNT was first introduced as a therapy for dystonia, many individuals developed antibodies and became resistant to its effects, with two main contributing reasons. Early preparations of BoNT contained some impurities that were highly immunogenic, and the lack of information on doses and dose intervals led to a trial-and-error approach, often with very frequent injections of very small amounts. Immunoresistance is now rare because modern preparations of BoNT are largely free of impurities, and most providers avoid frequent booster doses.[90] Currently, other reasons for secondary resistance are more common. Several studies have shown that secondary resistance most commonly reflects inadequate dosing or targeting, often because of unrecognized evolution of the individual's condition over time with increased severity or number of muscles involved.[56,73,89]

Clinical tests of functional resistance should be conducted when primary or secondary resistance is suspected. There are numerous studies reporting a high frequency of "neutralizing antibodies" or "blocking antibodies" in individuals treated with BoNT.[3,10,20,23,37,51,62,64,72,77] However, the correlation between these antibody tests and clinical response is poor. Many individuals may have good clinical responses despite high antibody titers. These tests therefore have limited value in assessing clinical resistance to BoNT.

A more useful clinical test is to inject BoNT into a region where the clinical response is easy to assess. One such test involves injecting 20–40 equivalent units of onabotulinumtoxinA into the extensor digitorum brevis, the muscle responsible for raising the four small toes of the foot.[46] Atrophy of this muscle is readily visualized 4 weeks later, and the effect can be quantified by comparing surface EMG between the treated and untreated foot. The main limitation is weakness of toe dorsiflexion. Alternative tests with less obvious side effects include injecting 10–25 equivalent units of BoNT into the frontalis in one or several sites and then assessing forehead wrinkling 4 weeks later, or injections into the medial brow targeting the corrugator/procerus and assessing the ability to frown.[10] These facial injections have few functional consequences, and the negative cosmetic appearance of facial asymmetry can be corrected by treating the other side if desired.

Discontinuation of Therapy

Although BoNT has proven efficacy for many types of dystonia, several studies have shown high rates of discontinuation.[14,44,55,59,64,67,90] Longitudinal studies from experienced centers have suggested that approximately one-third of patients with cervical dystonia and blepharospasm eventually stop therapy. Discontinuation is even higher (approximately half of all treated patients) for focal hand dystonia or more complex dystonias.[59,64,67]

There are many potential reasons for discontinuation. Discontinuation may occur early (after only 1–2 treatments) or later (after many cycles of successful treatment). Early discontinuation may reflect inadequate counseling regarding the need to customize dose patterns over 2–3 treatment cycles, unrealistic expectations, or unexpectedly troublesome side effects. Later discontinuation reflects a variety of reasons including insufficient efficacy, recurrent side effects, dislike of injections, and practical considerations such as travel and cost.[14,29,68,90]

SYNOPSIS AND FUTURE PROSPECTS

BoNT is one of the most versatile therapies that can be used for many different types of dystonia. In experienced hands, good long-term outcomes can be expected for the majority of individuals with dystonia. Therapeutic efficacy and unwanted side effects may be influenced by numerous variables including the type and severity of dystonia being treated, the BoNT dose, the volume and timing of injections, the localization of injections, muscle activity before or after injection, adjunctive use of zinc or physical therapy, and others. However, the exact impact of many of these variables on dystonia remains unproved because conclusive studies in the relevant populations addressing functionally meaningful outcomes and side effects are lacking and further studies are needed.

Historically, many treated individuals became resistant to therapy because of the development of antibodies. Fortunately, antibody-mediated resistance is now relatively rare so other reasons need to be explored when an individual with good responses appears to become less responsive. A substantial portion of individuals discontinue therapy, even when they are not resistant. Further studies of the reasons for discontinuation are needed to improve treatment outcomes and long-term adherence.

There are substantial ongoing efforts aimed at further improving BoNT therapies. One major area of improvement relates to educating clinicians regarding existing therapeutics for the ideal muscle targets, doses, and reinjection intervals. Another relates to bioengineering the BoNT molecule itself to improve molecular targeting or duration of action. Therefore, the value of BoNT therapy is likely to continue to grow in the future.

REFERENCES

1. Albanese A, Abbruzzese G, Dressler D, Duzynski W, Khatkova S, Marti MJ, et al. Practical guidance for CD management involving treatment of botulinum toxin: A consensus statement. J Neurol 2015;262:2201–2213.
2. Albanese A, Bentivoglio AR, Colosimo C, Galardi G, Maderna L, Tonali P. Pretarsal injections of botulinum toxin improve blepharospasm in previously unresponsive patients. J Neurol Neurosurg Psychiatry 1996;60:693–694.
3. Albrecht P, Jansen A, Lee JI, Moll M, Ringelstein M, Rosenthal D, et al. High prevalence of neutralizing antibodies after long-term botulinum neurotoxin therapy. Neurology 2019;92:e48–e54.
4. Alter KE, Wilson NA. *Botulinum Toxin Dosing Manual.* Demos; 2021.
5. Anandan C, Jankovic J. Botulinum toxin in movement disorders: An update. Toxins 2021;13:42.

6. Antonucci F, Rossi C, Gianfranceschi L, Rossetto O, Caleo M. Long-distance retrograde effects of botulinum neurotoxin A. J Neurosci 2008;28:3689–3696.
7. Aramideh M, Ongerboer de Visser BW, Brans JW, Koelman JH, Speelman JD. Pretarsal application of botulinum toxin for treatment of blepharospasm. J Neurol Neurosurg Psychiatry 1995;59:309–311.
8. Baizabal-Carvallo JF, Jankovic J, Feld J. Flu-like symptoms and associated immunological response following therapy with botulinum toxins. Neurotox Res 2013;24:298–306.
9. Baizabal-Carvallo JF, Jankovic J, Pappert E. Flu-like symptoms following botulinum toxin therapy. Toxicon 2011;58:1–7.
10. Bellows S, Jankovic J. Immunogenicity associated with botulinum toxin treatment. Toxins 2019;11:491.
11. Bielamowicz S, Ludlow CL. Effects of botulinum toxin on pathophysiology in spasmodic dysphonia. Ann Otol Rhinol Laryngol 2000;109:194–203.
12. Blitzer A, Brin MF, Stewart CF. Botulinum toxin management of spasmodic dysphonia (laryngeal dystonia): A 12-year experience in more than 900 patients. Laryngoscope 2015;125:1751–1757.
13. Bohn E, Goren K, Switzer L, Falck-Ytter Y, Fehlings D. Pharmacological and neurosurgical interventions for individuals with cerebral palsy and dystonia: A systematic review update and meta-analysis. Dev Med Child Neurol 2021;63:1038–1050.
14. Boyce MJ, McCambridge AB, Bradnam LV, Canning CG, De Oliveira CQ, Verhagen AP. Botulinum toxin and conservative treatment strategies in people with cervical dystonia: An online survey. J Neural Transm 2024;131:43–51.
15. Caleo M, Spinelli M, Colosimo F, Matak I, Rossetto O, Lackovic Z, Restani L. Transynaptic action of botulinum neurotoxin type A at central cholinergic boutons. J Neurosci 2018;38:10329–10337.
16. Cani I, Latorre A, Cordivari C, Balint B, Bhatia KP. Brachial neuritis after botulinum toxin injections for cervical dystonia: A need for a reappraisal? Mov Disord Clin Pract 2019;6:160–165.
17. Castagna A, Albanese A. Management of cervical dystonia with botulinum neurotoxins and EMG/ultrasound guidance. Neurol Clin Pract 2019;9:64–73.
18. Castelao M, Marques RE, Duarte GS, Rodrigues FB, Ferreira J, Sampaio C, et al. Botulinum toxin type A therapy for cervical dystonia. Cochrane Database Syst Rev 2017;12:CD003633.
19. Chen R, Karp BI, Goldstein SR, Bara-Jimenez W, Yaseen Z, Hallett M. Effect of muscle activity immediately after botulinum toxin injection for writer's cramp. Mov Disord 1999;14:307–312.
20. Chinnapongse RB, Lew MF, Ferreira JJ, Gullo KL, Nemeth PR, Zhang Y. Immunogenicity and long-term efficacy of botulinum toxin type B in the treatment of cervical dystonia: Report of 4 prospective, multicenter trials. Clin Neuropharmacol 2012;35:215–223.
21. Cohen JL. Scientific skepticism and new discoveries: An analysis of a report of zinc/phytase supplementation and the efficacy of botulinum toxins in treating cosmetic facial rhytides, hemifacial spasm and benign essential blepharospasm. J Cosmet Laser Ther 2014;16:258–262.
22. Cohen LG, Hallett M, Geller BD, Hochberg F. Treatment of focal dystonias of the hand with botulinum toxin injections. J Neurol Neurosurg Psychiatry 1989;52:355–363.
23. Coleman C, Hubble J, Schwab J, Beffy JL, Picaut P, Morte C. Immunoresistance in cervical dystonia patients after treatment with abobotulinumtoxinA. Int J Neurosci 2012;122:358–362.
24. Colosimo C, Charles D, Misra VP, Maisonobe P, Om S, Interest in CD 2 Study Group. How satisfied are cervical dystonia patients after 3 years of botulinum toxin type A treatment? Results from a prospective, long-term observational study. J Neurol 2019;266:3038–3046.
25. Colosimo C, Charles D, Misra VP, Maisonobe P, Om S, Interest in CD 2 Study Group. Cumulative effects of long-term treatment with abobotulinumtoxinA in cervical dystonia: Findings from a prospective, observational study. J Neurol Sci 2020;416:117015.
26. Colosimo C, Tiple D, Berardelli A. Efficacy and safety of long-term botulinum toxin treatment in craniocervical dystonia: A systematic review. Neurotox Res 2012;22:265–273.
27. Comella CL. Systematic review of botulinum toxin treatment for oromandibular dystonia. Toxicon 2018;147:96–99.
28. Comella C, Bhatia K. An international survey of patients with cervical dystonia. J Neurol 2015;262:837–848.
29. Comella C, Ferreira JJ, Pain E, Azoulai M, Om S. Patient perspectives on the therapeutic profile of botulinum neurotoxin type A in cervical dystonia. J Neurol 2021;268:903–912.
30. Dadgardoust PD, Rosales RL, Asuncion RM, Dressler D. Botulinum neurotoxin a therapy efficacy and safety for oromandibular dystonia: A meta-analysis. J Neural Transm (Vienna) 2019;126:141–148.
31. Dashtipour K, Chen JJ, Espay AJ, Mari Z, Ondo W. OnabotulinumtoxinA and abobotulinumtoxinA dose conversion: A systematic literature review. Mov Disord Clin Pract 2016;3:109–115.
32. De Pauw J, Van der Velden K, Meirte J, Van Daele U, Truijen S, Cras P, et al. The effectiveness of physiotherapy for cervical dystonia: A systematic literature review. J Neurol 2014:261:1857–1865.
33. Duarte GS, Rodrigues FB, Marques RE, Castelao M, Ferreira J, Sampaio C, et al. Botulinum toxin type A therapy for blepharospasm. Cochrane Database Syst Rev 2020;11:CD004900.
34. Eleopra R, Tugnoli V, De Grandis D. The variability in the clinical effect induced by botulinum toxin type A: The role of muscle activity in humans. Mov Disord 1997;12:89–94.
35. Esposito M, Fasano A, Crisci C, Dubbioso R, Iodice R, Santoro L. The combined treatment with orbital and pretarsal botulinum toxin injections in the management of poorly responsive blepharospasm. Neurol Sci 2013;35:397–400.
36. Evidente VG, Pappert EJ. Botulinum toxin therapy for cervical dystonia: The science of dosing. Tremor Other Hyperkinet Mov 2014;4:273.
37. Fabbri M, Leodori G, Fernandes RM, Bhidayasiri R, Marti MJ, Colosimo C, Ferreira JJ. Neutralizing antibody and Botulinum toxin therapy: A systematic review and meta-analysis. Neurotox Res 2015;25:105–117.
38. Faham M, Ahmadi A, Silverman E, Harouni GG, Dabirmoghaddam P. Quality of life after botulinum toxin injection in patients with adductor spasmodic dysphonia: A systematic review and meta-analysis. J Voice 2021;35:271–283.

39. Fasano A, Paramanandam V, Jog M. Use of abobotulinumtoxinA in adults with cervical dystonia: A systematic literature review. Toxins (Basel) 2020;12:470.
40. Ferreira JJ, Colosimo C, Bhidayasiri R, Marti MJ, Maisonobe P, Om S. Factors influencing secondary non-response to botulinum toxin type A injections in cervical dystonia. Parkinsonism Relat Disord 2015;21:111–115.
41. Fezza J, Burns J, Woodward J, Truong D, Hedges T, Verma A. A cross-sectional structured survey of patients receiving botulinum toxin type A treatment for blepharospasm. J Neurol Sci 2016;367:56–62.
42. Fleming BM, Schwab EL, Nouer SS, Wan JY, LeDoux MS. Prevalence, predictors, and perceived effectiveness of complementary, alternative and integrative medicine in adult-onset primary dystonia. Parkinsonism Relat Disord 2012;18:936–940.
43. George EB, Cotton AC, Shneyder N, Jinnah HA. A strategy for managing flu-like symptoms after botulinum toxin injections. J Neurol 2018;265:1932–1933.
44. Gill CE, Manus ND, Pelster MW, Cook JA, Title W, Molinari AL, Charles D. Continuation of long-term care for cervical dystonia at an academic movement disorders clinic. Toxins (Basel) 2013;5:776–783.
45. Girlanda P, Quartarone A, Sinicropi S, Nicolosi C, Messina C. Unilateral injection of botulinum toxin in blepharospasm: Single fiber electromyography and blink reflex study. Mov Disord 1996;11:27–31.
46. Gordon PH, Gooch CL, Greene PE. Extensor digitorum brevis test and resistance to botulinum toxin type A. Muscle Nerve 2002;26:828–831.
47. Hallett M. Explanation of timing of botulinum neurotoxin effects, onset and duration, and clinical ways of influencing them. Toxicon 2015;107:64–67.
48. Hallett M. Mechanism of action of botulinum neurotoxin: Unexpected consequences. Toxicon 2018;147:73–76.
49. Hallett M, Albanese A, Dressler D, Segal KR, Simpson DM, Truong D, Jankovic J. Evidence-based review and assessment of botulinum neurotoxin for the treatment of movement disorders. Toxicon 2013;67:94–114.
50. Hallett M, Glocker FX, Deuschl G. Mechanism of action of botulinum toxin. Ann Neurol 1994;36:449–450.
51. Hefter H, Urer B, Brauns R, Rosenthal D, Meuth SG, Lee JI, et al. The complex relationship between antibody titers and clinical outcome in botulinum toxin type A long-term treated patients with cervical dystonia. J Neurol 2022;269:5991–6002.
52. Hok P, Veverka T, Hlustik P, Nevrly M, Kanovsky P. The central effects of botulinum toxin in dystonia and spasticity. Toxins 2021;13:155.
53. Jabbari B. History of botulinum toxin treatment in movement disorders. Tremor Other Hyperkinet Mov 2016;6:394.
54. Jankovic J. Botulinum toxin: State of the art. Mov Disord 2017;32:1131–1138.
55. Jinnah HA, Comella CL, Perlmutter J, Lungu C, Hallett M, Dystonia Coalition I. Longitudinal studies of botulinum toxin in cervical dystonia: Why do patients discontinue therapy? Toxicon 2018;147:89–95.
56. Jinnah HA, Goodmann E, Rosen AR, Evatt M, Freeman A, Factor S. Botulinum toxin treatment failures in cervical dystonia: Causes, management, and outcomes. J Neurol 2016;263:1188–1194.
57. Jost W, Valerius KP. *Atlas of Botulinum Toxin Injection: Dosage, Localization, Application*, 3rd ed. Quintessence; 2019.
58. Kanovsky P, Rosales RL. Debunking the pathophysiological puzzle of dystonia--with special reference to botulinum toxin therapy. Parkinsonism Relat Disord 2011;17 Suppl 1:S11–14.
59. Karp BI, Cole RA, Cohen LG, Grill S, Lou JS, Hallett M. Long-term botulinum toxin treatment of focal hand dystonia. Neurology 1994;44:70–76.
60. Kollewe K, Mohammadi B, Kohler S, Pickenbrock H, Dengler R, Dressler D. Blepharospasm: Long-term treatment with either Botox(R), Xeomin(R) or Dysport(R). J Neural Transm 2015;122:427–431.
61. Koshy JC, Sharabi SE, Feldman EM, Hollier LH, Jr., Patrinely JR, Soparkar CN. Effect of dietary zinc and phytase supplementation on botulinum toxin treatments. J Drugs Dermatol 2012;11:507–512.
62. Lange O, Bigalke H, Dengler R, Wegner F, deGroot M, Wohlfarth K. Neutralizing antibodies and secondary therapy failure after treatment with botulinum toxin type A: Much ado about nothing? Clin Neuropharmacol 2009;32:213–218.
63. Lebeda FJ, Cer RZ, Stephens RM, Mudunuri U. Temporal characteristics of botulinum neurotoxin therapy. Expert Rev Neurother 2010;10:93–103.
64. Lee JI, Jansen A, Samadzadeh S, Kahlen U, Moll M, Ringelstein M, et al. Long-term adherence and response to botulinum toxin in different indications. Ann Clin Transl Neurol 2021;8:15–28.
65. Leplow B, Eggebrecht A, Pohl J. Treatment satisfaction with botulinum toxin: A comparison between blepharospasm and cervical dystonia. Patient Prefer Adherence 2017;11:1555–1563.
66. Loudovici-Krug D, Derlien S, Best N, Gunther A. Physiotherapy for cervical dystonia: A systematic review of randomised controlled trials. Toxins 2022;14:784.
67. Lungu C, Karp BI, Alter K, Zolbrod R, Hallett M. Long-term follow-up of botulinum toxin therapy for focal hand dystonia: Outcome at 10 years or more. Mov Disord 2011;26:750–753.
68. Marciniec M, Szczepanska-Szerej A, Rejdak K. Cervical dystonia: Factors deteriorating patient satisfaction of long-term treatment with botulinum toxin. Neurol Res 2020;4:987–991.
69. Marsh WA, Monroe DM, Brin MF, Gallagher CJ. Systematic review and meta-analysis of the duration of clinical effect of onabotulinumtoxinA in cervical dystonia. BMC Neurol 2014;14:91.
70. Misra VP, Ehler E, Zakine B, Maisonobe P, Simonetta-Moreau M, Interest in CD 2 Study Group. Factors influencing response to Botulinum toxin type A in patients with idiopathic cervical dystonia: Results from an international observational study. BMJ Open 2012;2:e000881.
71. Mitsikostas DD, Dekundy A, Hanschmann A, Althaus M, Scheschonka A, Pagan F, Jankovic J. Duration and onset of effect of incobotulinumtoxinA for the treatment of blepharospasm in botulinum toxin-naive subjects. Curr Med Res Opin 2021:37:1761–1768.
72. Naumann M, Boo LM, Ackerman AH, Gallagher CJ. Immunogenicity of botulinum toxins. J Neural Transm 2013;120:275–290.
73. Nijmeijer SW, Koelman JH, Standaar TS, Postma M, Tijssen MA. Cervical dystonia: Improved treatment response to botulinum toxin after referral to a tertiary centre and the use of polymyography. Parkinsonism Relat Disord 2013;19:533–538.

74. Ojo OO, Fernandez HH. Is it time for flexibility in botulinum inter-injection intervals? Toxicon 2015;107:72–76.
75. Pirio Richardson S, Jinnah HA. New approaches to discovering drugs that treat dystonia. Expert Opin Drug Discov 2019;10:893–900.
76. Prudente CN, Zetterberg L, Bring A, Bradnam L, Kimberley TJ. Systematic review of rehabilitation in focal dystonias: Classification and recommendations. Mov Disord Clin Pract 2018;5:237–245.
77. Rahman E, Banerjee PS, Asghar A, Gupta NK, Mosahebi A. Botulinum toxin type A immunogenicity across multiple indications: An overview systematic review. Plast Reconstr Surg 2022;149:837–848.
78. Ramirez-Castaneda J, Jankovic J, Comella C, Dashtipour K, Fernandez HH, Mari Z. Diffusion, spread, and migration of botulinum toxin. Mov Disord 2013;28:1775–1783.
79. Rana AQ, Shah R. Combination of blepharospasm and apraxia of eyelid opening: A condition resistant to treatment. Acta Neurol Belg 2012;112:95–96.
80. Rayess YA, Awaida CJ, Jabbour SF, Ballan AS, Sleilati FH, Abou Zeid SM, Nasr MW. Botulinum toxin for benign essential blepharospasm: A systematic review and an algorithmic approach. Rev Neurol 2021;177:107–114.
81. Rosales RL, Dressler D. On muscle spindles, dystonia and botulinum toxin. Eur J Neurol 2010;17 Suppl 1:71–80.
82. Satila H. Over 25 years of pediatric botulinum toxin treatments: What have we learned from injection techniques, doses, diluations, and recovery from repeated injections? Toxins 2020;12:440.
83. Scaglione F. Conversion ratio between Botox, Dysport, and Xeomin in clinical practice. Toxins 2016;8:65.
84. Scorr LM, Factor SA, Perez-Parra S, Kaye R, Paniello RC, Norris SA, et al. Oromandibular dystonia: A clinical examination of 2,020 cases. Front Neurol 2021;12:700714.
85. Sethi KD, Rodriguez R, Olayinka B. Satisfaction with botulinum toxin treatment: A cross-sectional survey of patients with cervical dystonia. J Med Econ 2012;15:419–423.
86. Simpson DM, Hallett M, Ashman EJ, Comella CL, Green MW, Gronseth GS, et al. Practice guideline update summary: Botulinum neurotoxin for the treatment of blepharospasm, cervical dystonia, adult spasticity, and headache: Report of the Guideline Development Subcommittee of the American Academy of Neurology. Neurology 2016;86:1818–1826.
87. Solish N, Carruthers J, Kaufman J, Rubio RG, Gross TM, Gallagher CJ. Overview of daxibotulinumtoxinA for injection: A novel formulation of botulinum toxin type A. Drugs 2021;81:2091–2101.
88. Truong D, Dressler D, Hallet M, Zachary C. *Manual of Botulinum Toxin*, 2nd ed. Cambridge University Press; 2014.
89. Tucker H, Osei-Poku F, Ashton D, Lally R, Jesuthasan A, Latorre A, et al. Management of secondary poor response to botulinum toxin in cervical dystonia: A multicenter audit. Mov Disord Clin Pract 2021;8:541–545.
90. Tyslerowicz M, Kiedrzynska W, Adamkiewicz B, Jost WH, Slawek J. Cervical dystonia - improving the effectiveness of botulinum toxin therapy. Neurol Neurochir Pol 2020;54:1–11.
91. van Esch BF, Wegner I, Stegeman I, Grolman W. Effect of botulinum toxin and surgery among spasmodic dysphonia patients. Otolaryngol Head Neck Surg 2017;156:238–254.
92. Wollner J, Weise D, Leplow B. Subjective versus objective symptom intensitites ratings in cervical dystonia and hemifacial spasm across a botulinum toxin neurotoxin cycle. Brain and Behav 2021;11:e02023.
93. Zoons E, Dijkgraaf MG, Dijk JM, van Schaik IN, Tijssen MA. Botulinum toxin as treatment for focal dystonia: A systematic review of the pharmaco-therapeutic and pharmaco-economic value. J Neurol 2012;259:2519–2526.

Chapter 31

Surgical Treatments for Dystonia

INTRODUCTION

The first approach to the treatment of dystonia usually involves oral medications (see Chapter 28, "Symptom-Targeted Oral Medications for Dystonia" and Chapter 29, "Special Interventions for Certain Types of Dystonia") and/or botulinum toxins (see Chapter 30, "Botulinum Toxin Treatment for Dystonia"). When these more conservative treatments are inadequate, surgical options are considered.

Over the years, a wide variety of surgical procedures have been offered to individuals with different types of dystonia.[15] Most of these surgical options are provided by specialized centers with highly trained teams. However, it is not uncommon for individuals with dystonia to learn about surgical options from acquaintances or the internet and then ask their primary care provider or general neurologist about them. As a result, it is useful for all clinicians to have a good working knowledge of these surgical options to guide counseling and referrals.

Placebo-controlled and double-blinded clinical trials are challenging for many surgical procedures. Although there are a few such trials assessing surgical interventions, much of the information regarding application comes from unblinded case reports and small series, usually from specialized centers with a high degree of expertise. It is important to acknowledge the sources and limitations of this type of evidence when considering this evidence during counseling.

Since numerous reviews describing the evidence for surgical treatments have been published already,[1,2,6,8,10,27,28,33,38] this chapter describes general principles of safety and efficacy for counseling purposes, along with some guidelines for the selection of surgical candidates for referrals. It focuses on surgical procedures with broad application in different types of dystonia. Only the most common surgical procedures that are still widely used are considered: deep brain stimulation (DBS) and ablative procedures. Special surgical procedures that are limited to specific subtypes of dystonia can be found in Chapter 5, "Cervical Dystonias," Chapter 6, "Craniofacial Dystonias," and Chapter 7, "Laryngeal Dystonias."

DEEP BRAIN STIMULATION

Overview

In recent years, DBS has become the most common surgical treatment for dystonia. Numerous reviews have been published, including several systematic reviews and meta-analyses.[1,2,6,8,10,27,28,33,38] DBS is most valuable for

Table 31.1 **Important aspects of counseling for deep brain stimulation surgery**

Factor	Consideration
Onset of benefits	Some benefits may be immediate, but full benefits be delayed by 3–12 months and often require multiple equipment adjustments
Degree of benefit	Varied, dependent on both individual clinical features and etiology. While occasional individuals experience near-complete reversal of dystonia, the more common outcome is partial improvement, and some experience no benefit.
Duration of benefit	Benefits last many years with no obvious waning of effect, unless underlying condition is progressive
Anticipated risks	Approximately one-quarter of individuals can expect some complication. The most common are infections, hardware malfunction or damage, or stroke
Follow-up	Regular follow-up is required for stimulator adjustments, battery replacement, and equipment checks.

individuals with types of dystonia that are challenging to treat with botulinum toxins or medications, such as generalized dystonia. However, it has also been used with success for individuals with focal or segmental dystonias.

In brief, the procedure involves the subcutaneous implantation of an impulse generator, usually in the chest just below the clavicle or sometimes in the flank. The device is attached to a wire that is tunneled under the skin to the top of the skull and the wire directed into the brain. The target is identified either by electrophysiological recordings or MRI. The most common target is the internal segment of the globus pallidus, although less common targets have included the subthalamic nucleus, thalamus, and sometimes other regions. After a recovery period of a few days to a few weeks, stimulation is started. While some benefit may occur immediately, full benefits often require several months, sometimes 6–12 months or longer. During this period, multiple adjustments may be made to the stimulator settings, including the amount and mode of current, and the use of different electrode contacts. This delay is important when counseling surgical candidates regarding expectations (Table 31.1).

Efficacy

Regarding efficacy, DBS is one of the few surgical options where rigorous and double-blinded clinical trials have been published. In one of the earliest trials, 40 individuals with isolated generalized or segmental dystonia studied across 10 centers underwent DBS targeting the internal pallidum, with half receiving active stimulation and the other half receiving sham stimulation.[24] Three months later, the stimulation group showed 39% improvements in severity of dystonia assessed by raters blinded to treatment group using the Burke-Fahn-Marsden dystonia motor rating scale, 38% improvements in disability as measured by the Burke-Fahn-Marsden disability scale, and 30% improvements in quality of life on the 36-item Short Form (SF-36). Another multicenter double-blind, placebo-controlled trial of 22 individuals with generalized dystonia undergoing DBS targeting the pallidum showed similar improvements over 3–12 months in dystonia severity, disability, and quality of life.[40] Placebo-controlled and blinded trials for focal or segmental cervical dystonia targeting the pallidum have revealed 26% improvement at 3 months[42] or 28% improvement at 6 months[19] assessed using Toronto Western Torticollis Rating Scale scores. A double-blind crossover study has also been reported for laryngeal dystonia.[12] In all of these blinded studies, individual responses varied widely, with some experiencing enormous benefits and others experiencing no benefit. DBS rarely eliminates dystonia. These heterogeneous and partial responses are important when counseling surgical candidates regarding expectations (Table 31.1).

In addition to these double-blind, placebo-controlled studies, numerous other studies involving DBS targeting the internal pallidum have been reported. In a meta-analysis encompassing a total of 523 individuals with various types of isolated dystonia reported across 24 different studies, the overall improvement in the Burke-Fahn-Marsden dystonia rating scale score was 67% (Figure 31.1).[27] Another meta-analysis focusing on DBS for cervical dystonia included 39 publications with 208 cases and showed an overall improvement of 59% using the Toronto Western Torticollis Rating Scale.[39] A third meta-analysis included 168 individuals with dyskinetic cerebral palsy reported in 13 different studies (Figure 31.2).[2] For cerebral palsy, overall improvement in

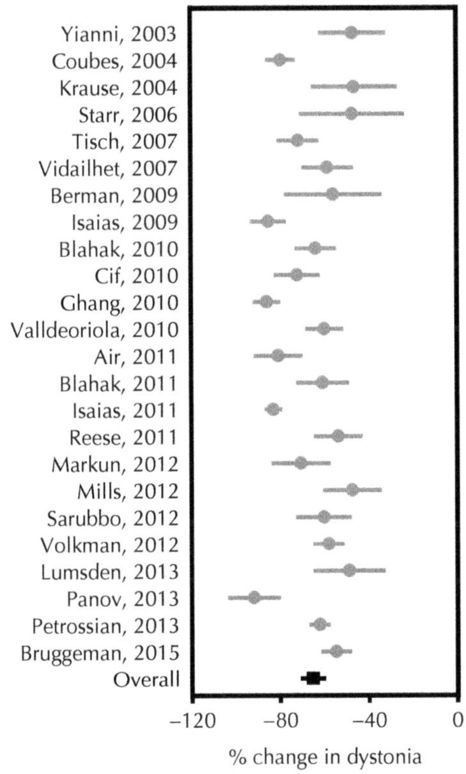

Figure 31.1. Meta-analysis of deep brain stimulation efficacy for isolated dystonias. This figure was adapted from a prior review that summarized the percentage of change in the Burke-Fahn Marsden Dystonia Rating Scale scores for 24 separate studies and a total of 523 patients with isolated dystonia.[27] The overall percentage of improvement averaged 67%.

the Burke-Fahn-Marsden scores averaged only 17%. All studies again showed significant variations in improvement among individual cases. These variations reflect many factors relating to the clinical characteristics of the individuals undergoing surgery, such as the severity and body distribution of dystonia; whether dystonia was fixed or mobile; age at operation and duration of illness; whether there were additional neurological signs not expected to benefit from DBS, such as spasticity or ataxia; and other features.

The subthalamic nucleus also appears to be an effective target, although fewer studies are available. In one prospective double-blind crossover study, simultaneous bilateral subthalamic and pallidal electrodes were implanted in 12 individuals with focal, multifocal, or generalized dystonia with similar results.[34] In long-term follow-up of 14 individuals, outcomes were similar whether DBS targeted the subthalamic nucleus, pallidum, or both together. Burke-Fahn-Marsden dystonia severity scale scores improved by a mean of 36%.[11]

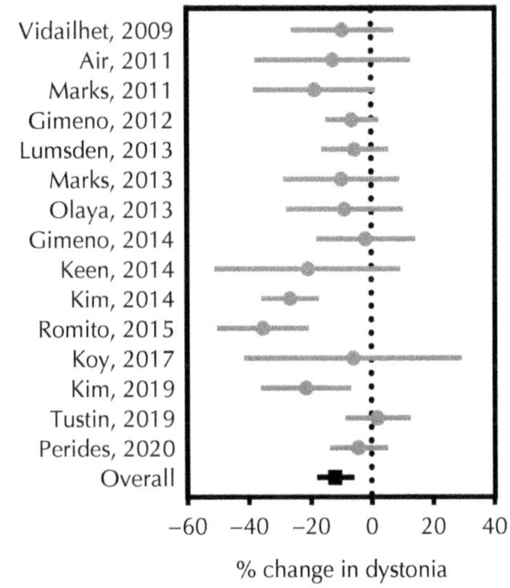

Figure 31.2. Meta-analysis of deep brain stimulation efficacy for cerebral palsy. This figure was adapted from a prior review that summarized the percentage of change in the Burke-Fahn Marsden Dystonia Rating Scale scores for 15 separate studies and a total of 168 cerebral palsy patients.[2] The overall percentage of improvement averaged 17%.

Benefits from subthalamic DBS were also reported for two series of 9 and 4 individuals with cervical dystonia.[20,30] A retrospective database comparison of 14 individuals treated with pallidal and 16 with subthalamic DBS for isolated dystonia found comparable results.[25] A prospective study of 15 individuals with blinded raters also reported benefits in 15 individuals with craniofacial dystonia.[43]

Predictors of Outcomes

Clinical features and etiology both have an impact on outcomes for DBS surgery. Early studies suggested that individuals with isolated dystonia routinely achieved better outcomes than those with more complex dystonia syndromes that included other neurological features. This view is now considered oversimplified because some types of isolated dystonia routinely respond poorly, while some combined dystonia syndromes respond quite well. Although results vary across different studies, the main clinical features that predict a good outcome for DBS include shorter duration of dystonia, mobile dystonia rather than fixed postures, appendicular (upper or lower limb) rather than axial (neck or trunk) location of dystonia, and lack of additional neurological features not expected to respond to surgery, such as spasticity or ataxia (Table 31.2). While age does

Table 31.2 **Factors influencing deep brain stimulation outcomes in dystonia**

Factor	Favorable outcome	Less favorable outcome
Temporal issues		
age at operation	Childhood-adulthood	<6 yrs of age, or very old
duration of illness	Shorter	Very long duration
Features of dystonia		
mobility	Mobile or phasic	Fixed or tonic
body location	Appendicular (arm, leg)	Axial (face, voice, neck)
progressive	Initial response good	Response may wane over time
Etiology		
brain MRI	Normal, or only minor changes	Severe structural abnormalities
responsible gene	(See Figure 31.3)	See Figure 31.3
Other features		
neurological	Pure dystonia (±tremor)	Spasticity, weakness, ataxia
psychiatric	Normal	Depression, anxiety
cognitive	Normal	Significant dementia

This table describes the most common factors thought to be relevant to prediction of good or bad outcomes in most cases. It provides general guidelines only, as many exceptions exist.

not appear to be a major determinant of efficacy, it is best to avoid young children because of the need to reposition of the electrode when the head and brain grow. It may also be best to avoid older adults where there are substantial additional comorbidities that may complicate surgery.

Etiology also plays an important role in outcomes. For example, outcomes for isolated dystonia depend on the underlying gene (Table 31.2 and Figure 31.3).[1,16,38] Good outcomes are typical for isolated dystonia caused by genetic variants in *TOR1A*. Good outcomes are also typical for variants in some genes where dystonia is combined with other features, such as *SCGE* (myoclonus-dystonia syndrome), *TAF1* (X-linked dystonia-parkinsonism), and *KMT2B*. However, outcomes have been uniformly poor for some genes, such as *ATP1A3* (rapid-onset dystonia-parkinsonism), so DBS should be avoided in these cases.[1,16,38] Outcomes for several genes are hard to predict, such as *THAP1*.[3] The reasons for varied responses with *THAP1* are not well understood. For other genes, variations in responses are better understood, such as *PANK2*. Individuals with

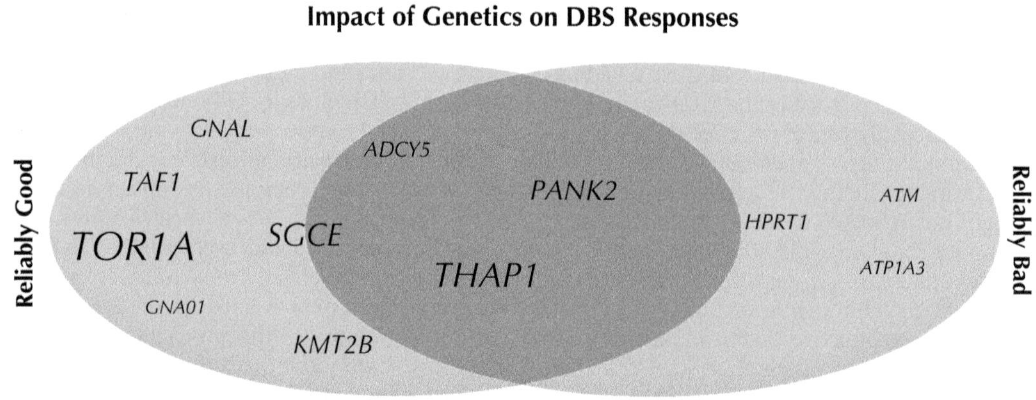

Figure 31.3. Impact of genetics on deep brain stimulation responses. Genes associated with reliable and good responses are shown toward the left, while genes associated with reliably poor responses are shown toward the right. The strength of the evidence varies according to the number of reported cases, shown as the size of the gene. The schematic provides only general guidelines because exceptions exist. For example, rare cases with *TOR1A* have poor response, although most have good response. This schematic was adapted from data provided in prior reviews.[1,38]

onset of this disease in early childhood (severe and progressive dystonia, spasticity, cognitive decline, seizures, retinopathy) do not respond as well as those with adolescent-onset disease (moderately progressive dystonia-parkinsonism).

For acquired forms of dystonia, etiology can also predict outcomes. For example, tardive dystonia secondary to neuroleptic exposure typically responds quite well to DBS, while responses for dystonic cerebral palsy secondary to neonatal hypoxia-ischemia are often limited.[9] In view of these observations, studies that address etiology are important for counseling surgical candidates (Table 31.1).

Outcomes are also related to the experience level of the surgical team. The ideal surgical team includes at least one neurosurgeon for operations, at least one neurologist for programming and medication adjustments, a psychologist or psychiatrist, and access to modern imaging methods. Several studies have shown many poor outcomes from less-experienced surgical teams might be avoided.[29,31] Some of the most common errors found from less-experienced teams include incorrect initial diagnoses, comorbidities that impede surgical treatment, improper placement of DBS leads, suboptimal programming, correctable side effects, and inadequate initial counseling regarding expected benefits.

Surgical Complications

In addition to counseling individuals regarding expected outcomes related to the clinical features and etiology of dystonia, counseling must also address safety. DBS is generally considered safe when performed at experienced centers. A systematic review of the safety of DBS for dystonia that included 592 cases reported across 21 studies revealed an overall complication rate of 26%.[17] The most common complications included infections (7.4%), stimulator malfunctions (5.7%), lead failures (4.2%), or lead migrations (3.0%). A meta-analysis that included 12,235 individuals in 66 studies using DBS for a variety of indications focused more specifically on infections.[18] Overall, approximately 5% of all individuals undergoing DBS had early infections relating to surgery or the immediate postsurgical period (Figure 31.4). Delayed infections related to indwelling hardware also occurred in 5% of all

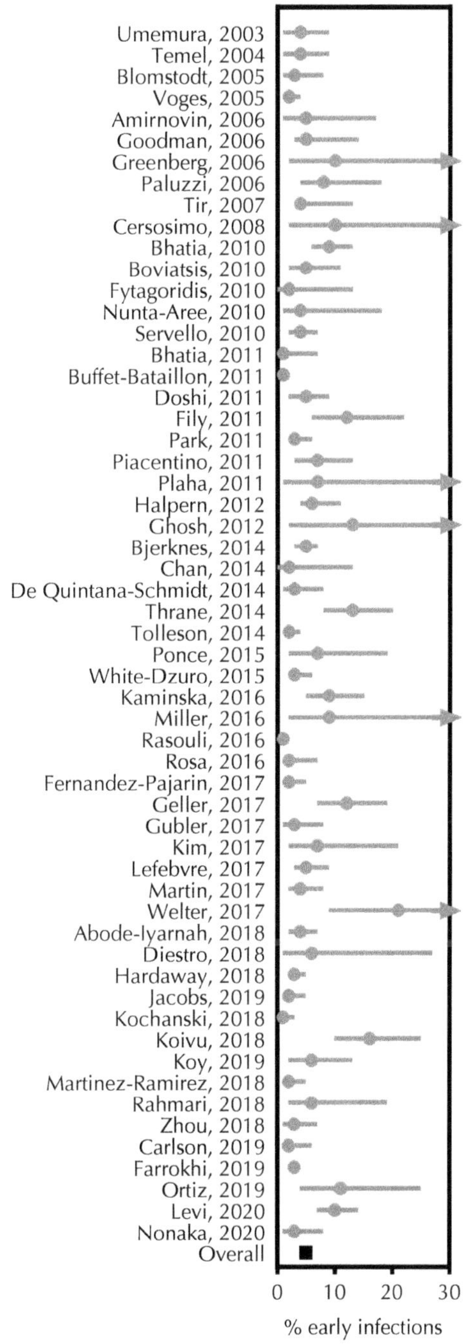

Figure 31.4. Meta-analysis of early infections following deep brain stimulation surgery. This figure was adapted from a prior review that summarized the percentage of individuals who had infections within 90 days of surgery for 66 separate studies and a total of 12,235 patients treated for all types of indications.[18] The overall risk of early infections was approximately 5%.

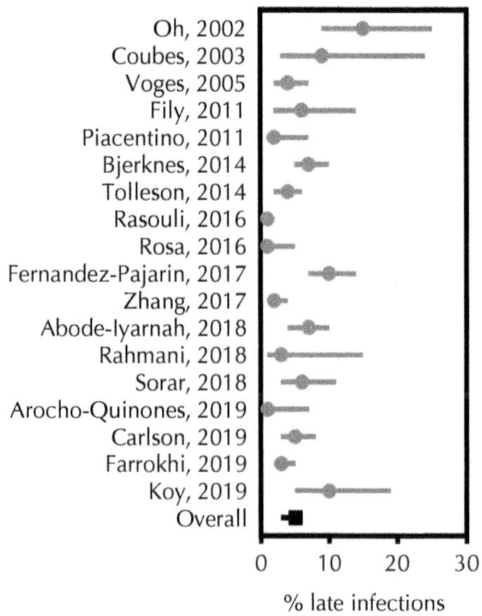

Figure 31.5. Meta-analysis of late infections following deep brain stimulation surgery. This figure was adapted from a prior review that summarized the percentage of individuals who had infections more than 90 days after surgery for 66 separate studies and a total of 12,235 patients treated for all types of indications.[18] The overall risk of late infections was approximately 5%.

cases (Figure 31.5). These infections may respond to antibiotics, but sometimes require removal of the hardware.

Finally, counseling should address the long-term prognosis (Table 31.1). Provided that complications are avoided or managed, long-term outcomes with DBS are good. Benefits last for many years without obvious lessening of effect unless the disorder is associated with an underlying neurodegenerative disorder.[32,35,41] Regular monitoring of the device is needed, and equipment failures may require additional operations. Battery changes are expected every few years as well, although modern rechargeable devices are increasingly used. Counseling of potential surgical candidates must therefore address the importance of routine checkups and sometimes the need for urgent intervention.

ABLATIVE APPROACHES

Before DBS was widely available, it was common to permanently ablate specific brain regions in individuals with dystonia.[7,21] Results of ablation were sometimes unpredictable, in part because of insufficient knowledge of brain regions most relevant for ablation and lack of appreciation that different etiological subgroups might require ablation of different targets. Continued advancements in understanding the varied etiologies and neuroanatomical bases for dystonia have led to improved targeting, with reliably good outcomes for some subtypes of dystonia.

The procedure involves making a permanent lesion in a small region of the brain. Radiofrequency or electrolytic lesions can be made by passing a temporary electrode to the target brain region, but more recently thermal lesions have become possible with focused ultrasound.[23] Although focused ultrasound is sometimes described as being preferable because it is less "invasive" than DBS, it is important to recognize that it still produces a permanent brain lesion, along with any potential side effects. Typical side effects depend on the location of the ablation but most often include sensory anomalies, dysphagia, and sometimes weakness.

Ablative procedures may be offered not only to individuals with generalized or segmental dystonia but also to individuals with focal dystonia and particularly task-specific dystonias.[5] For individuals with generalized or segmental dystonia, the most common target has been the internal segment of the globus pallidus, the same target used for DBS. Small thalamic lesions have proved safe and effective for task-specific dystonias involving the upper limb, such as musician's dystonia.[13,14,37] Benefits from ablation seem to be similar to those for DBS.

While DBS remains the most common surgical option offered to individuals with dystonia, ablative strategies may be preferable in some circumstances (Table 31.3).[37] The effect of ablation is relatively durable, an aspect that has both advantages and disadvantages. The main disadvantage is the possibility of a permanent side effect. In comparison, undesired side effects of DBS can often be reversed because the equipment is tunable and removable. On the other hand, some advantages of ablation include the lack of requirement for maintenance of indwelling hardware, with the associated lower risks for equipment failure or hardware infections. Ablative strategies may be preferable in particularly young or thin individuals who cannot tolerate subcutaneous implantation of an impulse generator because of its size. Ablative procedures may also be preferable for individuals who cannot afford DBS surgery and subsequent

Table 31.3 **Comparison of deep brain stimulation and ablation**

Comparison	Deep brain stimulation	Ablation
Technical aspects		
Adjustable	Yes	No
Reversible	Yes	No
Indwelling hardware	Yes	No
Risks		
Infection	5–10%	Very low
Hardware malfunction	5–10%	Very low
Side effects reversible	Usually	Usually not
Very young	Higher risk of complication	No change in risk
Very thin	Higher risk of complication	No change in risk
Nature of dystonia		
Generalized/segmental	Well-established	Less-established
Task-specific	Less-utilized	Well-established
Status dystonicus	Challenging	More feasible
Rapidly progressive	Challenging	More feasible

maintenance, individuals who live too far from an experienced center to return for regular management, or individuals who may be unreliable when it comes to regular checkups. Ablation may also be a reasonable option as a palliative procedure for individuals with severe dystonia, such as status dystonicus, where DBS is a challenge. It may also be a good option as a palliative procedure for severely progressive disorders when the affected individual and family may want to avoid constant need to return for medical care.

SYNOPSIS AND FUTURE PROSPECTS

The initial approach to treatment of dystonia usually involves medications and botulinum toxins. When these appear insufficient, there are surgical options. The most commonly used approach involves DBS, although ablative strategies appear to be equally effective and may be preferable under certain circumstances. The efficacy of surgery varies widely, and outcomes are influenced by both clinical features and the etiology of dystonia. Complications are not uncommon. They occur in approximately one-quarter of all DBS operations, sometimes shortly after surgery and sometimes after several months or years. All surgical options should be provided by skilled teams with experience to address the many immediate and long-term complications. In experienced hands, surgical options can provide a safe and effective approach to treatment of many different types of dystonia.

Ongoing research has led to constant improvements in devices and strategies for surgical treatments of dystonia. There have been enormous advances in understanding the types of individuals who respond best and in possible novel target sites, including those outside of the basal ganglia.[4,26,36] There have also been enormous advances in the devices, including smaller impulse generators, rechargeable generators, electrodes that permit controlling not only the amount but the direction of current, and stimulation patterns that adapt to the clinical features of the disorder.[22] Experience with focused ultrasound for making non-invasive permanent ablations is currently limited in dystonia, but it has seen considerable growth in other disorders, such as tremor. It is likely that further developments in this strategy may become more widely used for dystonia in the near future.

REFERENCES

1. Artusi CA, Dwivedi A, Romagnolo A, Bortolani S, Marsili L, Imbalzano G, et al. Differential response to pallidal deep brain stimulation among monogenic dystonias: Systematic review and meta-analysis. J Neurol Neurosurg Psychiatry 2020;91:426–433.
2. Bohn E, Goren K, Switzer L, Falck-Ytter Y, Fehlings D. Pharmacological and neurosurgical interventions for individuals with cerebral palsy and dystonia: A systematic review update and meta-analysis. Dev Med Child Neurol 2021;63:1038–1050.
3. Bruggemann N, Kuhn A, Schneider SA, Kamm C, Wolters A, Krause P, et al. Short- and long-term outcome

of chronic pallidal neurostimulation in monogenic isolated dystonia. Neurology 2015;84:895–903.
4. Cajigas I, Morrison MA, Luciano MS, Starr PA. Cerebellar deep brain stimulation for the treatment of movement disorders in cerebral palsy. J Neurosurg 2023:1–10.
5. Centen LM, Oterdoom DLM, Tijssen MAJ, Lesman-Leegte I, van Egmond ME, van Dijk JMC. Bilateral pallidotomy for dystonia: A systematic review. Mov Disord 2021;36:547–557.
6. Chen W, Fan H, Lu G. The efficacy and predictors of using GPi-DBS to treat early-onset dystonia: An individual patient analysis. Neural Plast 2021;2021:9924639.
7. Cury RG, Kalia SK, Shah BB, Jimenez-Shahed J, Prashanth LK, Moro E. Surgical treatment of dystonia. Expert Rev Neurother 2018;18:477–492.
8. Elkaim LM, Alotaibi NM, Sigal A, Alotaibi HM, Lipsman N, Kalia SK, et al. Deep brain stimulation for pediatric dystonia: A meta-analysis with individual participant data. Dev Med Child Neurol 2019;61:49–56.
9. Fehlings D, Brown L, Harvey A, Himmelmann K, Lin JP, Macintosh A, et al. Pharmacological and neurosurgical interventions for managing dystonia in cerebral palsy: A systematic review. Dev Med Child Neurol 2018;60:356–366.
10. Hale AT, Monsour MA, Rolston JD, Naftel RP, Englot DJ. Deep brain stimulation in pediatric dystonia: A systematic review. Neurosurg Rev 2018;43:873–880.
11. Hock AN, Jensen SR, Svaerke KW, Brennum J, Jespersen B, Bergdal O, et al. A randomised double-blind controlled study of deep brain stimulation for dystonia in STN or GPi - A long term follow-up after up to 15 years. Parkinsonism Relat Disord 2022;96:74–79.
12. Honey CR, Kruger MT, Almeida T, Rammage LA, Tamber MS, Morrison MD, et al. Thalamic deep brain stimulation for spasmodic dysphonia: A phase I prospective randomized double-blind crossover trial. Neurosurgery 2021;89:45–52.
13. Horisawa S, Taira T, Goto S, Ochiai T, Nakajima T. Long-term improvement of musician's dystonia after stereotactic ventrooralthalamotomy. Ann Neurol 2013;74:648–654.
14. Horisawa S, Ochiai T, Goto S, Nakajima T, Takeda N, Fukui A, et al. Safety and long-term efficacy of ventro-oral thalamotomy for focal hand dystonia: A retrospective study of 171 patients. Neurology 2019;92:e371–e377.
15. Jinnah HA. Medical and surgical treatments for dystonia. Neurol Clin 2020;38:325–348.
16. Jinnah HA, Alterman R, Klein C, Krauss JK, Moro E, Vidailhet M, Raike R. Deep brain stimulation for dystonia: A novel perspective on the value of genetic testing. J Neural Transm (Vienna) 2017;124:417–430.
17. Jitkritsadakul O, Bhidayasiri R, Kalia SK, Hodaie M, Lozano AM, Fasano A. Systematic review of hardware-related complications of Deep Brain Stimulation: Do new indications pose an increased risk? Brain Stimul 2017;10:967–976.
18. Kantzanou M, Korfias S, Panourias I, Sakas DE, Karalexi MA. Deep brain stimulation-related surgical site infections: A systematic review and meta-analysis. Neuromodulation 2021;24:197–211.
19. Kiss ZH, Doig-Beyaert K, Eliasziw M, Tsui J, Haffenden A, Suchowersky O. The Canadian multicentre study of deep brain stimulation for cervical dystonia. Brain 2007;130:2879–2886.
20. Kleiner-Fisman G, Liang GS, Moberg PJ, Ruocco AC, Hurtig HI, Baltuch GH, et al. Subthalamic nucleus deep brain stimulation for severe idiopathic dystonia: Impact on severity, neuropsychological status, and quality of life. J Neurosurg 2007;107:29–36.
21. Krack P, Martinez-Fernandez R, Del Alamo M, Obeso JA. Current applications and limitations of surgical treatments for movement disorders. Mov Disord 2017;32:36–52.
22. Krauss JK, Lipsman N, Aziz T, Boutet A, Brown P, Chang JW, et al. Technology of deep brain stimulation: Current status and future directions. Nat Rev Neurol 2021;17:75–87.
23. Krishna V, Sammartino F, Rezai A. A review of the current therapies, challenges, and future directions of transcranial focused ultrasound technology: Advances in diagnosis and treatment. JAMA Neurol 2018;75:246–254.
24. Kupsch A, Benecke R, Muller J, Trottenberg T, Schneider GH, Poewe W, et al. Pallidal deep-brain stimulation in primary generalized or segmental dystonia. N Engl J Med 2006;355:1978–1990.
25. Lin S, Wu Y, Li H, Zhang C, Wang T, Pan Y, et al. Deep brain stimulation of the globus pallidus internus versus the subthalamic nucleus in isolated dystonia. J Neurosurg 2019;132:721–732.
26. Miterko LN, Baker KB, Beckinghausen J, Bradnam LV, Cheng MY, Cooperrider J, et al. Consensus paper: Experimental neurostimulation of the cerebellum. Cerebellum 2019;18:1064–1097.
27. Moro E, LeReun C, Krauss JK, Albanese A, Lin JP, Walleser Autiero S, et al. Efficacy of pallidal stimulation in isolated dystonia: A systematic review and meta-analysis. Eur J Neurol 2017;24:552–560.
28. Odorfer TM, Volkmann J. Deep brain stimulation for focal or segmental craniocervical dystonia in patients who have failed botulinum neurotoxin therapy-A narrative review of the literature. Toxins 2023;15:606.
29. Okun MS, Tagliati M, Pourfar M, Fernandez HH, Rodriguez RL, Alterman RL, Foote KD. Management of referred deep brain stimulation failures: A retrospective analysis from 2 movement disorders centers. Arch Neurol 2005;62:1250–1255.
30. Ostrem JL, Racine CA, Glass GA, Grace JK, Volz MM, Heath SL, Starr PA. Subthalamic nucleus deep brain stimulation in primary cervical dystonia. Neurology 2011;76:870–878.
31. Pauls KAM, Krauss JK, Kampfer CE, Kuhn AA, Schrader C, Sudmeyer M, et al. Causes of failure of pallidal deep brain stimulation in cases with pre-operative diagnosis of isolated dystonia. Parkinsonism Relat Disord 2017;43:38–48.
32. Reese R, Gruber D, Schoenecker T, Bazner H, Blahak C, Capelle HH, et al. Long-term clinical outcome in Meige syndrome treated with internal pallidum deep brain stimulation. Mov Disord 2011;26:691–698.
33. Rodrigues FB, Duarte GS, Prescott D, Ferreira J, Costa J. Deep brain stimulation for dystonia. Cochrane Database Syst Rev 2019;1:CD012405.
34. Schjerling L, Hjermind LE, Jespersen B, Madsen FF, Brennum J, Jensen SR, et al. A randomized double-blind crossover trial comparing subthalamic and pallidal deep brain stimulation for dystonia. J Neurosurg 2013;119:1537–1545.
35. Tagliati M, Krack P, Volkmann J, Aziz T, Krauss JK, Kupsch A, Vidailhet AM. Long-term management of

DBS in dystonia: Response to stimulation, adverse events, battery changes, and special considerations. Mov Disord 2011;26 Suppl 1:S54–62.

36. Tai CH, Tseng SH. Cerebellar deep brain stimulation for movement disorders. Neurobiolo Dis 2022;175:105899.
37. Taira T, Horisawa S, Takeda N, Ghate P. Stereotactic radiofrequency lesioning for movement disorders. Prog Neurol Surg 2018;33:107–119.
38. Tisch S, Kumar KR. Pallidal deep brain stimulation for monogenic dystonia: The effect of gene on outcome. Front Neurol 2021;11:630391.
39. Tsuboi T, Wong JK, Almeida L, Hess CW, Wagle Shukla A, Foote KD, et al. A pooled meta-analysis of GPi and STN deep brain stimulation outcomes for cervical dystonia. J Neurol 2020;267:1278–1290.
40. Vidailhet M, Vercueil L, Houeto JL, Krystkowiak P, Lagrange C, Yelnik J, et al. Bilateral, pallidal, deep-brain stimulation in primary generalised dystonia: A prospective 3 year follow-up study. Lancet Neurol 2007;6:223–229.
41. Volkmann J, Wolters A, Kupsch A, Muller J, Kuhn AA, Schneider GH, et al. Pallidal deep brain stimulation in patients with primary generalised or segmental dystonia: 5-year follow-up of a randomised trial. Lancet Neurol 2012;11:1029–1038.
42. Volkmann J, Mueller J, Deuschl G, Kuhn AA, Krauss JK, Poewe W, et al. Pallidal neurostimulation in patients with medication-refractory cervical dystonia: A randomised, sham-controlled trial. Lancet Neurol 2014;13:875–884.
43. Zhan S, Sun F, Pan Y, Liu W, Huang P, Cao C, et al. Bilateral deep brain stimulation of the subthalamic nucleus in primary Meige syndrome. J Neurosurg 2018;128:897–902.

Chapter 32

Physiotherapy and Complementary Medicine for Dystonia

INTRODUCTION

The defining feature of dystonia is excessive muscle contractions causing abnormal movements and postures, often accompanied by muscle spasms and pain. These features of dystonia resemble other more common musculoskeletal problems, which are often treated with physiotherapy (PT). As a result, PT frequently is offered to individuals with dystonia, often before the diagnosis leads to more specific therapies. Even after the diagnosis of dystonia is made, PT continues to be offered to affected individuals because these methods appear intuitively useful to both affected individuals and clinical providers.

There is an enormous literature on PT for many types of dystonia. Despite its popularity, evidence for the value of each of the many interventions is surprisingly mixed, with disagreement regarding best practices even among experts. One of the major reasons for the plethora of strategies is that different techniques are obviously needed for different types of dystonia, such as generalized dystonia or cerebral palsy, focal cervical or hand dystonia, or dystonia affecting the ability to speak. However, even within a specific type of dystonia such as cervical dystonia, numerous different PT strategies have been proposed. Because there are so many different strategies, often with very small numbers of cases or unblinded study designs, it is challenging to compare studies and reach generalizable conclusions.

This chapter first summarizes the theoretical basis for the many different PT strategies that have been proposed for different types of dystonia. It then addresses the most common strategies used for individual types of dystonia including generalized dystonia (including cerebral palsy), cervical dystonia, limb dystonia, and speech or voice therapy for dystonias affecting verbal communication. Also considered are other forms of complementary and alternative medicine (CAM). The chapter concludes with some practical recommendations that may be followed in the absence of definitive evidence for these treatment interventions, along with some suggestions for future work that may be useful for better understanding the role of PT and other forms of CAM for dystonia.

PHYSIOTHERAPY

Heterogeneity of Physiotherapy Methods

Strategies for PT in dystonia have varied enormously. Some strategies rely on rest and relaxation or even complete immobilization. Other strategies rely instead on intensive exercise and muscle strengthening. These apparently opposite strategies are driven by different hypotheses regarding the etiopathogenesis of dystonia (see Chapter 24, "Dystonia Physiology").

A systematic review of PT across different types of adult-onset focal dystonia grouped the many different methods used into six main categories, with some overlap (Table 32.1).[27] Although this review focused on adult-onset focal dystonias, many of the principles can be applied also to pediatric or generalized dystonias. The first and most common category of *movement practice* is based on the theory that motor retraining might correct an otherwise abnormal movement. Some form of movement practice was included in nearly all the PT trials reviewed. The category of *training with constraint* is based on the concept that excessive movements characteristic of dystonia may be corrected by restraining them while simultaneously retraining more normal movements. The category of *sensory reorganization* is based on physiological studies of dystonia suggesting abnormal sensorimotor integration in dystonia, where abnormal sensory input or abnormal perception of sensory input is thought to distort motor responses. Thus, resetting of sensory feedback by immobilization or more finely retraining sensory inputs by learning braille may be beneficial for retuning the sensorimotor pathways. The category of *normalization of muscle activity with external methods* involves methods that help the individual learn to reestablish normal motor patterns using biofeedback from electromyography (EMG), visual or auditory cues, transcutaneous nerve stimulation, vibration, kinesiotaping, or other methods. The category of *neuromodulation with training* combines retraining with external methods thought to alter neuronal excitability, such as transcranial magnetic stimulation or transcranial direct current stimulation. The last category is *compensatory strategies*, in which an affected individual is trained to perform a task in a novel way that does not provoke dystonia.

Most (but not all) of the studies reviewed described positive results with a variety of outcomes to assess efficacy, such as motor scales for severity of dystonia or motor performance, patient-reported measures, and quality of life.[27] However, the overall quality of the evidence supporting the use of these methods was rated as low or very low using the GRADE system for evidence-based medicine (Table 32.2). The most common reason for the low ratings was small sample sizes among the studies, with many individual case reports or very small series of cases. Another common limitation was the lack of an appropriate control group for comparisons. Other study limitations included lack of objective measurement outcomes, lack of blinding or randomization, clinical heterogeneity of affected individuals studied, procedural heterogeneity for the intervention, and use of combined interventions without understanding the effects of each intervention when used individually.

Table 32.1 **Categories of physiotherapy techniques**

Category	Description
Movement practice	Intensive motor training to restore normal voluntary movement
Training with constraint	Limiting adventitious movements in unaffected joints during training to support normal voluntary movement
Sensory reorganization	Techniques presumed to aid in the restoration of distorted sensorimotor cortical maps
External methods	Normalization of motor activity through active or passive external devices
Neuromodulation with training	Combination of movement practice with methods thought to alter neuronal excitability
Compensatory strategies	Replacement of abnormal motor activity with compensatory or alternative motor strategies

Adapted from a prior report.[27]

Table 32.2 **GRADE levels of evidence**

Quality rating	Explanation	Example study methods
High	Further research is unlikely to change confidence in the estimate of effect	Randomized trials or double-upgraded observational studies
Moderate	Further research is likely to have an important impact in confidence in the estimate of effect and may change the estimate	Downgraded randomized trials or upgraded observational studies
Low	Further research is very likely to have an impact in confidence in the estimate of effect and is likely to change the estimate	Observational studies or double downgraded randomized trials
Very low	Any estimate of effect is uncertain	Case reports or series, triple downgraded randomized trials, downgraded observational studies

Downgrade examples include limitations to study quality, inconsistencies, uncertainty about directness, and imprecise or sparse data or high probability of bias. Upgrade examples include strong evidence of association based on consistent evidence from two or more studies, evidence of a dose-effect, all plausible confounders would have reduced the effect. Adapted from prior reports.[16,27]

Physiotherapy for Generalized Dystonia

Physiotherapy is probably most extensively used in the generalized dystonias and particularly in cerebral palsy. It is widely accepted that stretching and/or strengthening exercises are valuable for preventing contractures in severe generalized dystonia with or without spasticity. An enormous number of clinical trials have been reported, with dozens of reviews. Most of these trials have focused on cerebral palsy, and they only rarely describe the clinical population's underlying distribution of motor features of spasticity, dystonia, or other motor problems. Some of these reviews focus on specific types of PT, such as general exercises, strength training, constraint-induced therapy, body vibration, or strategies assisted by using aquatic resources, robots, horses, or virtual reality. Other reviews focus on improvements in specific functions such as gross motor function, the ability to walk, skilled use of the upper limbs, speaking, or sitting.

One particularly thorough review summarized results from 15 different types of interventions described in 34 different systematic reviews.[8] A moderate level of evidence was found to support specific types of interventions such as constraint-induced therapies for the upper limb, goal-direction functional training, and gait training. There was also evidence that some types of interventions were not effective and should no longer be recommended. For many other interventions, the evidence was conflicting, and no clear recommendations could be made.

A more recent comprehensive review considered 43 systematic reviews, four expert guidelines, and three primary studies.[13] A high level of evidence was found in support of constraint-induced and bimanual therapies, with low levels of evidence for several other methods. The current overall recommendations include a multidisciplinary approach that is tailored to the specific abilities and needs of the affected individual and family. Despite the sometimes profound motor impairments, any activity that promotes an increased level of physical activity seems to be beneficial, especially if it is done in a goal-directed manner.

Physiotherapy for Cervical Dystonia

There are numerous reports of PT for cervical dystonia. A systematic review from 2014 summarized results from 16 studies including six clinical trials, four case series, and six case reports.[9] Different methods were used, including relaxation therapy, multimodal physical techniques, EMG biofeedback, and vibration or transcutaneous nerve stimulation. Potential benefits were assessed in different ways including rating scales for abnormal movements, pain, or quality of life. The conclusion was that multimodal physical therapy may provide benefits when used together with botulinum toxins, but the strength of the evidence was limited by the small numbers of subjects studied and the lack of blinding.

A second systematic review from 2022 summarized some additional studies, limiting to randomized controlled trials (Table 32.3).[21] The conclusion was that PT did not have an obvious impact on motor signs but may improve disability and quality of life. The strength of the evidence was again considered limited by the small size of most trials and lack of blinding.

Physiotherapy may be particularly useful for cervical dystonia under certain circumstances (see Chapter 5, "Cervical Dystonias"). One of these is severe, untreated cervical dystonia with a very abnormal head posture, such as extreme laterocollis. Success with botulinum toxin therapy may be aided by a simultaneous effort to manually correct the head posture by stretching tight neck muscles and strengthening those that have been weakened by being chronically overstretched. In this setting botulinum toxin injections alone may be insufficient. Another circumstance is individuals undergoing treatment with botulinum toxins who have short-duration responses, where there may be a need for some additional intervention during wearing-off periods. A third may involve individuals who get discouraged or depressed, where PT may provide an improved sense of self-efficacy.

Physiotherapy for Limb Dystonia

There are many studies of PT for focal hand dystonias, most notably writer's cramp and musician's dystonia. Once again, many different strategies have been applied, with many different endpoints for determining efficacy. One systematic review summarized the effects of nine independent studies of musicians with hand dystonia using various neuromuscular re-education strategies including constraint-inducted therapy, sensorimotor learning or retuning, and slow-down exercises.[12] Evidence to support these interventions for improving dystonia was classified as moderate, although the benefits are often not sufficient to restore a level of function satisfactory to professional musicians.

Another systematic review addressed behavioral techniques for nine different studies of adult-onset focal dystonias, including three studies of writer's cramp and three studies of golfer's dystonia (yips).[2] Methodological shortcomings led the authors to conclude that evidence for

Table 32.3 **Randomized controlled trials for cervical dystonia**

Study	Cases	Intervention	Main results
Tassorelli[29]	40	BoNT vs BoNT plus PT (exercises, stretching, massage)	No significant differences between groups for TWSTRS or Tsui scores; improved pain and ADLs and lower BoNT requirements in PT group
Boyce[4]	20	CD-specific relaxation and exercise and vs non-specific whole-body relaxation (with or without BoNT)	Non-significant trend towards reduced TWSTRS and improved depression in focused PT group
Stankovic[28]	14	PT with or without BoNT	Both groups had improved Tsui scores, only BoNT group had improved TWSTRS scores
Van den Dool[31]	96	CD-specific PT vs standard PT, both combined with BoNT	Both groups improved with no significant differences in TWSTRS scores; specific PT group had greater perceived benefits and lower treatment costs
Hu[17]	16	Unsatisfactory BoNT responders with or without PT (manual manipulations)	TWSTRS scores were better with PT than without PT
Dec-Cweik[10]	25	Three group cross-over study; BoNT alone, BoNT + kinesiotaping, BoNT+sham taping	Significant improvement in symptoms in all groups; quality of life improved only in kinesiotaping group

Adapted from a prior report.[21]

efficacy in these conditions was only limited, but relaxation methods could nevertheless be recommended. It is worth noting that some studies have advocated limb immobilization as a treatment for focal hand dystonia,[25,26] while others have discouraged its use, noting that immobilization itself can sometimes trigger dystonia.[24,32]

Speech and Voice Therapy for Laryngeal Dystonia

Individuals with laryngeal dystonia may receive various forms of voice therapy, often in combination with botulinum toxin treatments. Similar to findings for other forms of dystonia, occasional individuals seem to benefit, but overall results are mixed, making it challenging to recommend any specific strategy.

Although voice therapy seems to have limited efficacy for laryngeal dystonia, it can be very helpful for muscle tension dysphonia (see Chapter 7, "Laryngeal Dystonias").[7,20] Muscle tension dysphonia is a distinct voice disorder that closely mimics laryngeal dystonia, but both voice disorders may coexist. Voice therapy can be curative for pure muscle tension dysphonia, and some experts advocate a trial of voice therapy to discriminate it from laryngeal dystonia.[19] The observation that laryngeal dystonia may coexist with muscle tension dysphonia may explain why some patients with a diagnosis of laryngeal dystonia respond at least in part to voice therapy.

COMPLEMENTARY AND ALTERNATIVE MEDICINE

Overview

Broadly defined, CAM refers to any intervention that generally falls outside the realm of conventional medicine. Numerous interventions are often considered under the CAM umbrella such as chiropractic manipulations, various exercises, massage, yoga or other forms of stretching, biofeedback, acupuncture or dry needling, relaxation or meditation techniques, detoxification, hypnosis, nutritional supplements, and others. Physiotherapy is sometimes also included under the CAM umbrella.

Many types of CAM are used by individuals with dystonia because many individuals with dystonia experience long delays between symptom onset and diagnosis, or they are not fully satisfied with conventional treatments. Because individuals with dystonia often experience muscle pulling and spasms, several popular techniques involve muscle exercises and stretching or massage. Many individuals also experience worsening of symptoms with stress or anxiety, making relaxation techniques attractive, too.[2]

There are very few systematic studies of CAM for the dystonias. One systematic review tabulated the many types of CAM studied in prior reports for various types of dystonia including cervical dystonia, writer's cramp, musician's dystonia, craniofacial dystonia, laryngeal dystonia, and generalized dystonia.[11] Although almost all the reports reviewed described positive outcomes for each type of CAM studied, the evidence for efficacy was considered weak for all of them. The main reasons for the weak evidence included observations that most studies were single case reports or unblinded, used outcome measures of uncertain value, or had no control or comparison group.

One meta-analysis assessed the value of acupuncture for reducing muscle tone in children with cerebral palsy across 15 separate studies.[33] All studies included a randomized design that compared standard physiotherapy to physiotherapy with acupuncture. None of the studies was conducted blind to treatment group. Both treatment groups showed significant improvements in muscle tone assessed with the Ashworth Scale and improvements in electromyographic measures.

Three other studies addressed CAM from the patient's perspective. A survey conducted using a German registry reported on the frequency and perceived efficacy of different types of CAM among 180 individuals with predominantly adult-onset focal dystonias.[18] In this population, 73% tried at least one CAM, with the vast majority trying more than one. Many of them used CAM along with botulinum toxin injections. Depending on the type of CAM, the percentage of individuals reporting at least some efficacy ranged from 4% to 62% (Figure 32.1A). Also depending on the type of CAM, up to 23% of individuals reported a negative effect, suggesting they are not always benign.

Another second study from America surveyed 389 individuals with mostly adult-onset focal dystonias.[14] A total of 53% reported trying at least one CAM, with the majority again trying more than one, often in combination with botulinum toxin. Affected individuals estimated average percentage improvements of 17–43% depending on the type of CAM (Figure 32.1B).

A third study from Australia surveyed 128 adults with cervical dystonia.[5] More than 50%

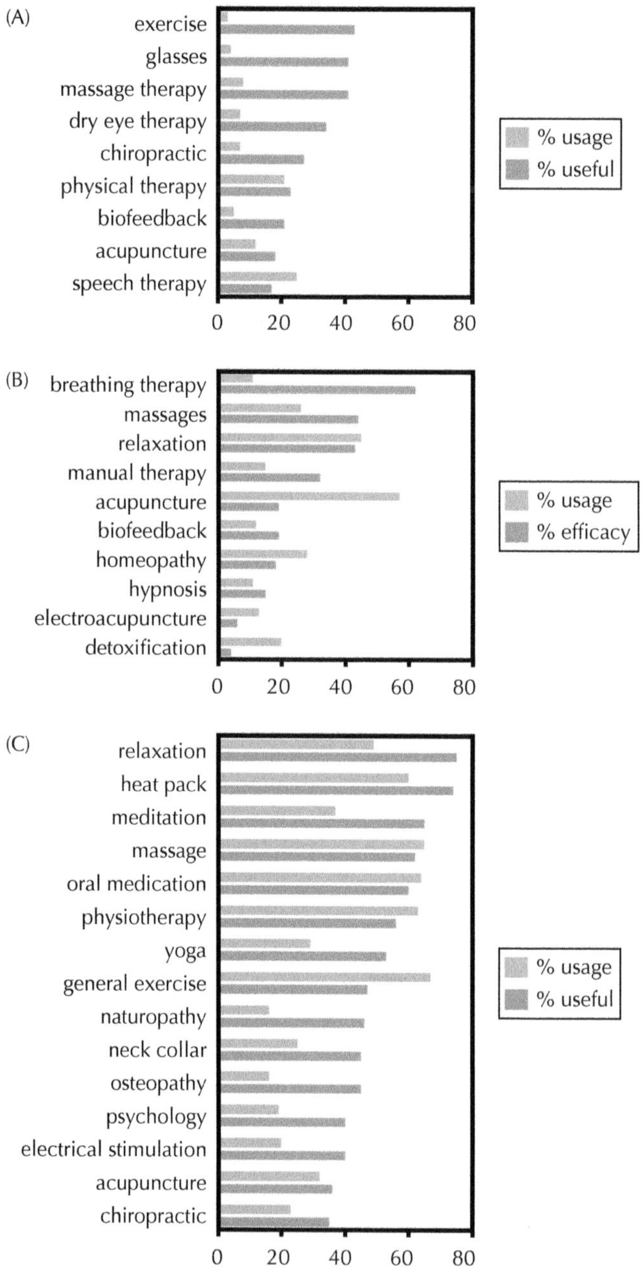

Figure 32.1. Complementary and alternative treatments used in dystonia. Three prior surveys of complementary and alternative treatments used by individuals with various types of dystonia were adapted to produce Panels A,[18] B,[14] and C.[5] The orange bars show the percentage of individuals who used the option listed, and the blue bars show the percentage of users who felt the option was at least partly effective. Some items may reflect usage by individuals with specific types of dystonia, such as laryngeal dystonia (speech therapy), blepharospasm (tinted glasses, dry eye therapy), or cervical dystonia (physiotherapy, massage).

of respondents reported at least some benefit from a variety of methods including heat packs, relaxation, massage, and PT or other forms of exercise (Figure 32.1C). Many individuals were using these methods alongside botulinum toxin therapies.

Cannabis and Related Derivatives

The term "cannabis" refers to a genus of plants, also sometimes called "hemp." Extracts from these plants contain hundreds of unique chemicals, including more than 80 that fall into a category known as *cannabinoids*. The best-known cannabinoid is tetrahydrocannabinol (THC), which is the main psychoactive ingredient in marijuana or hashish. Cannabis and related cannabinoids have become increasingly available to the public as products that may be smoked, chewed as gummies or other substances, swallowed as pills or elixirs, or put on the skin as creams and ointments. The increased availability has led to an increase in enthusiasm for using them for a variety of ailments, with a parallel increase in clinical studies aimed at evaluating their safety and efficacy.

A variety of different synthetic cannabinoids thought to be less psychoactive than THC (cannabidiol, dronabinol, nabilone, and nabiximols) have been subject to clinical trials in numerous medical conditions. Movement disorders have been studied particularly intensively because of high levels of cannabinoid receptors in brain regions that control movement, including both the basal ganglia and cerebellum. One systematic review evaluated 152 randomized controlled trials of all types of cannabinoids across all medical conditions.[3] Evidence for therapeutic efficacy depended on the medical condition and the type of cannabinoid tested. A high level of evidence to support therapeutic use was found only for cannabidiol in epilepsy. However, there was moderate supportive evidence for using some cannabinoids in other conditions including cannabidiol (Parkinson disease), dronabinol (chronic pain, low appetite, Tourette syndrome), and nabiximols (chronic pain, spasticity, sleep). Evidence to support their use in other conditions, including dystonia, was insufficient to make any recommendation. Another systematic review focusing only on movement disorders also found no clear support for the use of cannabinoids in dystonia.[23]

For dystonia, there are only two randomized controlled trials. One study found no benefit of nabilone in 15 adults with severe segmental or generalized dystonia evaluated using the Burke-Fahn-Marsden dystonia rating scale.[15] Another study found no benefit for nine adults with cervical dystonia evaluated using the Toronto Western Torticollis Rating Scale.[34] Despite these negative clinical trials, many individuals with dystonia ask about cannabinoids, or they try them on their own. For example, one survey study that included 158 subjects with voice disorders where the majority had laryngeal dystonia revealed that 54% had tried cannabinoids at least once.[22] Approximately half of these individuals rated the effect as "somewhat effective" and elected to continue using the drugs. However, 46% rated these drugs as "ineffective" and discontinued. Another study suggested that a subgroup of individuals with broad patterns of dystonia may benefit more than those with focal dystonia.[1]

PRACTICAL RECOMMENDATIONS AND EVIDENCE-BASED MEDICINE

It is common practice that recommendations for the application of conventional medicines and procedures be driven by good evidence for safety and efficacy. The field of evidence-based medicine has emerged to evaluate the evidence, with specific criteria guiding the strength of any recommendations (Table 32.2).[16] However, these criteria were developed for common disorders, not rare disorders like dystonia.

Unfortunately, PT methods and CAM only rarely satisfy criteria for reaching the strongest recommendations in dystonia. One of the reasons for this failure is that these criteria call for clinical trials with large numbers of individuals, a requirement that is a challenge for rare disorders such as dystonia. Most PT trials in dystonia include only small numbers of subjects. Another criterion for judging the evidence is that multiple similar trials should show similar results. Due to limited resources for rare disease research, redundant trials are only rarely conducted. A third criteria is that one of the most favored clinical trial designs is placebo-controlled, double-blinded, and randomized. This type of design is particularly challenging for PT, where a true placebo condition is rarely available, and it is nearly impossible to blind the provider and recipient to the intervention. The final challenge is that the best measures of the success of PT are not entirely clear. Physiotherapy may not have an impact on the motor features of dystonia, but it may impact non-motor features such as pain, sense of self-efficacy, or quality of life. In view of all these considerations, it has been argued that the conventional criteria used for recommendations from evidence-based medicine should not be applied to PT, and some other measure of success may be needed.[27]

There is reasonably strong evidence in favor of PT for generalized dystonia and particularly cerebral palsy. In view of the absence of definitive evidence for the value of PT in other types of dystonia, clinical providers take very different approaches. Some do not recommend any type of PT, citing the lack of definitive evidence and importance of reserving limited medical resources only for proven interventions. Others take a more wholistic approach, offering PT to most individuals and continuing it for those where it seems useful. These differences of opinion translate into different behaviors worldwide. A survey of clinical providers in Europe revealed that PT for cervical dystonia was readily accessible in only 12 of 24 countries, yet PT was viewed as an integral part of the standard of care in some countries, such as Sweden and the Netherlands.[30]

Another approach that is useful to aid decisions regarding recommendations for PT is to consider what affected individuals may want. There are very few methodical studies regarding patient preferences, although some estimates may be obtained from the percentage of affected individuals using PT. A survey of 389 individuals in the United States with different types of dystonia revealed that 20% were using some form of PT.[14] For cervical dystonia, an international survey with 1,071 respondents from 38 countries revealed that 31% were using some form of PT.[6] Another survey of 131 individuals with different types of dystonia in Germany revealed that 73% were using some type of PT, and its efficacy was rated as very good or good by 34% and moderate in 46%.[18] A study of 128 adults with cervical dystonia revealed 66% preferred some type of PT, and 36% reported benefit.[5]

Although more methodical studies of the patient perspective are clearly needed, these observations reveal that a substantial portion of individuals with dystonia are using some form of PT, often in concert with botulinum toxins or other treatments. This relatively high level of utilization suggests that patients find value in PT.

SUMMARY AND FUTURE PROSPECTS

The many subtypes of dystonia have each been treated with sometimes very different types of PT and also other forms of CAM. There is good evidence for the use of certain types of PT for generalized dystonia and particularly cerebral palsy, where clear recommendations have been forthcoming. For most other types of dystonia, the medical evidence for recommending different forms of PT appears to be inconclusive when judged using normal criteria established for evidence-based medicine. However, whether the criteria used for evidence-based medicine are appropriate for PT in dystonia can been questioned. In contrast with this equivocal evidence are observations that many affected individuals request some form of PT, and many report PT to be useful and continue. In view of these somewhat conflicting sources of information regarding the value of PT, habits for recommending PT vary widely among different clinical providers.

In the absence of conclusive evidence, a good strategy is to offer PT according to the preferences of individual patients. It is important to recognize that all subtypes of dystonia are uncommon, and physiotherapists rarely receive specialized training in how to address them. It is important that physiotherapists familiarize themselves with the unique needs of individuals with dystonia because some exercises or manipulations may be counterproductive. Physiotherapy may be particularly valuable in three circumstances. One is severe untreated cervical dystonia where botulinum toxin alone may be insufficient. Another is individuals who have short-duration responses to botulinum toxin and need some alternative to address problems that emerge during the wearing-off period. A third is individuals who have substantial pain or who get discouraged and depressed, where PT can provide a sense of self-efficacy that may be valuable.

Clearly, further research is needed to refine understanding of which PT strategies might be most useful for each different type of dystonia. The role of other forms of CAM in treatment remains undefined, but surveys of affected individuals imply some benefits for certain options. Obviously, the best approach may not be the same for cervical dystonia as it is for laryngeal dystonia or hand dystonia in a musician, so future studies may need to address individual subtypes more specifically.

REFERENCES

1. Anis S, Faust-Socher A, Sverdlov D, Lassman S, Hezi N, Anis O, et al. A single-center real-life study on the use of medical cannabis in patients with dystonia. Front Neurol 2023;14:1218300.
2. Bernstein CJ, Ellard DR, Davies G, Hertenstein E, Tang NK, Underwood M, Sandhu H. Behavioural interventions for people living with adult-onset primary dystonia: A systematic review. BMC Neurol 2016;16:40.
3. Bilbao A, Spanagel R. Medical cannabinoids: A pharmacology-based systematic review and meta-analysis for all relevant medical indications. BMC Med 2022;20:259.
4. Boyce MJ, Canning CG, Mahant N, Morris J, Latimer J, Fung VS. Active exercise for individuals with cervical dystonia: A pilot randomized controlled trial. Clin Rehabil 2012;27:226–235.
5. Boyce MJ, McCambridge AB, Bradnam LV, Canning CG, De Oliveira CQ, Verhagen AP. Botulinum toxin and conservative treatment strategies in people with cervical dystonia: An online survey. J Neural Transm 2024;131:43–51.
6. Comella C, Bhatia K. An international survey of patients with cervical dystonia. J Neurol 2015;262:837–848.
7. da Cunha Pereira G, de Oliveira Lemos I, Dalbosco Gadenz C, Cassol M. Effects of voice therapy on muscle tension dysphonia: A systematic literature review. J Voice 2018;32:546–552.
8. Das SP, Ganesh GS. Evidence-based approach to physical therapy in cerebral palsy. Indian J Orthop 2019;53:20–34.
9. De Pauw J, Van der Velden K, Meirte J, Van Daele U, Truijen S, Cras P, et al. The effectiveness of physiotherapy for cervical dystonia: A systematic literature review. J Neurol 2014;261:1857–1865.
10. Dec-Cwiek M, Porebska K, Sawczynska K, Kubala M, Witkowska M, Zmijewska K, et al. KinesioTaping after botulinum toxin type A for cervical dystonia in adult patients. Brain Behav 2022;12:e2541.
11. Delnooz CC, Horstink MW, Tijssen MA, van de Warrenburg BP. Paramedical treatment in primary dystonia: A systematic review. Mov Disord 2009;24:2187–2198.
12. Enke AM, Poskey GA. Neuromuscular re-education programs for musicians with focal hand dystonia: A systematic review. Med Probl Perform Art 2018;33:137–145.
13. Faccioli S, Pagliano E, Ferrari A, Maghini C, Siani MF, Sgherri G, et al. Evidence-based management and motor rehabilitation of cerebral palsy children and adolescents: A systematic review. Front Neurol 2023;14:1171224.
14. Fleming BM, Schwab EL, Nouer SS, Wan JY, LeDoux MS. Prevalence, predictors, and perceived effectiveness of complementary, alternative and integrative medicine in adult-onset primary dystonia. Parkinsonism Relat Disord 2012;18:936–940.
15. Fox SH, Kellett M, Moore AP, Crossman AR, Brotchie JM. Randomised, double-blind, placebo-controlled trial to assess the potential of cannabinoid receptor stimulation in the treatment of dystonia. Mov Disord 2002;17:145–149.
16. Guyatt GH, Oxman AD, Vist GE, Kunz R, Falck-Ytter Y, Alonso-Coello P, et al. GRADE: An emerging consensus on rating quality of evidence and strength of recommendations. BMJ 2008;336:924–926.
17. Hu W, Rundle-Gonzalez V, Kulkarni SJ, Martinez-Ramirez D, Almeida L, Okun MS, Wagle Shukla A. A randomized study of botulinum toxin versus botulinum toxin plus physical therapy for treatment of cervical dystonia. Parkinsonism Relat Disord 2019;63:195–198.
18. Junker J, Oberwittler C, Jackson D, Berger K. Utilization and perceived effectiveness of complementary and alternative medicine in patients with dystonia. Mov Disord 2004;19:158–161.
19. Kodama N, Sanuki T, Miyamoto T, Tashiro J. Effects and differences of voice therapy on spasmodic dysphonia and muscle tension dysphonia: A retrospective pilot study. J Voice 2024;38:129–135.
20. Lester-Smith RA, Miller CH, Cherney LR. Behavioral therapy for temor or dystonia affecting voice in speakers with hyperkinetic dysarthria: A systematic review. J Voice 2023;37:561–573.
21. Loudovici-Krug D, Derlien S, Best N, Gunther A. Physiotherapy for cervical dystonia: A systematic review of randomised controlled trials. Toxins 2022;14:784.
22. Millman N, van der Woerd B, Sund LT, Johns M. Cannabinoid use in the treatment of laryngeal dystonia and vocal tremor: A pilot investigation. J Voice 2023;S0892-1997(23)00158-3. doi:10.1016/j.jvoice.2023.05.006.
23. Oikonomou P, Jost WH. Randomized controlled trials on the use of cannabis-based medicines in movement disorders: A systematic review. J Neural Transm 2022;129:1247–1256.
24. Okun MS, Nadeau SE, Rossi F, Triggs WJ. Immobilization dystonia. J Neurol Sci 2002;201:79–83.
25. Pesenti A, Barbieri S, Priori A. Limb immobilization for occupational dystonia: A possible alternative treatment for selected patients. Adv Neurol 2004;94:247–254.
26. Priori A, Pesenti A, Cappellari A, Scarlato G, Barbieri S. Limb immobilization for the treatment of focal occupational dystonia. Neurology 2001;57:405–409.
27. Prudente CN, Zetterberg L, Bring A, Bradnam L, Kimberley TJ. Systematic review of rehabilitation in focal dystonias: Classification and recommendations. Mov Disord Clin Pract 2018;5:237–245.
28. Stankovic I, Colovic H, Zivkovic V, Stamenovic J, Stankovic A, Zlatanovic D, et al. The effect of physical therapy in the treatment of patients with cervical dystonia with or without concomitant use of botulinum toxin. Vojnosanit Pregl 2018;75.
29. Tassorelli C, Mancini F, Balloni L, Pacchetti C, Sandrini G, Nappi G, Martignoni E. Botulinum toxin and neuromotor rehabilitation: An integrated approach to idiopathic cervical dystonia. Mov Disord 2006;21:2240–2243.
30. Valadas A, Contarino MF, Albanese A, Bhatia KP, Falup-Pecurariu C, Forsgren L, et al. Management of dystonia in Europe: A survey of the European network for the study of the dystonia syndromes. Eur J Neurol 2016;23:772–779.

31. van den Dool J, Visser B, Koelman JH, Engelbert RH, Tijssen MA. Cervical dystonia: Effectiveness of a standardized physical therapy program; study design and protocol of a single blind randomized controlled trial. BMC Neurol 2013;13:85.
32. van Rooijen DE, Geraedts EJ, Marinus J, Jankovic J, van Hilten JJ. Peripheral trauma and movement disorders: A systematic review of reported cases. J Neurol Neurosurg Psychiatry 2011;82:892–898.
33. Yuanjie Y, Jianyi X, Jinyan X, Mao H, Siyang Y, Zhenjin Y. Acupuncture in the treatment of abnormal muscle tone in children with cerebral palsy: A meta-analysis. Behav Neurol 2023;2023:4662788.
34. Zadikoff C, Wadia PM, Miyasaki J, Chen R, Lange AE, So J, Fox SH. Cannabinoid, CB1 agonists in cervical dystonia: Failure in a phase Iia randomized controlled trial. Basal Ganglia 2011;2:91–95.

Index

For the benefit of digital users, terms that are indexed as spanning two pages (e.g., 52–53) may, on occasion, appear on only one of those pages.

Tables and figures are indicated by an italic *t* and *f* following the page number.